Targeting Wnt Signaling in Cancer: Opportunities Abound If We Can Avoid the Sword of Damocles

Targeting Wnt Signaling in Cancer: Opportunities Abound If We Can Avoid the Sword of Damocles

Editors

**Michael Kahn
Keane Lai**

MDPI • Basel • Beijing • Wuhan • Barcelona • Belgrade • Manchester • Tokyo • Cluj • Tianjin

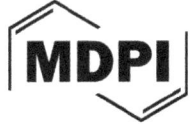

Editors
Michael Kahn
Beckman Research Institute of City of Hope
USA

Keane Lai
Beckman Research Institute of City of Hope
USA

Editorial Office
MDPI
St. Alban-Anlage 66
4052 Basel, Switzerland

This is a reprint of articles from the Special Issue published online in the open access journal *Cancers* (ISSN 2072-6694) (available at: https://www.mdpi.com/journal/cancers/special_issues/Targeting_Wnt).

For citation purposes, cite each article independently as indicated on the article page online and as indicated below:

LastName, A.A.; LastName, B.B.; LastName, C.C. Article Title. *Journal Name* **Year**, *Volume Number*, Page Range.

ISBN 978-3-0365-3517-3 (Hbk)
ISBN 978-3-0365-3518-0 (PDF)

© 2022 by the authors. Articles in this book are Open Access and distributed under the Creative Commons Attribution (CC BY) license, which allows users to download, copy and build upon published articles, as long as the author and publisher are properly credited, which ensures maximum dissemination and a wider impact of our publications.

The book as a whole is distributed by MDPI under the terms and conditions of the Creative Commons license CC BY-NC-ND.

Contents

About the Editors vii

Preface to "Targeting Wnt Signaling in Cancer: Opportunities Abound If We Can Avoid the
Sword of Damocles" ix

Taybor W. Parker, Aaron J. Rudeen and Kristi L. Neufeld
Oncogenic Serine 45-Deleted β-Catenin Remains Susceptible to Wnt Stimulation and APC Regulation in Human Colonocytes
Reprinted from: *Cancers* **2020**, *12*, 2114, doi:10.3390/cancers12082114 1

Lan Lan, Jiajun Liu, Minli Xing, Amber R. Smith, Jinan Wang, Xiaoqing Wu, Carl Appelman, Ke Li, Anuradha Roy, Ragul Gowthaman, John Karanicolas, Amber D. Somoza, Clay C. C. Wang, Yinglong Miao, Roberto De Guzman, Berl R. Oakley, Kristi L. Neufeld and Liang Xu
Identification and Validation of an *Aspergillus nidulans* Secondary Metabolite Derivative as an Inhibitor of the Musashi-RNA Interaction
Reprinted from: *Cancers* **2020**, *12*, 2221, doi:10.3390/cancers12082221 19

Sam O. Kleeman and Simon J. Leedham
Not All Wnt Activation Is Equal: Ligand-Dependent versus Ligand-Independent Wnt Activation in Colorectal Cancer
Reprinted from: *Cancers* **2020**, *12*, 3355, doi:10.3390/cancers12113355 37

José Manuel González-Sancho, María Jesús Larriba and Alberto Muñoz
Wnt and Vitamin D at the Crossroads in Solid Cancer
Reprinted from: *Cancers* **2020**, *12*, 3434, doi:10.3390/cancers12113434 53

Sanith Cheriyamundath and Avri Ben-Ze'ev
Wnt/β-Catenin Target Genes in Colon Cancer Metastasis: The Special Case of L1CAM
Reprinted from: *Cancers* **2020**, *12*, 3444, doi:10.3390/cancers12113444 73

Aldona Kasprzak
Angiogenesis-Related Functions of Wnt Signaling in Colorectal Carcinogenesis
Reprinted from: *Cancers* **2020**, *12*, 3601, doi:10.3390/cancers12123601 87

Moon Jong Kim, Yuanjian Huang and Jae-Il Park
Targeting Wnt Signaling for Gastrointestinal Cancer Therapy: Present and Evolving Views
Reprinted from: *Cancers* **2020**, *12*, 3638, doi:10.3390/cancers12123638 127

Keane K. Y. Lai, Xiaohui Hu, Keisuke Chosa, Cu Nguyen, David P. Lin, Keith K. Lai, Nobuo Kato, Yusuke Higuchi, Sarah K. Highlander, Elizabeth Melendez, Yoshihiro Eriguchi, Patrick T. Fueger, Andre J. Ouellette, Nyam-Osor Chimge, Masaya Ono and Michael Kahn
p300 Serine 89: A Critical Signaling Integrator and Its Effects on Intestinal Homeostasis and Repair
Reprinted from: *Cancers* **2021**, *13*, 1288, doi:10.3390/cancers13061288 155

Bang Manh Tran, Dustin James Flanagan, Gregor Ebert, Nadia Warner, Hoanh Tran, Theodora Fifis, Georgios Kastrappis, Christopher Christophi, Marc Pellegrini, Joseph Torresi, Toby James Phesse and Elizabeth Vincan
The Hepatitis B Virus Pre-Core Protein p22 Activates Wnt Signaling
Reprinted from: *Cancers* **2020**, *12*, 1435, doi:10.3390/cancers12061435 177

Yekaterina Krutsenko, Aatur D. Singhi and Satdarshan P. Monga
β-Catenin Activation in Hepatocellular Cancer: Implications in Biology and Therapy
Reprinted from: *Cancers* **2021**, *13*, 1830, doi:10.3390/cancers13081830 . . . . **191**

Mingtian Che, Soo-Mi Kweon, Jia-Ling Teo, Yate-Ching Yuan, Laleh G. Melstrom, Richard T. Waldron, Aurelia Lugea, Raul A. Urrutia, Stephen J. Pandol and Keane K. Y. Lai
Targeting the CBP/β-Catenin Interaction to Suppress Activation of Cancer-Promoting Pancreatic Stellate Cells
Reprinted from: *Cancers* **2020**, *12*, 1476, doi:10.3390/cancers12061476 . . . . **207**

Tetsuya Sekita, Tesshi Yamada, Eisuke Kobayashi, Akihiko Yoshida, Toru Hirozane, Akira Kawai, Yuko Uno, Hideki Moriyama, Masaaki Sawa, Yuichi Nagakawa, Akihiko Tsuchida, Morio Matsumoto, Masaya Nakamura, Robert Nakayama and Mari Masuda
Feasibility of Targeting Traf2-and-Nck-Interacting Kinase in Synovial Sarcoma
Reprinted from: *Cancers* **2020**, *12*, 1258, doi:10.3390/cancers12051258 . . . . **221**

Alexander Chehrazi-Raffle, Tanya B. Dorff, Sumanta K. Pal and Yung Lyou
Wnt/β-Catenin Signaling and Immunotherapy Resistance: Lessons for the Treatment of Urothelial Carcinoma
Reprinted from: *Cancers* **2021**, *13*, 889, doi:10.3390/cancers13040889 . . . . **239**

Anja Kafka, Anja Bukovac, Emilija Brglez, Ana-Marija Jarmek, Karolina Poljak, Petar Brlek, Kamelija Žarković, Niko Njirić and Nives Pećina-Šlaus
Methylation Patterns of *DKK1*, *DKK3* and *GSK3β* Are Accompanied with Different Expression Levels in Human Astrocytoma
Reprinted from: *Cancers* **2021**, *13*, 2530, doi:10.3390/cancers13112530 . . . . **253**

Paul Takam Kamga, Giada Dal Collo, Adriana Cassaro, Riccardo Bazzoni, Pietro Delfino, Annalisa Adamo, Alice Bonato, Carmine Carbone, Ilaria Tanasi, Massimiliano Bonifacio and Mauro Krampera
Small Molecule Inhibitors of Microenvironmental Wnt/β-Catenin Signaling Enhance the Chemosensitivity of Acute Myeloid Leukemia
Reprinted from: *Cancers* **2020**, *12*, 2696, doi:10.3390/cancers12092696 . . . . **271**

About the Editors

Michael Kahn, Ph.D., is professor and chair of the Department of Molecular Medicine at the Beckman Research Institute of City of Hope. Prof. Kahn's research program is focused on the integration of basic science with translational medicine. His lab utilizes a forward chemical genomic strategy to identify and validate novel pharmacologic tools to study complex signaling pathways in development and disease. Utilizing a proprietary chemical library, his lab identified the first specific CBP/β-catenin antagonist ICG-001, which has been fundamental in studies involving both normal somatic stem cell and cancer stem cell biology. From a translational perspective, these studies led to the development of the second-generation CBP/β-catenin antagonist, Wnt modulating drug, PRI-724. These efforts resulted in clinical trials of PRI-724 in colon and pancreatic cancer, leukemia and liver fibrosis. His lab is currently continuing basic research investigations concerning differential Kat3 coactivator usage (i.e., CBP versus p300) in somatic stem cell biology and cancer, regenerative medicine, and aging. Another area of interest to his lab is the endogenous mechanisms that control the differential usage of these coactivators and the role that the N-termini play as a nexus for the integration of a number of additional signaling pathways (e.g., STAT1/2, nuclear receptor family, RAR/RXR, Vit D) with the Wnt signaling cascade. Prof. Kahn is also applying the forward chemical genomic strategy to additional critical signaling cascades with the broader goal of developing novel small-molecule therapeutics.

Keane Lai, M.D., is principal investigator in the Department of Molecular Medicine at the Beckman Research Institute of City of Hope. Dr. Lai's lab was the first to demonstrate the functional significance of the obscure gene midnolin in liver cancer. In addition to focusing on characterization of the role of midnolin in liver pathobiology, Dr. Lai's lab studies the role of Wnt/β-catenin signaling in the liver and pancreas.

Preface to "Targeting Wnt Signaling in Cancer: Opportunities Abound If We Can Avoid the Sword of Damocles"

Dysregulation of Wnt signaling is known to be associated with various cancers. As such, identification of novel Wnt pathway targets in cancer and better characterization of already-known targets present exciting, emerging opportunities for cancer treatment. In this Special Issue, we feature papers that discuss the role of Wnt signaling and associated targets in cancer metabolism, tumor immune response, and the tumor microenvironment. Papers discussing a range of Wnt-mediated cancers, including those of the colon, liver, pancreas, synovium, bladder, etc. are included.

Michael Kahn, Keane Lai
Editors

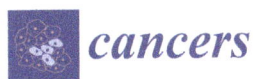

Article

Oncogenic Serine 45-Deleted β-Catenin Remains Susceptible to Wnt Stimulation and APC Regulation in Human Colonocytes

Taybor W. Parker, Aaron J. Rudeen and Kristi L. Neufeld *

Department of Molecular Biosciences, University of Kansas, Lawrence, KS 66049, USA; parkertw@ku.edu (T.W.P.); aaron.rudeen@ku.edu (A.J.R.)
* Correspondence: klneuf@ku.edu; Tel.: +1-785-864-5079

Received: 11 June 2020; Accepted: 28 July 2020; Published: 30 July 2020

Abstract: The Wnt/β-catenin signaling pathway is deregulated in nearly all colorectal cancers (CRCs), predominantly through mutation of the tumor suppressor *Adenomatous Polyposis Coli* (*APC*). *APC* mutation is thought to allow a "just-right" amount of Wnt pathway activation by fine-tuning β-catenin levels. While at a much lower frequency, mutations that result in a β-catenin that is compromised for degradation occur in a subset of human CRCs. Here, we investigate whether one such "stabilized" β-catenin responds to regulatory stimuli, thus allowing β-catenin levels conducive for tumor formation. We utilize cells harboring a single mutant allele encoding Ser45-deleted β-catenin (β-catΔS45) to test the effects of Wnt3a treatment or APC-depletion on β-catΔS45 regulation and activity. We find that APC and β-catΔS45 retain interaction with Wnt receptors. Unexpectedly, β-catΔS45 accumulates and activates TOPflash reporter upon Wnt treatment or APC-depletion, but only accumulates in the nucleus upon APC loss. Finally, we find that β-catenin phosphorylation at GSK-3β sites and proteasomal degradation continue to occur in the absence of Ser45. Our results expand the current understanding of Wnt/β-catenin signaling and provide an example of a β-catenin mutation that maintains some ability to respond to Wnt, a possible key to establishing β-catenin activity that is "just-right" for tumorigenesis.

Keywords: Wnt signaling; just-right signaling; APC; β-catenin; colorectal cancer

1. Introduction

Discovered nearly 40 years ago, the Wnt signaling pathway has proven essential for many cellular functions, including proliferation, polarity, developmental cell-fate determination, and tissue homeostasis [1]. Consequently, the Wnt pathway is often deregulated in cancer and other diseases. Normal colon tissue homeostasis is dependent on well-controlled Wnt signaling, as Wnt pathway components are mutated in over 90% of colorectal cancers (CRCs) [2–4].

The key downstream effector molecule in the Wnt pathway is the transcription cofactor β-catenin. In the absence of a Wnt signal, a cytoplasmic β-catenin destruction complex efficiently catalyzes the proteasome-mediated degradation of β-catenin. The core components of the complex include two scaffolding proteins, Adenomatous Polyposis Coli (APC) and Axin, as well as two kinases, GSK-3β and CK1-α [5]. In the absence of ligands, the complex binds and phosphorylates β-catenin, leading to β-TrCP-mediated ubiquitination and proteasomal degradation [6–8]. Binding of Wnt to membrane-bound coreceptors Frizzled and LRP5/6 results in inhibition of the β-catenin destruction complex through an incompletely resolved mechanism, followed by β-catenin accumulation, nuclear translocation, and activation of the Wnt transcriptional program [9,10].

In canonical Wnt signaling, β-catenin destruction is initiated through a dual-kinase mechanism. First, CK1-α phosphorylates Ser45 of β-catenin (Figure 1A,B) [8,11]. Next, phospho-Ser45 primes

GSK-3β activity, which typically requires a phospho-Ser or threonine and the S/T-X-X-X-pS/pT motif [12–14]. Three sites on β-catenin are then primed and phosphorylated hierarchically, beginning with Thr41, then Ser37, and finally Ser33, as each phosphorylating event primes the next (see Figure 1). Phosphorylation of Ser33 and Ser37 generates a WD40-like binding site for β-TrCP, the substrate recognition subunit of the E3 ubiquitin ligase SCF$^{β-TrCP}$ which ubiquitinates β-catenin and marks it for degradation by the proteasome [7,15–18]. A mutation that eliminates any one of the phosphorylation sites is thought to stabilize β-catenin, making it resistant to destruction and able to activate downstream Wnt signaling.

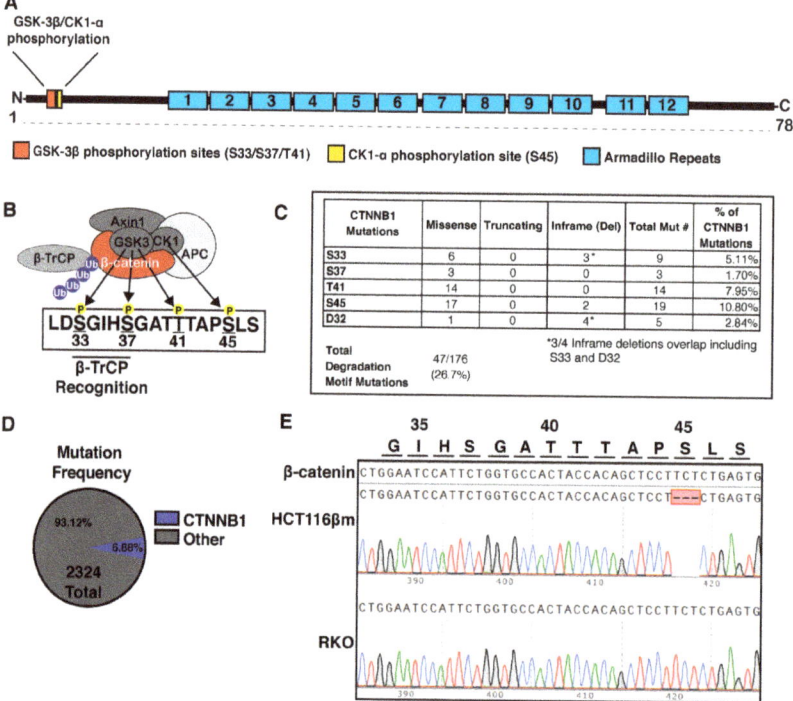

Figure 1. β-catenin phospho-regulation by the β-catenin destruction complex. (**A**) Diagram of β-catenin structure, indicating the N-terminal GSK-3β phosphorylation sites (Ser33/Ser37/T41), the CK1-α phosphorylation site (Ser45), and the 12 armadillo repeats. (**B**) Schematic of the β-catenin destruction complex composed of Axin, Adenomatous Polyposis Coli (APC), GSK-3β, and CK1-α, which bind and phosphorylate β-catenin at Ser45, Thr41, Ser37, and Ser33. Phosphorylation at Ser33/Ser37 creates a β-TrCP recognition site. (**C**) Mutation frequency of destruction complex phosphorylation sites among *CTNNB1* mutations. (**D**) Mutation frequency of *CTNNB1* among 2324 colorectal cancer patients using cBioPortal. (**E**) Sanger sequencing and alignment of *CTNNB1* around the destruction complex phosphorylation sites in HCT116βm and RKO colon cancer cell lines.

Mutations in the tumor suppressor *Adenomatous Polyposis Coli* (*APC*) occur early in the development of over 80% of CRCs. The vast majority of *APC* mutations lead to the expression of truncated APC protein that retains some ability to interact with and regulate β-catenin. The "just right" model rationalizes the limited range of APC truncations observed in CRCs as facilitating a precise level of β-catenin for optimal cellular proliferation—not too much or too little [19]. In addition to a scaffolding function, other APC activities have been suggested to contribute to Wnt signaling. For example, APC can interact with nuclear β-catenin, leading to repression of Wnt target genes through several proposed mechanisms:

providing access to the transcriptional corepressor CtBP or E3 ligase β-TrCP, sequestration of β-catenin from the transcriptional coactivator LEF-1/TCF, or facilitating β-catenin's nuclear export [20–24]. APC can maintain interaction with β-catenin following Wnt stimulation and appears critical for trafficking the destruction complex to the Wnt receptors [25,26]. Additionally, APC has been postulated to promote β-catenin ubiquitination. APC truncation commonly found in human CRCs renders cells unable to appropriately ubiquitinate β-catenin and target it for proteasomal degradation [25,27,28]. A region of APC just C-terminal to sites of common truncations appears to be sufficient for the rescue of β-catenin ubiquitination [25,28].

CRCs without *APC* mutations commonly have mutations in genes encoding other components of the Wnt pathway. The key downstream effector molecule in Wnt signaling, the β-catenin gene, *CTNNB1*, is mutated in ~12% of CRCs lacking an *APC* mutation (Table S1). It is curious why mutations that protect β-catenin from degradation are not more prevalent in CRC, as this would be a direct path to β-catenin mediated transcription. It is possible that mutations that completely stabilize β-catenin do not support cell viability. In this event, β-catenin mutations may also act in a "just-right" manner to precisely tune the amount of β-catenin for optimal levels of Wnt activation. Another, not mutually exclusive, possibility is that destroying β-catenin is not the only critical tumor-suppressive role for APC, and that additional APC-mediated processes such as cytoskeletal arrangement, β-catenin localization, and cellular orientation during cell division must be affected to initiate adenoma formation.

Mutations that eliminate the GSK-3β or CK1-α phosphorylation sites are reported to "stabilize" β-catenin, making it resistant to regulation by the destruction complex and thus resistant to regulation by Wnt signaling [5]. Cells expressing β-catenin containing a Ser45 deletion or S33Y substitution are reported to display constitutively active Wnt signaling [29]. HCT116 cells, which express two versions of β-catenin (a wild-type and a Ser45-deleted) show elevated Wnt reporter activity when treated with Wnt, however, this was explained by the retained ability to regulate the wild-type β-catenin [25]. While the prevailing notion has maintained that oncogenic *CTNNB1* mutations result in an abolished response to Wnt, new evidence suggests otherwise. In hepatocellular carcinoma (HCC) cells, Rebouissou and colleagues reported that S45 mutations are only weakly activating and they concluded that S45 mutation alone is not sufficient to drive liver tumorigenesis [30]. Our own analysis of 351 liver cancers using cBioPortal confirmed that patients with S45 mutations showed elevated expression of Wnt target genes *Axin2*, *GLUL*, and *LGR5*, but not to the levels seen in patients with mutations in D32-S37 (Table S2). We recently demonstrated that colon cancer cells expressing only mutant β-catenin (Ser45del, termed β-catΔS45) still show the redistribution of both the destruction complex and β-catΔS45 toward a localized Wnt ligand [26]. Phosphorylation at the GSK-3β sites (Ser33/Ser37/Thr41) was previously reported to occur in the absence of Ser45 [31]. These results indicate that the presence of β-catΔS45 does not render cells completely unresponsive to Wnt and raises additional questions about the mechanism underlying β-catenin regulation.

Here, we sought to further test the "just-right" model of β-catenin mutation proposed for hepatocellular carcinoma by Rebouissou et al. by examining the effect of a β-catΔS45 mutation on the Wnt response in HCT116βm cells which harbor a single *CTNNB1* allele encoding a Ser45 deletion [32]. Ser45 modifications are seen in 10.8% of CRCs with β-catenin alterations and are considered to be stabilizing (Figure 1C). We demonstrate for the first time that HCT116βm cells accumulate β-catΔS45 when treated with Wnt3a or when depleted for APC and also display increased downstream Wnt transcriptional activation. However, β-catΔS45 nuclear translocation is only elevated in cells depleted for APC and not by Wnt3a treatment alone. We also find that β-catΔS45 is phosphorylated on the S33/S37/T41 residues, albeit somewhat less than wild-type β-catenin. It has been proposed that "just-right" signaling could result from *CTNNB1* mutation as well as *APC* mutation [33]. Our work demonstrates that β-catΔS45 is regulated by the destruction complex and responds to Wnt by accumulating and becoming more active in promoting Wnt target gene transcription. Further, these results implicate additional roles for APC in β-catenin regulation beyond those as a destruction complex scaffold.

2. Results

2.1. Phosphorylation Sites Important For B-Catenin Destruction Are Mutated in a Subset of Colorectal Cancers

Over-active Wnt signaling has been linked to many malignancies. In liver and endometrial cancer, *CTNNB1* mutations are common while *APC* mutations are rare [34]. In the majority of CRCs, mutations in *APC*, a key member of the β-catenin destruction complex, predominate. In CRCs without *APC* mutation, the Wnt pathway is often activated by other means, such as mutation of another pathway component. To assess the frequency of *CTNNB1* mutation in CRCs, we utilized four datasets from cBioPortal (DFCI, Genentech, MSKCC, and TCGA) and found that β-catenin mutations occurred in 160/2324 of patients (6.88%; Figure 1D) [4,35–39]. Of these β-catenin mutations, 47/176 were in the degradation motif sites (Figure 1C). Mutations within exon 3 of *CTNNB1* are considered drivers of tumorigenesis and account for 57/176 of the analyzed mutations [40]. Additionally, 91/176 mutations (51.7%) occurred within the armadillo repeat regions, which are thought to interact with APC, Axin, and LEF-1 [41–43]. We note that mutations outside of exon 3 may be passenger mutations and also find that truncating events that are unlikely to activate Wnt/β-catenin signaling account for 32/176 mutations. The "just-right" signaling hypothesis has been proposed as a means for the cell to regulate levels of Wnt activity through mutation of the *APC* gene. We wondered if mutations of the effector protein, β-catenin, also invoke a similar "just-right" response, allowing a specific level of Wnt regulation.

2.2. Generation of a Novel Anti-APC IgY Antibody

Current commercially available antibodies for the analysis of APC have limited applications and specificity [44,45]. To expand the repertoire of antibody species, we generated a chicken polyclonal antibody using the same central region of APC (amino acids 1001–1326) which we had successfully used to generate rabbit antisera [46]. The new IgY antibody was purified from yolk extracts and tested by Western immunoblot (Figure S1). The major band detected by the purified antibody migrated with an apparent molecular weight of 310 kDa with only faint signals for the smaller sized bands. When compared against a commercially available APC antibody, our chicken antibody shows a robust signal. Using siRNA to efficiently knockdown APC, we confirm that the 310 kDa band is reduced upon APC-depletion. This new tool will allow specific detection of APC, simultaneously with other proteins detected using mouse or rabbit antibodies.

2.3. B-CatδS45 Associates With a Locally-Applied Wnt-3a Ligand

Using immunofluorescence microscopy, we previously established that β-catΔS45 localizes toward a Wnt cue in HCT116βm cells [26]. We initially verified that a single allele encoding β-catenin is present in HCT116βm cells by performing Sanger sequencing, using RKO cells, another CRC cell line, which express only wild-type β-catenin as a control (Figure 1E). To test for a physical interaction between Wnt and β-catΔS45, Wnt3a-conjugated beads were applied to HCT116βm cells and then used to "pull down" associated proteins from cell lysates (Figure 2A). APC associated with Wnt-beads more than with the Unloaded-beads (Figure 2B). β-catΔS45 also associated more with the Wnt-beads than with the Unloaded-beads (Figure 2C). These data demonstrate that a core component of the destruction complex and a "stabilized" β-catenin both respond to a Wnt3a cue by localizing to the membrane, presumably through interactions with Frizzled and LRP5/6 coreceptors.

2.4. Wnt3a Exposure or APC-Depletion Increases Level of B-CatδS45 Protein

We previously reported that β-catenin destruction complex localization toward a Wnt cue was APC-dependent and appeared to correlate with an increased level of β-catenin in cells harboring fully intact Wnt signaling pathways [26]. Whether Wnt influences β-catΔS45 protein levels has yet to be determined. The β-catΔS45 protein expressed in HCT116βm cells lacks the site of CK1-α phosphorylation and is therefore generally assumed to be compromised for phosphorylation by GSK-3β and subsequent proteasome-mediated destruction. Notably, treatment with Wnt3a resulted in a 1.57-fold increase in total β-catΔS45 compared to untreated cells (Figure 3A–C). This unexpected result indicates that HCT116βm cells at least partially respond to Wnt by further stabilizing β-catΔS45 and therefore, β-catenin degradation can occur independently of Ser45. We efficiently depleted 90–95% of APC in HCT116βm cells with small interfering RNA (siAPC; Figure 3A,C). This APC-depletion led to a 1.47-fold increase in total β-catΔS45 protein level, while APC-depletion combined with Wnt3a treatment led to a 1.31-fold increase (Figure 3B). All of these increases were significant when compared to control-siRNA-treated cells (NT siRNA). These data indicate that cells exposed to Wnt ligand are able to further increase β-catΔS45 levels and that APC participates in β-catΔS45 destruction. Because APC-depletion together with Wnt treatment did not result in β-catΔS45 protein levels greater than either condition alone, it seems likely that these two components function in the same pathway to control β-catΔS45 protein levels.

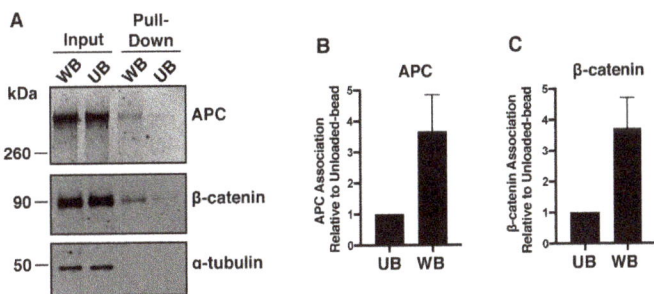

Figure 2. Wnt-beads pull-down APC and β-catΔS45. (**A**) HCT116βm cells treated with Wnt-beads or Unloaded-beads were lysed and proteins were pulled-down with the beads. Both APC and β-catΔS45 were detected in the Wnt-bead pull-down but not the Unloaded-bead pull-down. (**B**) Quantification of APC pulled-down by Wnt-beads compared to Unloaded-beads from three independent experiments. (**C**) Quantification of β-catΔS45 pulled-down by Wnt-beads compared to Unloaded-beads from three independent experiments. Protein levels that were pulled-down by beads were divided by the respective input protein levels and normalized to the Unloaded-bead to demonstrate fold change. Error bars, standard deviation (SD)Full blots, Figure S2).

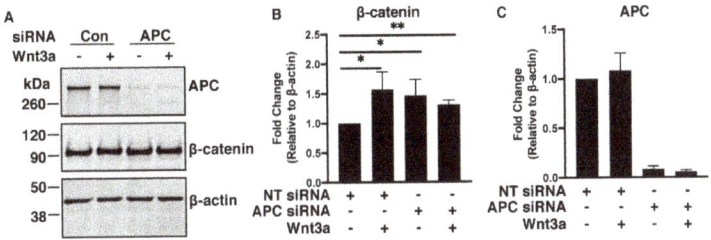

Figure 3. β-catΔS45 accumulates upon Wnt-3a treatment or APC-depletion. (**A**) Western blot of HCT116βm cells transfected with control-siRNA or APC-siRNA and treated in the presence or absence of 125 ng Wnt3a. (**B**) Relative fold-change of β-catenin relative to β-actin and normalized to control-siRNA without Wnt. Data averaged from four independent experiments. Error bars, SD; Statistical analysis by *t*-test: * $p < 0.05$; ** $p < 0.01$. (**C**) Quantification of APC fold-change relative to β-actin and normalized to control-siRNA without Wnt.

2.5. Wnt Signaling Is Activated in HCT116βm Cells Following APC-Depletion or Wnt3a Exposure

In cells with an intact Wnt signaling pathway, cellular β-catenin accumulation is followed by β-catenin's nuclear translocation and interaction with the transcription cofactor TCF-4 to activate Wnt target genes. HCT116βm cells harbor an activated Wnt pathway, demonstrated through increased TOPflash compared to isogenic cells only expressing wild-type β-catenin [32]. We wondered if the increased level of cellular β-catenin following Wnt exposure or APC-depletion would result in further increases in nuclear β-catenin activity. To test this, we cotransfected HCT116βm cells with TOPflash Wnt luciferase reporter plasmid and then depleted APC with siRNA, in the presence or absence of Wnt3a. Wnt3a treatment resulted in a three-fold increase and APC-depletion led to a 2.2-fold increase in Wnt reporter activity (Figure 4A). Unexpectedly, cells both depleted for APC and exposed to Wnt3a displayed a four-fold increase in Wnt reporter activity (Figure 4A). In RKO cells, which possess an intact Wnt signaling pathway, Wnt treatment resulted in an 8.2-fold increase in Wnt reporter activity (Figure 4B). However, in RKO cells with CRISPR/Cas9-deleted APC or in DLD1 cells that express endogenous truncated APC, Wnt3a presentation had no effect on Wnt reporter activity (Figure 4B).

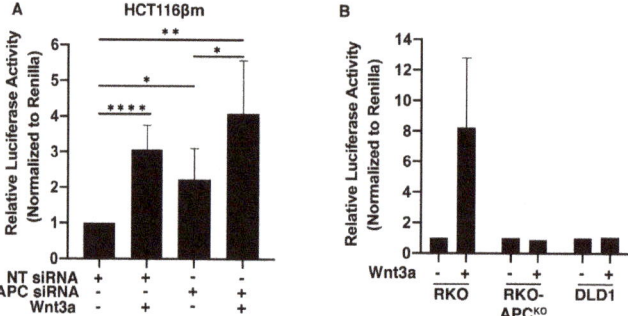

Figure 4. The Wnt transcriptional program is induced in HCT116βm upon Wnt-3a treatment or APC-depletion. (**A**) HCT116βm cells were cotransfected with pTOPflash and pRenilla luciferase reporter plasmids as well as control-siRNA or APC-siRNA, and subsequently treated with 125 ng Wnt3a for 24 h. Data averaged from seven individual experiments. Relative luciferase activity determined by the TOPflash/Renilla ratio of each group, followed by normalization to the control. Error bars, SD; Statistical analysis by t-test: * $p < 0.05$; ** $p < 0.01$; **** $p < 0.0001$. (**B**) TOPflash reporter assay in RKO, RKO-APC^{KO}, and DLD-1 colorectal cancer cell lines. Data for RKO averaged from four individual experiments, and RKO-APC^{KO} and DLD1 are from one experiment. Error bars, SD.

Combined, these data indicate that β-catΔS45 is still regulated by Wnt signaling, despite being able to evade Ser45 phosphorylation by CK1-α. Interestingly, cells with APC knock-out or mutant APC are resistant to further Wnt reporter activation, presumably due to maximal levels of pathway activation (Figure 4B) [25]. Yet, HCT116βm cells containing a stabilized β-catΔS45 are responsive to APC-depletion, even more responsive to Wnt addition, and show the most Wnt reporter activation when APC-depletion is combined with Wnt stimulation. This finding suggests that Wnt3a presentation and APC loss may stimulate Wnt reporter activity in an additive manner. This additive response may indicate the involvement of multiple pathways.

2.6. β-catΔS45 Increases Nuclear Localization Upon APC Loss, But Not Upon Wnt Exposure

APC-depletion has revealed a mechanism to regulate β-catΔS45 activity that appears distinct from that of Wnt stimulation. To explain this, we turned to other potential APC functions. Notably, APC is reported to be involved in sequestration, trafficking, and nuclear-cytoplasmic shuttling of proteins as well as Wnt-induced membrane localization of the destruction complex. We therefore considered the possibility that APC aids in the sequestration or trafficking of β-catΔS45, despite the ability of β-catΔS45 to evade destruction-complex-mediated Ser45 phosphorylation. We found that cells treated with Wnt displayed no changes in the ratio of nuclear to cytoplasmic β-catΔS45 compared to control cells (Figure 5A,B). However, upon APC-depletion, β-catΔS45 shifted into the nucleus, displaying an increased nuclear/cytoplasmic ratio and increased level of nuclear β-catenin compared to control (Figure 5A–C). Altered nuclear morphology observed in APC-depleted cells is consistent with previous reports that APC loss can lead to apoptosis [47,48]. The ratio of nuclear to cytoplasmic β-catΔS45 seen with APC-depletion did not further increase with added Wnt treatment (Figure 5B). Although still more nuclear than in control cells, the percent of change in nuclear β-catΔS45 in APC-depleted cells that were also treated with Wnt was significantly less than in cells only depleted of APC (Figure 5C). These data indicate that regulation of a "stabilized" β-catΔS45 is not merely through a degradation mechanism, but also may involve cytoplasmic sequestration or nuclear export, facilitated by APC.

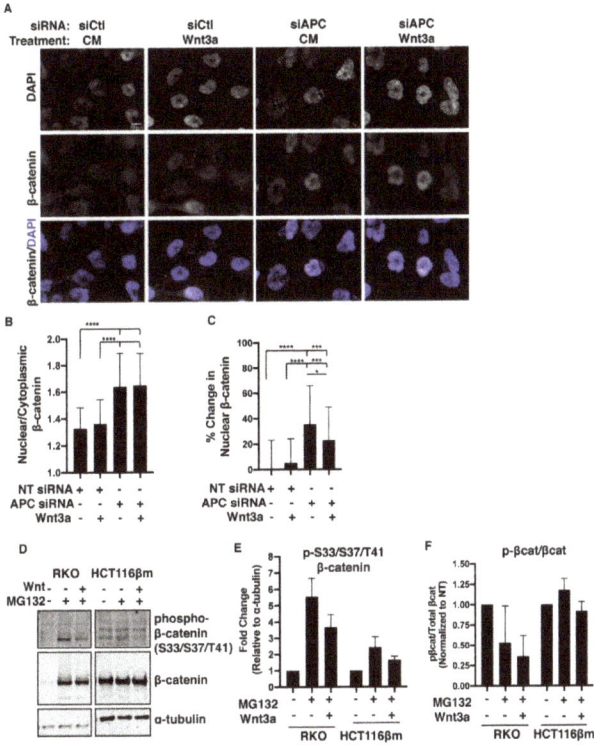

Figure 5. β-catΔS45 nuclear localization is controlled by APC and continues to be susceptible to GSK-3β phosphorylation and proteasomal degradation. (**A**) HCT116βm cells transfected with control-siRNA or APC-siRNA were treated with 125 ng Wnt3a and β-catenin localization was visualized by immunofluorescent detection. (**B**) Ratio of nuclear to cytoplasmic β-catenin quantified from immunofluorescent staining. Data representative of at least 36 individual cells per group (from two independent experiments). Error bars, SD; Statistical analysis by *t*-test: * $p < 0.05$, *** $p < 0.001$, **** $p < 0.0001$. (**C**) Percent change in nuclear β-catenin. Percent of nuclear β-catenin was calculated by dividing nuclear β-catenin by total β-catenin. Using nuclear β-catenin percentage, the percent change was calculated by comparing it to control. (**D**) RKO and HCT116βm cells were treated with 10 mM MG132 in the presence or absence of 25 ng/mL Wnt3a for 4 h prior to lysis. Western blot utilizing anti-phospho-Ser33/Ser37/Thr41-β-catenin or anti-β-catenin antibodies. (**E**) Quantification of the fold change of Ser33/Ser37/Thr41-phosphorylated β-catenin. Data averaged from two independent experiments. Error bars, SD. (**F**) Quantification of the ratio of phosphorylated-β-catenin to total β-catenin in RKO and HCT116βm cells following treatment with MG132 +/− Wnt3a. Data averaged from two independent experiments. Error bars, SD.

Assessment of β-catΔS45 nuclear and cytoplasmic localization showed that Wnt treatment alone does not affect nuclear translocation. However, APC-knockdown or Wnt treatment plus APC-knockdown caused a dramatic increase in nuclear β-catΔS45 compared to control. Of note, through assessment of β-catenin level (Figure 3), β-catΔS45 activity (Figure 4), and β-catΔS45 nuclear translocation (Figure 5), we found that increases in the level and nuclear localization of β-catΔS45 did not always translate into increased activity. Using these different data sets, we normalized the TOPflash values to the level of nuclear β-catΔS45 to estimate activity per unit of nuclear β-catΔS45. This analysis revealed that, though there was little change in nuclear β-catΔS45 levels, Wnt treatment alone resulted in a near doubling of the β-catΔS45 activity (1.92-fold) compared to untreated cells. In contrast, APC-depletion resulted in more β-catenin protein and nuclear localization but did not alter the activity per β-catΔS45 unit (1.05-fold) compared to untreated cells. The combination of APC-depletion and Wnt treatment resulted in elevated β-catenin protein and nuclear localization, similar to that observed with only APC-depletion. Finally, the activity per β-catΔS45 unit was much higher (2.5-fold) in combination-treated cells than that of untreated cells or only APC-depleted cells.

2.7. β-catΔS45 Is Phosphorylated at the GSK-3β Sites and Is Susceptible to Proteasomal Degradation

Solely considering the destruction complex, it is perplexing that APC-depletion or Wnt exposure would impact the protein level of a "stabilized" β-catenin. Previously, it was reported that β-catΔS45 is phosphorylated at the GSK-3β sites Ser33/Ser37/Thr41 [31]. However, it was unknown whether β-catΔS45 is also degraded by the proteasome. We detected more total β-catenin and phospho-Ser33/Ser37/Thr41-β-catenin when RKO cells were treated with an MG132 proteasome inhibitor (Figure 5D,E). This was expected, since RKO cells have an intact β-catenin destruction complex. The ratio of p-β-catenin to total β-catenin decreased in RKO cells treated with MG132 (Figure 5F). This decrease is potentially due to the large increase in total β-catenin level (~14-fold), and may reflect saturated destruction complexes unable to phosphorylate all of the accumulated β-catenin, as previously proposed [25]. We also detected phospho-β-catΔS45 in HCT116βm cells, thus confirming previous reports (Figure 5D) [31]. MG132 treatment resulted in increased total β-catΔS45 and phospho-β-catΔS45 levels, indicative of proteasomal degradation (Figure 5E). However, we did not observe a decreased ratio of p-β-catΔS45/β-catΔS45 in HCT116βm cells treated with both MG132 and Wnt (Figure 5F). Together, these data support a proposed mechanism in which cells containing a deletion of the CK1-α phosphorylation site are able to maintain some β-catenin regulation through the potential alternative priming of GSK-3β-mediated phosphorylation and through proteasomal degradation. Of note, this ability to respond to Wnt ligand distinguishes β-catΔS45-mutant colorectal cancer cells from the APC-mutant colorectal cancer cells (Figure 4B).

2.8. APC Truncation But Not β-Catenin Mutation Results in Elevated Wnt Target Gene Expression in Human Colorectal Cancers

Having demonstrated that β-catΔS45 still shows evidence of regulation by Wnt and APC, we turned our attention back to human colorectal cancer patient samples. Using cBioPortal, we queried the TCGA (PanCancer Atlas) dataset for expression of Wnt target genes in colon cancers with various categories of *APC* or *CTNNB1* mutations. mRNA levels for demonstrated Wnt targets *Axin2*, *Myc*, and *Lgr5* were significantly elevated in CRC tumors with *APC* mutations that result in protein truncation vs. samples lacking these truncating *APC* mutations, designated as wild-type (Figure 6A). Therefore, expression patterns for these three genes can provide a surrogate marker for β-catenin signaling in the patient tissue samples. In contrast, *CCND1* and *GLUL*, which have also been described as Wnt targets, showed no expression changes that correlated with *APC* status.

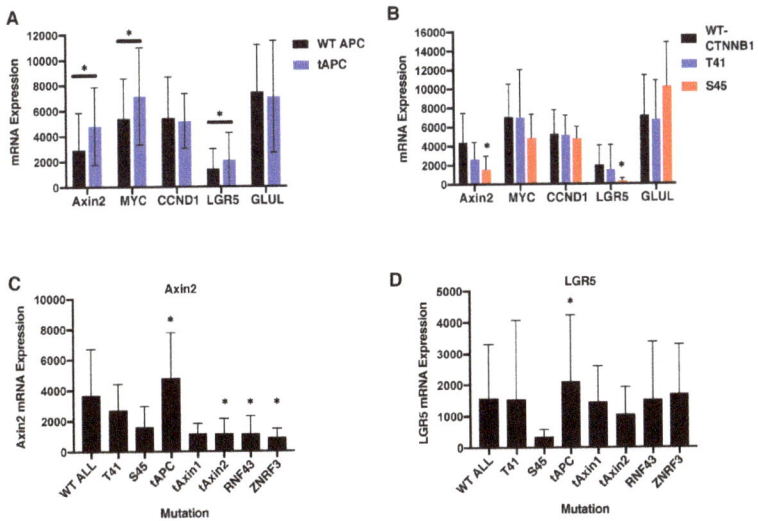

Figure 6. Wnt target gene activation in colorectal cancers with truncating APC mutations. Wnt target gene mRNA expression was determined from 524 colorectal cancer patients using cBioPortal and is displayed as RSEM. *CCND1* encodes CyclinD1 and *GLUL* encodes Glutamate–Ammonia Ligase. (**A**) mRNA expression in 374 patients with truncating "driver" *APC* mutations and 150 with wild-type *APC* or missense mutations (all included in the wild-type category). (**B**) mRNA expression for 491 patients with wild-type *CTNNB1*, 7 with Ser45 mutations, and 6 with Thr41 mutations. For (**C**) and (**D**) 426 colorectal cancer patient samples were queried for levels of Wnt target AXIN2 or *LGR5* RNA, respectively. Samples were categorized by mutation status of *CTNNB1* or truncating driver mutations in β-catenin regulatory genes. WT ALL samples had no driver mutations in any Wnt-related category queried. Error is presented as SD. * indicates *p*-value calculated with paired student *T*-test < 0.0005 in (**A**) and < 0.05 in (**B–D**) for each pair combination. For (**C**) and (**D**), n values of each group were as follows: WT All (101), T41 (6), S45 (7), tAPC (374), tAxin1 (5), tAxin2 (19), RNF43 (36), and ZNRF3 (8).

Using a similar approach, sample groups were established based on *CTNNB1* status (Figure 6B). There were seven samples with Ser45 mutations (deletions or substitution of Phe or Pro) and six with T41 mutations (Ala or Ile substitution). In liver cancers, these mutations were categorized as having "weak" and "moderate" β-catenin activity, respectively [30]. Other *CTNNB1* mutations were not present in enough patient samples to analyze. Relative to samples with wild-type *CTNNB1*, none of the Wnt target gene markers showed significant upregulation in either the Ser45- or Thr41-mutant group. Rather, the mRNA level for the β-catenin activity reporters that were elevated with *APC* truncating mutation was either unchanged or decreased in patients with *CTNNB1* mutations when compared to patients with wild-type *CTNNB1*. Over 70% of the colorectal cancer patient samples with wild-type *CTNNB1* displayed truncating *APC* mutations and another 9% displayed mutations in one or more other genes involved in β-catenin destruction (*Axin1, Axin2, RNF43,* and *ZNRF3*). To ensure that mutations in these other β-catenin regulators were not influencing Wnt target gene expression in our "wild-type" samples presented in Figure 6A,B, the RNA levels were reanalyzed taking into account the status of these various Wnt regulatory genes (Figure 6C,D). Once again, the mRNA levels for β-catenin activity reporters *AXIN2* and *LGR5* were either unchanged or decreased in patients with *CTNNB1* mutations when compared to patients that were wild-type for all of these β-catenin regulator genes. Though these results were consistent with our in vitro data, they contradict results from a similar analysis of liver cancers [30] and (Table S2). We conclude that in colon cancers, the Ser45 mutation does not appear to increase Wnt signaling and that the effects of *CTNNB1* mutations are not the same in the liver and colon.

3. Discussion

The Wnt/β-catenin pathway is typically described as signaling in a linear manner; Wnt ligand binds the Frizzled and LRP5/6 coreceptors, leading to inhibition of the β-catenin destruction complex and subsequent β-catenin stabilization, accumulation, and nuclear translocation. Mutation to a downstream component such as APC or β-catenin is thought to activate the pathway and render it unresponsive to regulation by upstream pathway components. The results presented here demonstrate that "downstream" components of the Wnt pathway can continue to be regulated by "upstream" components despite the presence of a stabilizing mutation. In the context of APC mutations, a "just-right" signaling hypothesis has been proposed in which APC mutations occur to allow a specific level of β-catenin that supports tumorigenesis. Our results support the notion that β-catenin itself may also be prone to just-right mutations that maintain some regulation of the β-catenin protein, limiting its accumulation and activity. As an initial proof of concept, we used the HCT116βm cell line which harbors a deletion of β-catenin Ser45, to assess the Wnt/Receptor/β-catΔS45 interaction and the changes in β-catΔS45 protein levels, activity, and localization upon Wnt3a stimulation or APC loss.

In agreement with our previous immunofluorescence data [26], we demonstrate that both β-catΔS45 and APC pull-down with a Wnt-bead, indicative of the interaction between Wnt ligand, receptor, β-catΔS45, and APC. Surprisingly, we find that Wnt3a treatment, APC knock-down, or treatment plus knockdown, results in elevated β-catΔS45 protein levels as well as increased TOPflash Wnt reporter activity. APC-depletion results in predominantly nuclear β-catΔS45, whereas Wnt treatment alone does not change the nuclear localization of β-catΔS45. Moreover, we confirm that β-catΔS45 can be phosphorylated at Ser33/Ser37/Thr41 and find that β-catΔS45 is regulated by the proteasome. Finally, we provide evidence that in colorectal cancer patient tissue, CTNNB1 mutations that eliminate Ser45 or Thr41 do not result in elevated β-catenin activity as assessed by Wnt target gene expression.

We propose the following expansion of the current Wnt signaling mechanism to explain our findings: (1) Wnt signaling leads to a secondary effect that further activates β-catenin in the nucleus, essentially amplifying the signal. An example of this would be that *LEF/TCF* is a Wnt target gene [49,50]. (2) APC inhibits the activity of this Wnt-induced β-catenin inducer. (3) APC promotes cytoplasmic localization of β-catenin, perhaps through cytoplasmic sequestration or nuclear to cytoplasmic shuttling. Our results are inconsistent with the role of APC in sequestering nuclear β-catenin or facilitating the nuclear import of β-catenin. (4) Wnt can also inhibit nuclear localization of β-catenin, independent of APC. (5) *CTNNB1* mutations to Thr41 or Ser45 in human CRC do not confer elevated Wnt signaling.

Our work is in agreement with previously published results by our lab and others, demonstrating that the interaction of APC with nuclear β-catenin leads to repression of Wnt target genes [20,21,23,24]. Further, it is intriguing that β-catΔS45 continues to be phosphorylated at GSK-3β sites and degraded by the proteasome, albeit less efficiently than wild-type β-catenin. The deletion of Ser45 may place Ser47 in close enough proximity (within five residues upon S45del) to T41 to act as a priming site for β-catenin phosphorylation [51]. Suggestive of alternative mechanisms for GSK-3β phosphorylation, S33/S37/T41 phosphorylation is also observed in LS174T cells containing a S45F substitution [25,31]. Finally, comparing our Wnt target gene mRNA expression analysis in human colon cancer tissue to similar analyses in liver cancer [30] and Table S2 reveals that Wnt signaling and the consequences of *CTNNB1* mutation are not the same in cancers of different tissues.

Colorectal cancer is generally assumed to be promoted by Wnt signal activation. Here, we provide insight into the mechanism by which β-catenin is regulated in the Wnt-on or Wnt-off states and also demonstrate that mutant β-catenin can be regulated by the Wnt pathway components. We find that *APC*-mutant cells are unresponsive to additional Wnt signaling, whereas cells expressing mutant β-catenin are responsive to extracellular Wnt ligand. It is likely that complete stabilization of β-catenin in colon epithelia would result in too much β-catenin protein and activity, thus impairing cell viability and potentially inducing apoptosis as previously demonstrated in mouse gut [48] and human epidermis [52]. Our finding that the Wnt/β-catenin signaling pathway does not act in a strictly linear fashion emphasizes the importance of a therapeutic strategy that targets multiple aspects of the pathway. Finally, we provide evidence that β-catΔS45 is still susceptible to regulation and that this mutation may act to provide "just-right" signaling for optimal tumorigenic capability in the colon.

4. Materials and Methods

4.1. Cell Culture and Treatments

HCT116βm, RKO, DLD1, and RKO-APC^{KO} cells were cultured in DMEM (with L-Glutamine and 4.5 g/L Glucose; without Sodium Pyruvate) supplemented with 10% fetal bovine serum (FBS) and were maintained at 37 °C and 5% CO_2. Wnt treatment was performed by adding recombinant Wnt-3a (Peprotech, Rocky Hill, NJ, USA; #315-20) at the indicated concentration/time prior to cell lysis or immunofluorescence analysis. For siRNA-mediated inhibition, HCT116βm cells were transfected using Lipofectamine 3000 (Invitrogen, Carlsbad, CA, USA) according to the manufacturer's instructions with 37.5 nM of each siRNA targeting human APC (Smartpool siRNAs 1-3: Dharmacon, Lafayette, CO, USA) or nontargeting siControl siRNA (Dharmacon). Cell media was changed one day following siRNA transfection, and cells were grown 48 h prior to Wnt treatment. MG-132 treatment was performed by the addition of 10 mM MG-132 to a final concentration of 10 µM in cell media for 4 h.

HCT116βm were derived from the parental HCT116 cell line (ATCC, Manassas, VA, USA) and kindly provided by Bert Vogelstein [32]. We received HCT116βm from Bert Vogelstein (who originally received HCT116 cells from ATCC) and passaged two times into Dulbecco's Modified Eagle Medium (DMEM)+10%FBS prior to preparing cell stocks. RKO and DLD1 cells were received from ATCC and passaged two times into DMEM + 10% FBS prior to preparing cell stocks. RKO-APC^{KO} cells were derived from the parental RKO cell line (ATCC) and kindly provided by Ethan Lee [53]. We passaged them two times into DMEM+ 10% FBS prior to preparing cell stocks.

4.2. Analysis of CTNNB1 Mutation Frequency and mRNA Expression of Wnt Target Genes

Mutation frequency of the *CTNNB1* gene was assessed using the cBioPortal [35,36]. Colorectal adenocarcinoma datasets from DFCI (Cell Reports 2016), Genentech (Nature 2012), MSKCC (Cancer Cell 2018), and TCGA (PanCancer Atlas) were queried for the *CTNNB1* and *APC* genes [37–39,54]. Of the 1287 total cases, 1225 had mutations data and were utilized for mutation frequency and mutual exclusivity determinations. The TCGA (PanCancer Atlas) dataset also contained RNAseq data which were queried for expression of Wnt target genes in colon cancers with various categories of *CTNNB1* mutations or "driver" mutations in *APC* or other β-catenin regulatory factors. Values were provided as RSEM (RNA-Seq by Expectation Maximization).

4.3. CTNNB1 Sanger Sequencing and Alignment

HCT116βm and RKO cells were harvested and DNA extraction was performed using the Qiagen (Hilden, Germany) DNeasy Blood and Tissue Kit according to the manufacturer's instructions. PCR amplification was performed using the following primers: 5'-cctcctaatggcttggtgaa-3'; 5'-caggacttgggaggtatcca-3'. Following amplification, PCR products were gel-purified and sequenced by Genewiz (South Plainfield, NJ, USA). Trace files and sequence alignment were analyzed using SnapGene, version 4 (Insightful Science).

4.4. Immobilization of Wnt Protein

Wnt3a was immobilized onto Dynabeads as described previously [55]. Briefly, 2.8 µm Dynabeads M-270 Carboxylic Acid (Invitrogen) were activated by NHS/EDC (Sigma, St. Louis, MO, USA, 50 mg/mL each in cold 25 mM MES pH 5) then washed three times with cold 25 mM, pH5 5 2-(*N*-morpholino)ethanesulfonic acid (MES) buffer. Wnt immobilization was performed by diluting 0.5 µg of purified Wnt3a protein in cold MES buffer and incubated at room temperature (RT) for 1 h. To quench nonreactive carboxylic acid groups, beads were incubated with 50 mM Tris pH 7.4 at RT for

15 min. Beads were washed twice in phosphate-buffered saline (PBS) pH 7.4 before final resuspension in 400 µL PBS/0.5% BSA and stored at 4 °C. Unloaded-beads were prepared in parallel by incubating 1 h in MES without Wnt. Wnt3a activity following bead immobilization was verified using a TOPflash luciferase reporter assay [56].

4.5. Immunoblotting

Cells were washed 1x in PBS prior to harvesting in preheated, high-salt sample lysis buffer (20% glycerol, 2% sodium dodecyl sulfate (SDS), 30% 10X PBS, 2.5% β-mercaptoethanol). Scraped cells were transferred to Eppendorf tubes, heated at 95 °C for 1 min, pulled through an insulin syringe three times, and heated again. Samples were separated on 7.5% SDS-PAGE (Bio-Rad, Hercules, CA, USA; TGX FastCast Acrylamide Kit) using Tris-Glycine running buffer and transferred to a nitrocellulose membrane (GE) with a 0.45 µm pore size. Antibodies were diluted in Odyssey Blocking Buffer TBS (LI-COR) as follows: anti-APC-M2 Chicken pAb (1:2000), anti-β-catenin mouse mAb (1:1000), anti-phospho-Ser33/Ser37/Thr41-β-catenin rabbit pAb (Cell Signaling Technology, Danvers, MA, USA; 1:500), anti-α-tubulin DM1A mouse mAb (Santa Cruz Biotechnology, Dallas, TX, USA; 1:1000), anti-β-actin mouse mAb (Sigma, 1:1000), and IRDye 680LT and 800CW anti-rabbit, anti-mouse, or anti-chicken secondary antibodies (1:150,000). Immunoblots were imaged on an LI-COR Odyssey CLx imaging system.

4.6. Wnt-Bead Pull-Down

Cells were grown in 6-well tissue culture plates and treated with 40 µL Unloaded-beads or Wnt-beads for 4 h. Following bead treatment, cells were briefly washed in 1x PBS prior to lysis in 200 µL lysis buffer (150 mM NaCl, 30 mM Tris pH 7.5, 1 mM EDTA, 1% Triton X-100, 10% glycerol, 0.1 mM PMSF, 0.5 mM DTT, and HALT protease and phosphatase inhibitors, Thermo Scientific, Waltham, MA, USA) [25,26]. Following the addition of the lysis buffer, cells were scraped into 1.5 mL tubes and rotated at 4 °C for 30 min. Beads were isolated using a magnet and the supernatant was transferred to a new tube. Beads were washed three times in 500 µL of cold lysis buffer. Following the last wash, beads were resuspended in 40 µL cold PBS and 20 µL 3X SDS sample buffer.

4.7. Generation of Anti-APC-M2 Chicken IgY Antibody

The central region of APC (amino acids 1001-1326, "APC-M2") was cloned and ligated into the pET28b (Novagen Millipore Sigma, Burlington, MA, USA) expression vector, which contains an N-terminal 6X-His tag. Sequence-verified plasmids were transformed into BL21-CodonPlus-(DE3)-RIPL *E. coli* cells (NEB) for expression. Cells were grown in standard LB broth containing 50 µg/mL kanamycin at 37 °C with shaking (225 rpm) and induced with 0.2 mM isopropyl-β-D-thiogalactopyranoside (IPTG) for protein expression when an OD of 0.4–0.6 was reached. Cells were allowed to express induced protein products for 3–4 h at 37 °C with shaking before harvested by centrifugation at 4000 rpm, 15 min, 4 °C. Cellular pellets were resuspended in a buffer containing 50 mM Tris pH 8.0, 50 mM NaCl, 50 mM imidazole, 10% glycerol, and HALT protease cocktail (Thermo). Cells were lysed by a French pressure cell (35,000 psi), and the insoluble cellular debris was removed by centrifugation at 16,000× *g* for 45 min, 4 °C. Supernatant was applied to a chelating sepharose fast-flow column (Amersham Biosciences, Little Chalfont, UK) charged with nickel chloride and pre-equilibrated in resuspension buffer. Protein retained on the column was washed with a 3-column volume (C.V.) salt gradient (50 mM potassium phosphate pH 8.0, 500 mM NaCl, 50 mM imidazole, 10% glycerol). Protein was eluted with an imidazole buffer gradient (50 mM Tris pH 8.0, 500 mM NaCl, 500 mM imidazole, 10% glycerol). Fractions containing recombinant protein were pooled and applied to a Superdex 200 size-exclusion column (Amersham Biosciences) pre-equilibrated with 50 mM Tris, pH 8.0, 150 mM NaCl, and 10% glycerol, 1 mM DTT, and 1 mM octyl β-D-gluctopyranoside. Fractions containing recombinant protein were pooled and concentrated with Amicon Ultra centrifugal filters (Millipore).

Recombinant APC antigen was shipped to Gallus Immunotech Inc. (now Exalpha Biologicals, Inc., Shirley, MA, USA) for injection into hens, and extraction of IgY-containing yolk extract. The anti-APC IgY was purified from the returned yolk extracts by affinity chromatography. Briefly, NHS-Sepharose (GE Healthcare, Chicago, IL, USA) was conjugated with APC-M2 antigen, purified as described above. 1M Tris (pH 8.0) and Tween-20 were added to the yolk extracts, to final concentrations of 10 mM and 0.2%, respectively. Buffered yolk extract was incubated with prepared APC-M2-conjugated NHS-Sepharose overnight at 4 °C. Columns were washed with multiple column volumes of PBS and PBS-T buffers. Anti-APC-M2 IgY was eluted from the column in 0.2 M glycine, pH 2.0. Fractions containing eluted anti-APC-M2 IgY were dialyzed into a buffer containing PBS at pH 7.4, 5% glycerol, and 0.01% sodium azide.

4.8. Luciferase Reporter Assay

Cells were seeded into 12-well plates 24 h prior to transfection. On the day of transfection, cell culture media was changed one hour prior to siRNA and plasmid transfection. Both reporter plasmids and siRNAs were transfected concurrently using Lipofectamine 3000 according to the manufacturer's instructions. Human APC-siRNA or control-siRNA was transfected as described above. For luciferase reporters, cells were cotransfected with TOPflash (450 ng) and Renilla (50 ng) expression plasmids. As a control, identical wells were transfected with FOPflash (450 ng) and Renilla (50 ng) expression plasmids to validate that a scrambled TCF-binding sequence does not result in increased reporter activity upon treatment. Following two days of APC-depletion, cells were treated with Wnt3a for 24 h and lysed using the Dual-Luciferase Reporter Assay System (Promega). Firefly luciferase signal was normalized to the Renilla luciferase signal, and data were normalized to control (set to 1).

4.9. Immunofluorescence and Analysis

Cells were briefly rinsed in PBS prior to fixation. Cells were fixed in 4% PFA in Brinkley's Buffer 1980 (80 mM PIPES pH 6.8, 1 mM $MgCl_2$, 1 mM EGTA) for 20 min at room temperature (RT) and washed two times in PBS prior to permeabilization in TBS + 0.2% Triton X-100 for 5 min. Cells were washed in TBS two times prior to incubation for 1 hour at RT in blocking buffer containing TBS + 0.2% Triton X-100, 1% BSA, and 3% Normal Goat Serum. Primary and secondary antibodies were incubated for 1 hour at RT. Cells were washed three times in TBS following primary and secondary antibody incubations. Mounting of coverslips was performed using Prolong Diamond Antifade Mountant with DAPI (Invitrogen). The anti-β-catenin mouse mAb (BD Transduction Laboratories, San Jose, CA, USA; #610154) was diluted 1:250 in blocking buffer. Stained cells were examined using an Axioplan microscope (Zeiss, Oberkochen, Germany) with a ×100 objective. Images of stained cells were captured using an Orca R^2 digital camera (Hamamatsu, Hamamatsu City, Shizuoka, Japan).

For calculation of the nuclear and cytoplasmic distribution of β-catenin, CellProfiler version 3.1.9 [57] was used to identify and measure the total and mean pixel intensities of β-catenin protein in cytoplasmic or nuclear compartments. Briefly, nuclei identification was first performed using the DAPI image, followed by cell identification by propagation. The cytoplasm was identified using the identified "total cells" and the identified nuclei to remove nuclei from the cytoplasmic calculation. Automated pipeline creation was performed using the following as a guide: [58].

4.10. Quantification and Statistical Analysis

Fluorescent-detection and quantification of immunoblots was performed using the LI-COR Odyssey CLx imaging system and Image Studio™ Lite software, version 5.2.5 (LI-COR, Lincoln, NE, USA). Graphs were generated using GraphPad Prism, version 8.4.3 (GraphPad Software, Inc.), and all statistical analyses were performed using a two-tailed, unpaired t-test in which a value of $p < 0.05$ is statistically significant.

5. Conclusions

Using data available on cBioPortal, we find that mutations to β-catenin occur in ~6% of human CRC and in 9% of CRCs lacking an APC mutation. Combined with our previously published data demonstrating that the β-catenin destruction complex relocalizes toward a Wnt cue in cells expressing mutant β-catenin, we hypothesized that "stabilizing" β-catenin mutations do not completely evade Wnt regulation. It has been previously proposed that *APC* mutations occur in a "just-right" fashion to allow optimal levels of β-catenin signaling for tumorigenesis. The current work demonstrates that stabilizing β-catenin mutations allow cells to respond to Wnt and are prone to regulation by APC. Wnt treatment and APC-depletion both induce increased β-catΔS45 protein and activity by the TOPflash reporter assay. Interestingly, we find that Wnt treatment does not increase the nuclear accumulation of β-catΔS45 whereas APC-depletion results in predominantly nuclear β-catΔS45 localization. This data supports a role for APC in cytoplasmic retention of β-catenin. Further, we verify that β-catΔS45 can be phosphorylated at the GSK-3β phosphorylation sites, despite the lack of a priming Ser45. Treatment with proteasome inhibitors results in β-catΔS45 accumulation, indicating that this "stabilized" protein is still able to be targeted to the proteasome. Our results indicate that a Wnt signal leads to secondary effects that further activate nuclear β-catenin and that APC may inhibit this activity by nuclear export and/or sequestration of β-catenin in the cytoplasm.

Supplementary Materials: The following are available online at http://www.mdpi.com/2072-6694/12/8/2114/s1, Figure S1: Validation of anti-APC-M2 chicken IgY antibody, Figure S2: Full-length Western blots, Table S1: Mutations analyzed from cBioPortal including data from: MSKCC, TCGA, DFCI, and Genentech, Table S2: Liver Cancer Patient Samples with various CTNNB1 mutations queried for Wnt target gene RNA level.

Author Contributions: Conceptualization, T.W.P. and K.L.N.; methodology, T.W.P., A.J.R., K.L.N.; software, T.W.P.; validation, T.W.P., A.J.R., and K.L.N.; formal analysis, T.W.P. and K.L.N.; investigation, T.W.P.; resources, K.L.N.; data curation, T.W.P. and K.L.N.; writing—original draft preparation, T.W.P.; writing—review and editing, T.W.P., A.J.R., and K.L.N.; visualization, T.W.P.; supervision, K.L.N.; project administration, K.L.N.; funding acquisition, K.L.N. All authors have read and agreed to the published version of the manuscript.

Funding: This research was funded by the National Science Foundation, IOS-1456538 and the National Institutes of Health, P30CA168524.

Acknowledgments: The authors thank E. Lee (Vanderbilt) for providing the RKO-APC^{KO} cell line. We thank B. Vogelstein (Johns Hopkins University) for providing the HCT116βm cell line. We are grateful to A. Lamb (University of Kansas) for use of lab equipment critical for developing the chicken IgY APC antibody.

Conflicts of Interest: The authors declare no conflicts of interest. The funders had no role in the design of the study; in the collection, analyses, or interpretation of data; in the writing of the manuscript, or in the decision to publish the results.

References

1. Logan, C.Y.; Nusse, R. The Wnt Signaling Pathway in Development and Disease. *Annu. Rev. Cell Dev. Biol.* **2004**, *20*, 781–810. [CrossRef]
2. Clevers, H. Wnt/β-Catenin Signaling in Development and Disease. *Cell* **2006**, *127*, 469–480. [CrossRef]
3. MacDonald, B.T.; Tamai, K.; He, X. Wnt/β-Catenin Signaling: Components, Mechanisms, and Diseases. *Dev. Cell* **2009**, *17*, 9–26. [CrossRef] [PubMed]
4. The Cancer Genome Atlas Network Comprehensive molecular characterization of human colon and rectal cancer. *Nature* **2012**, *487*, 330–337. [CrossRef] [PubMed]
5. Stamos, J.L.; Weis, W.I. The β-Catenin Destruction Complex. *Cold Spring Harb. Perspect. Biol.* **2013**, *5*, a007898. [CrossRef]
6. Aberle, H.; Bauer, A.; Stappert, J.; Kispert, A.; Kemler, R. beta-catenin is a target for the ubiquitin-proteasome pathway. *EMBO J.* **1997**, *16*, 3797–3804. [CrossRef]
7. Kitagawa, M.; Hatakeyama, S.; Shirane, M.; Matsumoto, M.; Ishida, N.; Hattori, K.; Nakamichi, I.; Kikuchi, A.; Nakayama, K.; Nakayama, K. An F-box protein, FWD1, mediates ubiquitin-dependent proteolysis of beta-catenin. *EMBO J.* **1999**, *18*, 2401–2410. [CrossRef]
8. Liu, C.; Li, Y.; Semenov, M.; Han, C.; Baeg, G.-H.; Tan, Y.; Zhang, Z.; Lin, X.; He, X. Control of β-Catenin Phosphorylation/Degradation by a Dual-Kinase Mechanism. *Cell* **2002**, *108*, 837–847. [CrossRef]

9. Bilić, J.; Huang, Y.-L.; Davidson, G.; Zimmermann, T.; Cruciat, C.-M.; Bienz, M.; Niehrs, C. Wnt Induces LRP6 Signalosomes and Promotes Dishevelled-Dependent LRP6 Phosphorylation. *Science* **2007**, *316*, 1619–1622. [CrossRef] [PubMed]
10. Tamai, K.; Semenov, M.; Kato, Y.; Spokony, R.; Liu, C.; Katsuyama, Y.; Hess, F.; Saint-Jeannet, J.-P.; He, X. LDL-receptor-related proteins in Wnt signal transduction. *Nature* **2000**, *407*, 530. [CrossRef]
11. Amit, S.; Hatzubai, A.; Birman, Y.; Andersen, J.S.; Ben-Shushan, E.; Mann, M.; Ben-Neriah, Y.; Alkalay, I. Axin-mediated CKI phosphorylation of β-catenin at Ser 45: A molecular switch for the Wnt pathway. *Genes Dev.* **2002**, *16*, 1066–1076. [CrossRef]
12. Fiol, C.J.; Mahrenholz, A.M.; Wang, Y.; Roeske, R.W.; Roach, P.J. Formation of protein kinase recognition sites by covalent modification of the substrate. Molecular mechanism for the synergistic action of casein kinase II and glycogen synthase kinase 3. *J. Biol. Chem.* **1987**, *262*, 14042–14048.
13. Frame, S.; Cohen, P.; Biondi, R.M. A Common Phosphate Binding Site Explains the Unique Substrate Specificity of GSK3 and Its Inactivation by Phosphorylation. *Mol. Cell* **2001**, *7*, 1321–1327. [CrossRef]
14. Hagen, T.; Vidal-Puig, A. Characterisation of the phosphorylation of β-catenin at the GSK-3 priming site Ser45. *Biochem. Biophys. Res. Commun.* **2002**, *294*, 324–328. [CrossRef]
15. Hart, M.; Concordet, J.-P.; Lassot, I.; Albert, I.; del los Santos, R.; Durand, H.; Perret, C.; Rubinfeld, B.; Margottin, F.; Benarous, R.; et al. The F-box protein β-TrCP associates with phosphorylated β-catenin and regulates its activity in the cell. *Curr. Biol.* **1999**, *9*, 207–211. [CrossRef]
16. Latres, E.; Chiaur, D.S.; Pagano, M. The human F box protein β-Trcp associates with the Cul1/Skp1 complex and regulates the stability of β-catenin. *Oncogene* **1999**, *18*, 849–854. [CrossRef] [PubMed]
17. Liu, C.; Kato, Y.; Zhang, Z.; Do, V.M.; Yankner, B.A.; He, X. β-Trcp couples β-catenin phosphorylation-degradation and regulates Xenopus axis formation. *Proc. Natl. Acad. Sci. USA* **1999**, *96*, 6273–6278. [CrossRef] [PubMed]
18. Winston, J.T.; Strack, P.; Beer-Romero, P.; Chu, C.Y.; Elledge, S.J.; Harper, J.W. The SCFβ-TRCP–ubiquitin ligase complex associates specifically with phosphorylated destruction motifs in IκBα and β-catenin and stimulates IκBα ubiquitination in vitro. *Genes Dev.* **1999**, *13*, 270–283. [CrossRef]
19. Albuquerque, C.; Breukel, C.; van der Luijt, R.; Fidalgo, P.; Lage, P.; Slors, F.J.M.; Leitão, C.N.; Fodde, R.; Smits, R. The 'just-right' signaling model: APC somatic mutations are selected based on a specific level of activation of the β-catenin signaling cascade. *Hum. Mol. Genet.* **2002**, *11*, 1549–1560. [CrossRef]
20. Neufeld, K.L.; Nix, D.A.; Bogerd, H.; Kang, Y.; Beckerle, M.C.; Cullen, B.R.; White, R.L. Adenomatous polyposis coli protein contains two nuclear export signals and shuttles between the nucleus and cytoplasm. *Proc. Natl. Acad. Sci. USA* **2000**, *97*, 12085–12090. [CrossRef]
21. Neufeld, K.L.; Zhang, F.; Cullen, B.R.; White, R.L. APC-mediated downregulation of -catenin activity involves nuclear sequestration and nuclear export. *EMBO Rep.* **2000**, *1*, 519–523. [CrossRef] [PubMed]
22. Rosin-Arbesfeld, R.; Townsley, F.; Bienz, M. The APC tumour suppressor has a nuclear export function. *Nature* **2000**, *406*, 1009. [CrossRef] [PubMed]
23. Rosin-Arbesfeld, R.; Cliffe, A.; Brabletz, T.; Bienz, M. Nuclear export of the APC tumour suppressor controls β-catenin function in transcription. *EMBO J.* **2003**, *22*, 1101–1113. [CrossRef] [PubMed]
24. Sierra, J.; Yoshida, T.; Joazeiro, C.A.; Jones, K.A. The APC tumor suppressor counteracts β-catenin activation and H3K4 methylation at Wnt target genes. *Genes Dev.* **2006**, *20*, 586–600. [CrossRef]
25. Li, V.S.W.; Ng, S.S.; Boersema, P.J.; Low, T.Y.; Karthaus, W.R.; Gerlach, J.P.; Mohammed, S.; Heck, A.J.R.; Maurice, M.M.; Mahmoudi, T.; et al. Wnt Signaling through Inhibition of β-Catenin Degradation in an Intact Axin1 Complex. *Cell* **2012**, *149*, 1245–1256. [CrossRef]
26. Parker, T.W.; Neufeld, K.L. APC controls Wnt-induced β-catenin destruction complex recruitment in human colonocytes. *Sci. Rep.* **2020**, *10*, 1–14. [CrossRef]
27. Su, Y.; Fu, C.; Ishikawa, S.; Stella, A.; Kojima, M.; Shitoh, K.; Schreiber, E.M.; Day, B.W.; Liu, B. APC Is Essential for Targeting Phosphorylated β-Catenin to the SCFβ-TrCP Ubiquitin Ligase. *Mol. Cell* **2008**, *32*, 652–661. [CrossRef]
28. Yang, J.; Zhang, W.; Evans, P.M.; Chen, X.; He, X.; Liu, C. Adenomatous Polyposis Coli (APC) Differentially Regulates β-Catenin Phosphorylation and Ubiquitination in Colon Cancer Cells. *J. Biol. Chem.* **2006**, *281*, 17751–17757. [CrossRef]

29. Morin, P.J.; Sparks, A.B.; Korinek, V.; Barker, N.; Clevers, H.; Vogelstein, B.; Kinzler, K.W. Activation of β-Catenin-Tcf Signaling in Colon Cancer by Mutations in β-Catenin or APC. *Science* **1997**, *275*, 1787–1790. [CrossRef]
30. Rebouissou, S.; Franconi, A.; Calderaro, J.; Letouzé, E.; Imbeaud, S.; Pilati, C.; Nault, J.-C.; Couchy, G.; Laurent, A.; Balabaud, C.; et al. Genotype-phenotype correlation of CTNNB1 mutations reveals different ß-catenin activity associated with liver tumor progression. *Hepatology* **2016**, *64*, 2047–2061. [CrossRef]
31. Wang, Z.; Vogelstein, B.; Kinzler, K.W. Phosphorylation of β-Catenin at S33, S37, or T41 Can Occur in the Absence of Phosphorylation at T45 in Colon Cancer Cells. *Cancer Res.* **2003**, *63*, 5234–5235. [PubMed]
32. Chan, T.A.; Wang, Z.; Dang, L.H.; Vogelstein, B.; Kinzler, K.W. Targeted inactivation of CTNNB1 reveals unexpected effects of β-catenin mutation. *Proc. Natl. Acad. Sci. USA* **2002**, *99*, 8265–8270. [CrossRef] [PubMed]
33. Albuquerque, C.; Bakker, E.R.M.; van Veelen, W.; Smits, R. Colorectal cancers choosing sides. *Biochim. Biophys. Acta BBA Rev. Cancer* **2011**, *1816*, 219–231. [CrossRef]
34. Kim, S.; Jeong, S. Mutation Hotspots in the β-Catenin Gene: Lessons from the Human Cancer Genome Databases. *Mol. Cells* **2019**, *42*, 8–16. [CrossRef] [PubMed]
35. Cerami, E.; Gao, J.; Dogrusoz, U.; Gross, B.E.; Sumer, S.O.; Aksoy, B.A.; Jacobsen, A.; Byrne, C.J.; Heuer, M.L.; Larsson, E.; et al. The cBio Cancer Genomics Portal: An Open Platform for Exploring Multidimensional Cancer Genomics Data. *Cancer Discov.* **2012**, *2*, 401–404. [CrossRef]
36. Gao, J.; Aksoy, B.A.; Dogrusoz, U.; Dresdner, G.; Gross, B.; Sumer, S.O.; Sun, Y.; Jacobsen, A.; Sinha, R.; Larsson, E.; et al. Integrative analysis of complex cancer genomics and clinical profiles using the cBioPortal. *Sci. Signal.* **2013**, *6*, pl1. [CrossRef]
37. Giannakis, M.; Mu, X.J.; Shukla, S.A.; Qian, Z.R.; Cohen, O.; Nishihara, R.; Bahl, S.; Cao, Y.; Amin-Mansour, A.; Yamauchi, M.; et al. Genomic Correlates of Immune-Cell Infiltrates in Colorectal Carcinoma. *Cell Rep.* **2016**, *15*, 857–865. [CrossRef]
38. Seshagiri, S.; Stawiski, E.W.; Durinck, S.; Modrusan, Z.; Storm, E.E.; Conboy, C.B.; Chaudhuri, S.; Guan, Y.; Janakiraman, V.; Jaiswal, B.S.; et al. Recurrent R-spondin fusions in colon cancer. *Nature* **2012**, *488*, 660–664. [CrossRef]
39. Yaeger, R.; Chatila, W.K.; Lipsyc, M.D.; Hechtman, J.F.; Cercek, A.; Sanchez-Vega, F.; Jayakumaran, G.; Middha, S.; Zehir, A.; Donoghue, M.T.A.; et al. Clinical Sequencing Defines the Genomic Landscape of Metastatic Colorectal Cancer. *Cancer Cell* **2018**, *33*, 125–136.e3. [CrossRef]
40. Gao, C.; Wang, Y.; Broaddus, R.; Sun, L.; Xue, F.; Zhang, W. Exon 3 mutations of CTNNB1 drive tumorigenesis: A review. *Oncotarget* **2017**, *9*, 5492–5508. [CrossRef]
41. Spink, K.E.; Fridman, S.G.; Weis, W.I. Molecular mechanisms of β-catenin recognition by adenomatous polyposis coli revealed by the structure of an APC–β-catenin complex. *EMBO J.* **2001**, *20*, 6203–6212. [CrossRef] [PubMed]
42. Xing, Y.; Clements, W.K.; Kimelman, D.; Xu, W. Crystal structure of a β-catenin/Axin complex suggests a mechanism for the β-catenin destruction complex. *Genes Dev.* **2003**, *17*, 2753–2764. [CrossRef] [PubMed]
43. Prieve, M.G.; Waterman, M.L. Nuclear Localization and Formation of β-Catenin–Lymphoid Enhancer Factor 1 Complexes Are Not Sufficient for Activation of Gene Expression. *Mol. Cell. Biol.* **1999**, *19*, 4503–4515. [CrossRef]
44. Brocardo, M.; Näthke, I.S.; Henderson, B.R. Redefining the subcellular location and transport of APC: New insights using a panel of antibodies. *EMBO Rep.* **2005**, *6*, 184–190. [CrossRef] [PubMed]
45. Davies, M.L.; Roberts, G.T.; Stuart, N.; Wakeman, J.A. Analysis of a panel of antibodies to APC reveals consistent activity towards an unidentified protein. *Br. J. Cancer* **2007**, *97*, 384–390. [CrossRef]
46. Wang, Y.; Azuma, Y.; Friedman, D.B.; Coffey, R.J.; Neufeld, K.L. Novel association of APC with intermediate filaments identified using a new versatile APC antibody. *BMC Cell Biol.* **2009**, *10*, 75. [CrossRef]
47. Ahmed, Y.; Hayashi, S.; Levine, A.; Wieschaus, E. Regulation of Armadillo by a Drosophila APC Inhibits Neuronal Apoptosis during Retinal Development. *Cell* **1998**, *93*, 1171–1182. [CrossRef]
48. Sansom, O.J.; Reed, K.R.; Hayes, A.J.; Ireland, H.; Brinkmann, H.; Newton, I.P.; Batlle, E.; Simon-Assmann, P.; Clevers, H.; Nathke, I.S.; et al. Loss of Apc in vivo immediately perturbs Wnt signaling, differentiation, and migration. *Genes Dev.* **2004**, *18*, 1385–1390. [CrossRef]
49. Bottomly, D.; Kyler, S.L.; McWeeney, S.K.; Yochum, G.S. Identification of β-catenin binding regions in colon cancer cells using ChIP-Seq. *Nucleic Acids Res.* **2010**, *38*, 5735–5745. [CrossRef]

50. Hatzis, P.; van der Flier, L.G.; van Driel, M.A.; Guryev, V.; Nielsen, F.; Denissov, S.; Nijman, I.J.; Koster, J.; Santo, E.E.; Welboren, W.; et al. Genome-Wide Pattern of TCF7L2/TCF4 Chromatin Occupancy in Colorectal Cancer Cells. *Mol. Cell. Biol.* **2008**, *28*, 2732–2744. [CrossRef]
51. Sutherland, C. What Are the Bona Fide GSK3 Substrates? Available online: https://www.hindawi.com/journals/ijad/2011/505607/ (accessed on 21 April 2020).
52. Olmeda, D.; Castel, S.; Vilaró, S.; Cano, A. β-Catenin Regulation during the Cell Cycle: Implications in G2/M and Apoptosis. *Mol. Biol. Cell* **2003**, *14*, 2844–2860. [CrossRef] [PubMed]
53. Saito-Diaz, K.; Benchabane, H.; Tiwari, A.; Tian, A.; Li, B.; Thompson, J.J.; Hyde, A.S.; Sawyer, L.M.; Jodoin, J.N.; Santos, E.; et al. APC Inhibits Ligand-Independent Wnt Signaling by the Clathrin Endocytic Pathway. *Dev. Cell* **2018**, *44*, 566–581.e8. [CrossRef] [PubMed]
54. Weinstein, J.N.; Collisson, E.A.; Mills, G.B.; Shaw, K.R.M.; Ozenberger, B.A.; Ellrott, K.; Shmulevich, I.; Sander, C.; Stuart, J.M. The Cancer Genome Atlas Pan-Cancer analysis project. *Nat. Genet.* **2013**, *45*, 1113–1120. [CrossRef]
55. Habib, S.J.; Chen, B.-C.; Tsai, F.-C.; Anastassiadis, K.; Meyer, T.; Betzig, E.; Nusse, R. A Localized Wnt Signal Orients Asymmetric Stem Cell Division in Vitro. *Science* **2013**, *339*, 1445–1448. [CrossRef] [PubMed]
56. Korinek, V.; Barker, N.; Morin, P.J.; van Wichen, D.; de Weger, R.; Kinzler, K.W.; Vogelstein, B.; Clevers, H. Constitutive Transcriptional Activation by a β-Catenin-Tcf Complex in APC−/− Colon Carcinoma. *Science* **1997**, *275*, 1784–1787. [CrossRef] [PubMed]
57. McQuin, C.; Goodman, A.; Chernyshev, V.; Kamentsky, L.; Cimini, B.A.; Karhohs, K.W.; Doan, M.; Ding, L.; Rafelski, S.M.; Thirstrup, D.; et al. CellProfiler 3.0: Next-generation image processing for biology. *PLoS Biol.* **2018**, *16*, e2005970. [CrossRef]
58. CellProfiler/Tutorials. Available online: https://github.com/CellProfiler/tutorials (accessed on 29 July 2020).

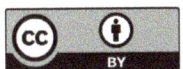

© 2020 by the authors. Licensee MDPI, Basel, Switzerland. This article is an open access article distributed under the terms and conditions of the Creative Commons Attribution (CC BY) license (http://creativecommons.org/licenses/by/4.0/).

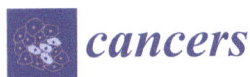

Article

Identification and Validation of an *Aspergillus nidulans* Secondary Metabolite Derivative as an Inhibitor of the Musashi-RNA Interaction

Lan Lan [1], Jiajun Liu [1], Minli Xing [2], Amber R. Smith [1], Jinan Wang [3], Xiaoqing Wu [1], Carl Appelman [1], Ke Li [1], Anuradha Roy [4], Ragul Gowthaman [3], John Karanicolas [5], Amber D. Somoza [6], Clay C. C. Wang [6,7], Yinglong Miao [3], Roberto De Guzman [1], Berl R. Oakley [1], Kristi L. Neufeld [1,8] and Liang Xu [1,9,*]

1. Departments of Molecular Biosciences, the University of Kansas, Lawrence, KS 66045, USA; lan@ku.edu (L.L.); gajun988@gmail.com (J.L.); arsmith1@stanford.edu (A.R.S.); wuxq@ku.edu (X.W.); carltonapps@gmail.com (C.A.); lk_jzs@xiyi.edu.cn (K.L.); rdguzman@ku.edu (R.D.G.); boakley@ku.edu (B.R.O.); klneuf@ku.edu (K.L.N.)
2. Bio-NMR Core Facility, the University of Kansas, Lawrence, KS 66045, USA; mlxing@umich.edu
3. Center for Computational Biology, the University of Kansas, Lawrence, KS 66045, USA; jawang@ku.edu (J.W.); ragul@umd.edu (R.G.); miao@ku.edu (Y.M.)
4. High Throughput Screening Laboratory, the University of Kansas, Lawrence, KS 66045, USA; anuroy@ku.edu
5. Program in Molecular Therapeutics, Fox Chase Cancer Center, Philadelphia, PA 19111, USA; John.Karanicolas@fccc.edu
6. Department of Chemistry, University of Southern California, Los Angeles, CA 90007, USA; amber.somoza@gmail.com (A.D.S.); clayw@usc.edu (C.C.C.W.)
7. Department of Pharmacology and Pharmaceutical Sciences, School of Pharmacy, University of Southern California, Los Angeles, CA 90007, USA
8. Department of Cancer Biology, the University of Kansas Cancer Center, Kansas City, KS 66160, USA
9. Department of Radiation Oncology, the University of Kansas Cancer Center, Kansas City, KS 66160, USA
* Correspondence: xul@ku.edu

Received: 1 April 2020; Accepted: 6 August 2020; Published: 8 August 2020

Abstract: RNA-binding protein Musashi-1 (MSI1) is a key regulator of several stem cell populations. MSI1 is involved in tumor proliferation and maintenance, and it regulates target mRNAs at the translational level. The known mRNA targets of MSI1 include *Numb*, *APC*, and $P21^{WAF-1}$, key regulators of Notch/Wnt signaling and cell cycle progression, respectively. In this study, we aim to identify small molecule inhibitors of MSI1–mRNA interactions, which could block the growth of cancer cells with high levels of MSI1. Using a fluorescence polarization (FP) assay, we screened small molecules from several chemical libraries for those that disrupt the binding of MSI1 to its consensus RNA. One cluster of hit compounds is the derivatives of secondary metabolites from *Aspergillus nidulans*. One of the top hits, Aza-9, from this cluster was further validated by surface plasmon resonance and nuclear magnetic resonance spectroscopy, which demonstrated that Aza-9 binds directly to MSI1, and the binding is at the RNA binding pocket. We also show that Aza-9 binds to Musashi-2 (MSI2) as well. To test whether Aza-9 has anti-cancer potential, we used liposomes to facilitate Aza-9 cellular uptake. Aza-9-liposome inhibits proliferation, induces apoptosis and autophagy, and down-regulates Notch and Wnt signaling in colon cancer cell lines. In conclusion, we identified a series of potential lead compounds for inhibiting MSI1/2 function, while establishing a framework for identifying small molecule inhibitors of RNA binding proteins using FP-based screening methodology.

Keywords: RNA-binding proteins; Musashi; drug discovery; Notch signaling; Wnt signaling; cancer therapy; fungi secondary metabolite derivative

1. Introduction

Post-transcriptional gene regulation occurs at the levels of pre-mRNA splicing and maturation, as well as mRNA transport, editing, storage, stability, and translation. This level of gene regulation is essential for normal development, but when dysregulated, contributes to diseases such as cancer. Post-transcriptional gene regulation is mediated by RNA-binding proteins, which are emerging new targets for cancer therapy.

One such RNA-binding protein is Musashi-1 (Msi1/MSI1), which was first identified in *Drosophila* and studied extensively for its role in sensory organ progenitor (SOP) cell lineage establishment [1]. In *Drosophila msi1* loss-of-function mutants, a SOP cell divides to produce two daughter cells with low Notch signaling rather than one daughter cell with relatively high Notch signaling and one with low Notch signaling [1]. In mammalian systems, MSI1 is expressed in multiple stem cell populations, including adult stem cells of the breast, colon, hair follicles, and brain [2–6]. MSI1 is overexpressed in a wide variety of cancers [4,7–15]; although it's specific function in tumorigenesis is largely unknown. Knocking down MSI1 reduces tumor progression in several cancer models [9,12] and overexpressing MSI1 in a rat intestinal crypt-derived cell line induces tumorigenesis in a mouse xenograft model [16]. These findings suggest that MSI1 can promote tumorigenesis and support MSI1 as a promising drug target for cancer therapy.

MSI1 appears to function by binding to the 3′UTR of target mRNAs and thereby regulating protein translation [17–20]. Targets whose translation is repressed by MSI1 include *NUMB*, *APC*, and *P21^{WAF-1}* [17,20–22]. In this study, we aimed to identify small molecules that disrupt the binding of MSI1 with target mRNAs. Novel small molecule inhibitors may be used in the future for treating patients with high MSI1 expression, while also serving as a tool to elucidate MSI1's role in cancer initiation and progression.

Previous efforts to identify small molecule inhibitors of protein-protein interactions have focused on proteins with well-defined binding pockets, while inhibitors of RNA-binding proteins were limited to proteins that bind to viral RNAs [23–25]. In an effort to identify small molecule inhibitors of MSI1, we employed a fluorescence polarization (FP) competition assay and screened nearly 2000 compounds, including those from three NCI (National Cancer Institute) libraries [26] and our in-house compounds. We identified a series of hit compounds including Aza-9, a semi-synthetic derivative of a secondary metabolite from *Aspergillus nidulans* [27] that inhibits MSI1 RNA binding activity. Surface plasmon resonance (SPR), nuclear magnetic resonance (NMR) spectroscopy, and RNA-IP assays demonstrate that Aza-9 binds to MSI1 directly.

Musashi-2 (MSI2) shares a high degree of sequence identity to MSI1 [28], functions redundantly in certain tissues, and is also overexpressed in many cancers [14,15,29–32]. We show here that Aza-9 binds to MSI2 as well. To test Aza-9 function in cells, we introduced liposomes to facilitate Aza-9 cellular entry. We show that with Aza-9-liposome treatment, colon cancer cells HCT-116 and DLD-1 undergo apoptosis/autophagy, cell cycle arrest and modest Notch/Wnt signaling down-regulation.

2. Results

2.1. FP Assay Optimization

We used an FP assay to identify compounds that disrupt the interaction of MSI1 with a target RNA, *Numb*. In our initial binding assays, we used 2 nM of RNA as specified in previous publications [33,34]. We measured the binding of different concentrations of protein G B1 domain-tagged MSI1 RNA-binding Domain1 (GB1-RBD1) to Fluorescein isothiocyanate (FITC)-labeled *Numb* RNA (*Numb*^{FITC}) or control RNA (*CTL*^{FITC}). As shown in Figure 1A, *Numb*^{FITC} but not *CTL*^{FITC} bound to GB1-RBD1 as indicated by the increased polarization value. We further tested binding by competing the RBD1-*Numb*^{FITC} complex with non-labeled *Numb* or control RNA. *Numb* RNA displaced the *Numb*^{FITC} from the protein–RNA complex at a much lower Ki than the control RNA (Figure 1B). This established binding between *Numb* RNA and GB1-RBD1 formed the basis for the following screening assay.

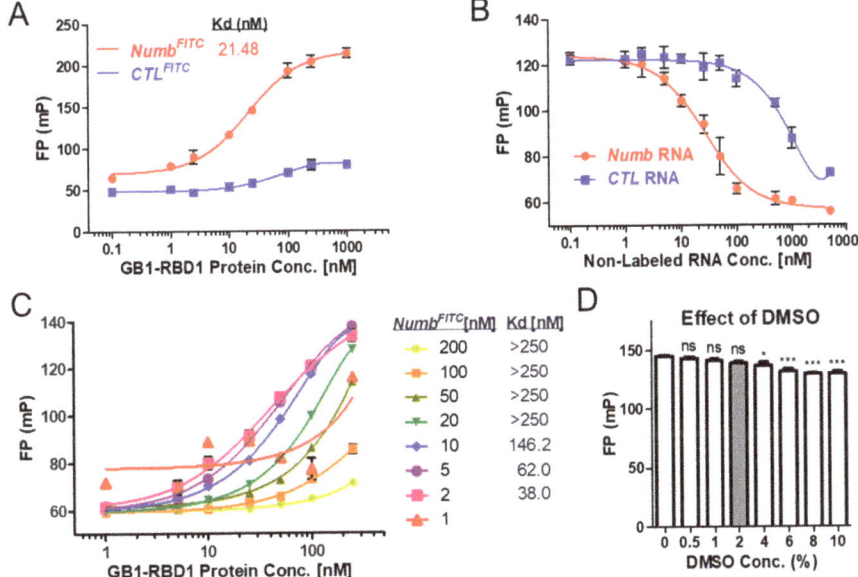

Figure 1. FP assay setup and optimization with MSI1 protein and *Numb* RNA. (**A**) Binding of the RNA binding domain 1 (aa 20–107) of MSI1 (GB1-RBD1) to *Numb* RNA. GB1-RBD1 binds to *Numb*^{FITC} RNA (5′-UAGGUAGUAGUUUUA-FITC-3′) but not to control oligo-FITC (*CTL*^{FITC} RNA). The concentration of FITC-tagged RNA used in the assay was 2 nM ($n > 3$). (**B**) RNA competition assay. Increasing concentrations of unlabeled *Numb* or *control* RNAs were added to preformed *Numb* RNA-protein complexes. (**C**) Optimization of protein and RNA concentration in FP assay. (**D**) Effect of DMSO on the stability of the FP assay system. ns: not significant; * $p < 0.05$; *** $p < 0.001$ versus no DMSO control (concentration 0).

To adapt our initial binding assay to a more robust screening method, we carried out several optimization steps. First, we titrated both the GB1-RBD1 protein (1 to 250 nM) and *Numb*^{FITC} RNA (1 to 200 nM). RNA concentrations less than 1 nM produced such low fluorescent signals that FP values were not stable. Figure 1C shows a dose response curve of RNA concentrations ≥ 1 nM. Optimal binding to RBD1 was achieved with 2–10 nM RNA, with an RBD1 equilibrium dissociation constant (Kd) value less than 250 nM. We chose 2 nM RNA for future assays based on the lowest Kd value of the protein (Figure 1C). Next, we tested whether the solvent, Dimethyl sulfoxide (DMSO), used for dissolving small molecules, is compatible with the binding assay. 0–2% of DMSO had no significant effect on the polarization values of the RBD1-numb^{FITC} complex after 2 h incubation (Figure 1D). Upon completion of assay optimization, we carried out a small library screening of small molecules.

2.2. Screening of Chemical Libraries

The screening was carried out in a 96-well format. We screened a total of 1920 small molecules from four different libraries (Figure 2A). Z′ factors assess the assay quality and measure the statistical effects; the assay window (ΔmP) calculates differences in polarization value between positive and negative controls. Using the negative (DMSO) and positive (Gn) controls, Z′ factors [35] and assay window were calculated and are shown in Figure 2B,C. We obtained an average Z′ of 0.79 ± 0.05 across all the plates and ΔmP of 74.8 ± 3.7, indicating the robustness of the assay [35]. Using median ± 3SD as the cut off, we obtained 32 hits and a hit rate of 2.03% (Figure 2D). One group of five compounds are sclerotiorin analogues with differences at C-5 and C-7 substituents (Figure 3). Examining the screened library, we identified six more compounds with similar scaffolds (Figure S1), which showed lower inhibition of RBD1-*Numb*^{FITC} complex or were completely negative. These six compounds were included in the later validation assays together with the five hit compounds to examine the structure–activity relationship (SAR).

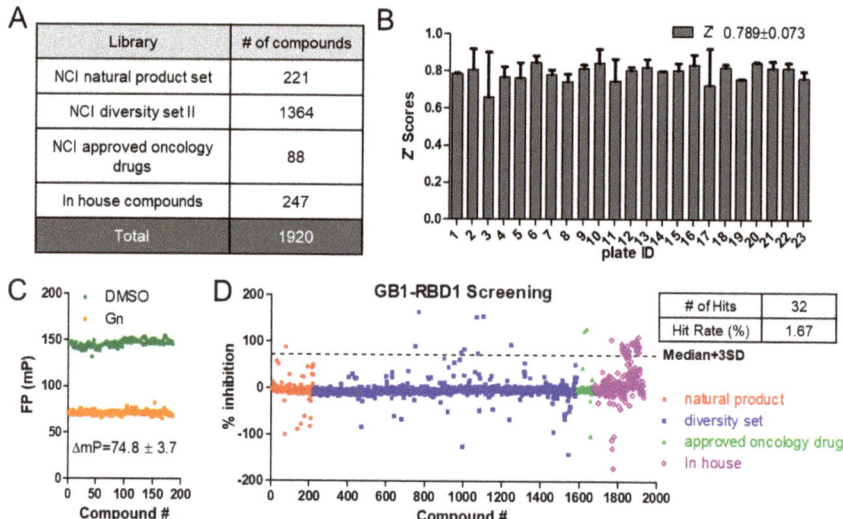

Figure 2. Screening of libraries. (**A**) Library composition. Our MSI1/*Numb* mRNA FP-based screening assay was carried out with 1920 compounds from the NCI (Diversity Set II, natural product set, and approved oncology drugs) and in-house libraries. (**B**) Z′ score across plates. (**C**) Positive and negative controls' values across plates. (**D**) Scattergram of the screening compounds. Median + 3SD was used as a threshold to pick the hits. Thirty-two hits were identified with a hit rate of 1.67%.

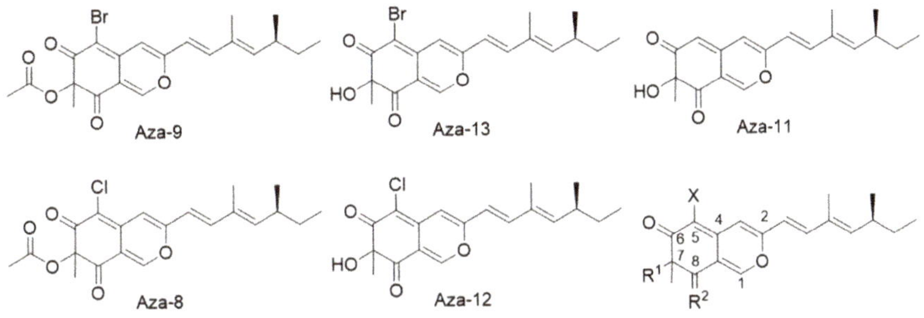

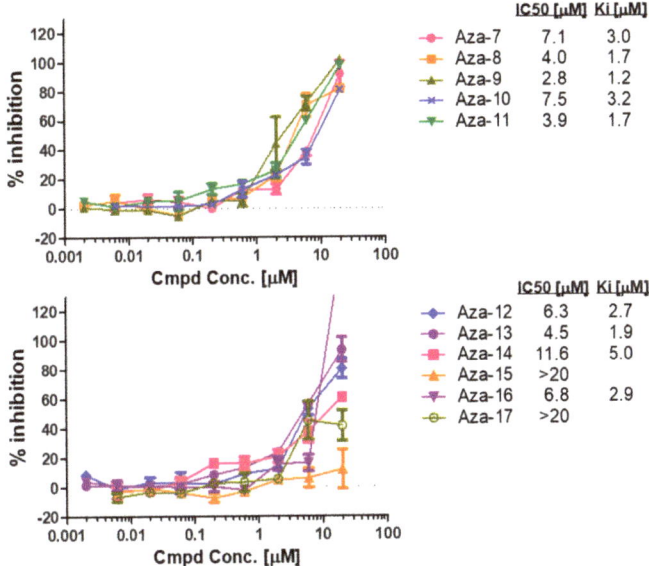

Figure 3. Structures of Azaphilone hits.

2.3. Hits Validation in an FP Dose-Response Test

To further examine the initial hits, we tested compounds with similar scaffolds shown in Figure 3 and Figure S1 in an FP dose-response assay. As shown in Figure 4, all compounds except Aza-15 and Aza-17 showed a dose-response effect in disrupting the RBD1-$Numb^{FITC}$ complex; Aza-9 showed the highest affinity towards GB1-RBD1. We thus focused our further validation studies on Aza-9.

Figure 4. FP dose-response validation compounds binding to RBD1 of MSI1. Ki values were calculated based on the Kd and the dose-response curves.

2.4. SPR Validation of Aza-9

An SPR assay with the protein GB1-RBD1 and not the RNA allowed us to evaluate the binding of the compound to the protein directly. As shown in Figure 5A, the SPR assay showed a dose-dependent binding of Aza-9 to GB1-RBD1.

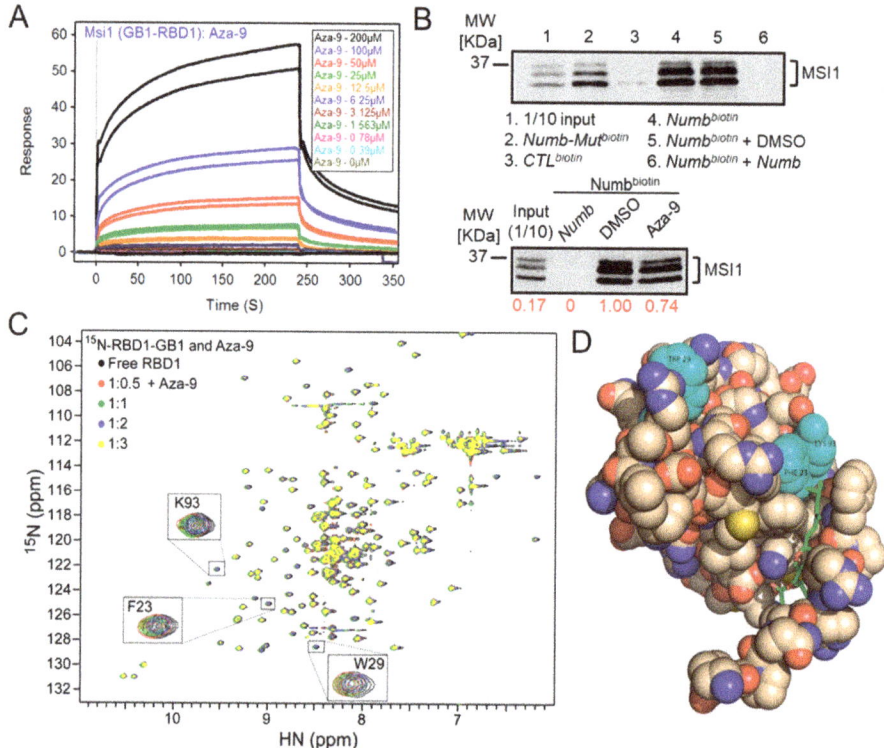

Figure 5. Validation of the top hit Aza-9. (**A**) SPR analyses of Aza-9 binding to immobilized GB1-RBD1. Sensorgram representing direct binding kinetics for Aza-9 are shown in response units (RUs) as a function of time with increasing concentrations (shown as colorful lines). (**B**) *Numb* RNA pulldown. (Top) *Numb*[biotin] (lane 4) can pull down MSI1 but not *CTL*[biotin] (lane 3); *Numb-Mut*[biotin] (lane 2) partially pulled down MSI1. Adding of unlabeled *Numb* RNA (lane 6) abolished the binding completely, while DMSO did not have an effect (lane 5). $n = 3$, one representative western blot is shown. (Bottom) 20 µM Aza-9 attenuated the binding between MSI1 and *Numb*[biotin] RNA. $n = 2$, one representative western blot is shown. (**C**) Overlay of 15N-HSQC (Heteronuclear single quantum coherence spectroscopy) spectra sections of MSI1-RBD1 (black), and MSI1-RBD1 bound to Aza-9 at different ratios. (**D**) Computational docking of Aza-9 bound to RBD1. The Aza-9 is shown in sticks, and the protein is represented as spheres. Three of MSI1-RBD1 RNA binding residues (W29, F23, and K93) that undergo significant peak shifts are highlighted in cyan.

2.5. RNA Pull-Down of Aza-9

To test whether Aza-9 disrupts the binding of MSI1 to *Numb* RNA in cells, we carried out an RNA pull-down assay using HCT-116 β/W cell lysate. Before we tested our compound in the assay, we tested whether biotinylated *Numb* RNA (*Numb*[biotin]) can pull down MSI1 protein from the cell lysate. We showed that *Numb*[biotin] pulled down MSI1 but *control*[biotin] could not (lane 3 versus lane 4, Figure 5B and Figure S4 top panel). Mutations in *Numb* (*Numb-mut*[biotin]) attenuated its binding to MSI1 (lane 2 versus lane 4, Figure 5B and Figure S4 top panel). As a positive control, we added non-labelled *Numb* RNA to the system, *Numb* RNA completely abolished the binding between *Numb*[biotin] and MSI1 (lane 6 versus lane 4, Figure 5B and Figure S4 top panel). A negative control DMSO solvent for our compounds did not affect the binding (lane 5 versus lane 4, Figure 5B and Figure S4 top panel). Next, we tested whether Aza-9 can attenuate MSI1 RNA binding. We showed that 20 µM Aza-9 can attenuate, at least in part, the binding between MSI1 and *Numb* RNA (Figure 5B and Figure S4, lower panel). Our data suggest that Aza-9 binds to MSI1 directly and decreases its RNA binding ability.

2.6. NMR Studies of Aza-9

To investigate further the binding of Aza-9 to MSI1-RBD1 and to identify the residues of MSI1-RBD1 that are affected upon binding of Aza-9, we used protein nuclear magnetic resonance (NMR). As described in our previous publication [36], using NMR, we successfully identified the RNA binding residues of MSI1-RBD1—W29, K93, F23, and F65 [37]. Upon titration of Aza-9 with ^{15}N-labeled MSI1-RBD1, residues 62, 64, 28, 94, 93, 22, 61, 23, 52, 95, 29, 40, and 68 experienced line broadening, indicating that these residues were affected by the binding of Aza-9 to MSI1-RBD1 (Figure 5C). When mapped onto the structure of MSI1-RBD1, many of the residues previously shown to bind to RNA are directly affected upon titration of Aza-9, along with the residues that are near the RNA-binding regions of MSI1-RBD1 (Figure 5C). Computational docking suggests a binding mode in which Aza-9 interacts with residues K93 and F23 in MSI1-RBD1 (Figure 5D). Binding of Aza-9 near K93 and F23 will compete with the aromatic packing of cognate RNA in the MSI1-RBD1. Our NMR results confirm that Aza-9 binds directly to MSI1-RBD1 and that this binding event occurs in the RNA binding pocket (Figure 5C). In parallel, computational docking provides a model consistent with these NMR observations and allows us to propose a specific binding mode for Aza-9.

2.7. Aza-9 Musashi-2 Binding

To test whether Aza-9 can be used as a dual inhibitor to block the RNA-binding ability of both Musashi proteins, we tested Aza-9 for Musashi-2 (MSI2) binding in FP and NMR assays as previously described [28]. We showed that Aza-9 disrupted the binding of MSI2-RBD1 and *Numb*^{FITC} RNA in FP (Figure 6A), and it induced reduction of NMR peak intensities when titrated with ^{15}N and ^{13}C ILV (Ile, Leu and Val) methyl labeled MSI2-RBD1. MSI2-RBD1 residues M23, F64, and K94 showed the most significant reduction in peak intensities (Figure 6B). These residues are in similar positions to F23, F65, and K93 in MSI1-RBD1 [36]. We mapped the peak intensity ratios lower than one standard deviation from the mean (Figure S2) to the structure of MSI2-RBD1. Residues with significant peak intensity reductions clustered around the RNA binding site, which is composed of the central four anti-parallel β sheets and surrounding loops (Figure 6C). The ILV ^{13}C methyl groups including I25δ1, V52γ1, and V67 γ2 showed significant reductions in peak intensities, and these residues clustered around the central anti-parallel β sheets (Figure S3). Our NMR results indicate that Aza-9 can directly interact with the RNA binding site, which consists of the central four anti-parallel β sheets and surrounding loops in both MSI1-RBD1 (Figure 5C) and MSI2-RBD1 (Figure 6B) and disrupts MSI1–RNA and MSI2–RNA interactions.

Carrying out the same docking calculation using MSI2-RBD1, we find again that Aza-9 adopts a very similar binding mode as for MSI1-RBD1. Aza-9 is bound near residues K94, M23, and V95 (shown in Figure 6D), consistent with the NMR results. Nearby residues connected through the backbone of the β sheets also include F64 and G26 (Figure 6B), which may respond in the NMR spectra either due to the effect of binding on the nearby sidechains or due to a slight change in the β sheet itself.

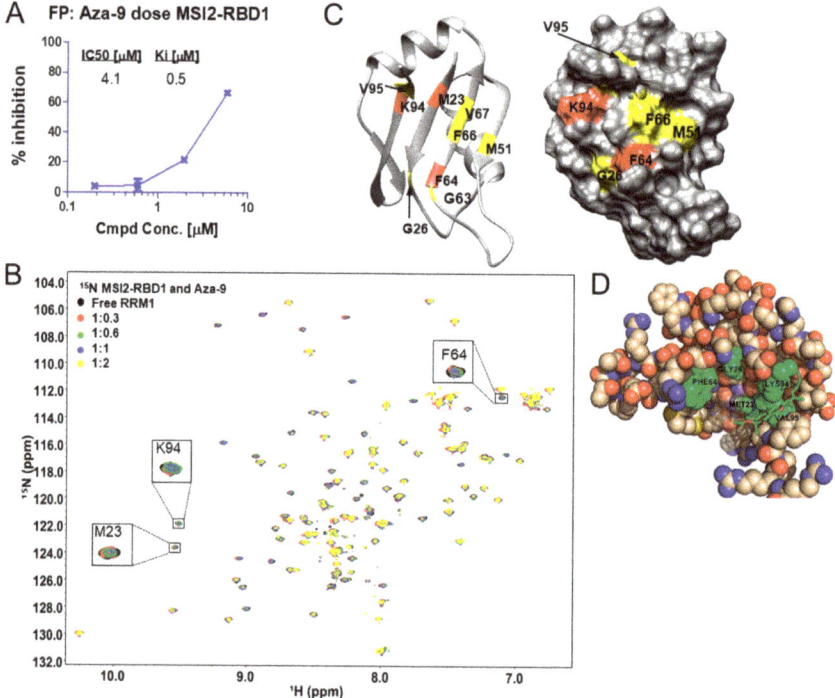

Figure 6. Aza-9 binds to MSI2-RBD1. (**A**) FP dose response of Aza-9 binding to MSI2-RBD1. (**B**) ^{1}H-^{15}N HSQC spectra of 80 μM ^{15}N and ^{13}C ILV methyl labeled MSI2-RBD1 with increasing molar ratios of AZA-9. (**C**) Mapping residues with peak intensity ratio lower than one standard deviation from the mean onto the structure of MSI2-RBD1. Residues with peak intensity ratio lower than 0.40 are colored red; residues with peak intensity ratios in the range of 0.40–0.54 are colored yellow. (**D**) Computational docking of Aza-9 bound to MSI2-RBD1. The Aza-9 is shown in sticks, and the protein is represented as spheres. Five of MSI2-RBD1 RNA binding residues (M23, G26, F64, V95, and K94) that undergo significant peak shifts are highlighted in green.

2.8. Aza-9-Liposome Inhibits Colon Cancer Cell Proliferation, Induces Apoptosis and Autophagy

In an 3-(4,5-dimethylthiazol-2-yl)-2,5-diphenyl tetrazolium bromide (MTT)-based cytotoxicity assay, free Aza-9 had no effect on the cell viability (Figure 7A), potentially due to poor cellular uptake (Figure 7B, upper left panel). We then used PEGylated liposomes to facilitate Aza-9 entry into the cells (Figure 7B, bottom panel compare to upper left panel). Compared to the free Aza-9, which has no effect at 300 μM, Aza-9-liposome (Aza-9-lip) killed colon cancer cell line HCT-116 with an IC50 around 90 μM (Figure 7A). Since liposomes showed toxicity to the cells at 300 μM but not at 100 μM (Figure 7A), we used 100 μM for both Aza-9-lip and liposomes in the following studies. Consistent with MTT, Aza-9-lip, but not liposomes, inhibited cell proliferation in a cell growth assay (Figure 7C). Cell cycle analysis showed that Aza-9-lip treatment also led to the accumulation of cells in G1 phase. (Figure 8A). To determine whether Aza-9-lip induces apoptosis and/or autophagy in the colon cancer cell lines, we first measured caspase-3 and PARP cleavage levels. As shown in Figure 8B and Figure S5, Aza-9-lip induced caspase-3 and PARP cleavage in HCT-116 and DLD-1 cells. Aza-9-lip caused an increase in sub-G1 population in both cells (Figure 8A), indication of apoptosis. Aza-9-lip also induced LC3 conversion and P62 degradation (Figure 8B and Figure S5), indicating autophagy induction and efficient autophagic flux. Taken together, these data indicate Aza-9-liposome inhibits colon cancer cell proliferation and induces apoptosis and autophagy.

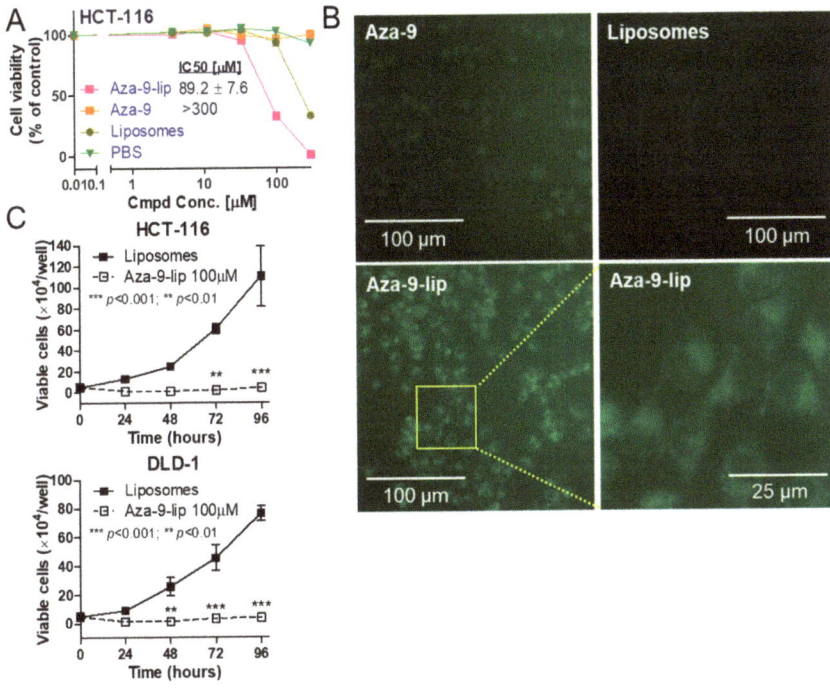

Figure 7. Aza-9-liposome (Aza-9-lip) inhibits colon cancer cell proliferation. (**A**) MTT-based cytotoxicity assay of Aza-9-lip, free Aza-9, liposomes, and PBS in colon cancer cell line HCT-116. Aza-9 had no effect on the cell viability due to poor cellular uptake. ($n = 3$, one representative experiment of three is shown.) (**B**) PEGylated liposomes facilitate Aza-9 entry into the cells. Aza-9 fluoresces in the green channel. Images of Aza-9-lip (100 µM), Aza-9 (100 µM), and liposomes were taken at 2 h after the treatment. (**C**) Aza-9-lip inhibits HCT-116 and DLD-1 cell growth. ($n = 3$, ** $p < 0.01$; *** $p < 0.001$ versus liposomes control. One representative experiment of three is shown.).

2.9. Aza-9-Liposome Down-Regulates Notch/Wnt Signaling in Colon Cancer Cell Lines

To investigate whether Aza-9 affects Musashi downstream pathways, we next tested the effects of Aza-9 on Notch/Wnt signaling. As shown in Figure 9A, Aza-9-lip significantly decreased the mRNA level of *AXIN2*, a direct downstream component of Wnt signaling. The levels of *SURVIVIN* mRNA, downstream of the Notch pathway, also decreased in DLD-1 but not HCT-116 cells, whereas SURVIVIN protein was decreased in both cell lines (Figure 9A,B and Figure S6). In addition, the down-regulation of *MSI1* was observed [16,22,36]. To our surprise, Wnt/Notch signaling downstream target gene *CYCLIN D1* (*CCND1*), mRNA and protein expression were increased. Direct targets APC and NUMB protein levels increased in both HCT-116 (Figure 9B and Figure S8) and RKO cells (Figures S7 and S8) as a consequence of translation de-repression when MSI function was blocked with treatment. We further tested Aza-9-lip in a functional Wnt reporter assay in HCT-116 cells. Aza-9-lip significantly decreased TOP/FOP reporter signal with (Figure S9) or without (Figure 9C) LiCl stimulation. Taken together, our data suggest that the effects of 100 µM Aza-9-lip on Wnt/Notch pathways are mediated, in part through SURVIVIN inhibition. We did not increase the concentration as higher concentrations of Aza-9-lip would have a more toxic influence from liposomes.

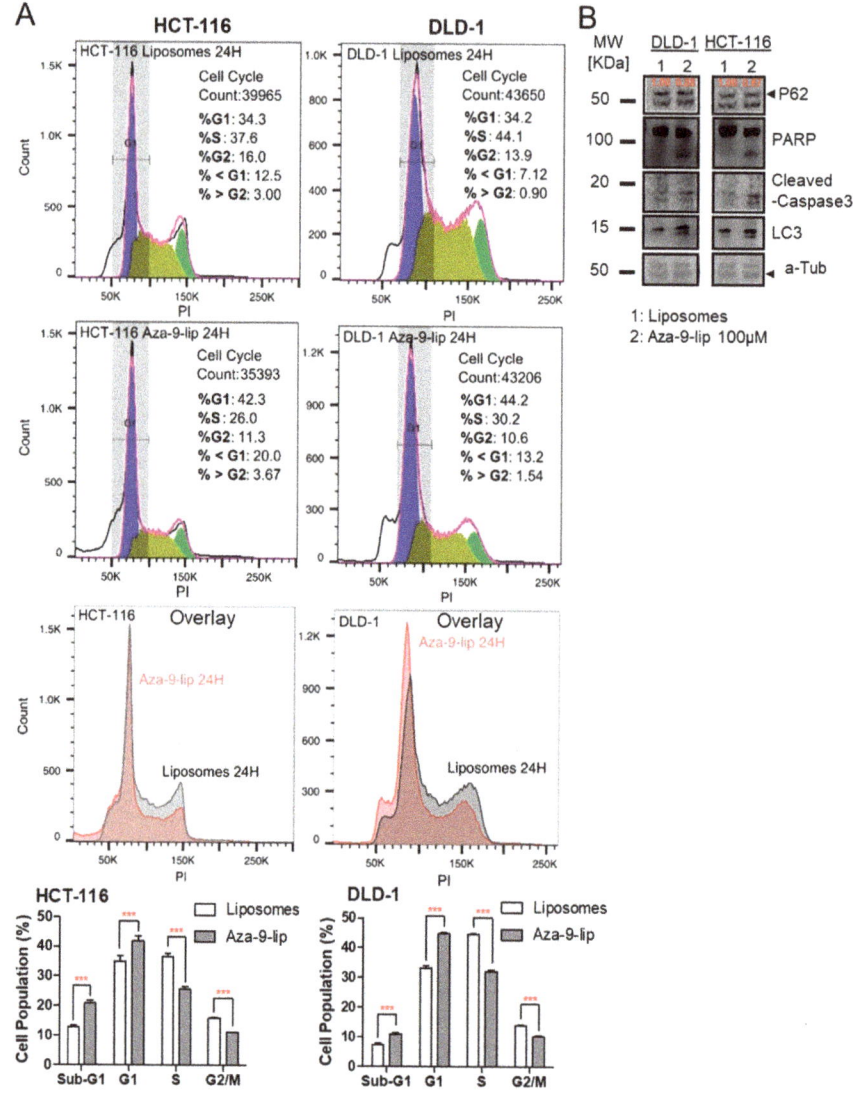

Figure 8. Aza-9-liposome (Aza-9-lip) induces apoptosis (or autophagy) and leads to cell cycle arrest. (**A**) Cell cycle analysis of 100 µM Aza-9-lip or liposomes treated DLD-1 or HCT-116 cells at 24 h. Aza-9-lip treatment led to an increased sub-G1 population, indication of apoptosis. Aza-9-lip treatment also induced a G1 block and led to cell cycle arrest. (Bar graph, $n = 3$, *** $p < 0.001$ versus liposomes control. Spectrums are from one representative treatment.) (**B**) Caspase-3/PARP cleavage, P62 degradation and LC3 conversion were observed in colon cancer cell lines treated with 100 µM Aza-9-lip for 24 h, cell lysate was subject to western blot for PARP cleavage, caspase-3 cleavage, and LC3 I/LC3II expression.

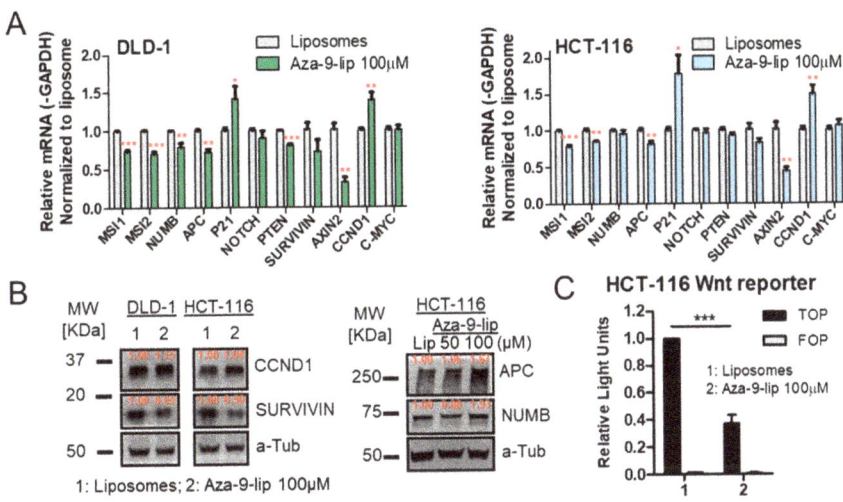

Figure 9. Aza-9-lip down-regulates Notch/Wnt signaling in colon cancer cell lines. (**A,B**) Notch/Wnt target genes expression changes upon Aza-9-lip treatment were examined in HCT-116 and DLD-1 cells by quantitative real-time PCR (**A**) and by western blot (**B,C**) Aza-9-lip inhibits Wnt/β-catenin reporter. HCT-116 cells were transfected with TOPflash or FOPflash reporter constructs. Cells were treated with Aza-9-lip or liposomes only for 24 h. All figures, $n = 3$; * $p < 0.05$; ** $p < 0.01$; *** $p < 0.001$ versus liposomes control.

3. Discussion

RNA binding proteins are considered "undruggable", potentially due to lack of a well-defined binding pocket for target RNA [38]. In this study, we used a fluorescence polarization-(FP) based competition assay to identify small molecules that directly inhibit MSI1–RNA interaction. After screening a small library of approximately 2000 compounds, we identified 39 initial hits, five of which are azaphilones. We used FP to test dose response of these five, together with other azaphilones in the library. We further validated one of our top hit, Aza-9, using SPR, NMR and *Numb* RNA-IP, showing that Aza-9 directly binds to MSI1 and inhibits MSI1–RNA interaction. We showed Aza-9 as a dual MSI1/2 inhibitor that inhibited MSI2–RNA interaction as well. In cells, Aza-9-liposome inhibited colon cancer cell growth, induced apoptosis/autophagy and led to G1 accumulation of cells, with a modest down-regulation of Notch/Wnt signaling.

There are reasons why RNA binding proteins are difficult to drug. Unlike many enzymes that have a defined binding pocket employing the "lock and key" scheme, regulatory RNA/DNA binding proteins have shallow binding pockets, and the binding events are not as tight and are less specific due to conformational flexibility. Targeting protein–protein interaction has yielded a list of small molecule compounds that are in clinical trials or in the clinic [39], while inhibitors of protein–RNA/DNA interaction are somewhat new. Our results, presented here as well as our previous publications, suggest that the RNA binding proteins are druggable [14,36,40–44]. In our study, we used an initial FP assay to screen for MSI1 inhibitors, and we validated the hits by three different assays, including SPR, NMR, and RNA-IP. Our assays are suitable for screening small molecule inhibitors of RNA-binding proteins and provide the foundation for large scale screening.

N-terminal RBDs of MSI1 and MSI2 share a high degree of similarity (~87%), thus we tested the binding of Aza-9 towards MSI2 and showed that Aza-9 disrupted the binding of MSI2 to *Numb* RNA in FP and that Aza-9 induced chemical shift perturbations in MSI2. MSI1 and MSI2 share similar roles in stem cells and in cancer initiation and progression, but they also have distinct roles [14,15,45–48]. Another previously identified Aza-9 target is HuR [44]. HuR is an RNA-binding protein that is overexpressed in a variety of cancers. One defined activity of HuR is to regulate MSI1 [49]. Aza-9 functions to inhibit both HuR and MSI1/2.

Although Aza-9 and the other azaphilones we have tested were produced semi-synthetically from asperbenzaldehyde, our semi-synthesis mimics a natural process. Aza-7 is identical to sclerotiorin, which is produced by a number of fungi [50–52], and has been reported to have anticancer activity [52]. Azaphilones are an interesting group of fungal natural products. More than 170 azaphilone compounds are produced by fungi, and they have a number of important biological activities. A substantial number of them have been reported to have anti-cancer activities [53].

With respect to our findings, an obvious question is why would fungi produce natural products that inhibit RNA–protein interactions? Fungi compete with other fungi, protozoans, and bacteria in their natural environments. Many organisms, including bacteria, produce extracellular RNAs that are thought to provide a variety of selective advantages [54]. It is quite conceivable that fungi have developed natural products to combat extracellular RNAs produced by their competitors.

An exciting aspect of the genomics era in natural products research is that we can now over-express genes to produce azaphilones and other valuable natural products. This allows us to produce natural products abundantly and cheaply. Furthermore, by interrupting biosynthetic pathways in organisms such as fungi, we can accumulate large amounts of intermediates such as asperbenzaldehyde and modify them semi-synthetically to increase their potency, efficacy, and medical value.

Investigation of Aza-9-liposome functions showed that Aza-9-liposome inhibited colon cancer cell growth, induced apoptosis/autophagy and led to G1 accumulation of cells, with a modest down-regulation of Notch/Wnt signaling. Our hypothesis is MSI1 and/or MSI2 block the translation of *NUMB*, *APC*, and *P21* mRNA, which leads to the up-regulation of both Notch and Wnt signaling pathways and promotes cell cycle progression. With Aza-9-liposome treatment, Aza-9 binds to MSI1/2, presumably releasing *NUMB*, *APC*, and *P21* mRNA from their translational repression. Increased level of NUMB, APC, and P21 proteins will block Notch/Wnt signaling and cell cycle progression, respectively. In colon cancers, Wnt signaling played a major role in the tumor initiation and progression. Two colon cancer cell lines HCT-116 and DLD-1 used in our study have different genetic profile of *APC* and *CTNNB1* genes that could lead to a different Wnt signaling response. For example, DLD-1 has a truncated APC thus cannot regulate β-catenin encoded by *CTNNB1* gene [55]. However, we observed similar response upon Aza-9-liposome treatment. A study on APC and β-catenin phosphorylation and ubiquitination showed that, although colon cancer cell lines SW480 DLD-1 and HT-29 all have truncated APC, β-catenin ubiquitination and degradation were inhibited in SW480 but not in DLD-1 and HT29 cells [56]. We think although APC is truncated in DLD-1, it can still regulate β-catenin. That's why we see a similar response upon Aza-9-liposome treatment in both cell lines. However, the same response in two different cell lines might be due to different mechanisms. In HCT-116 cells with a full-length APC, we observed increased APC protein level with treatment, the same increase was observed in RKO cells with the full-length APC. We believe that the increased APC level is responsible for the β-catenin sequestering or degradation, which lead to down-regulation of Wnt signaling. In DLD-1 cells, truncated APC protein levels were decreased slightly upon treatment, 0.97 (50 μM Aza-9-liposome) and 0.89 (100 μM Aza-9-liposome) compared to liposome only (1.00) (data not shown). Other mechanisms in addition to the β-catenin ubiquitination and degradation might account for the decrease in Wnt/Notch signaling we observed in DLD-1 cells. In the future, we will carry our further target validation studies and examination of other MSI targets including but not limited to *SMAD3* and *TGFβR1* [29,57].

In this study, we prepared PEGylated liposomal Aza-9, which facilies cellular uptake of Aza-9. One of our future directions is structure-based optimization of Aza-9 by introducing hydrophilic substituents or shortening the hydrophobic tail, with the aim of improving cell penetration and cytotoxicity to cancer cells with high levels of Musashi family proteins.

4. Materials and Methods

4.1. Cell Cultures and Reagents

Human colon cancer cell lines HCT-116, DLD-1, and RKO were obtained from American Type Culture Collection (ATCC) and are as described by Lan et al. [36,40]. Cell growth, MTT, cell cycle analysis, western blot analysis, RT-PCR, and quantitative real-time PCR were carried out according to our previous publications [36,58–62]. For western blot analysis with Aza-9-liposome treatment, samples were collected after 24 h; for quantitative real-time PCR, samples were collected after 48 h. The primer sequences, the primary and the secondary antibodies used were from Lan et al. [36]. Fluorescent and live cell imaging was carried out using EVOS FL Auto Cell Imaging System (Invitrogen, Thermo Fisher Scientific, Waltham, MA, USA), and images were cropped and processed using ImageJ (NIH).

4.2. Compound Libraries

The chemical libraries used in the initial screening contained three chemical libraries from the National Cancer Institute (NCI) [26] and our own in-house compounds. NCI libraries consist of a (1) natural products set; (2) diversity set II; (3) approved oncology drugs set. Compounds from NCI are stored at −20 °C in 96-well plates at the concentration of 10 mM in DMSO. The in-house compounds are stored as 20 mM DMSO stocks and diluted to 0.5 mM to use in the one-dose initial screening. For the NCI chemicals, 0.1 µL of 10 mM stock was deposited into A2-H11 of each plate in duplicate, 0.1 µL DMSO was placed into A1-H1, and our positive control Gossypolone (10 mM) (0.1 µL) was placed into A12-H12. For our in-house compounds, we first diluted the chemical stocks to 0.5 mM, and then placed 2 µL of each chemical into each individual well. A total of 100 µL RBD1-$Numb^{FITC}$ complex was added to each well.

4.3. Overexpression and Purification of MSI1-RBD1 and MSI2-RBD1 Proteins

pET21a-GB1-RBD1 (MSI1-RBD1) plasmids encoding the *Homo sapiens* RNA binding domain 1 (RBD1, residues 20-107) of MSI1 were constructed with Mus musculus cDNAs under T7 promoter. MSI1-RBD1 proteins were expressed in *Escherichia coli* and purified, as previously described [63]. Protein concentrations were determined using the Bradford assay (Bio-Rad, Hercules, CA, USA). Purification of MSI2-RBD1 protein was carried out according to the previous publication [28,36,40].

4.4. FP, SPR, NMR, and Computer Modeling

FP, SPR and NMR assays were carried out according to the previous publication [28,36,40]. For computer modeling of Aza-9 to MSI1/2, the AutoDock4.2.6 program was used for predicting the binding mode. The NMR structure of MSI1-RBD1 in complex with RNA (PDB: 2RS2) and the NMR structure of apo MSI2-RBD1 (PDB: 6C8U) were used as the receptor structure. The MSI1 RBD1–RNA interface and corresponding site in MSI2-RBD1 was used as the starting point for the docking calculations. The initial three-dimensional model of the Aza-9 compound was generated using the BABEL program and was used as starting coordinates to define the ligand structure. For docking, a grid box of size 40 × 44 × 56 A with 0.375 A spacing was centered at residue F23 in MSI1-RBD1 (or F24 in MSI2-RBD1). A total of 200 docking runs were carried out using the Lamarckian genetic algorithm. The docked conformation with the lowest energy was selected as the final conformation.

4.5. RNA Pull-Down

RNA pull-downs were carried out according to manufacturer's protocol with modifications (Roche, Basel, Switzerland). Briefly, HCT-116 β/W cells were plated on 100 mm dish on day 1. The next day, cells were treated with Aza-9 (20 µM) or DMSO for 6 h, and cell lysates were collected using buffer 1 from IP kit (Roche). Protein concentrations were measured for each sample, and streptavidin beads were added for preclearance and incubated at 4 °C for 3 h. After preclearance, for each sample,

500 µg of total protein was transferred to a new tube. For positive control, unlabeled *Numb* (final concentration: 5 µM) was added and incubated in 4 °C. After 0.5 h, heat-shocked biotinylated-*Numb* (final concentration: 500 nM) was added to each sample and incubated at 4 °C for 2 h, after which 50 µL of streptavidin beads were added and incubated for 2–16 h. Beads were washed three times (Roche), and protein sample buffer was added to the beads and boiled for 5 min. Supernatants were taken and loaded in SDS gels for western blot.

4.6. Wnt Luciferase Reporter Assay

HCT-116 cells were plated at a density of 4×10^4 cells per well in a 48-well dish the day prior to transfection. Cells were transfected with 0.125 µg of either TOPflash or FOPflash reporter constructs and a pRL-TK Renilla luciferase plasmid to control for transfection efficiency and cell number. Transfections were performed with Lipofectamine 3000 (Invitrogen, Thermo Fisher Scientific, Waltham, MA, USA), according to the manufacturer's instructions. The next day, cells were stimulated with or without 20 mM LiCl and treated with Aza-9-lip or liposomes control. Cells were harvested and assayed using the Dual-Glo Luciferase Assay (Promega, Fitchburg, WI, USA) 24 h after treatment. All firefly luciferase values were normalized to Renilla control.

5. Conclusions

In our effort to screening for Musashi-1 inhibitors, we identified a cluster of hit compounds that are the derivatives of secondary metabolites from *Aspergillus nidulans*. One of the top hits, Aza-9, was further validated by SPR, NMR, and RNA-IP, which demonstrated that Aza-9 binds directly to MSI1–RNA binding pocket. We also showed that Aza-9 binds to Musashi-2 (MSI2) as well. To test whether Aza-9 has anti-cancer potential, we used liposomes to facilitate Aza-9 cellular uptake. Aza-9-liposome inhibits proliferation, induces apoptosis and autophagy, and down-regulates Notch and Wnt signaling in colon cancer cell lines. In conclusion, we identified a series of potential lead compounds for inhibiting MSI1/2 function, while establishing a framework for identifying small molecule inhibitors of RNA-binding proteins using FP-based screening methodology.

Supplementary Materials: The following are available online at http://www.mdpi.com/2072-6694/12/8/2221/s1, Figure S1: Structures of other azaphilones in the screening, Figure S2: Plot of relative peak intensity for all nonoverlapping MSI2-RRM1 resonances in the ligand bound form versus free state (I1:0.3/I1:0), Figure S3: Aza-9 titration against 13C ILV methyl labeled MSI2-RRM1, Figure S4: Figure 5B supplemental, Figure S5: Figure 8B supplemental, Figure S6: Figure 9B supplemental, Figure S7: MSI direct targets APC and NUMB protein levels increased in RKO cells with Aza-9-liposome treatment, Figure S8: Figure 9B right panel and Figure S7 Supplemental, Figure S9: Aza-9-lip inhibits Wnt/β-catenin reporter. HCT-116 cells were transfected with TOPflash or FOPflash reporter constructs. Cells were treated with Aza-9-lip or liposomes only for 24 h in the presence of 20 mM LiCl.

Author Contributions: Conceptualization, L.L. and L.X.; methodology, L.L.; software, J.W., R.G., J.K., and Y.M.; validation, L.L.; formal analysis, L.L.; investigation, L.L., J.L., M.X, A.R.S., J.W., X.W., C.A., K.L., A.R., and A.D.S.; resources, K.L., A.R., A.D.S., and C.C.C.W.; data curation, L.L.; writing—original draft preparation, L.L.; writing—review and editing, L.L., M.X., A.R.S., J.W., X.W., R.G., J.K., R.D.G., B.R.O., and K.L.N.; visualization, L.L., M.X., A.R.S., J.W., and R.G.; supervision, L.X.; project administration, L.X.; funding acquisition, B.R.O., C.C.C.W., K.L.N., R.D.G., and L.X. All authors have read and agreed to the published version of the manuscript.

Funding: This study was supported in part by National Institutes of Health grants R01 CA178831 and CA191785, P01GM084077 from the National Institute of General Medical Science (to B.R.O. and C.C.C.W.); the University of Kansas Bold Aspiration Strategic Initiative Award and National Cancer Institute Cancer Center Support Grant P30 CA168524 (to L.X., K.N.); Kansas Bioscience Authority Rising Star Award (to L.X.); NIH grant AI074856 (to R.N.D.); NIH COBRE at KU CCET Pilot Project (P30 RR030926 to K.N.) and the Irving S. Johnson Fund of the University of Kansas Endowment (to B.R.O.).

Acknowledgments: The authors thank the NCI/DTP Open Chemical Repository (http://dtp.cancer.gov) for providing the compound libraries.

Conflicts of Interest: The authors declare no conflict of interest. The funders had no role in the design of the study; in the collection, analyses, or interpretation of data; in the writing of the manuscript, or in the decision to publish the results.

References

1. Nakamura, M.; Okano, H.; Blendy, J.A.; Montell, C. Musashi, a neural RNA-binding protein required for Drosophila adult external sensory organ development. *Neuron* **1994**, *13*, 67–81. [CrossRef]
2. Sugiyama-Nakagiri, Y.; Akiyama, M.; Shibata, S.; Okano, H.; Shimizu, H. Expression of RNA-binding protein Musashi in hair follicle development and hair cycle progression. *Am. J. Pathol.* **2006**, *168*, 80–92. [CrossRef] [PubMed]
3. Potten, C.S.; Booth, C.; Tudor, G.L.; Booth, D.; Brady, G.; Hurley, P.; Ashton, G.; Clarke, R.; Sakakibara, S.; Okano, H. Identification of a putative intestinal stem cell and early lineage marker; musashi-1. *Differentiation* **2003**, *71*, 28–41. [CrossRef] [PubMed]
4. Toda, M.; Iizuka, Y.; Yu, W.; Imai, T.; Ikeda, E.; Yoshida, K.; Kawase, T.; Kawakami, Y.; Okano, H.; Uyemura, K. Expression of the neural RNA-binding protein Musashi1 in human gliomas. *Glia* **2001**, *34*, 1–7. [CrossRef] [PubMed]
5. Kaneko, Y.; Sakakibara, S.; Imai, T.; Suzuki, A.; Nakamura, Y.; Sawamoto, K.; Ogawa, Y.; Toyama, Y.; Miyata, T.; Okano, H. Musashi1: An evolutionarily conserved marker for CNS progenitor cells including neural stem cells. *Dev. Neurosci.* **2000**, *22*, 139–153. [CrossRef] [PubMed]
6. Sakakibara, S.; Imai, T.; Hamaguchi, K.; Okabe, M.; Aruga, J.; Nakajima, K.; Yasutomi, D.; Nagata, T.; Kurihara, Y.; Uesugi, S.; et al. Mouse-Musashi-1, a neural RNA-binding protein highly enriched in the mammalian CNS stem cell. *Dev. Biol.* **1996**, *176*, 230–242. [CrossRef] [PubMed]
7. Wang, X.Y.; Yu, H.; Linnoila, R.I.; Li, L.; Li, D.; Mo, B.; Okano, H.; Penalva, L.O.; Glazer, R.I. Musashi1 as a potential therapeutic target and diagnostic marker for lung cancer. *Oncotarget* **2013**, *4*, 739–750. [CrossRef]
8. Glazer, R.I.; Vo, D.T.; Penalva, L.O. Musashi1: An RBP with versatile functions in normal and cancer stem cells. *Front. Biosci.* **2012**, *17*, 54–64. [CrossRef]
9. Wang, X.-Y.; Penalva, L.; Yuan, H.; Linnoila, R.I.; Lu, J.; Okano, H.; Glazer, R. Musashi1 regulates breast tumor cell proliferation and is a prognostic indicator of poor survival. *Mol. Cancer* **2010**, *9*, 221. [CrossRef]
10. Fan, L.-F.; Dong, W.-G.; Jiang, C.-Q.; Xia, D.; Liao, F.; Yu, Q.-F. Expression of putative stem cell genes Musashi-1 and β1-integrin in human colorectal adenomas and adenocarcinomas. *Int. J. Colorectal Dis.* **2010**, *25*, 17–23. [CrossRef]
11. Ito, T.; Kwon, H.Y.; Zimdahl, B.; Congdon, K.L.; Blum, J.; Lento, W.E.; Zhao, C.; Lagoo, A.; Gerrard, G.; Foroni, L.; et al. Regulation of myeloid leukaemia by the cell-fate determinant Musashi. *Nature* **2010**, *466*, 765–768. [CrossRef] [PubMed]
12. Sureban, S.M.; May, R.; George, R.J.; Dieckgraefe, B.K.; McLeod, H.L.; Ramalingam, S.; Bishnupuri, K.S.; Natarajan, G.; Anant, S.; Houchen, C.W. Knockdown of RNA Binding Protein Musashi-1 Leads to Tumor Regression In Vivo. *Gastroenterology* **2008**, *134*, 1448–1458. [CrossRef] [PubMed]
13. Ye, F.; Zhou, C.; Cheng, Q.; Shen, J.; Chen, H. Stem-cell-abundant proteins Nanog, Nucleostemin and Musashi1 are highly expressed in malignant cervical epithelial cells. *BMC Cancer* **2008**, *8*, 108. [CrossRef] [PubMed]
14. Kudinov, A.E.; Karanicolas, J.; Golemis, E.A.; Boumber, Y. Musashi RNA-binding proteins as cancer drivers and novel therapeutic targets. *Clin. Cancer Res.* **2017**. [CrossRef]
15. Kharas, M.G.; Lengner, C.J. Stem Cells, Cancer, and MUSASHI in Blood and Guts. *Trends Cancer* **2017**, *3*, 347–356. [CrossRef]
16. Rezza, A.; Skah, S.; Roche, C.; Nadjar, J.; Samarut, J.; Plateroti, M. The overexpression of the putative gut stem cell marker Musashi-1 induces tumorigenesis through Wnt and Notch activation. *J. Cell Sci.* **2010**, *123*, 3256–3265. [CrossRef]
17. Takahashi, T.; Suzuki, H.; Imai, T.; Shibata, S.; Tabuchi, Y.; Tsuchimoto, K.; Okano, H.; Hibi, T. Musashi-1 post-transcriptionally enhances phosphotyrosine-binding domain-containing m-Numb protein expression in regenerating gastric mucosa. *PLoS ONE* **2013**, *8*, e53540. [CrossRef]
18. Kuwako, K.; Kakumoto, K.; Imai, T.; Igarashi, M.; Hamakubo, T.; Sakakibara, S.; Tessier-Lavigne, M.; Okano, H.J.; Okano, H. Neural RNA-binding protein Musashi1 controls midline crossing of precerebellar neurons through posttranscriptional regulation of Robo3/Rig-1 expression. *Neuron* **2010**, *67*, 407–421. [CrossRef]
19. Charlesworth, A.; Wilczynska, A.; Thampi, P.; Cox, L.L.; MacNicol, A.M. Musashi regulates the temporal order of mRNA translation during Xenopus oocyte maturation. *EMBO J.* **2006**, *25*, 2792–2801. [CrossRef]

20. Imai, T.; Tokunaga, A.; Yoshida, T.; Hashimoto, M.; Mikoshiba, K.; Weinmaster, G.; Nakafuku, M.; Okano, H. The neural RNA-binding protein Musashi1 translationally regulates mammalian numb gene expression by interacting with its mRNA. *Mol. Cell. Biol.* **2001**, *21*, 3888–3900. [CrossRef]
21. Battelli, C.; Nikopoulos, G.N.; Mitchell, J.G.; Verdi, J.M. The RNA-binding protein Musashi-1 regulates neural development through the translational repression of p21WAF-1. *Mol. Cell. Neurosci.* **2006**, *31*, 85–96. [CrossRef] [PubMed]
22. Spears, E.; Neufeld, K.L. Novel double-negative feedback loop links Adenomatous polyposis coli and Musashi in colon epithelia. *J. Biol. Chem.* **2011**, *286*, 4946–4950. [CrossRef] [PubMed]
23. Warui, D.M.; Baranger, A.M. Identification of small molecule inhibitors of the HIV-1 nucleocapsid-stem-loop 3 RNA complex. *J. Med. Chem.* **2012**, *55*, 4132–4141. [CrossRef] [PubMed]
24. Mei, H.Y.; Mack, D.P.; Galan, A.A.; Halim, N.S.; Heldsinger, A.; Loo, J.A.; Moreland, D.W.; Sannes-Lowery, K.A.; Sharmeen, L.; Truong, H.N.; et al. Discovery of selective, small-molecule inhibitors of RNA complexes—I. The Tat protein/TAR RNA complexes required for HIV-1 transcription. *Bioorg. Med. Chem.* **1997**, *5*, 1173–1184. [CrossRef]
25. Zapp, M.L.; Stern, S.; Green, M.R. Small molecules that selectively block RNA binding of HIV-1 Rev protein inhibit Rev function and viral production. *Cell* **1993**, *74*, 969–978. [CrossRef]
26. In the Open Chemical Repository Collection. Available online: https://dtp.cancer.gov/organization/dscb/default.htm (accessed on 8 July 2020).
27. Somoza, A.D.; Lee, K.H.; Chiang, Y.M.; Oakley, B.R.; Wang, C.C. Reengineering an azaphilone biosynthesis pathway in Aspergillus nidulans to create lipoxygenase inhibitors. *Org. Lett.* **2012**, *14*, 972–975. [CrossRef]
28. Lan, L.; Xing, M.; Douglas, J.T.; Gao, P.; Hanzlik, R.P.; Xu, L. Human oncoprotein Musashi-2 N-terminal RNA recognition motif backbone assignment and identification of RNA-binding pocket. *Oncotarget* **2017**, *8*, 106587–106597. [CrossRef]
29. Kudinov, A.E.; Deneka, A.; Nikonova, A.S.; Beck, T.N.; Ahn, Y.H.; Liu, X.; Martinez, C.F.; Schultz, F.A.; Reynolds, S.; Yang, D.H.; et al. Musashi-2 (MSI2) supports TGF-beta signaling and inhibits claudins to promote non-small cell lung cancer (NSCLC) metastasis. *Proc. Natl. Acad. Sci. USA* **2016**, *113*, 6955–6960. [CrossRef]
30. Shan, W.; Ning, L.; Maryam, Y.; Angela, N.-D.; Fan, L.; Kimberly, P.; Shilpa, R.; Gerard, M.; Yarden, K.; Brian, D.G.; et al. Transformation of the intestinal epithelium by the MSI2 RNA-binding protein. *Nat. Commun.* **2015**, *6*. [CrossRef]
31. Kharas, M.G.; Lengner, C.J.; Al-Shahrour, F.; Bullinger, L.; Ball, B.; Zaidi, S.; Morgan, K.; Tam, W.; Paktinat, M.; Okabe, R.; et al. Musashi-2 regulates normal hematopoiesis and promotes aggressive myeloid leukemia. *Nat. Med.* **2010**, *16*, 903–908. [CrossRef]
32. Griner, L.N.; Reuther, G.W. Aggressive myeloid leukemia formation is directed by the Musashi 2/Numb pathway. *Cancer Biol. Ther.* **2010**, *10*, 979–982. [CrossRef] [PubMed]
33. Aviv, T.; Lin, Z.; Lau, S.; Rendl, L.M.; Sicheri, F.; Smibert, C.A. The RNA-binding SAM domain of Smaug defines a new family of post-transcriptional regulators. *Nat. Struct. Biol.* **2003**, *10*, 614–621. [CrossRef] [PubMed]
34. Pagano, J.M.; Clingman, C.C.; Ryder, S.P. Quantitative approaches to monitor protein-nucleic acid interactions using fluorescent probes. *RNA* **2011**, *17*, 14–20. [CrossRef] [PubMed]
35. Zhang, J.H.; Chung, T.D.; Oldenburg, K.R. A Simple Statistical Parameter for Use in Evaluation and Validation of High Throughput Screening Assays. *J. Biomol. Screen.* **1999**, *4*, 67–73. [CrossRef] [PubMed]
36. Lan, L.; Appelman, C.; Smith, A.R.; Yu, J.; Larsen, S.; Marquez, R.T.; Liu, H.; Wu, X.; Gao, P.; Roy, A.; et al. Natural product (−)-gossypol inhibits colon cancer cell growth by targeting RNA-binding protein Musashi-1. *Mol. Oncol.* **2015**. [CrossRef] [PubMed]
37. Ohyama, T.; Nagata, T.; Tsuda, K.; Kobayashi, N.; Imai, T.; Okano, H.; Yamazaki, T.; Katahira, M. Structure of Musashi1 in a complex with target RNA: The role of aromatic stacking interactions. *Nucleic Acids Res.* **2012**, *40*, 3218–3231. [CrossRef] [PubMed]
38. Gowthaman, R.; Deeds, E.J.; Karanicolas, J. Structural properties of non-traditional drug targets present new challenges for virtual screening. *J. Chem. Inf. Model.* **2013**, *53*, 2073–2081. [CrossRef] [PubMed]
39. Nero, T.L.; Morton, C.J.; Holien, J.K.; Wielens, J.; Parker, M.W. Oncogenic protein interfaces: Small molecules, big challenges. *Nat. Rev. Cancer* **2014**, *14*, 248–262. [CrossRef]

40. Lan, L.; Liu, H.; Smith, A.R.; Appelman, C.; Yu, J.; Larsen, S.; Marquez, R.T.; Wu, X.; Liu, F.Y.; Gao, P.; et al. Natural product derivative Gossypolone inhibits Musashi family of RNA-binding proteins. *BMC Cancer* **2018**, *18*, 809. [CrossRef]
41. Wu, X.; Lan, L.; Wilson, D.M.; Marquez, R.T.; Tsao, W.C.; Gao, P.; Roy, A.; Turner, B.A.; McDonald, P.; Tunge, J.A.; et al. Identification and Validation of Novel Small Molecule Disruptors of HuR-mRNA Interaction. *ACS Chem. Biol.* **2015**, *10*, 1476–1484. [CrossRef]
42. Hong, S. RNA Binding Protein as an Emerging Therapeutic Target for Cancer Prevention and Treatment. *J. Cancer Prev.* **2017**, *22*, 203–210. [CrossRef] [PubMed]
43. Minuesa, G.; Antczak, C.; Shum, D.; Radu, C.; Bhinder, B.; Li, Y.; Djaballah, H.; Kharas, M.G. A 1536-well fluorescence polarization assay to screen for modulators of the MUSASHI family of RNA-binding proteins. *Comb. Chem. High Throughput Screen.* **2014**, *17*, 596–609. [CrossRef] [PubMed]
44. Kaur, K.; Wu, X.; Fields, J.K.; Johnson, D.K.; Lan, L.; Pratt, M.; Somoza, A.D.; Wang, C.C.C.; Karanicolas, J.; Oakley, B.R.; et al. The fungal natural product azaphilone-9 binds to HuR and inhibits HuR-RNA interaction in vitro. *PLoS ONE* **2017**, *12*, e0175471. [CrossRef] [PubMed]
45. Fox, R.G.; Park, F.D.; Koechlein, C.S.; Kritzik, M.; Reya, T. Musashi signaling in stem cells and cancer. *Annu. Rev. Cell Dev. Biol.* **2015**, *31*, 249–267. [CrossRef] [PubMed]
46. Sutherland, J.M.; McLaughlin, E.A.; Hime, G.R.; Siddall, N.A. The musashi family of RNA binding proteins: Master regulators of multiple stem cell populations. *Adv. Exp. Med. Biol.* **2013**, *786*, 233–245. [CrossRef] [PubMed]
47. Sakakibara, S.; Nakamura, Y.; Yoshida, T.; Shibata, S.; Koike, M.; Takano, H.; Ueda, S.; Uchiyama, Y.; Noda, T.; Okano, H. RNA-binding protein Musashi family: Roles for CNS stem cells and a subpopulation of ependymal cells revealed by targeted disruption and antisense ablation. *Proc. Natl. Acad. Sci. USA* **2002**, *99*, 15194–15199. [CrossRef]
48. Li, N.; Yousefi, M.; Nakauka-Ddamba, A.; Li, F.; Vandivier, L.; Parada, K.; Woo, D.H.; Wang, S.; Naqvi, A.S.; Rao, S.; et al. The Msi Family of RNA-Binding Proteins Function Redundantly as Intestinal Oncoproteins. *Cell Rep.* **2015**, *13*, 2440–2455. [CrossRef]
49. Vo, D.T.; Abdelmohsen, K.; Martindale, J.L.; Qiao, M.; Tominaga, K.; Burton, T.L.; Gelfond, J.A.; Brenner, A.J.; Patel, V.; Trageser, D.; et al. The oncogenic RNA-binding protein Musashi1 is regulated by HuR via mRNA translation and stability in glioblastoma cells. *Mol. Cancer Res.* **2012**, *10*, 143–155. [CrossRef]
50. Curtin, T.P.; Reilly, J. Sclerotiorine, $C_{20}H_{20}O_5Cl$, a chlorine-containing metabolic product of Penicillium sclerotiorum van Beyma. *Biochem. J.* **1940**, *34*, 1418.1–1421. [CrossRef]
51. Chidananda, C.; Rao, L.J.; Sattur, A.P. Sclerotiorin, from Penicillium frequentans, a potent inhibitor of aldose reductase. *Biotechnol. Lett.* **2006**, *28*, 1633–1636. [CrossRef]
52. Giridharan, P.; Verekar, S.A.; Khanna, A.; Mishra, P.D.; Deshmukh, S.K. Anticancer activity of sclerotiorin, isolated from an endophytic fungus Cephalotheca faveolata Yaguchi, Nishim. & Udagawa. *Indian J. Exp. Biol.* **2012**, *50*, 464–468. [PubMed]
53. Osmanova, N.; Schultze, W.; Ayoub, N. Azaphilones: A class of fungal metabolites with diverse biological activities. *Phytochem. Rev.* **2010**, *9*, 315–342. [CrossRef]
54. Ozoline, O.N.; Jass, J. Editorial: Secretion and signalling of bacterial RNAs. *FEMS Microbiol. Lett.* **2019**, *366*. [CrossRef] [PubMed]
55. Chan, T.A.; Wang, Z.; Dang, L.H.; Vogelstein, B.; Kinzler, K.W. Targeted inactivation of CTNNB1 reveals unexpected effects of beta-catenin mutation. *Proc. Natl. Acad. Sci. USA* **2002**, *99*, 8265–8270. [CrossRef]
56. Yang, J.; Zhang, W.; Evans, P.M.; Chen, X.; He, X.; Liu, C. Adenomatous polyposis coli (APC) differentially regulates beta-catenin phosphorylation and ubiquitination in colon cancer cells. *J. Biol. Chem.* **2006**, *281*, 17751–17757. [CrossRef]
57. Minuesa, G.; Albanese, S.K.; Xie, W.; Kazansky, Y.; Worroll, D.; Chow, A.; Schurer, A.; Park, S.M.; Rotsides, C.Z.; Taggart, J.; et al. Small-molecule targeting of MUSASHI RNA-binding activity in acute myeloid leukemia. *Nat. Commun.* **2019**, *10*, 2691. [CrossRef]
58. Lian, J.; Wu, X.; He, F.; Karnak, D.; Tang, W.; Meng, Y.; Xiang, D.; Ji, M.; Lawrence, T.S.; Xu, L. A natural BH3 mimetic induces autophagy in apoptosis-resistant prostate cancer via modulating Bcl-2-Beclin1 interaction at endoplasmic reticulum. *Cell Death Differ.* **2011**, *18*, 60–71. [CrossRef]

59. Meng, Y.; Tang, W.; Dai, Y.; Wu, X.; Liu, M.; Ji, Q.; Ji, M.; Pienta, K.; Lawrence, T.; Xu, L. Natural BH3 mimetic (-)-gossypol chemosensitizes human prostate cancer via Bcl-xL inhibition accompanied by increase of Puma and Noxa. *Mol. Cancer Ther.* **2008**, *7*, 2192–2202. [CrossRef]
60. Wu, X.; Li, M.; Qu, Y.; Tang, W.; Zheng, Y.; Lian, J.; Ji, M.; Xu, L. Design and synthesis of novel Gefitinib analogues with improved anti-tumor activity. *Bioorg. Med. Chem.* **2010**, *18*, 3812–3822. [CrossRef]
61. Li, L.; Hao, X.; Qin, J.; Tang, W.; He, F.; Smith, A.; Zhang, M.; Simeone, D.M.; Qiao, X.T.; Chen, Z.N.; et al. Antibody Against CD44s Inhibits Pancreatic Tumor Initiation and Post-Radiation Recurrence in Mice. *Gastroenterology* **2014**. [CrossRef]
62. Li, L.; Tang, W.; Wu, X.; Karnak, D.; Meng, X.; Thompson, R.; Hao, X.; Li, Y.; Qiao, X.T.; Lin, J.; et al. HAb18G/CD147 promotes pSTAT3-mediated pancreatic cancer development via CD44s. *Clin. Cancer Res.* **2013**, *19*, 6703–6715. [CrossRef] [PubMed]
63. Estrada, D.F.; Boudreaux, D.M.; Zhong, D.; St Jeor, S.C.; De Guzman, R.N. The Hantavirus Glycoprotein G1 Tail Contains Dual CCHC-type Classical Zinc Fingers. *J. Biol. Chem.* **2009**, *284*, 8654–8660. [CrossRef] [PubMed]

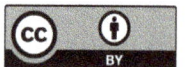

© 2020 by the authors. Licensee MDPI, Basel, Switzerland. This article is an open access article distributed under the terms and conditions of the Creative Commons Attribution (CC BY) license (http://creativecommons.org/licenses/by/4.0/).

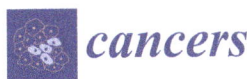

Review

Not All Wnt Activation Is Equal: Ligand-Dependent versus Ligand-Independent Wnt Activation in Colorectal Cancer

Sam O. Kleeman [1,2] and Simon J. Leedham [2,*]

1. Cold Spring Harbor Laboratory, Cold Spring Harbor, NY 11724, USA; skleeman@cshl.edu
2. Intestinal Stem Cell Biology Lab, Wellcome Trust Centre Human Genetics, University of Oxford, Oxford OX3 7BN, UK
* Correspondence: simonl@well.ox.ac.uk

Received: 16 October 2020; Accepted: 12 November 2020; Published: 13 November 2020

Simple Summary: Colorectal cancer is the third most common cause of cancer-related deaths. The Wnt signaling pathway is activated by genetic mutations in most patients with colorectal cancer. A number of different types of Wnt pathway mutation have been described: some increase the sensitivity of tumor cells to Wnt ligands produced by stromal cells (ligand-dependent), while others drive downstream activation of the pathway (ligand-independent). Ligand-dependent tumors are of particular interest as there are a number of emerging treatment options, such as porcupine inhibitors, that can specifically target these tumors. In this review, we discuss what is known about these different types of Wnt activating mutations. We propose that ligand-dependent tumors should be viewed as a separate subset of colorectal cancer with its own biomarkers, prognosis and targeted therapies.

Abstract: Wnt signaling is ubiquitously activated in colorectal tumors and driver mutations are identified in genes such as APC, CTNNB1, RNF43 and R-spondin (RSPO2/3). Adenomatous polyposis coli (APC) and CTNNB1 mutations lead to downstream constitutive activation (ligand-independent), while RNF43 and RSPO mutations require exogenous Wnt ligand to activate signaling (ligand-dependent). Here, we present evidence that these mutations are not equivalent and that ligand-dependent and ligand-independent tumors differ in terms of underlying Wnt biology, molecular pathogenesis, morphology and prognosis. These non-overlapping characteristics can be harnessed to develop biomarkers and targeted treatments for ligand-dependent tumors, including porcupine inhibitors, anti-RSPO3 antibodies and asparaginase. There is emerging evidence that these therapies may synergize with immunotherapy in ligand-dependent tumors. In summary, we propose that ligand-dependent tumors are an underappreciated separate disease entity in colorectal cancer.

Keywords: Wnt; signaling; colorectal; cancer; porcupine; R-spondin; serrated; immunotherapy

1. Introduction

Metastatic colorectal cancer (CRC) is a lethal malignancy with a five-year survival of less than 15% [1]. Patients with metastatic CRC are treated with combination cytotoxic chemotherapy alongside monoclonal antibodies targeting angiogenesis or epidermal growth factor receptor (EGFR) [2]. There is a need to develop new therapeutic strategies for metastatic cancer, especially in light of evidence showing rapid increases in CRC incidence affecting younger patients [3]. Molecular profiling of CRC has shown considerable disease heterogeneity, suggesting that patients might benefit from precision medicine, in which treatments are personalized for their tumor profile [4]. For example, immunotherapy targeting PD-1/PD-L1 signaling is only active in hypermutated tumors, while anti-EGFR antibodies are only effective in tumors without downstream mutations [5–7].

Colorectal cancer is characterized by near-ubiquitous activation of the Wnt signaling pathway [8]. The Wnt pathway is an evolutionarily conserved mechanism for intercellular communication, with essential roles in embryogenesis and adult tissue development [9]. In the colonic crypt, Wnt signaling is necessary to maintain the adult intestinal stem cell niche and epithelial homeostasis [10]. Colorectal tumors are dependent upon aberrant Wnt signaling to maintain stemness and a de-differentiated phenotype and genetic Wnt inhibition leads to rapid tumor regression [11]. Additionally, Wnt signaling can protect cells from immune surveillance, thus restricting anti-tumoral immunity [12,13]. Altogether, this suggests that the Wnt pathway could be a viable therapeutic target for patients with CRC.

Colorectal tumors are thought to evolve through the sequential acquisition of mutations driving progression from a normal founder cell to adenoma and then carcinoma [14]. Adenomas can be histologically classified as either conventional, such as tubular or tubulovillous (TVA), or serrated, such as sessile serrated lesions (SSL) or traditional serrated adenomas (TSA) [15]. Serrated adenomas are characterized histologically by a saw-tooth morphology. The cell-of-origin for TVA is likely the crypt-based columnar stem cell [16] while the cell-of-origin for serrated lesions is unknown, but may derive from ectopic crypt foci in the rare traditional serrated adenoma subtype [17].

Here, we present evidence for a new model of CRC in which Wnt pathway activation can take one of two distinct trajectories, ligand-dependent (LD) and ligand-independent (LI), with implications spanning tumor biology, screening, diagnosis and treatment. We will first outline the Wnt signaling pathway in the normal colon and types of recurrent Wnt mutations in CRC. We will then discuss morphological and molecular biomarkers that can be used to identify LD tumors in the clinic. Finally, we will argue that this model has the potential to transform the landscape of precision medicine in CRC.

2. Wnt Signaling Pathway

The Wnt signaling pathway in normal colon crypts is summarized in Figure 1. Briefly, canonical Wnt ligands are secreted by the cells in the stem cell niche following O-acylation by porcupine [18,19]. Wnt ligands bind to Frizzled (FZD) and lipoprotein receptor-related protein (LRP) receptor complexes on the plasma membrane of neighboring cells [20]. Both Wnt ligand secretion and binding to FZD depend upon acylation of Wnt ligands [21]. The downstream effector of Wnt signaling is the transcriptional co-activator β-catenin (CTNNB1). In the absence of Wnt ligands, CTNNB1 is degraded by the action of a destruction complex containing adenomatous polyposis coli (APC), axin-like protein (AXIN1/2), glycogen synthase kinase (GSK3) and casein kinase (CSNK1A) [22]. Wnt ligand binding inhibits the destruction complex, thus stabilizing CTNNB1 and activating expression of Wnt target genes. An additional level of regulation comes from E3 ubiquitin ligases ring finger protein 43 (RNF43) and zinc and ring finger 3 (ZNRF3), which constitutively degrade FZD to repress Wnt signaling [23]. R-spondin (RSPO) ligands bind to leucine-rich repeat-containing G protein-coupled (LGR) receptors, inhibiting RNF43/ZNRF3 and substantially amplifying Wnt signaling [24]. There are four homologous human RSPO ligands (RSPO1-4) and, while all four can bind to LGR-family receptors, the EC_{50} for activation of Wnt signaling varies 100-fold, with RSPO2 and RSPO3 demonstrating the highest potency (0.02–0.05 nM) [25]. R-spondins are produced by stromal cells adjacent to the stem cell niche [26]. Consistent with this, R-spondin signaling is necessary to maintain the stem cell niche, both in vivo and as part of organoid culture systems [24,27,28]. Wnt target genes, such as notum palmitoleoyl-protein carboxylesterase (NOTUM) and AXIN2 are negative regulators of Wnt signaling, functioning as negative feedback loops to fine-tune and limit downstream signaling [29]. AXIN2 is an inducible component of the destruction complex, while NOTUM works in the extracellular space to deacetylate and inactivate Wnt ligands [30].

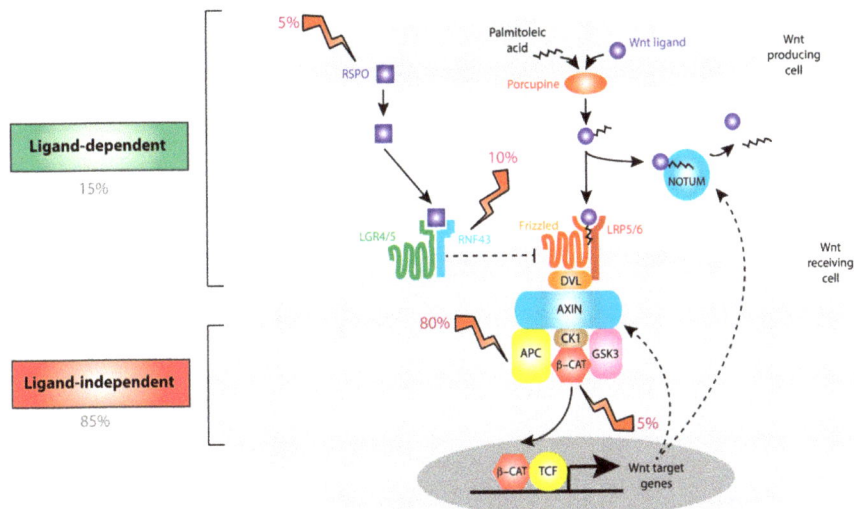

Figure 1. Overview of Wnt signaling pathway. Wnt ligands secreted from stromal cells are activated by porcupine-mediated post-translational modification and bind to Frizzled (FZD) receptors on Wnt receiving cells. This functions to inhibit a destruction complex containing axin-like protein (AXIN)1/2 and adenomatous polyposis coli (APC) thus disinhibiting β-catenin (CTNNB1), the master transcriptional regulator of Wnt singaling. Frizzled receptors are degraded due to the action of ring finger protein 43 (RNF43), which is in turn inhibited by binding of R-spondin (RSPO) ligands to leucine-rich repeat-containing G protein-coupled (LGR) family receptors, thus augmenting Wnt signaling tone. Wnt pathway activation is regulated at multiple levels by negative feedback loops, including those mediated by AXIN2 and notum palmitoleoyl-protein carboxylesterase (NOTUM). Recurrent mutations in CTNNB1 and APC result in ligand-independent pathway activation while mutations in RSPO and RNF43 depend upon binding of Wnt ligands to Frizzled receptors. GSK: glycogen synthase kinase; LRP: lipoprotein receptor-related protein.

3. Ligand-Dependent and Ligand-Independent Alterations in Colorectal Cancer

Large-scale sequencing studies in CRC have established the presence of pervasive Wnt pathway mutations. Recurrent mutations include loss-of-function mutations in APC and RNF43, and gain-of-function mutations in CTNNB1 and RSPO2/3 (Figure 1, Table 1) [8,31,32]. Consistent with driver mutation status, in vivo modeling indicates that these mutations can be sufficient for colorectal tumorigenesis [33–36]. For tumor suppressors APC and RNF43, we only consider protein-truncating mutations or deletions as potential driver alterations [37]. ZNRF3 is a homolog of RNF43 but truncating mutations are rare in colorectal tumors, potentially reflecting its comparably low mRNA expression in normal colon and colorectal tumors [8,38]. This is in contrast to the situation in murine intestine, in which Znrf3 and Rnf43 gene expression is comparable, and loss-of-function alterations in both Znrf3 and Rnf43 are necessary to activate Wnt signaling [36,39].

While *APC* and *CTNNB1* alterations drive downstream, constitutive activation of the Wnt pathway that is independent of Wnt ligand binding (ligand-independent, LI), *RSPO* and *RNF43* alterations disrupt the synergistic RSPO axis and by doing so, amplify endogenous and otherwise intact, Wnt ligand signaling (ligand-dependent, LD). APC mutations are characteristically nonsense or frameshift alterations affecting the "mutation cluster region", often with a second "hit" from loss of heterozygosity [40]. CTNNB1 mutations are gain-of-function missense mutations affecting specific amino acid residues that are phosphorylation sites for components of the destruction complex [41].

Table 1. Driver Wnt alterations in colorectal cancer. Prevalence refers to the frequency of each mutation in the subset of colorectal tumors with a detectable driver Wnt alteration, as derived from [42]. Loss-of-function alterations in APC and RNF43 are frequently accompanied by loss of heterozygosity (LOH) affecting the second allele [13].

Mutation Type	Gene	Type of Alteration	Prevalence in CRC
Ligand-dependent	RNF43	Loss-of-function - Nonsense - Frameshift	10%
	R-spondin (RSPO2, RSPO3)	Gain-of-function - Stromal overexpression - Epithelial gene fusions	8%
Ligand-independent	APC	Loss-of-function - Nonsense - Frameshift	81%
	CTNNB1	Gain-of-function - Missense (affecting codons 31–35, 37, 40, 41, 45, 383 and 387)	2%

RSPO mutations induce R-spondin ligand overexpression either from epithelial cells (autocrine), as RSPO fusion genes [42]. R-spondin gain-of-function is only observed for RSPO2 and RSPO3, consistent with their enhanced potency to induce Wnt signaling in vitro [25]. RSPO3 fusion genes commonly result in the replacement of RSPO3 exon one and promoter with that of a gene with higher basal expression, resulting in a functional epithelial-expressed protein [32]. A wide range of fusion partners have been identified including PTPRK, EIF3E, NRIP1 and PIEZO1 [43,44], all of which are associated with relatively high constitutive gene expression [38]. RSPO fusions cannot be reliably identified even from whole-genome sequencing due to large inconsistency in genomic alterations, while the transcript breakpoints are more stereotypical [32]. Alternatively, in a rare subset of colorectal tumors, we identified R-spondin overexpression in the absence of RSPO fusions or any other detectable Wnt driver alteration [42]. In situ hybridization demonstrated high stromal RSPO3 expression in these tumors, implicating a role for paracrine R-spondin signaling driven by stromal overexpression [42]. RSPO3 overexpression in the absence of gene fusions has been previously detected in lung cancer, where it was associated with RSPO3 hypomethylation [45]. The concept that RSPO overexpression can derive from either epithelial or stromal sources is consistent with previous evidence that RSPO3 expression is significantly and positively correlated with stromal expression signatures [46]. RNF43 mutations are mostly recurrent frameshift mutations at amino acid positions 117 and 659 that result in a truncated gene product [31]. These recurrent mutations occur at tandem repeats called microsatellites whose stability is dependent upon proficient mismatch repair (MMR) [47]. As a result, these mutations tend to occur in tumors with MMR deficiency, detected as microsatellite instability (MSI), which is often caused by promoter hypermethylation of MLH1 [8,48].

Recently, there has been some controversy about whether the RNF43 G659Vfs*41 mutation demonstrably leads to impaired protein function. In vitro transfection experiments have indicated that this mutant RNF43 protein retains the ability to bind R-spondin and repress Frizzled [49]. However, this alteration is associated with significantly reduced RNF43 expression, potentially consistent with nonsense-mediated decay [49], and CRISPR-Cas9 editing of the endogenous RNF43 locus to mimic the G659Vfs*41 mutation, was sufficient to increase cell surface Frizzled expression [50]. Furthermore, the G659Vfs*41 mutation occurs substantially more often than would be expected by chance in microsatellite-unstable tumors, indicating strong positive selection [31,51].

It is important to note that driver Wnt alterations affecting APC, CTNNB1, RNF43 and RSPO in pre-cancerous polyps and tumors show marked mutual exclusivity [42]. There are two logical implications from this: firstly, these alterations are redundantly able to activate Wnt signaling. Secondly, there may be selection against the accumulation of driver alterations in more than one gene.

This is consistent with the "just right" theory of Wnt signaling: that there is an optimal level of Wnt activation to drive tumorigenesis. It has been observed that there is a non-random distribution of second "hit" mutations in APC that is consistent with selection for APC genotypes that retain some CTNNB1 repression [52]. Additionally, ectopic expression of R-spondin in APC-mutant mice results in reduced proliferation and increased apoptosis [53], consistent with evidence that Wnt can directly promote apoptosis [54].

4. Mutation Selection in Lesion Subtypes

Molecular profiling in pre-cancerous polyps has shown that ligand-dependent alterations are predominantly seen in the serrated pathway (Figure 2) [44,55]. A total of 55% of TSAs have ligand-dependent alterations, namely truncating RNF43 mutations or RSPO fusions (mostly PTPRK-RSPO3) [44]. In sessile serrated lesions (SSL), mutations in the Wnt signaling pathway are not thought to be initiating lesions as Wnt disruption is observed predominantly in dysplastic rather than non-dysplastic lesions. A total of 50% of SSLs had ligand-dependent RNF43 mutations [55], whereas APC mutations are much rarer in serrated lesions, being detected in 13% and 9% of TSAs and dysplastic SSLs, respectively [44,55]. In contrast, conventional adenomas have a high frequency (>85%) of ligand-independent alterations [56]. APC mutation is sufficient to initiate adenoma pathogenesis [57] and no ligand-dependent alterations have been reported in conventional adenomas [44].

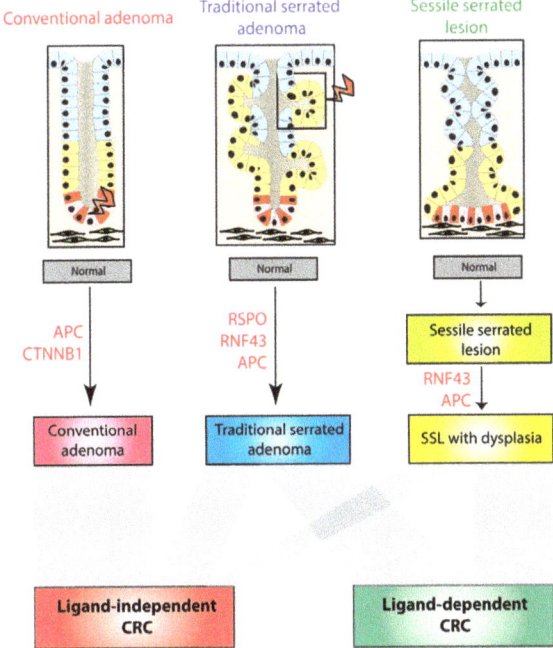

Figure 2. Molecular pathogenesis of different colorectal precursor subtypes. Colorectal cancer develops from three types of pre-cancerous polyps: conventional and serrated adenomas—divided into traditional serrated adenomas (TSAs) and sessile serrated lesions (SSLs). Conventional adenomas are driven by ligand-independent mutations that likely arise in the crypt base columnar (CBC) stem cells. TSAs arise from APC, RSPO or RNF43 mutations, possibly in ectopic crypts. SSL pathogenesis is characterized by the late acquisition of APC or RNF43 mutations, concurrent with the onset of the detectable dysplasia. Ligand-dependent CRC arises from TSAs and SSLs while ligand-independent CRC arises from all three types of polyp (bottom panel).

Altogether, this raises the possibility that different intestinal lesions follow distinct molecular carcinogenesis pathways. These different evolutionary trajectories appear to result in the selection of either ligand-dependent or independent mutations. This may also partly explain the mutual exclusivity of Wnt driver mutations discussed above. Why polyp subtypes acquire apparent obligatory Wnt disruption through these different mechanisms is unknown, but may be influenced by the variable cell-of-origin in different lesion subtypes (Figure 2). Indeed, APC mutations induce tumorigenesis in vivo if introduced into the LGR5+ intestinal stem cell but not transit-amplifying cells [16], while RSPO fusions significantly co-occur with loss-of-function mutations in the Bone morphogenic protein (BMP) signaling pathway that are known to induce ectopic crypt formation [58,59]. These data would also suggest that RSPO-mutant colorectal tumors are wholly derived from TSAs.

5. Negative Regulation of Wnt Signaling

In some ways, it is surprising that despite multiple levels of negative feedback, ligand-dependent mutations, which act upstream in an otherwise normal pathway, can induce activation of Wnt signaling at all. Ligand-dependent pathway activation would be expected to induce physiological expression of Wnt negative regulators such as AXIN2 or NOTUM, which would function to proportionately constrain activation of the pathway. In contrast, ligand-independent alterations result in downstream, constitutive activation that is uncoupled from the action of negative regulators. We have recently shown that tumors with ligand-dependent alterations are associated with significant repression of Wnt negative regulators, especially AXIN2 [42]. This repression may be at least partly explained by AXIN2 methylation [60]. This raises the possibility that ligand-dependent Wnt activation requires two "hits"—firstly a driver mutation affecting RNF43 or RSPO, and secondly, epigenetic downregulation of Wnt negative regulators. Indeed, serrated adenomas which are enriched for ligand dependent mutations, have lower AXIN2 expression and increased AXIN2 methylation compared to conventional tubulovillous adenomas [61,62], as do MSI-high cancers that progress via this pathway [45,53]. AXIN2 expression is also decreased in an in vivo model of ligand-dependent tumors, generated by orthotopic engraftment of CRISPR-edited organoids [63]. Furthermore, ectopic expression of AXIN2, leading to re-activation of Wnt negative feedback in an RNF43-mutant cell line (HCT116) resulted in rapid cell death [60,61]. In fact, AXIN2 is not the only Wnt negative regulator known to be silenced by promoter hypermethylation in colorectal cancer: hypermethylation has been detected in negative regulators including WIF1, SFRP1/2/4, DKK1–3 and NOTUM [42,62,64]. These genes are predominantly hypermethylated in ligand-dependent or microsatellite-unstable tumors. This suggests that repression of negative regulators is a more global phenomenon in ligand-dependent CRC, with loss of negative feedback mechanisms at multiple levels of the Wnt signaling pathway.

6. Application of AXIN2 as a Biomarker for Ligand-Dependent Wnt Biology

Our finding that ligand-dependent tumors exhibit suppressed expression of negative regulators of Wnt can be harnessed to utilize AXIN2 as a single-gene biomarker to distinguish between ligand-dependent and ligand-independent tumors at the point of diagnosis. This is particularly important as otherwise ligand-dependent tumors would need to be identified from expensive and time-consuming analysis of paired DNA (for APC, CTNNB1 and RNF43) and RNA sequencing (RSPO fusions). Paired DNA and RNA sequencing is simply not practical for routine diagnostic assessment in the clinic, both in terms of cost and the relatively high failure rate of sequencing (>10%) from diagnostic clinical samples [65].

We recently demonstrated that AXIN2 mRNA expression could be used as a discriminatory biomarker with an area under the curve (AUC) greater than 0.93 in three independent cohorts, indicating excellent diagnostic performance. This analysis incorporated both RNA sequencing and microarray profiling to assay gene expression in resection and biopsy specimens [42]. The diagnostic performance corresponded to sensitivity and specificity >90%. We also demonstrated similar results with high-throughput AXIN2 profiling by quantitative real-time polymerase chain reaction (qRT-PCR). These findings were recently supported by the use of an organoid biobank derived from patients with colorectal cancer, in which organoids with RSPO fusions or RNF43 mutations exhibited lower AXIN2 expression than APC-mutant organoids [58]. Our analysis of paired qRT-PCR and immunohistochemistry for AXIN2 showed that there was only weak correlation between AXIN2 mRNA and scored AXIN2 protein expression, suggesting that AXIN2 may undergo significant translational regulation, as has been described previously [66]. This would suggest that profiling of AXIN2 mRNA expression would be the preferred approach to translate this biomarker into the clinic.

It is worth noting that AXIN2 gene expression is widely used as a read-out of global Wnt pathway activation [67] and our findings suggest that this should be interpreted with caution, as AXIN2 expression can be confounded by the type of acquired Wnt disrupting pathway mutation. This confounding has important implications for the interpretation of analyses that have demonstrated inverse correlations between AXIN2 (used as a read-out of Wnt activation) and immune infiltration [13]. Tumors with low AXIN2 expression are enriched with RNF43-mutant MSI-high tumors that have enhanced anti-tumoral immune responses, thought to result from an increased neoantigen load [68]. As a result, the inverse relationship between AXIN2 and immune infiltration may be partly explained by increased mutational load in RNF43-mutant ligand-dependent tumors, rather than reduced Wnt activation.

In summary, the distinction between ligand-dependent and ligand-independent tumors is clinically-actionable because tumors can be robustly discriminated using a low-cost single-gene molecular biomarker.

7. Non-Overlapping Clinicopathological Features of Ligand-Dependent Tumors

Consistent with altered Wnt pathway biology and an altered trajectory through the serrated pathway, ligand-dependent tumors have non-overlapping morphological and clinical characteristics with ligand-independent tumors, reflecting an underappreciated separate disease entity in colorectal cancer. Using manual and automated digital pathological approaches, we have demonstrated that ligand-dependent tumors are enriched with mucin [13,42]. Mucin is a high molecular-weight glycoprotein that is secreted by goblet cells and forms a key component of the mucous layer that provides physical protection in the gastrointestinal tract [69]. Mucinous differentiation has long been recognized in a subset of colorectal tumors (around 10%) and is diagnosed in tumors where mucin comprises >50% of the tumor volume [70]. Indeed, mucinous differentiation is associated with microsatellite instability, implicating a link with RNF43-mutant tumors. We have demonstrated that computational-scored mucin area alone could discriminate between ligand-dependent and ligand-independent tumors with an AUC > 0.75. Based on our findings, we propose that mucinous differentiation may well either be induced by ligand-dependent Wnt signaling or reflect the association with the serrated pathway. Consistent with the former hypothesis, the induction of ligand-dependent alterations in organoids is sufficient to generate orthotopic colon tumors with mucinous differentiation [63]. Furthermore, RNF43 mutations in biliary malignancies are associated with mucin hypersecretion [71]. Altogether, this suggests that mucin content, which is routinely scored by histopathologists, can be used as a phenotypic biomarker for ligand-dependent tumors with good diagnostic performance.

In our comparison of ligand-dependent and ligand-independent tumors in a pooled cohort of over 600 tumors with available outcome data, we did not identify any significant differences in prognosis [42]. However, this is likely to mask, considerably, the prognostic heterogeneity between the subsets of ligand-dependent tumors. One way to examine this is to compare specific subsets with their consensus molecular subtype (CMS) classifications, as this study was well-powered to identify prognostic associations incorporating over 2000 patients [72]. Ligand-dependent tumors appear to lie on a continuum between RNF43-mutant tumors which mostly classify as CMS1 (associated with good prognosis) and tumors with stromal RSPO overexpression which mostly classify as CMS4 (associated with poor prognosis). Consistent with this, we observed a high frequency of tumor budding and enriched desmoplastic stroma in tumors with stromal RSPO overexpression, both of which are associated with poor prognosis [73,74]. Of note, mucinous differentiation is associated with marginally reduced overall survival [75]. These data suggest that the prognostic implications of ligand-dependent Wnt biology are likely to be highly heterogenous.

8. Selective Vulnerabilities in Ligand-Dependent Tumors

Downstream ligand-independent Wnt signaling has proved difficult to target in solid tumors, reflecting challenges in designing small-molecule inhibitors to inhibit constitutive pathway activation through transcription factors such as beta-catenin [76]. In contrast, from a conceptual and experimental standpoint, ligand-dependent Wnt activation is inherently "druggable" through deprivation of extracellular ligand (Wnt or R-spondin) or attenuation of negative regulator suppression with demethylating agents (Figure 3) [27,60,77]. Furthermore, emerging evidence would indicate that these selective vulnerabilities in ligand-dependent tumors could synergize with immunotherapy targeting PD-1/PD-L1 signaling in tumors [78]. This makes ligand-dependent tumors a fascinating subset of colorectal cancer, with the real possibility of new transformative treatments.

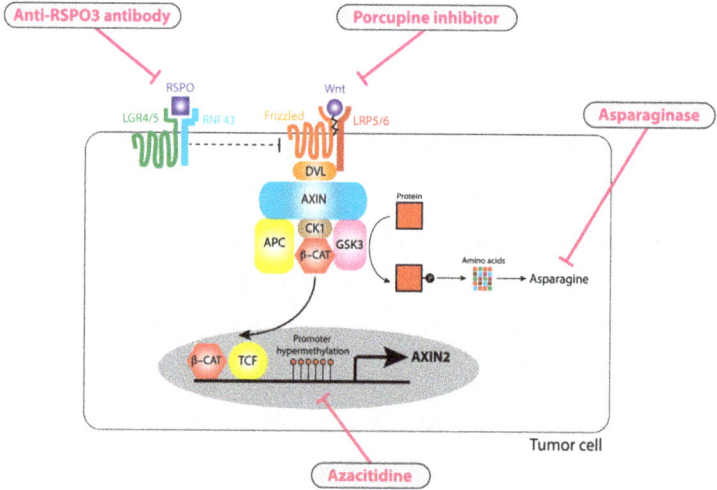

Figure 3. Target therapies for ligand-dependent tumors. All ligand-dependent tumors require Wnt ligands for pathway activation and so are sensitive to porcupine inhibitors that impair Wnt ligand activation. RSPO3 overexpression can be antagonized by anti-RSPO3 antibodies. Ligand-dependent GSK3 inhibition results in reduced proteasomal degradation to generate amino acids such as asparagine, making tumor cells sensitive to asparagine depletion with asparaginase treatment. Ligand-dependent tumors are characterized by AXIN2 repression which can be antagonized with licensed demethylating agents such as azacitidine.

By definition, ligand-dependent Wnt alterations can only induce downstream Wnt pathway activation in the presence of Wnt ligand. As a result, depletion and inactivation of Wnt ligand by inhibition of porcupine is a viable therapeutic approach for ligand-dependent tumors. In vitro models of ligand-dependent tumors, including organoids with RNF43 mutations [79] and cell lines with RSPO fusions [46], are exquisitely sensitive to porcupine inhibitors. This has also been demonstrated in various in vivo settings, including xenografts with RSPO fusions [77] and autochthonous Rnf43/Znrf3-null intestinal tumors [80]. Porcupine inhibition is associated with marked repression of Wnt pathway activity, reduced tumor size and substantial remodeling the transcriptomic landscape that includes increased intestinal differentiation [77,80]. Porcupine inhibitors have entered early-phase clinical trials (NCT01351103, NCT03447470, NCT03507998). Preliminary evidence from a phase 1 trial identified a partial response in one patient with a detectable RNF43 mutation [81] while porcupine inhibition was associated with reduced AXIN2 expression, suggesting on-target effects [82].

However, in vitro modeling of porcupine inhibition in ligand-dependent CRC cell lines has identified selection for resistance mutations, such as loss-of-function alterations to AXIN1, leading to loss of function of the destruction complex and downstream constitutive pathway activation [46]. It is worth noting that AXIN2 repression seen in ligand-dependent tumors does not result in downstream pathway activation because of redundancy with AXIN1. AXIN1 is a constitutive component of the destruction complex and not a Wnt pathway target. This would suggest that AXIN1 inactivation alone would not be sufficient to drive Wnt pathway activation unless AXIN2 was concurrently repressed—we would hypothesize that this situation could only arise in ligand-dependent tumors. This might explain the relatively low frequency (<0.05%) of truncating AXIN1 mutations seen in CRC [8].

In tumors with epithelial RSPO fusions, the autocrine signaling loop can be blocked by an anti-RSPO3 antibody. For example, treatment with anti-RSPO3 antibody has been shown to result in inhibition of xenograft tumor growth with tumor regression in some cases [27,83–85]. As with porcupine inhibitors, this was associated with evidence of increased intestinal differentiation on morphological and transcriptomic analysis [27,83]. This differentiated phenotype was associated with reduced expression of stem cell markers and key Wnt targets such as LGR5 and ASCL2. A phase 1 trial of an anti-RSPO3 antibody in patients with metastatic colorectal cancer was associated with partial responses in some patients, although this was not clearly associated with baseline RSPO3 expression [86]. In addition, while it has not been formally tested, it is entirely plausible that anti-RSPO3 therapy would also be effective for tumors with stromal RSPO overexpression.

The Wnt pathway plays a critical role in bone homeostasis [87] and unsurprisingly inhibition of ligand-dependent Wnt signaling via porcupine inhibitors or anti-RSPO3 antibodies results in on-target bone toxicity, including reduced bone strength and pathological fractures [86,88,89]. Consistent with this, porcupine-null mice have widespread bone defects, while germline loss-of-function Wnt ligand mutations in humans are associated with high fracture risk [90–92]. Preliminary evidence has shown that bone toxicity could be reduced with co-administration of denosumab, which inhibits bone degradation [89]. Altogether, concerns about resistance and on-target toxicity would likely limit the use of direct Wnt inhibitions (porcupine, anti-RSPO3) to short durations of time, likely in conjunction with other treatments.

In light of evidence that ligand-dependent tumors may depend upon repression of negative regulators, possibly via promoter hypermethylation [42], demethylating agents could be a viable therapeutic strategy in ligand-dependent tumors. Demethylation treatment with azacitidine in HCT116, a colorectal cancer cell line with an RNF43 mutation and comparatively low AXIN2 expression, resulted in increased AXIN2 expression and increased cell death [60,93]. Azacitidine is an approved treatment for myelodysplastic syndrome with a well-established toxicity profile suggesting that this would be a feasible treatment for ligand-dependent CRC [94].

Unexpectedly, recent work in acute myeloid leukemia found that asparaginase treatment was synthetically lethal with inhibition of GSK3 [95]. Asparaginase functions to deaminate and so degrade the nonessential amino acid asparagine, which is required for leukemic cell growth [96]. GSK3 mediates ubiquitination of a wide range of proteins, such as APC, and resulting proteasomal degradation provides a source of asparagine in the cell. Asparaginase treatment has a relatively favorable toxicity profile and is licensed for acute myeloid leukemia [97]. In contrast to ligand-independent alterations, which act downstream and by-pass GSK3, ligand-dependent mutations directly lead to inhibition of GSK3 (Figure 1) through activation of the canonical Wnt pathway, thus explaining a unique selective vulnerability for asparaginase treatment in ligand-dependent tumors. Specifically, asparaginase treatments were highly toxic for organoids with RSPO fusions but had no activity against organoids with APC or CTNNB1 mutations [98]. Treatment of mice with subcutaneous implantation of RSPO-mutant organoids was associated with marked tumor regression and prolonged progression-free survival, with no evidence of early therapy resistance [98]. No benefit was seen for implanted APC-mutant organoids. Altogether, these data would suggest that asparaginase could be a viable and well-tolerated treatment for patients with ligand-dependent CRC.

In summary, ligand-dependent Wnt biology is associated with a range of therapeutic vulnerabilities that could be exploited as effective anti-cancer therapy.

9. Combination Therapy for Ligand-Dependent Tumors

Considering that direct inhibition of the Wnt pathway is unlikely to be feasible for extended periods of time, it is important to consider how treatments for ligand-dependent tumors might synergize with existing anti-cancer therapy. Wnt pathway activation is often detected as a marker of resistance to cytotoxic chemotherapy [99]. Resistance to paclitaxel, which is a type of cytotoxic chemotherapy that inhibits microtubule detachment from centrosomes, is associated with Wnt pathway activation, detected as increased CTNNB1 protein expression. Considering that Wnt functions as a regulator of centrosome separation [100], it is feasible that Wnt activation could directly promote survival of tumor cells. Consistent with this, anti-Wnt treatments such as anti-RSPO3 antibodies synergize with paclitaxel in patient-derived xenografts with RSPO3 fusions [84].

More generally, inhibition of Wnt signaling in ligand-dependent tumors is consistently shown to skew cells from a stem-like phenotype to a more differentiated phenotype [27,101,102]. Resistance to cancer radiotherapy and chemotherapy is often driven by acquisition of stem-like phenotypes, with enrichment of tumor cells that are able to repopulate a tumor on transplantation, often termed cancer stem cells [103,104]. This suggests that short courses of Wnt pathway inhibitors could be synergistic with a wide range of existing and innovative drug regimens, especially if Wnt inhibitors are early in the treatment schedule.

The Wnt signaling pathway appears to play a role in protecting cells from immune surveillance. As a result, there is considerable interest in the combination of immunotherapy that targets PD-L1/PD-1 signaling and direct inhibition of the Wnt signaling pathway. Signaling through the PD-1 receptor is thought to promote an exhausted phenotype in cytotoxic T cells that impairs effective anti-tumoral immunity [105]. While immunotherapy has demonstrated activity in diverse tumor types, it has proved ineffective in unselected patients with CRC [5]. There are multiple lines of evidence that the Wnt signaling pathway can directly promote an immune suppressive environment [106]. Early data from trials of porcupine inhibitors have shown evidence for increased expression of activated immune signatures [82]. Furthermore, porcupine inhibition was synergistic with anti-CTLA4 immunotherapy in a murine melanoma model [107]. Altogether, this raises the question of whether anti-Wnt therapies would act synergistically with immunotherapy in colorectal tumors and this hypothesis is under active investigation in several early-phase clinical trials (NCT01351103, NCT02521844, NCT02675946).

Furthermore, as discussed above, the microsatellite-unstable subset of colorectal tumors ligand-dependent tumors is enriched with tumors, which have enhanced responses to immunotherapy [6]. Unexpectedly, a recent analysis incorporating a large cohort of patients with colorectal cancer who were treated with immunotherapy, demonstrated that RNF43-mutant tumors responded significantly better to immunotherapy than would have been expected from their mutational burden [108]. This is an exciting finding that raises the possibility the ligand-dependent Wnt biology might be independently associated with responses to immunotherapy and warrants further investigation in additional cohorts.

10. Outlook—Landscape of Precision Medicine in CRC

Approximately 15% of colorectal tumors have ligand-dependent alterations in the Wnt signaling pathway, affecting RNF43 or RSPO2/3. This unique Wnt biology is associated with a range of specific therapeutic vulnerabilities, especially to depletion of Wnt ligand by porcupine inhibitors. There is a strong theoretical basis for the combination of immunotherapy with a time-limited course of porcupine inhibition. Inhibitors of ligand-dependent Wnt signaling are known to be ineffectual in tumors with ligand-independent alterations such as APC mutations [79]. As a result, due to the low frequency of ligand-dependent alterations, clinical trials of these selective treatments will fail in unselected patients.

Precision medicine depends upon the ability to stratify patients into clinically meaningful subsets, followed by targeting with biologically appropriate therapies. It is contingent on the existence of biomarkers specific for each subset that can be feasibly adopted into routine clinic practice. We propose that AXIN2 is one such biomarker and could be measured at low cost from routine clinical specimens. It can be measured by high-throughput qRT-PCR and does not require costly and time-consuming DNA and RNA sequencing. On the basis of AXIN2 expression, it would be possible to identify patients with ligand-dependent Wnt biology who could then be targeted with effective personalized therapies. In summary, we propose that the concept of ligand-dependent tumors as an individual disease entity has the potential to revolutionize precision medicine and improve the outcomes for patients with colorectal cancer.

Author Contributions: S.O.K. and S.J.L. co-wrote the manuscript. All authors have read and agreed to the published version of the manuscript.

Funding: This work was supported by Wellcome Trust Senior Clinical Research Fellowship (206314/Z/17/Z).

Conflicts of Interest: The authors declare no conflict of interest.

References

1. Siegel, R.L.; Miller, K.D.; Sauer, A.G.; Fedewa, S.A.; Butterly, L.F.; Anderson, J.C.; Cercek, A.; Smith, R.A.; Jemal, A. Colorectal cancer statistics, 2020. *CA Cancer J. Clin.* **2020**, *70*, 145–164. [CrossRef] [PubMed]
2. Cutsem, E.V.; Cervantes, A.; Nordlinger, B.; Arnold, D.; Group, E.G.W. Metastatic colorectal cancer: ESMO Clinical Practice Guidelines for diagnosis, treatment and follow-up. *Ann. Oncol.* **2014**, *25*, iii1–iii9. [CrossRef] [PubMed]
3. Araghi, M.; Soerjomataram, I.; Bardot, A.; Ferlay, J.; Cabasag, C.J.; Morrison, D.S.; De, P.; Tervonen, H.; Walsh, P.M.; Bucher, O.; et al. Changes in colorectal cancer incidence in seven high-income countries: A population-based study. *Lancet Gastroenterol. Hepatol.* **2019**, *4*, 511–518. [CrossRef]
4. Dienstmann, R.; Vermeulen, L.; Guinney, J.; Kopetz, S.; Tejpar, S.; Tabernero, J. Consensus molecular subtypes and the evolution of precision medicine in colorectal cancer. *Nat. Rev. Cancer* **2017**, *17*, 79–92. [CrossRef] [PubMed]
5. Brahmer, J.R.; Tykodi, S.S.; Chow, L.Q.M.; Hwu, W.-J.; Topalian, S.L.; Hwu, P.; Drake, C.G.; Camacho, L.H.; Kauh, J.; Odunsi, K.; et al. Safety and Activity of Anti–PD-L1 Antibody in Patients with Advanced Cancer. *N. Engl. J. Med.* **2012**, *366*, 2455–2465. [CrossRef]
6. Overman, M.J.; McDermott, R.; Leach, J.L.; Lonardi, S.; Lenz, H.-J.; Morse, M.A.; Desai, J.; Hill, A.; Axelson, M.; Moss, R.A.; et al. Nivolumab in patients with metastatic DNA mismatch repair-deficient or microsatellite instability-high colorectal cancer (CheckMate 142): An open-label, multicentre, phase 2 study. *Lancet Oncol.* **2017**, *18*, 1182–1191. [CrossRef]
7. Xie, Y.-H.; Chen, Y.-X.; Fang, J.-Y. Comprehensive review of targeted therapy for colorectal cancer. *Signal Transduct. Target. Ther.* **2020**, *5*, 22. [CrossRef]
8. Muzny, D.M.; Bainbridge, M.N.; Chang, K.; Dinh, H.H.; Drummond, J.A.; Fowler, G.; Kovar, C.L.; Lewis, L.R.; Morgan, M.B.; Newsham, I.F.; et al. Comprehensive molecular characterization of human colon and rectal cancer. *Nature* **2012**, *487*, 330–337. [CrossRef]
9. Wiese, K.E.; Nusse, R.; Amerongen, R. Van Wnt signalling: Conquering complexity. *Development* **2018**, *145*, dev165902. [CrossRef]
10. Fevr, T.; Robine, S.; Louvard, D.; Huelsken, J. Wnt/β-Catenin Is Essential for Intestinal Homeostasis and Maintenance of Intestinal Stem Cells. *Mol. Cell Biol.* **2007**, *27*, 7551–7559. [CrossRef]
11. Dow, L.E.; O'Rourke, K.P.; Simon, J.; Tschaharganeh, D.F.; van Es, J.H.; Clevers, H.; Lowe, S.W. Apc Restoration Promotes Cellular Differentiation and Reestablishes Crypt Homeostasis in Colorectal Cancer. *Cell* **2015**, *161*, 1539–1552. [CrossRef] [PubMed]
12. Spranger, S.; Bao, R.; Gajewski, T.F. Melanoma-intrinsic β-catenin signalling prevents anti-tumour immunity. *Nature* **2015**, *523*, 231–235. [CrossRef] [PubMed]
13. Grasso, C.S.; Giannakis, M.; Wells, D.K.; Hamada, T.; Mu, X.J.; Quist, M.; Nowak, J.A.; Nishihara, R.; Qian, Z.R.; Inamura, K.; et al. Genetic mechanisms of immune evasion in colorectal cancer. *Cancer Discov.* **2018**, *8*, 730–749. [CrossRef] [PubMed]

14. Fearon, E.R.; Vogelstein, B. A genetic model for colorectal tumorigenesis. *Cell* **1990**, *61*, 759–767. [CrossRef]
15. Bettington, M.; Walker, N.; Clouston, A.; Brown, I.; Leggett, B.; Whitehall, V. The serrated pathway to colorectal carcinoma: Current concepts and challenges. *Histopathology* **2013**, *62*, 367–386. [CrossRef]
16. Barker, N.; Ridgway, R.A.; Van Es, J.H.; Van De Wetering, M.; Begthel, H.; Born, M.V.D.; Danenberg, E.; Clarke, A.R.; Sansom, O.J.; Clevers, H. Crypt stem cells as the cells-of-origin of intestinal cancer. *Nat. Cell Biol.* **2009**, *457*, 608–611. [CrossRef]
17. Davis, H.; Irshad, S.; Bansal, M.; Rafferty, H.; Boitsova, T.; Bardella, C.; Jaeger, E.; Lewis, A.; Freeman-Mills, L.; Giner, F.C.; et al. Aberrant epithelial GREM1 expression initiates colonic tumorigenesis from cells outside the stem cell niche. *Nat. Med.* **2015**, *21*, 62–70. [CrossRef]
18. Takada, R.; Satomi, Y.; Kurata, T.; Ueno, N.; Norioka, S.; Kondoh, H.; Takao, T.; Takada, S. Monounsaturated Fatty Acid Modification of Wnt Protein: Its Role in Wnt Secretion. *Dev. Cell* **2006**, *11*, 791–801. [CrossRef]
19. Shoshkes-Carmel, M.; Wang, Y.J.; Wangensteen, K.J.; Tóth, B.; Kondo, A.; Massasa, E.E.; Itzkovitz, S.; Kaestner, K.H. Subepithelial telocytes are an important source of Wnts that supports intestinal crypts. *Nature* **2018**, *557*, 242–246. [CrossRef]
20. Niehrs, C. The complex world of WNT receptor signalling. *Nat. Rev. Mol. Cell Biol.* **2012**, *13*, 767–779. [CrossRef]
21. Janda, C.Y.; Waghray, D.; Levin, A.M.; Thomas, C.; Garcia, K.C. Structural Basis of Wnt Recognition by Frizzled. *Science* **2012**, *337*, 59–64. [CrossRef] [PubMed]
22. Stamos, J.L.; Weis, W.I. The β-Catenin Destruction Complex. *Cold Spring Harb. Perspect. Biol.* **2013**, *5*, a007898. [CrossRef] [PubMed]
23. De Lau, W.; Peng, W.C.; Gros, P.; Clevers, H. The R-spondin/Lgr5/Rnf43 module: Regulator of Wnt signal strength. *Genes Dev.* **2014**, *28*, 305–316. [CrossRef] [PubMed]
24. Yan, K.S.; Janda, C.Y.; Chang, J.; Zheng, G.X.Y.; Larkin, K.A.; Luca, V.C.; Chia, L.A.; Mah, A.T.; Han, A.; Terry, J.M.; et al. Non-equivalence of Wnt and R-spondin ligands during Lgr5+ intestinal stem-cell self-renewal. *Nature* **2017**, *545*, 238–242. [CrossRef] [PubMed]
25. Park, S.; Cui, J.; Yu, W.; Wu, L.; Carmon, K.S.; Liu, Q.J. Differential activities and mechanisms of the four R-spondins in potentiating Wnt/β-catenin signaling. *J. Biol. Chem.* **2018**, *293*, 9759–9769. [CrossRef]
26. Greicius, G.; Kabiri, Z.; Sigmundsson, K.; Liang, C.; Bunte, R.; Singh, M.K.; Virshup, D.M. PDGFRα+ pericryptal stromal cells are the critical source of Wnts and RSPO3 for murine intestinal stem cells in vivo. *Proc. Natl. Acad. Sci. USA* **2018**, *115*, 201713510. [CrossRef]
27. Storm, E.E.; Durinck, S.; Melo, F.D.S.E.; Tremayne, J.; Kljavin, N.M.; Tan, C.; Ye, X.; Chiu, C.; Pham, T.; Hongo, J.-A.; et al. Targeting PTPRK-RSPO3 colon tumours promotes differentiation and loss of stem-cell function. *Nat. Cell Biol.* **2016**, *529*, 97–100. [CrossRef]
28. Sato, T.; Stange, D.E.; Ferrante, M.; Vries, R.G.; Van Es, J.H.; Brink, S.V.D.; Van Houdt, W.J.; Pronk, A.; Van Gorp, J.; Siersema, P.D.; et al. Long-term Expansion of Epithelial Organoids From Human Colon, Adenoma, Adenocarcinoma, and Barrett's Epithelium. *Gastroenterology* **2011**, *141*, 1762–1772. [CrossRef]
29. Filipovich, A.; Gehrke, I.; Poll-Wolbeck, S.J.; Kreuzer, K. Physiological inhibitors of Wnt signaling. *Eur. J. Haematol.* **2011**, *86*, 453–465. [CrossRef]
30. Kakugawa, S.; Langton, P.F.; Zebisch, M.; Howell, S.A.; Chang, T.-H.; Liu, Y.; Feizi, T.; Bineva, G.; O'Reilly, N.; Snijders, A.P.; et al. Notum deacylates Wnt proteins to suppress signalling activity. *Nature* **2015**, *519*, 187–192. [CrossRef]
31. Giannakis, M.; Hodis, E.; Mu, X.J.; Yamauchi, M.; Rosenbluh, J.; Cibulskis, K.; Saksena, G.; Lawrence, M.S.; Qian, Z.R.; Nishihara, R.; et al. RNF43 is frequently mutated in colorectal and endometrial cancers. *Nat. Genet.* **2014**, *46*, 1264–1266. [CrossRef] [PubMed]
32. Seshagiri, S.; Stawiski, E.W.; Durinck, S.; Modrusan, Z.; Storm, E.E.; Conboy, C.B.; Chaudhuri, S.; Guan, Y.; Janakiraman, V.; Jaiswal, B.S.; et al. Recurrent R-spondin fusions in colon cancer. *Nature* **2012**, *488*, 660–664. [CrossRef] [PubMed]
33. Han, T.; Schatoff, E.M.; Murphy, C.; Zafra, M.P.; Wilkinson, J.E.; Elemento, O.; Dow, L.E. R-Spondin chromosome rearrangements drive Wnt-dependent tumour initiation and maintenance in the intestine. *Nat. Commun.* **2017**, *8*, 15945. [CrossRef]
34. Harada, N.; Tamai, Y.; Ishikawa, T.; Sauer, B.; Takaku, K.; Oshima, M.; Taketo, M.M. Intestinal polyposis in mice with a dominant stable mutation of the β-catenin gene. *EMBO J.* **1999**, *18*, 5931–5942. [CrossRef]

35. Pollard, P.; Deheragoda, M.; Segditsas, S.; Lewis, A.; Rowan, A.; Howarth, K.; Willis, L.; Nye, E.; McCart, A.; Mandir, N.; et al. The Apc1322T Mouse Develops Severe Polyposis Associated with Submaximal Nuclear β-Catenin Expression. *Gastroenterology* **2009**, *136*, 2204–2213.e13. [CrossRef]

36. Koo, B.-K.; Spit, M.; Jordens, I.; Low, T.Y.; Stange, D.E.; Van De Wetering, M.; Van Es, J.H.; Mohammed, S.; Heck, A.J.R.; Maurice, M.M.; et al. Tumour suppressor RNF43 is a stem-cell E3 ligase that induces endocytosis of Wnt receptors. *Nat. Cell Biol.* **2012**, *488*, 665–669. [CrossRef]

37. Vogelstein, B.; Papadopoulos, N.; Velculescu, V.E.; Zhou, S.; Diaz, L.A.; Kinzler, K.W. Cancer Genome Landscapes. *Science* **2013**, *339*, 1546–1558. [CrossRef] [PubMed]

38. Melé, M.; Ferreira, P.G.; Reverter, F.; DeLuca, D.S.; Monlong, J.; Sammeth, M.; Young, T.R.; Goldmann, J.M.; Pervouchine, D.D.; Sullivan, T.J.; et al. The human transcriptome across tissues and individuals. *Science* **2015**, *348*, 660–665. [CrossRef] [PubMed]

39. Carninci, P.; Kasukawa, T.; Katayama, S.; Gough, J.; Frith, M.C.; Maeda, N.; Oyama, R.; Ravasi, T.; Lenhard, B.; Wells, C.; et al. The Transcriptional Landscape of the Mammalian Genome. *Science* **2005**, *309*, 1559–1563. [CrossRef]

40. Mori, Y.; Nagse, H.; Ando, H.; Horii, A.; Ichii, S.; Nakatsuru, S.; Aoki, T.; Miki, Y.; Mori, T.; Nakamura, Y. Somatic mutations of the APC gene in colorectal tumors: Mutation cluster region in the APC gene. *Hum. Mol. Genet.* **1992**, *1*, 229–233. [CrossRef]

41. Gao, C.; Wang, Y.; Broaddus, R.; Sun, L.; Xue, F.; Zhang, W. Exon 3 mutations of CTNNB1 drive tumorigenesis: A review. *Oncotarget* **2017**, *9*, 5492–5508. [CrossRef] [PubMed]

42. Kleeman, S.O.; Koelzer, V.H.; Jones, H.J.; Vazquez, E.G.; Davis, H.; East, J.E.; Arnold, R.; Koppens, M.A.; Blake, A.; Domingo, E.; et al. Exploiting differential Wnt target gene expression to generate a molecular biomarker for colorectal cancer stratification. *Gut* **2020**, *69*, 1092–1103. [CrossRef] [PubMed]

43. Hashimoto, T.; Ogawa, R.; Yoshida, H.; Taniguchi, H.; Kojima, M.; Saito, Y.; Sekine, S. EIF3E–RSPO2 and PIEZO1–RSPO2 fusions in colorectal traditional serrated adenoma. *Histopathology* **2019**, *75*, 266–273. [CrossRef] [PubMed]

44. Sekine, S.; Yamashita, S.; Tanabe, T.; Hashimoto, T.; Yoshida, H.; Taniguchi, H.; Kojima, M.; Shinmura, K.; Saito, Y.; Hiraoka, N.; et al. Frequent PTPRK–RSPO3 fusions and RNF43 mutations in colorectal traditional serrated adenoma. *J. Pathol.* **2016**, *239*, 133–138. [CrossRef] [PubMed]

45. Gong, X.; Yi, J.; Carmon, K.S.; Crumbley, C.A.; Xiong, W.; Thomas, A.; Fan, X.; Guo, S.; An, Z.; Chang, J.T.; et al. Aberrant RSPO3-LGR4 signaling in Keap1-deficient lung adenocarcinomas promotes tumor aggressiveness. *Oncogene* **2015**, *34*, 4692–4701. [CrossRef]

46. Picco, G.; Petti, C.; Centonze, A.; Torchiaro, E.; Crisafulli, G.; Novara, L.; Acquaviva, A.; Bardelli, A.; Medico, E. Loss of AXIN1 drives acquired resistance to WNT pathway blockade in colorectal cancer cells carrying RSPO3 fusions. *EMBO Mol. Med.* **2017**, *9*, 293–303. [CrossRef]

47. Ellegren, H. Microsatellites: Simple sequences with complex evolution. *Nat. Rev. Genet.* **2004**, *5*, 435–445. [CrossRef]

48. Maruvka, Y.E.; Mouw, K.W.; Karlic, R.; Parasuraman, P.; Kamburov, A.; Polak, P.; Haradhvala, N.J.; Hess, J.M.; Rheinbay, E.; Brody, Y.; et al. Analysis of somatic microsatellite indels identifies driver events in human tumors. *Nat. Biotechnol.* **2017**, *35*, 951–959. [CrossRef]

49. Tu, J.; Park, S.; Yu, W.; Zhang, S.; Wu, L.; Carmon, K.; Liu, Q.J. The most common RNF43 mutant G659Vfs*41 is fully functional in inhibiting Wnt signaling and unlikely to play a role in tumorigenesis. *Sci. Rep.* **2019**, *9*, 18557. [CrossRef]

50. Yu, J.; Yuso, P.A.B.M.; Woutersen, D.T.; Goh, P.; Harmston, N.; Smits, R.; Epstein, D.; Virshup, D.M.; Madan, B. The functional landscape of patient-derived RNF43 mutations predicts sensitivity to Wnt inhibiton. *Cancer Res.* **2020**. [CrossRef]

51. Hause, R.J.; Pritchard, C.C.; Shendure, J.; Salipante, S.J. Classification and characterization of microsatellite instability across 18 cancer types. *Nat. Med.* **2016**, *22*, 1342–1350. [CrossRef] [PubMed]

52. Albuquerque, C.; Breukel, C.; van der Luijt, R.; Fidalgo, P.; Lage, P.; Slors, F.J.M.; Leitão, C.N.; Fodde, R.; Smits, R. The 'just-right' signaling model: APC somatic mutations are selected based on a specific level of activation of the β-catenin signaling cascade. *Hum. Mol. Genet.* **2002**, *11*, 1549–1560. [CrossRef] [PubMed]

53. Lähde, M.; Heino, S.; Högström, J.; Kaijalainen, S.; Anisimov, A.; Flanagan, D.; Kallio, P.; Leppänen, V.-M.; Ristimäki, A.; Ritvos, O.; et al. Expression of R-spondin1 in Apc Min/+ Mice Reduces Growth of Intestinal Adenomas by Altering Wnt and TGFB Signaling. *Gastroenterology* **2020**. [CrossRef]

54. Biechele, T.L.; Kulikauskas, R.M.; Toroni, R.A.; Lucero, O.M.; Swift, R.D.; James, R.G.; Robin, N.C.; Dawson, D.W.; Moon, R.T.; Chien, A.J. Wnt/{beta}-Catenin Signaling and AXIN1 Regulate Apoptosis Triggered by Inhibition of the Mutant Kinase BRAFV600E in Human Melanoma. *Sci. Signal* **2012**, *5*, ra3. [CrossRef] [PubMed]
55. Hashimoto, T.; Yamashita, S.; Yoshida, H.; Taniguchi, H.; Ushijima, T.; Yamada, T.; Saito, Y.; Ochiai, A.; Sekine, S.; Hiraoka, N. WNT Pathway Gene Mutations Are Associated With the Presence of Dysplasia in Colorectal Sessile Serrated Adenoma/Polyps. *Am. J. Surg. Pathol.* **2017**, *41*, 1188–1197. [CrossRef] [PubMed]
56. Borowsky, J.; Dumenil, T.; Bettington, M.; Pearson, S.-A.; Bond, C.; Fennell, L.; Liu, C.; McKeone, D.; Rosty, C.; Brown, I.; et al. The role of APC in WNT pathway activation in serrated neoplasia. *Mod. Pathol.* **2018**, *31*, 495–504. [CrossRef]
57. Lamlum, H.; Papadopoulou, A.; Ilyas, M.; Rowan, A.; Gillet, C.; Hanby, A.; Talbot, I.; Bodmer, W.; Tomlinson, I. APC mutations are sufficient for the growth of early colorectal adenomas. *Proc. Natl. Acad. Sci. USA* **2000**, *97*, 2225–2228. [CrossRef]
58. Yan, H.H.N.; Siu, H.C.; Ho, S.L.; Yue, S.S.K.; Gao, Y.; Tsui, W.Y.; Chan, D.; Chan, A.S.; Wong, J.W.H.; Man, A.H.Y.; et al. Organoid cultures of early-onset colorectal cancers reveal distinct and rare genetic profiles. *Gut* **2020**. [CrossRef]
59. Perekatt, A.O.; Shah, P.P.; Cheung, S.; Jariwala, N.; Wu, A.; Gandhi, V.; Kumar, N.; Feng, Q.; Patel, N.; Chen, L.; et al. SMAD4 suppresses WNT-driven de-differentiation and oncogenesis in the differentiated gut epithelium. *Cancer Res.* **2018**, *78*. [CrossRef]
60. Koinuma, K.; Yamashita, Y.; Liu, W.; Hatanaka, H.; Kurashina, K.; Wada, T.; Takada, S.; Kaneda, R.; Choi, Y.L.; Fujiwara, S.-I.; et al. Epigenetic silencing of AXIN2 in colorectal carcinoma with microsatellite instability. *Oncogene* **2006**, *25*, 139–146. [CrossRef]
61. Muto, Y.; Maeda, T.; Suzuki, K.; Kato, T.; Watanabe, F.; Kamiyama, H.; Saito, M.; Koizumi, K.; Miyaki, Y.; Konishi, F.; et al. DNA methylation alterations of AXIN2 in serrated adenomas and colon carcinomas with microsatellite instability. *BMC Cancer* **2014**, *14*, 466. [CrossRef] [PubMed]
62. Murakami, T.; Mitomi, H.; Saito, T.; Takahashi, M.; Sakamoto, N.; Fukui, N.; Yao, T.; Watanabe, S. Distinct WNT/β-catenin signaling activation in the serrated neoplasia pathway and the adenoma-carcinoma sequence of the colorectum. *Mod. Pathol.* **2015**, *28*, 146–158. [CrossRef] [PubMed]
63. Lannagan, T.R.M.; Lee, Y.K.; Wang, T.; Roper, J.; Bettington, M.L.; Fennell, L.; Vrbanac, L.; Jonavicius, L.; Somashekar, R.; Gieniec, K.; et al. Genetic editing of colonic organoids provides a molecularly distinct and orthotopic preclinical model of serrated carcinogenesis. *Gut* **2019**, *68*, 684. [CrossRef] [PubMed]
64. Belshaw, N.J.; Elliott, G.O.; Foxall, R.J.; Dainty, J.R.; Pal, N.; Coupe, A.; Garg, D.; Bradburn, D.M.; Mathers, J.C.; Johnson, I.T. Profiling CpG island field methylation in both morphologically normal and neoplastic human colonic mucosa. *Br. J. Cancer* **2008**, *99*, 136–142. [CrossRef]
65. Zehir, A.; Benayed, R.; Shah, R.H.; Syed, A.; Middha, S.; Kim, H.R.; Srinivasan, P.; Gao, J.; Chakravarty, D.; Devlin, S.M.; et al. Mutational landscape of metastatic cancer revealed from prospective clinical sequencing of 10,000 patients. *Nat. Med.* **2017**, *23*, 703–713. [CrossRef]
66. Hughes, T.A.; Brady, H.J.M. Regulation of axin2 expression at the levels of transcription, translation and protein stability in lung and colon cancer. *Cancer Lett.* **2006**, *233*, 338–347. [CrossRef]
67. Jho, E.; Zhang, T.; Domon, C.; Joo, C.-K.; Freund, J.-N.; Costantini, F. Wnt/β-Catenin/Tcf Signaling Induces the Transcription of Axin2, a Negative Regulator of the Signaling Pathway. *Mol. Cell Biol.* **2002**, *22*, 1172–1183. [CrossRef]
68. Giannakis, M.; Mu, X.J.; Shukla, S.A.; Qian, Z.R.; Cohen, O.; Nishihara, R.; Bahl, S.; Cao, Y.; Amin-Mansour, A.; Yamauchi, M.; et al. Genomic Correlates of Immune-Cell Infiltrates in Colorectal Carcinoma. *Cell Rep.* **2016**, *15*, 857–865. [CrossRef]
69. Kim, Y.S.; Ho, S.B. Intestinal Goblet Cells and Mucins in Health and Disease: Recent Insights and Progress. *Curr. Gastroenterol. Rep.* **2010**, *12*, 319–330. [CrossRef]
70. Luo, C.; Cen, S.; Ding, G.; Wu, W. Mucinous colorectal adenocarcinoma: Clinical pathology and treatment options. *Cancer Commun.* **2019**, *39*, 1–13. [CrossRef]
71. Tsai, J.; Liau, J.; Yuan, C.; Cheng, M.; Yuan, R.; Jeng, Y. RNF43 mutation frequently occurs with GNAS mutation and mucin hypersecretion in intraductal papillary neoplasms of the bile duct. *Histopathology* **2017**, *70*, 756–765. [CrossRef] [PubMed]

72. Guinney, J.; Dienstmann, R.; Wang, X.; De Reyniès, A.; Schlicker, A.; Soneson, C.; Marisa, L.; Roepman, P.; Nyamundanda, G.; Angelino, P.; et al. The consensus molecular subtypes of colorectal cancer. *Nat. Med.* **2015**, *21*, 1350–1356. [CrossRef] [PubMed]
73. Koelzer, V.H.; Zlobec, I.; Lugli, A. Tumor budding in colorectal cancer—ready for diagnostic practice? *Hum. Pathol.* **2016**, *47*, 4–19. [CrossRef] [PubMed]
74. Sis, B.; Sarioglu, S.; Sokmen, S.; Sakar, M.; Kupelioglu, A.; Fuzun, M. Desmoplasia measured by computer assisted image analysis: An independent prognostic marker in colorectal carcinoma. *J. Clin. Pathol.* **2005**, *58*, 32. [CrossRef]
75. Verhulst, J.; Ferdinande, L.; Demetter, P.; Ceelen, W. Mucinous subtype as prognostic factor in colorectal cancer: A systematic review and meta-analysis. *J. Clin. Pathol.* **2012**, *65*, 381. [CrossRef]
76. Cui, C.; Zhou, X.; Zhang, W.; Qu, Y.; Ke, X. Is β-Catenin a Druggable Target for Cancer Therapy? *Trends Biochem. Sci.* **2018**, *43*, 623–634. [CrossRef]
77. Madan, B.; Ke, Z.; Harmston, N.; Ho, S.Y.; Frois, A.O.; Alam, J.; Jeyaraj, D.A.; Pendharkar, V.; Ghosh, K.; Virshup, I.H.; et al. Wnt addiction of genetically defined cancers reversed by PORCN inhibition. *Oncogene* **2016**, *35*, 2197–2207. [CrossRef]
78. Wang, B.; Tian, T.; Kalland, K.-H.; Ke, X.; Qu, Y. Targeting Wnt/β-Catenin Signaling for Cancer Immunotherapy. *Trends Pharmacol. Sci.* **2018**, *39*, 648–658. [CrossRef]
79. Van de Wetering, M.; Francies, H.E.; Francis, J.M.; Bounova, G.; Iorio, F.; Pronk, A.; van Houdt, W.; van Gorp, J.; Taylor-Weiner, A.; Kester, L.; et al. Prospective Derivation of a Living Organoid Biobank of Colorectal Cancer Patients. *Cell* **2015**, *161*, 933–945. [CrossRef]
80. Koo, B.-K.; Van Es, J.H.; Born, M.V.D.; Clevers, H. Porcupine inhibitor suppresses paracrine Wnt-driven growth of Rnf43;Znrf3-mutant neoplasia. *Proc. Natl. Acad. Sci. USA* **2015**, *112*, 7548–7550. [CrossRef]
81. Janku, F.; Connolly, R.; Lorusso, P.; De Jonge, M.; Vaishampayan, U.; Rodon, J.; Argilés, G.; Myers, A.; Schmitz, S.-F.H.; Ji, Y.; et al. Abstract C45: Phase I study of WNT974, a first-in-class Porcupine inhibitor, in advanced solid tumors. *Clin. Trials* **2015**, *14*, C45. [CrossRef]
82. Rodon, J.; Argilés, G.; Connolly, R.M.; Vaishampayan, U.; De Jonge, M.; Garralda, E.; Giannakis, M.; Smith, D.C.; Dobson, J.R.; McLaughlin, M.; et al. Abstract CT175: Biomarker analyses from a phase I study of WNT974, a first-in-class Porcupine inhibitor, in patients (pts) with advanced solid tumors. *Clin. Trials* **2018**, *78*, CT175. [CrossRef]
83. Chartier, C.; Raval, J.; Axelrod, F.; Bond, C.; Cain, J.; Dee-Hoskins, C.; Ma, S.; Fischer, M.M.; Shah, J.; Wei, J.; et al. Therapeutic Targeting of Tumor-Derived R-Spondin Attenuates -Catenin Signaling and Tumorigenesis in Multiple Cancer Types. *Cancer Res.* **2015**, *76*, 713–723. [CrossRef] [PubMed]
84. Fischer, M.M.; Yeung, V.P.; Cattaruzza, F.; Hussien, R.; Yen, W.-C.; Murriel, C.; Evans, J.W.; O'Young, G.; Brunner, A.L.; Wang, M.; et al. RSPO3 antagonism inhibits growth and tumorigenicity in colorectal tumors harboring common Wnt pathway mutations. *Sci. Rep.* **2017**, *7*, 15270. [CrossRef] [PubMed]
85. Li, C.; Cao, J.; Zhang, N.; Tu, M.; Xu, F.; Wei, S.; Chen, X.; Xu, Y. Identification of RSPO2 Fusion Mutations and Target Therapy Using a Porcupine Inhibitor. *Sci. Rep.* **2018**, *8*, 14244. [CrossRef] [PubMed]
86. Bendell, J.; Eckhardt, G.S.; Hochster, H.S.; Morris, V.K.; Strickler, J.; Kapoun, A.M.; Wang, M.; Xu, L.; McGuire, K.; Dupont, J.; et al. 68 Initial results from a phase 1a/b study of OMP-131R10, a first-in-class anti-RSPO3 antibody, in advanced solid tumors and previously treated metastatic colorectal cancer (CRC). *Eur. J. Cancer* **2016**, *69*, S29–S30. [CrossRef]
87. Monroe, D.G.; McGee-Lawrence, M.E.; Oursler, M.J.; Westendorf, J.J. Update on Wnt signaling in bone cell biology and bone disease. *Gene* **2012**, *492*, 1–18. [CrossRef]
88. Funck-Brentano, T.; Nilsson, K.H.; Brommage, R.; Henning, P.; Lerner, U.H.; Koskela, A.; Tuukkanen, J.; Cohen-Solal, M.; Movérare-Skrtic, S.; Ohlsson, C. Porcupine inhibitors impair trabecular and cortical bone mass and strength in mice. *J. Endocrinol.* **2018**, *238*, 13–23. [CrossRef]
89. Tan, D.; Ng, M.; Subbiah, V.; Messersmith, W.; Teneggi, V.; Diermayr, V.; Ethirajulu, K.; Yeo, P.; Gan, B.H.; Lee, L.H.; et al. 71O Phase I extension study of ETC-159 an oral PORCN inhibitor administered with bone protective treatment, in patients with advanced solid tumours. *Ann. Oncol.* **2018**, *29*, ix23–ix24. [CrossRef]
90. Barrott, J.J.; Cash, G.M.; Smith, A.P.; Barrow, J.R.; Murtaugh, L.C. Deletion of mouse Porcn blocks Wnt ligand secretion and reveals an ectodermal etiology of human focal dermal hypoplasia/Goltz syndrome. *Proc. Natl. Acad. Sci. USA* **2011**, *108*, 12752–12757. [CrossRef]

91. Fahiminiya, S.; Majewski, J.; Mort, J.; Moffatt, P.; Glorieux, F.H.; Rauch, F. Mutations in WNT1 are a cause of osteogenesis imperfecta. *J. Med. Genet.* **2013**, *50*, 345. [CrossRef]
92. Zheng, H.-F.; Tobias, J.H.; Duncan, E.L.; Evans, D.M.; Eriksson, J.; Paternoster, L.; Yerges-Armstrong, L.M.; Lehtimäki, T.; Bergström, U.; Kähönen, M.; et al. WNT16 Influences Bone Mineral Density, Cortical Bone Thickness, Bone Strength, and Osteoporotic Fracture Risk. *PLoS Genet.* **2012**, *8*, e1002745. [CrossRef]
93. Tsai, H.-C.; Li, H.; Van Neste, L.; Cai, Y.; Robert, C.; Rassool, F.V.; Shin, J.J.; Harbom, K.M.; Beaty, R.; Pappou, E.; et al. Transient Low Doses of DNA-Demethylating Agents Exert Durable Antitumor Effects on Hematological and Epithelial Tumor Cells. *Cancer Cell* **2012**, *21*, 430–446. [CrossRef]
94. Howell, P.M.; Liu, Z.; Khong, H.T. Demethylating Agents in the Treatment of Cancer. *Pharm* **2010**, *3*, 2022–2044. [CrossRef]
95. Hinze, L.; Pfirrmann, M.; Karim, S.; Degar, J.; McGuckin, C.; Vinjamur, D.; Sacher, J.; Stevenson, K.E.; Neuberg, D.S.; Orellana, E.; et al. Synthetic Lethality of Wnt Pathway Activation and Asparaginase in Drug-Resistant Acute Leukemias. *Cancer Cell* **2019**, *35*, 664–676.e7. [CrossRef]
96. Rizzari, C.; Conter, V.; Starý, J.; Colombini, A.; Moericke, A.; Schrappe, M. Optimizing asparaginase therapy for acute lymphoblastic leukemia. *Curr. Opin. Oncol.* **2013**, *25*, S1–S9. [CrossRef]
97. Pieters, R.; Hunger, S.P.; Boos, J.; Rizzari, C.; Silverman, L.; Baruchel, A.; Goekbuget, N.; Schrappe, M.; Pui, C. L-asparaginase treatment in acute lymphoblastic leukemia. *Cancer* **2011**, *117*, 238–249. [CrossRef]
98. Hinze, L.; Labrosse, R.; Degar, J.; Han, T.; Schatoff, E.M.; Schreek, S.; Karim, S.; McGuckin, C.; Sacher, J.R.; Wagner, F.; et al. Exploiting the Therapeutic Interaction of WNT Pathway Activation and Asparaginase for Colorectal Cancer Therapy. *Cancer Discov.* **2020**, *10*, 1690–1705. [CrossRef]
99. Mohammed, M.K.; Shao, C.; Wang, J.; Wei, Q.; Wang, X.; Collier, Z.; Tang, S.; Liu, H.; Zhang, F.; Huang, J.; et al. Wnt/β-catenin signaling plays an ever-expanding role in stem cell self-renewal, tumorigenesis and cancer chemoresistance. *Genes Dis.* **2016**, *3*, 11–40. [CrossRef]
100. Mbom, B.C.; Siemers, K.A.; Ostrowski, M.A.; Nelson, W.J.; Barth, A.I.M. Nek2 phosphorylates and stabilizes β-catenin at mitotic centrosomes downstream of Plk1. *Mol. Biol. Cell* **2014**, *25*, 977–991. [CrossRef]
101. Kabiri, Z.; Greicius, G.; Zaribafzadeh, H.; Hemmerich, A.; Counter, C.M.; Virshup, D.M. Wnt signaling suppresses MAPK-driven proliferation of intestinal stem cells. *J. Clin. Investig.* **2018**, *128*, 3806–3812. [CrossRef] [PubMed]
102. Clarke, M.F.; Dick, J.E.; Dirks, P.B.; Eaves, C.J.; Jamieson, C.H.M.; Jones, D.L.; Visvader, J.; Weissman, I.L.; Wahl, G.M. Cancer Stem Cells—Perspectives on Current Status and Future Directions: AACR Workshop on Cancer Stem Cells. *Cancer Res.* **2006**, *66*, 9339–9344. [CrossRef] [PubMed]
103. Todaro, M.; Alea, M.P.; Stefano, A.B.D.; Cammareri, P.; Vermeulen, L.; Iovino, F.; Tripodo, C.; Russo, A.; Gulotta, G.; Medema, J.P.; et al. Colon Cancer Stem Cells Dictate Tumor Growth and Resist Cell Death by Production of Interleukin-4. *Cell Stem Cell* **2007**, *1*, 389–402. [CrossRef] [PubMed]
104. Bao, S.; Wu, Q.; McLendon, R.E.; Hao, Y.; Shi, Q.; Hjelmeland, A.B.; Dewhirst, M.W.; Bigner, D.D.; Rich, J.N. Glioma stem cells promote radioresistance by preferential activation of the DNA damage response. *Nature* **2006**, *444*, 756–760. [CrossRef] [PubMed]
105. Keir, M.E.; Butte, M.J.; Freeman, G.J.; Sharpe, A.H. PD-1 and Its Ligands in Tolerance and Immunity. *Annu. Rev. Immunol.* **2008**, *26*, 677–704. [CrossRef]
106. Galluzzi, L.; Spranger, S.; Fuchs, E.; López-Soto, A. WNT Signaling in Cancer Immunosurveillance. *Trends Cell Biol.* **2018**, *29*, 44–65. [CrossRef]
107. Holtzhausen, A.; Zhao, F.; Evans, K.S.; Tsutsui, M.; Orabona, C.; Tyler, D.S.; Hanks, B.A. Melanoma-Derived Wnt5a Promotes Local Dendritic-Cell Expression of IDO and Immunotolerance: Opportunities for Pharmacologic Enhancement of Immunotherapy. *Cancer Immunol. Res.* **2015**, *3*, 1082–1095. [CrossRef]
108. Jun, T.; Qing, T.; Dong, G.; Signaevski, M.; Hopkins, J.F.; Frampton, G.M.; Albacker, L.A.; Cordon-Cardo, C.; Samstein, R.; Pusztai, L.; et al. Cancer-specific associations of driver genes with immunotherapy outcome. *Biorxiv* **2020**. [CrossRef]

Publisher's Note: MDPI stays neutral with regard to jurisdictional claims in published maps and institutional affiliations.

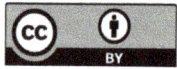

© 2020 by the authors. Licensee MDPI, Basel, Switzerland. This article is an open access article distributed under the terms and conditions of the Creative Commons Attribution (CC BY) license (http://creativecommons.org/licenses/by/4.0/).

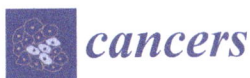

Review

Wnt and Vitamin D at the Crossroads in Solid Cancer

José Manuel González-Sancho [1,2,3]**, María Jesús Larriba** [1,3,4] **and Alberto Muñoz** [1,3,4,]*

1. Instituto de Investigaciones Biomédicas "Alberto Sols", Consejo Superior de Investigaciones Científicas, Universidad Autónoma de Madrid, 28029 Madrid, Spain; josemanuel.gonzalez@uam.es (J.M.G.-S.); mjlarriba@iib.uam.es (M.J.L.)
2. Departamento de Bioquímica, Facultad de Medicina, Universidad Autónoma de Madrid, 28029 Madrid, Spain
3. Centro de Investigación Biomédica en Red de Cáncer (CIBERONC), 28029 Madrid, Spain
4. Instituto de Investigación Sanitaria del Hospital Universitario La Paz—IdiPAZ (Hospital Universitario La Paz—Universidad Autónoma de Madrid), 28029 Madrid, Spain
* Correspondence: amunoz@iib.uam.es

Received: 29 October 2020; Accepted: 17 November 2020; Published: 19 November 2020

Simple Summary: The Wnt/β-catenin signaling pathway is aberrantly activated in most colorectal cancers and less frequently in a variety of other solid neoplasias. Many epidemiological and experimental studies and some clinical trials suggest an anticancer action of vitamin D, mainly against colorectal cancer. The aim of this review was to analyze the literature supporting the interference of Wnt/β-catenin signaling by the active vitamin D metabolite 1α,25-dihydroxyvitamin D_3. We discuss the molecular mechanisms of this antagonism in colorectal cancer and other cancer types. Additionally, we summarize the available data indicating a reciprocal inhibition of vitamin D action by the activated Wnt/β-catenin pathway. Thus, a complex mutual antagonism between Wnt/β-catenin signaling and the vitamin D system seems to be at the root of many solid cancers.

Abstract: Abnormal activation of the Wnt/β-catenin pathway is common in many types of solid cancers. Likewise, a large proportion of cancer patients have vitamin D deficiency. In line with these observations, Wnt/β-catenin signaling and 1α,25-dihydroxyvitamin D_3 (1,25(OH)$_2$$D_3$), the active vitamin D metabolite, usually have opposite effects on cancer cell proliferation and phenotype. In recent years, an increasing number of studies performed in a variety of cancer types have revealed a complex crosstalk between Wnt/β-catenin signaling and 1,25(OH)$_2$$D_3$. Here we review the mechanisms by which 1,25(OH)$_2$$D_3$ inhibits Wnt/β-catenin signaling and, conversely, how the activated Wnt/β-catenin pathway may abrogate vitamin D action. The available data suggest that interaction between Wnt/β-catenin signaling and the vitamin D system is at the crossroads in solid cancers and may have therapeutic applications.

Keywords: wnt; β-catenin; vitamin D; cancer; colon cancer

1. Introduction

1.1. Wnt

Wnt proteins are extracellular signaling molecules that control many key processes during embryonic development and regulate the homeostasis of adult tissues, mainly by modulating the survival, self-renewal, and proliferation of stem cells. They are secreted by a variety of cell types and typically have a short range of action, mediating communication between neighboring cells. Wnt proteins bind to cell surface receptors, of which several classes have been described. Specific Wnt-receptor combinations and cellular contexts determine which of the existing Wnt signaling pathways is engaged [1].

The Wnt/β-catenin pathway is triggered by Wnt binding to cell membrane receptors of the Frizzled and low-density lipoprotein receptor-related protein (LRP) families. In the absence of a Wnt ligand, β-catenin protein is mainly located at cell-cell contacts and free cytoplasmic β-catenin is kept low because of a proteolytic destruction machinery. A complex containing the tumor suppressor proteins APC (*adenomatous polyposis coli*) and axin, and the kinases casein kinase 1 (CK1) and glycogen synthase kinase-3β (GSK-3β) targets β-catenin for N-terminal phosphorylation and subsequent ubiquitination and proteasome-mediated degradation. Wnt binding to Frizzled and LRP5/6 leads to inhibition of the β-catenin destruction complex and, therefore, to the accumulation of β-catenin in the cytoplasm. A proportion of β-catenin enters the nucleus and binds to transcription factors of the LEF/TCF family acting as a co-activator and regulating the expression of a large variety of genes. Wnt target genes are cell and tissue type-dependent and affect many cellular functions and processes, such as cell proliferation, stemness, migration, and invasion. Some of these targets include the *c-MYC* and *CCND1*/cyclin D1 oncogenes, the Wnt inhibitors *DKK1* and *NKD1/2*, and the Wnt effector *LEF1*. In addition, the Wnt inhibitor *AXIN2* is the most ubiquitously regulated β-catenin target gene [1–3].

Wnt/β-catenin signaling is highly dependent on the number of Frizzled receptor molecules present on the cell surface. Vertebrates have evolved a complex regulatory mechanism to control the amount of Frizzled on the plasma membrane that involves three types of proteins: leucine-rich repeat-containing G-protein coupled receptors (LGR4-6), their extracellular ligands R-spondins (RSPO1-4), and the E3 transmembrane ubiquitin ligases ZNRF3 and RNF43 [4,5]. In the absence of RSPO, Frizzled receptors are targeted for degradation by ZNRF3/RNF43-mediated ubiquitination, which results in low Frizzled membrane concentration and, therefore, in attenuated Wnt signaling. In contrast, RSPO binding to LGR4-6 sequesters ZNRF3/RNF43 in a ternary complex and prevents ubiquitin tagging of Frizzled. Thus, RSPOs are responsible for the accumulation of Frizzled receptors on the cell surface and the potentiation of Wnt/β-catenin signaling in target cells [6–8].

Dysregulation of Wnt/β-catenin signaling is involved in human diseases including cancer. In many types of cancer, e.g., colorectal, breast, and liver carcinoma, melanoma and leukemia, β-catenin constitutively accumulates within the nucleus of tumor cells [9–13]. In fact, aberrant activation of the Wnt/β-catenin pathway is the most common event in human colorectal cancer (CRC) [14,15] in which massive sequencing has estimated that over 94% of primary colon tumors carry mutations in one or more genes involved in this pathway [16]. Truncation mutations and allelic losses in the tumor suppressor gene *APC* are present in around 80% of sporadic CRC cases, whereas a small proportion carries mutations in *AXIN2* or *CTNNB1*/β-catenin genes. Moreover, chromosomal rearrangements in R-spondin family members *RSPO2* and *RSPO3* have been found in 10% of human CRC leading to enhanced Wnt signaling [17,18]. In addition, *RNF43* is mutated in a proportion of mismatch repair-deficient colon tumors. Alterations in genes encoding components of the Wnt/β-catenin pathway are frequently mutually exclusive, which confirms that aberrant activation of this pathway is a hallmark of CRC. Mutations in *CTNNB1*/β-catenin or *AXIN2* have been reported in other human tumors, e.g., hepatocellular carcinomas [19–21], whereas overexpression of Wnt factors/receptors or silencing of extracellular Wnt inhibitors are the preferred mechanisms of Wnt/β-catenin sustained activation in other cancers, e.g., breast and lung cancers [22–27].

1.2. Vitamin D

Vitamin D_3 (cholecalciferol) is a natural seco-steroid whose main source is non-enzymatic production in human skin from UV-B exposed 7-dehydrocholesterol, an abundant cholesterol precursor [28,29]. Vitamin D_3 from skin production and from dietary uptake is hydroxylated in the liver to 25-hydroxyvitamin D_3 (25(OH)D_3, calcidiol), a stable compound that is used as a biomarker for the vitamin D status of a person [29–31]. Subsequent hydroxylation of 25(OH)D_3 at carbon 1, which occurs mainly in the kidneys but also in several types of epithelial and immune cells, renders 1,25-dihydroxyvitamin D_3 (1,25(OH)$_2D_3$, calcitriol). This is the most active vitamin D_3 metabolite and a high affinity ligand for the vitamin D receptor (VDR) [29,31,32].

VDR is a member of the nuclear receptor superfamily of transcription factors, which includes receptors for other hormones such as estrogen, progesterone or glucocorticoids, as well as a number of orphan receptors. Nuclear receptors present a highly conserved ligand-binding domain, which in the case of VDR fixes 1,25(OH)$_2$D$_3$ or its synthetic analogues with high specificity [33]. Binding of 1,25(OH)$_2$D$_3$ to VDR promotes the formation of complexes with RXR, the receptor for 9-*cis*-retinoic acid, and the binding of these VDR/RXR heterodimers to DNA. This leads to epigenetic changes that affect the transcription rate of hundreds of target genes involved in many cellular processes, including proliferation, differentiation and survival [29,31]. Moreover, a proportion of VDR molecules locate in the cytoplasm of some cell types where, on ligand binding, they trigger rapid, non-genomic, modulatory effects on signaling pathways by acting on kinases, phosphatases, and ion channels [34,35].

Current evidence indicates that 1,25(OH)$_2$D$_3$ and its derivatives modulate signaling pathways that affect cell survival, growth, and differentiation [29,36,37], key processes that are dysregulated in human cancers. One of these signaling routes is the Wnt/β-catenin pathway. This review will focus on the crosstalk between Wnt and vitamin D in solid tumors.

2. Antagonism of Wnt/β-Catenin Signaling by 1,25(OH)$_2$D$_3$ in Solid Cancers

2.1. Colorectal Cancer

Four decades ago, an epidemiological study hinted at the protective effects of vitamin D$_3$ against CRC by indicating that high UVB exposure or life at lower latitudes, both of which result in higher vitamin D$_3$ synthesis, lead to lower incidence of CRC [38]. Since then, a large number of epidemiological studies, experimental work performed in cultured cells and animal models, and also some, but not all, vitamin D$_3$ supplementation human clinical trials have strongly suggested that 1,25(OH)$_2$D$_3$ has anticancer effects, particularly in CRC [31,37,39–44].

Our group was a pioneer in demonstrating that 1,25(OH)$_2$D$_3$ antagonizes the Wnt/β-catenin signaling pathway in colon carcinoma cells [45], a mechanism that could at least partly account for the protective effects of vitamin D$_3$ observed in epidemiological and animal studies. Previously, other groups had reported a crosstalk between Wnt signaling and other nuclear receptors, such as those for retinoid acid and androgen [46,47].

Results from our laboratory showed that 1,25(OH)$_2$D$_3$ interferes with Wnt/β-catenin signaling in human colon carcinoma cells by at least three mechanisms (Figure 1). Firstly, ligand-activated nuclear VDR binds and sequesters β-catenin, which prevents its binding to LEF/TCF transcription factors and thus blocks β-catenin/TCF-mediated transcription of Wnt target genes [45]. VDR/β-catenin physical interaction was later confirmed in this and other cell systems and involves the C-terminal region of β-catenin and the activator function-2 domain of VDR [48]. Interestingly, wild-type APC potentiates VDR/β-catenin binding [49]. Lithocholic acid, a low affinity VDR ligand, also prompts this interaction, although less efficiently than 1,25(OH)$_2$D$_3$ [49].

Secondly, 1,25(OH)$_2$D$_3$ induces the expression of E-cadherin protein, which sequesters newly synthesized β-catenin at subcortical cell-cell adherens junctions, thus avoiding its translocation to the nucleus and β-catenin/TCF-mediated transcription [45]. Our data suggest that the small GTPase RhoA, the protease inhibitor cystatin D, the regulator of tyrosine kinase receptor signaling Sprouty-2, and the histone demethylase JMJD3 are involved in this mechanism [34,50–52]. Induction of E-cadherin by 1,25(OH)$_2$D$_3$ and concomitant inhibition of the Wnt/β-catenin pathway have also been reported in other cell types [53]. However, 1,25(OH)$_2$D$_3$ can antagonize Wnt/β-catenin signaling in colon carcinoma cells that do not express E-cadherin, which implies that this mechanism is not strictly required [45].

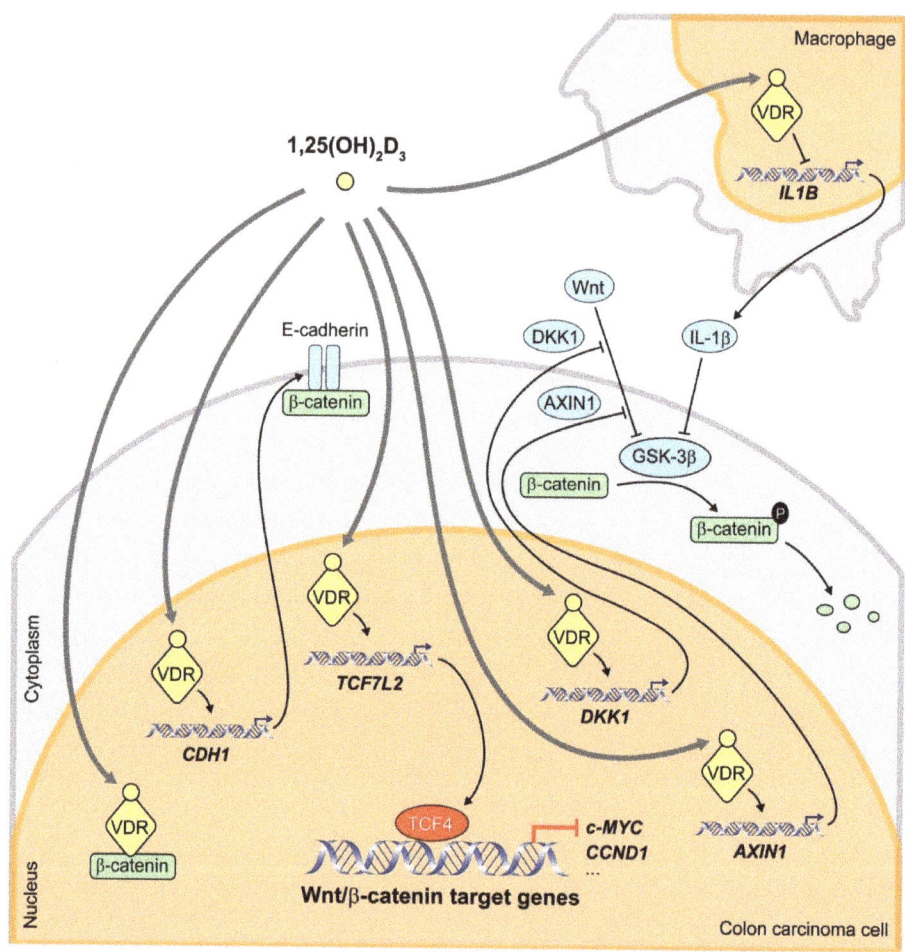

Figure 1. Schematic representation of the mechanisms by which 1,25(OH)$_2$D$_3$ interferes the Wnt/β-catenin signaling pathway in human CRC cells. 1,25(OH)$_2$D$_3$ binds to its high affinity receptor VDR inducing the formation of β-catenin/VDR complexes and thus preventing that of transcriptionally active β-catenin/TCF4 complexes. In addition, 1,25(OH)$_2$D$_3$ increases the transcription of the *CDH1* gene encoding E-cadherin, which sequesters newly synthesized β-catenin protein at the subcortical adherens junctions. Furthermore, 1,25(OH)$_2$D$_3$ upregulates the expression of the negative regulators of the Wnt/β-catenin pathway *TCF7L2* (encoding TCF4), *DKK1* and *AXIN1*. 1,25(OH)$_2$D$_3$ also antagonizes the pathway by reducing the secretion by nearby macrophages of IL-1β, which inhibits GSK-3β activity in CRC cells leading to an increase in β-catenin levels.

Thirdly, 1,25(OH)$_2$D$_3$ promotes the expression of Dickkopf 1 (DKK1), a member of a family of extracellular inhibitors of the Wnt/β-catenin pathway [54]. DKK1 can inhibit Wnt/β-catenin signaling by two mechanisms. On the one hand, DKK1 direct binding to LRP5/6 blocks Wnt-LRP interaction [55]. On the other, DKK1 can engage a ternary complex with LRP5/6 and Kremen receptors, which prompts rapid endocytosis and removal of LRP5/6 from the plasma membrane [56]. In addition to a Wnt inhibitor, *DKK1* is a β-catenin/TCF target gene [57–59]. Although most CRC carry mutations that activate the Wnt/β-catenin pathway downstream of DKK1, evidence suggests that this extracellular inhibitor has antitumor effects that are independent of β-catenin/TCF transcriptional activity [60–62].

Supporting the relevance of DKK1 in CRC, we and others have demonstrated that DKK1 expression is frequently downregulated in this neoplasia [59], in part due to gene promoter hypermethylation [62–64]. Moreover, the expression levels of VDR and DKK1 in human CRC biopsies directly correlate [54], and dietary vitamin D intake is inversely associated with *DKK1* promoter methylation in a large cohort of CRC patients [65].

DKK4 is another member of the Dickkopf family of Wnt extracellular inhibitors, although it is a weaker Wnt antagonist than DKK1. We reported that 1,25(OH)$_2$D$_3$ downregulates the expression of DKK4 in both human colon and breast cancer cells. Accordingly, a significant inverse correlation between DKK4 and VDR expression exists in human CRC biopsies [66]. Unexpectedly, overexpression of DKK4 in human CRC cells enhances their migratory, invasive, and angiogenic potential [66]. These effects are probably unrelated to Wnt/β-catenin inhibition and imply additional mechanisms of action of DKK4. In this regard, we and others found that DKK4 transcripts are overexpressed in human CRC samples and in biopsies from patients with inflammatory bowel disease [66–68]. These data suggest that downregulation of DKK4 by 1,25(OH)$_2$D$_3$ may be another mechanism for the antitumor action of 1,25(OH)$_2$D$_3$ in CRC.

The *c-MYC* oncogene is a well-known β-catenin/TCF target gene that is frequently deregulated in human cancers and activates genetic programs that orchestrate biological processes to promote cell growth and proliferation [69]. Therefore, targeting the function of MYC oncoproteins holds the promise of achieving new, effective anticancer therapies that can be applied to a broad range of tumors [70]. In particular, mutational and integrative analyses have stressed the essential role of *c-MYC* in CRC [16]. A study reported by Meyer and colleagues using chromatin immunoprecipitation assays followed by high-throughput DNA sequencing (ChIP-Seq) in the CRC cell line LS180 concluded that β-catenin/TCF4 and VDR/RXR heterodimers colocalize at 74 sites near a limited set of genes that included *c-MYC* and *c-FOS* oncogenes [71]. These data strongly suggest a direct action of both complexes at these gene *loci*. In fact, 1,25(OH)$_2$D$_3$ effects on *c-MYC* gene expression may count as another mechanism of crosstalk between 1,25(OH)$_2$D$_3$ and Wnt/β-catenin signaling pathways. Firstly, ligand-activated VDR represses *c-MYC* expression by direct interaction with two vitamin D response elements (VDRE) in the promoter region [71,72]. Secondly, the antagonism exerted by 1,25(OH)$_2$D$_3$ on Wnt/β-catenin signaling impairs the transcription of *c-MYC* mediated by β-catenin/TCF complexes through their binding to several Wnt responsive elements (WRE) at the *c-MYC* promoter [45,73].

Some authors have proposed additional mechanisms of 1,25(OH)$_2$D$_3$ crosstalk with Wnt/β-catenin signaling in CRC cells (Figure 1). Beildeck and colleagues showed that 1,25(OH)$_2$D$_3$ increases TCF4 expression in several human CRC cell lines. The effect is indirect but completely dependent on VDR [74]. Tang and colleagues have reported that TCF4 functions as a transcriptional repressor that restricts CRC cell growth [75]. Therefore, 1,25(OH)$_2$D$_3$/VDR-mediated upregulation of TCF4 possibly has a protective effect on CRC. Furthermore, 1,25(OH)$_2$D$_3$/VDR induces expression of the negative regulator of the Wnt/β-catenin pathway AXIN1 in CRC cells through a VDRE localized in the regulatory region of the gene [76]. In addition, Gröschel and colleagues found that 1,25(OH)$_2$D$_3$ reduces nuclear β-catenin levels in LT97 colon microadenoma cells and thus downregulates the expression of Wnt target genes such as *BCL2*, *CCND1*/cyclin D1, *SNAI1*, *CD44*, and *LGR5* [77]. Moreover, in healthy colon of mice fed a high vitamin D diet, β-catenin protein expression is decreased and the same effect is observed for TCF4 [77], which contrasts with the results of Beildeck and colleagues [74].

Kaler and colleagues described a paracrine mechanism that involves not only a crosstalk between 1,25(OH)$_2$D$_3$ and Wnt/β-catenin signaling pathways but also between carcinoma cells and the tumor microenvironment (Figure 1). They demonstrated that colon carcinoma cells induce the release of interleukin-1β (IL-1β) from macrophagic THP-1 cells in a process that requires constitutive activation of STAT1 [78]. Secreted IL-1β then acts on colon carcinoma cells where it triggers the inactivation of GSK-3β and thus the stabilization of β-catenin and subsequent expression of Wnt target genes. 1,25(OH)$_2$D$_3$ interrupts this crosstalk by blocking the constitutive activation of STAT1 and thus the production of IL-1β in macrophages in a VDR-dependent manner, which hampers the ability of macrophages to activate Wnt/β-catenin signaling in CRC cells [78]. The possibility that this mechanism works in vivo with tumor-associated macrophages is highly interesting.

Our group has also studied the interplay between 1,25(OH)$_2$D$_3$ and Wnt3A (an activator of the Wnt/β-catenin pathway) in human colon fibroblasts. Both agents strongly modulate the gene expression profile and phenotype of these cells. However, in contrast to the antagonism exerted by 1,25(OH)$_2$D$_3$ on the Wnt/β-catenin pathway in colon carcinoma cells, they have a partially overlapping effect. Both compounds inhibit fibroblast proliferation and migration, but while 1,25(OH)$_2$D$_3$ reduces, Wnt3A increases fibroblast capacity to remodel the extracellular matrix [79]. In addition, in contrast to the effects observed in established colon carcinoma cell lines, 1,25(OH)$_2$D$_3$ does not affect the expression of key genes of the Wnt/β-catenin pathway (*AXIN2*, *CCND1*, *DKK1* and *c-MYC*) in human colon tumor or normal organoids derived from CRC patients, where only the *DKK4* Wnt/β-catenin target gene is repressed by 1,25(OH)$_2$D$_3$ [80]. This shows that antagonism of the Wnt/β-catenin pathway is not a universal action of 1,25(OH)$_2$D$_3$ in tumor contexts. Moreover, 1,25(OH)$_2$D$_3$ cooperates with Wnt factors in the differentiation of bone (osteoblasts), skin (keratinocytes) and brain (neuronal precursors) cells under physiologic conditions [81,82]. Together, available data indicate a mostly repressive action of 1,25(OH)$_2$D$_3$ on overactivation of the Wnt/β-catenin pathway with different effects in particular scenarios.

The interplay between 1,25(OH)$_2$D$_3$ and Wnt/β-catenin signaling in CRC has also been studied in vivo in animal models and patients. Our group showed that the 1,25(OH)$_2$D$_3$ analogue EB1089 reduces the growth of xenografts generated by human CRC cells in immunosuppressed mice. In line with data obtained in cell cultures, this inhibition is associated with an increase of E-cadherin and DKK1 levels, and a decrease of β-catenin nuclear content and of the expression of the β-catenin/TCF target gene *ENC1* in the xenografts [54,83,84]. Likewise, the antitumor action of 1,25(OH)$_2$D$_3$ on chemically induced mouse intestinal tumors is concomitant with increased expression of E-cadherin and the inhibition of β-catenin/TCF target genes such as *c-Myc* and *Ccnd1*/cyclin D1 in the intestinal crypts of these animals [85,86]. Concordantly, Xu and colleagues reported that 1,25(OH)$_2$D$_3$ and two of its analogues reduce the tumor load in the *Apc*$^{min/+}$ mouse model of intestinal tumorigenesis associated with an increase of E-cadherin protein and a decrease of nuclear β-catenin levels and of the expression of the Wnt target genes *c-Myc* and *Tcf1* [87].

A Western-style diet that is high in fat and low in calcium and vitamin D is a risk factor for gastrointestinal carcinogenesis. This diet increases the frequency of intestinal tumors in normal mice and speeds up tumor formation in mouse models for intestinal cancer [88]. Several groups have shown that a Western-style diet alters components of the Wnt/β-catenin pathway in intestinal epithelial cells of normal mice [88,89]. These effects can be reversed by calcium and vitamin D supplementation, which prevents the increase of β-catenin/TCF transcriptional activity and reduces the expression of β-catenin, Ephb2 and Frizzled-2, -5, and -10 [89,90].

Vdr knockout mice have also been used to study the role of the vitamin D pathway on CRC. Larriba and colleagues [91] and Zheng and colleagues [92] generated *Apc*$^{min/+}$ *Vdr*$^{-/-}$ mice and discovered that the absence of Vdr results in a higher tumor load and an increased number of premalignant lesions. Interestingly, nuclear staining of β-catenin and expression of Wnt target genes *Ccnd1*/cyclin D1 and *Lef1* are higher in *Apc*$^{min/+}$ *Vdr*$^{-/-}$ than in *Apc*$^{min/+}$ *Vdr*$^{+/+}$ mice. This suggests that *Vdr* inactivation facilitates intestinal tumorigenesis fostered by Wnt/β-catenin activation [91,92].

Remarkably, in a randomized, double-blinded, placebo-controlled clinical trial, Bostick's group reported that vitamin D supplements increase the expression of APC, E-cadherin and other differentiation markers, and decrease that of β-catenin in the upper part of the crypt of normal rectal mucosa from sporadic colorectal adenoma patients [93–96]. In addition, a recent study with 67 CRC patients has revealed that a high circulating 25(OH)D$_3$ level associates with low promoter methylation of secreted frizzled-related protein 2 (*SFRP2*) gene that encodes a soluble inhibitor of the Wnt/β-catenin pathway [97]. These data support an inhibitory effect of vitamin D on Wnt signaling in the human colon in vivo.

2.2. Other Solid Tumors

Although Wnt signaling was first described as inducing breast tumors in mice [98] and Wnt/β-catenin signaling is activated in a proportion of multiple subtypes of human breast cancers [10,99], the typical mutations in components of the pathway found in CRC (*APC*, *CTNNB1*, *AXIN2*) are rare in breast carcinomas [27]. The elevated level of nuclear β-catenin and Wnt signaling in these tumors may be due to high expression of Wnt factors in the tumor environment, loss of APC, Wnt inhibitors (DKK1, SFRPs), and/or E-cadherin expression by epigenetic modification/gene silencing, or alterations in the expression of other genes that encode constituents of the pathway (*RSPO2*, *FZD6*) [27].

Notably, nuclear β-catenin accumulation in a subset of triple-negative and basal-like breast cancer subtypes has been associated with a poor patient outcome [10,99]. Our group has shown that 1,25(OH)$_2$D$_3$ downregulates the expression of myoepithelial/basal markers, such as P-cadherin, smooth muscle α-actin, and α6 and β4 integrins in a panel of breast carcinoma cells, and that $Vdr^{-/-}$ mice express higher levels of P-cadherin and smooth muscle α-actin in the mammary gland than *wt* littermates [100]. These results suggest that 1,25(OH)$_2$D$_3$/VDR antagonizes the Wnt/β-catenin pathway in breast cancer cells, which might protect against the triple-negative and basal-like phenotype. In line with this, 1,25(OH)$_2$D$_3$ induces DKK1 expression and reduces β-catenin transcriptional activity in R7 murine breast cancer cells, and *Vdr* deletion and 1,25(OH)$_2$D$_3$ treatment increases and inhibits, respectively, the tumor expression of several Wnt/β-catenin target genes in breast cancer mouse models [101,102]. The capacity of 1,25(OH)$_2$D$_3$ to inhibit spheroid formation by breast cancer stem cells is overcome by β-catenin overexpression, which suggests that inhibition of the Wnt/β-catenin pathway is essential for this action of 1,25(OH)$_2$D$_3$ [101]. Furthermore, Zheng and colleagues have reported that VDR overexpression in a stem cell-enriched subpopulation of MCF-7 breast cancer cells inhibits Wnt/β-catenin signaling and increases cell sensitivity to tamoxifen [103]. Surprisingly, however, in another study the stable knockdown of *VDR* expression leads to attenuation of the Wnt/β-catenin pathway in MDA-MB-231 breast cancer cells: cytoplasmic and nuclear levels of β-catenin are reduced with the subsequent downregulation of its target genes *AXIN2*, *CCND1*/cyclin D1, *IL6*, and *IL8* [104].

Long non-coding RNA colon cancer-associated transcript 2 (*CCAT2*) is upregulated in ovarian cancer cells and promotes epithelial-mesenchymal transition (EMT) at least partially through the Wnt/β-catenin pathway. CCAT2 knockdown represses the expression of β-catenin and the activity of TCF/LEF factors and inhibits EMT by upregulating E-cadherin and downregulating N-cadherin, Snail1, and Twist1 [105]. Of note, 1,25(OH)$_2$D$_3$ inhibits CCAT2 expression in ovarian cancer cells concomitantly with a reduction in cell proliferation, migration, and invasion. This is linked to decreased binding of TCF4 to the *c-MYC* promoter and, thus, to repression of c-MYC protein expression [106]. Thus, inhibition of CCAT2 represents a novel mechanism of Wnt/β-catenin antagonism by 1,25(OH)$_2$D$_3$. In addition, Srivastava and colleagues have shown that 1,25(OH)$_2$D$_3$/VDR can deplete ovarian cancer stem cells via inhibition of the Wnt/β-catenin pathway [107].

A recent study has investigated whether 1,25(OH)$_2$D$_3$ can affect Wnt/β-catenin signaling in human uterine leiomyoma primary cells using a Wnt pathway PCR array. Up to 75% of the β-catenin/TCF target genes analyzed are repressed by 1,25(OH)$_2$D$_3$. Similarly, 1,25(OH)$_2$D$_3$ inhibits the expression of 73.3% and 77.2% of the Wnt-related genes involved in tissue polarity and cell migration, and in cell cycle, cell growth and proliferation, respectively [108]. These results suggest that not only Wnt/β-catenin but probably also Wnt non-canonical pathways are inhibited by 1,25(OH)$_2$D$_3$ in this cellular context.

1,25(OH)$_2$D$_3$ and its analogue TX527 increase β-catenin protein levels in the nucleus and at the plasma membrane in a Kaposi's sarcoma cellular model and potentiate β-catenin/VDR interaction. The net outcome is downregulation of the β-catenin/TCF target genes *c-MYC*, *MMP9* and *CCND1*/cyclin D1. Moreover, VE-cadherin protein and *DKK1* RNA levels are increased [109]. As in Kaposi's sarcoma cells, 1,25(OH)$_2$D$_3$ augments the level of total β-catenin (both cytoplasmic and nuclear pools), while it reduces that of phosphorylated β-catenin in renal cell carcinoma cells [110]. More importantly, 1,25(OH)$_2$D$_3$ enhances VDR/β-catenin interaction while attenuating β-catenin/TCF binding. Accordingly, 1,25(OH)$_2$D$_3$ downregulates the expression of *CCND1*/cyclin D1 and *AXIN2* genes. In addition, 1,25(OH)$_2$D$_3$ upregulates E-cadherin expression and blocks TGFβ1-induced nuclear translocation of ZEB1, Snail1 and Twist1, which contributes to the suppression of EMT and the inhibition of cell migration and invasion [110]. Thus, the effects of 1,25(OH)$_2$D$_3$ on Kaposi's sarcoma and renal cell carcinoma cells are largely in agreement with those observed on CRC cells. Distinctly, in pancreatic carcinoma cells, the 1,25(OH)$_2$D$_3$ analogue calcipotriol inhibits Wnt/β-catenin signaling by a different mechanism: the promotion of lysosomal degradation of the Wnt membrane receptor LRP6 [111].

Concomitant with an increase in Wnt/β-catenin signaling, global and epidermal-specific *Vdr* deletion predispose mice to either chemical [112] or long-term UVB-induced [113,114] skin tumor formation. 1,25(OH)$_2$D$_3$ enhances β-catenin binding to E-cadherin at the plasma membrane, which promotes epidermal cell differentiation. Moreover, VDR competes with LEF/TCF to recruit β-catenin to gene promoters [115,116] and both 1,25(OH)$_2$D$_3$ and VDR suppress β-catenin-stimulated LEF1/TCF-driven reporter activity [116,117]. The 1,25(OH)$_2$D$_3$ analogue EB1089 prevents the development of β-catenin-induced trichofolliculomas, while β-catenin activation in the absence of Vdr results in basal cell carcinomas [115]. Recently, Muralidhar and colleagues analyzed 703 primary melanoma transcriptomes and found that high tumor *VDR* expression is associated with upregulation of pathways mediating antitumor immunity and downregulation of proliferative pathways, notably Wnt/β-catenin [118]. Functional validation in vitro showed that 1,25(OH)$_2$D$_3$ inhibits the expression of Wnt/β-catenin pathway genes. These results suggest that 1,25(OH)$_2$D$_3$/VDR inhibits the pro-proliferative and immunosuppressive Wnt/β-catenin pathway in melanoma and that this is associated with less metastatic disease and stronger host immune responses [118].

Salehi-Tabar and colleagues have reported that *VDR* knockdown induces, while 1,25(OH)$_2$D$_3$ inhibits, β-catenin binding to and activation of *c-MYC* promoter in head and neck squamous cell carcinoma [119]. In this neoplasia, two vitamin D hydroxyderivatives, 20(OH)D$_3$ and 1,20(OH)$_2$D$_3$, interfere with β-catenin nuclear translocation [120]. In a recent study, Rubin and colleagues analyzed the antitumor effects of 1,25(OH)$_2$D$_3$ and mitotane, the only chemotherapeutic agent available for adrenocortical carcinoma treatment. These authors reported a reduction in adrenocortical carcinoma cell growth and migration in response to either of the two agents, which is stronger when they are combined [121]. 1,25(OH)$_2$D$_3$ triggers a decrease in β-catenin RNA and nuclear protein levels, and both 1,25(OH)$_2$D$_3$ and mitotane induce RNA expression of the Wnt inhibitor *DKK1*, with a more marked effect with the combined treatment, although neither of them can reduce expression of the Wnt target gene *c-MYC* [121].

Vitamin D deficiency has been shown to promote hepatocellular carcinoma growth in *Smad3*$^{+/-}$ mice via upregulation of toll-like receptor 7 expression and β-catenin activation and, accordingly, vitamin D supplementation reduced β-catenin levels [122]. In contrast, Matsuda and colleagues reported that neither dietary supplements of vitamin D nor treatment with vitamin D analogues affect tumor formation or growth in a mouse model of hepatocarcinogenesis induced by mutant β-catenin and *c-MET* overexpression. Hence, they questioned the utility of vitamin D for hepatocellular carcinoma therapy in that setting [123].

In summary, available data show that 1,25(OH)$_2$D$_3$ and its analogues interfere with Wnt/β-catenin signaling in a variety of human solid tumors using mechanisms that mostly resemble those observed in CRC cells (Table 1).

Table 1. Mechanisms of Wnt/β-catenin pathway interference by 1,25(OH)$_2$D$_3$ in solid cancers.

Cancer Type	Mechanism of Antagonism	Reference
Colorectal carcinoma	Increase of VDR/β-catenin interaction	[45]
	Upregulation of *CDH1*/E-cadherin	[34,45,50–52,83,85,87]
	Reduction of nuclear β-catenin	[45,77,84,87]
	Upregulation of *DKK1*	[54]
	Upregulation of *TCF7L2*/TCF4	[74]
	Upregulation of *AXIN1*	[76]
	Repression of *IL1B* (macrophages)	[78]
Breast carcinoma	Upregulation of *CDH1*/E-cadherin	[53]
	Reduction of active β-catenin	[102]
	Upregulation of *DKK1*	[102]
Ovarian carcinoma	Repression of *CCAT2* lncRNA	[106]
Kaposi's sarcoma	Increase of VDR/β-catenin interaction	[109]
	Upregulation of VE-cadherin	[109]
	Upregulation of *DKK1*	[109]
Renal carcinoma	Increase of VDR/β-catenin interaction	[110]
	Upregulation of *CDH1*/E-cadherin	[110]
Pancreatic carcinoma	Increase of LRP6 lysosomal degradation	[111]
Head and neck squamous cell carcinoma	Reduction of nuclear β-catenin	[120]
Adrenocortical carcinoma	Reduction of nuclear β-catenin	[121]
	Upregulation of *DKK1*	[121]
Hepatocellular carcinoma	Reduction of β-catenin level	[122]

3. Antagonism of 1,25(OH)$_2$D$_3$/VDR Signaling by the Wnt/β-Catenin Pathway

The abovementioned data indicate that 1,25(OH)$_2$D$_3$ antagonizes Wnt/β-catenin signaling in several neoplasias. However, the interplay between both pathways is a two-way road, that is, activation of the Wnt/β-catenin pathway may also result in 1,25(OH)$_2$D$_3$/VDR inhibition.

VDR is the only high affinity receptor for 1,25(OH)$_2$D$_3$ and mediates most if not all 1,25(OH)$_2$D$_3$ effects. Thus, cellular VDR expression is the main determinant of 1,25(OH)$_2$D$_3$ action and its downregulation leads to 1,25(OH)$_2$D$_3$ unresponsiveness. VDR is expressed in most normal human cell types and tissues, but also in cancer cell lines and tumors of diverse origins. In line with the antitumor effects of 1,25(OH)$_2$D$_3$ observed in several neoplasias, high VDR expression in human cancer is usually a hallmark of good prognosis [29,31,36,37,124]. VDR expression and activity is regulated transcriptionally, posttranscriptionally by several microRNAs (miRs), and posttranslationally (via phosphorylation, ubiquitination, acetylation, and sumoylation) [125].

3.1. Repression of VDR by Snail Transcription Factors

Wnt/β-catenin signaling is known to promote EMT through upregulation of the expression and activity of key EMT transcription factors such as Snail1, Snail2, Zeb1 and Twist1 by several mechanisms [126,127]. Snail1 and Snail2 are phosphorylated by GSK-3β and tagged for β-TrCP-mediated ubiquitination and subsequent proteasomal degradation [128–130]. Thus, GSK-3β inhibition in response to Wnt/β-catenin signaling results in Snail1 and Snail2 protein stabilization. Inhibition of GSK-3β also increases *SNAI1* transcription via NFκB activation [131]. Furthermore, the Wnt/β-catenin target gene *AXIN2* contributes to Snail1 protein stabilization in breast cancer cells by regulating GSK-3β localization. When levels of AXIN2 increase in response to β-catenin/TCF signaling, GSK-3β is exported from the nuclear compartment leaving Snail1 in its non-phosphorylated transcriptionally active form [132]. In addition, induction of *SNAI2* RNA levels by Wnt3 has been described in breast cancer cells [133].

Interestingly, Snail1 and Snail2 are the best-characterized transcriptional repressors of the human *VDR* gene. Our group demonstrated that Snail1 represses the expression of *VDR* by two mechanisms [83] (Figure 2). On the one hand, Snail1 inhibits *VDR* gene transcription by binding to three E-box sequences in its promoter. On the other, Snail1 reduces *VDR* RNA half-life. As a consequence, Snail1 strongly decreases the level of VDR RNA and protein and the cellular response to 1,25(OH)$_2$D$_3$ [83,84]. Moreover, forced expression of Snail1 in human CRC cells prevents the upregulation of E-cadherin and the subsequent cell differentiation triggered by 1,25(OH)$_2$D$_3$. Therefore, by repressing *VDR* and *CDH1*/E-cadherin genes, Snail1 abolishes 1,25(OH)$_2$D$_3$ action and favors the accumulation of β-catenin in the nucleus and the transcription of β-catenin/TCF target genes [83,84]. Later, Snail2 was found to also inhibit *VDR* gene expression in CRC cells through the same E-boxes in the promoter used by Snail1 (Figure 2). Actually, both transcription factors present an additive repressive effect on the *VDR* gene [134]. *SNAI1* and/or *SNAI2* upregulation is observed in 76% of human CRC and is associated with *VDR* downregulation [83,134–136]. Not surprisingly, the lowest *VDR* RNA levels are found in tumors with upregulation of both *SNAI1* and *SNAI2* genes [134]. *VDR* expression is also reduced in normal colonic tissue surrounding the tumor, which suggests that Snail1 expression in tumor cells promotes the secretion of factors that reduce *VDR* expression in neighboring normal cells [137]. In addition to CRC cells, Snail1 and Snail2 also repress *VDR* gene expression and antagonize the antitumor action of 1,25(OH)$_2$D$_3$ in human osteosarcoma and breast cancer cells [138,139]. Knackstedt and colleagues showed that downregulation of Vdr observed in the colon of a colitis mouse model is associated with an increase in the expression of Snail1 and Snail2 [140]. Altogether, these results support that activation of the Wnt/β-catenin pathway upregulates Snail1 and Snail2, which antagonizes 1,25(OH)$_2$D$_3$/VDR signaling by inhibiting *VDR* gene expression.

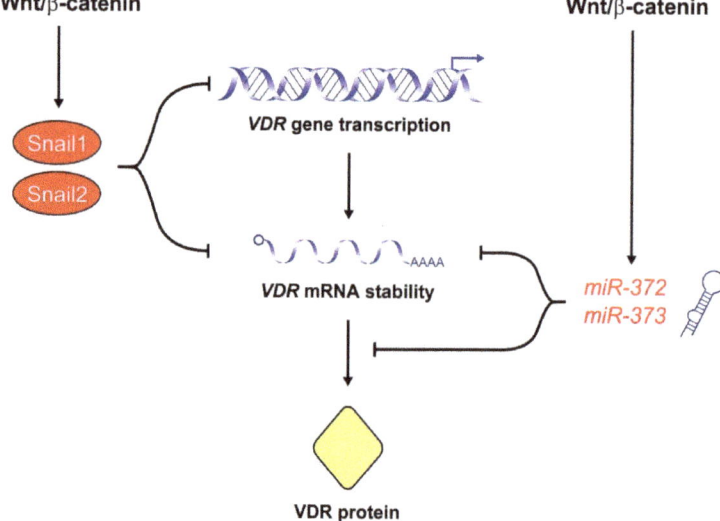

Figure 2. The Wnt/β-catenin signaling pathway represses VDR expression. A major mechanism of this effect is the upregulation of Snail1 and Snail2, which repress *VDR* gene transcription and decrease VDR RNA half-life. The Wnt/β-catenin pathway also antagonizes 1,25(OH)$_2$D$_3$/VDR signaling by the upregulation of *miR-372* and *miR-373*, which reduce the level of VDR RNA and protein.

3.2. Posttranscriptional Repression of VDR by miRNAs

A novel, recently described mechanism of Wnt/β-catenin-mediated antagonism of 1,25(OH)$_2$D$_3$/VDR signaling involves the *miR-372/373* cluster (Figure 2). *miR-372/373* expression is induced by β-catenin/TCF in several human cancer cell lines through three TCF/LEF binding sites located in its promoter region [141]. Accordingly, this cluster of stem cell-specific miRs is dysregulated in various cancers, particularly in CRC due to the constitutive activation of the Wnt/β-catenin pathway [142–144]. Wang and colleagues have shown that overexpression of *miR-372/373* enhances the stemness of CRC cells and promotes their self-renewal, chemotherapy resistance and invasive potential [145].

These authors found that overexpression of *miR-372/373* results in upregulation of stemness-related pathways, e.g., Nanog and Hedgehog and, conversely, downregulation of differentiation-related pathways, e.g., NFκB, MAPK/ERK, and VDR. Interestingly, they demonstrated that *miR-372/373* overexpression leads to reduced expression of VDR RNA and protein in CRC cells, which contributes to the maintenance of the cancer stem cell phenotype [145]. These data suggest that the Wnt/β-catenin pathway also inhibits VDR expression through the induction of *miR-372/373*.

4. Conclusions

The Wnt/β-catenin pathway is frequently overactivated in cancer and promotes tumorigenesis, which makes it an attractive candidate for therapeutic intervention. The active vitamin D metabolite $1,25(OH)_2D_3$, a major regulator of the human genome, cooperates with the Wnt/β-catenin pathway in the physiological control of tissues and organs such as bone, skin, and brain. Conversely, $1,25(OH)_2D_3$ attenuates aberrant activation of the Wnt/β-catenin pathway that takes place in most CRC and in a variable proportion of other solid tumors. To do this, $1,25(OH)_2D_3$ modulates a series of genes and mechanisms acting at different levels of the Wnt/β-catenin pathway that vary among cancer types. $1,25(OH)_2D_3$ does not completely block the pathway but rather reduces its overactivation. This probably helps to maintain the physiological effects of Wnt/β-catenin in healthy organs, with few toxic side-effects. As expected from two crucial regulators of the organism and its necessary homeostasis, $1,25(OH)_2D_3$ action is counterbalanced by Wnt factors.

The multilevel antagonistic action of $1,25(OH)_2D_3$ on aberrantly activated Wnt/β-catenin signaling strongly supports the therapeutic utility of vitamin D compounds in cancer prevention and treatment.

Author Contributions: Conceptualization, A.M.; writing-original draft preparation, J.M.G.-S.; writing—review and editing, M.J.L. and A.M.; artwork, M.J.L. All authors have read and agreed to the published version of the manuscript.

Funding: The work in the authors' laboratory is funded by the Agencia Estatal de Investigación (PID2019-104867RB-I00/AEI/10.13039/501100011033), the Agencia Estatal de Investigación—Fondo Europeo de Desarrollo Regional (SAF2016-76377-R, MINECO/AEI/FEDER, EU), the Ministerio de Economía y Competitividad (SAF2017-90604-REDT/NuRCaMeIn), and the Instituto de Salud Carlos III—Fondo Europeo de Desarrollo Regional (CIBERONC; CB16/12/00273).

Acknowledgments: We thank Lucille Banham and Javier Pérez for their valuable assistance in the preparation of the English manuscript and the artwork, respectively.

Conflicts of Interest: The authors declare no conflict of interest. The funders had no role in the writing of the manuscript or in the decision to publish it.

References

1. Nusse, R.; Clevers, H. Wnt/beta-catenin signaling, disease, and emerging therapeutic modalities. *Cell* **2017**, *169*, 985–999. [CrossRef] [PubMed]
2. Shang, S.; Hua, F.; Hu, Z.W. The regulation of beta-catenin activity and function in cancer: Therapeutic opportunities. *Oncotarget* **2017**, *8*, 33972–33989. [CrossRef] [PubMed]
3. Zhan, T.; Rindtorff, N.; Boutros, M. Wnt signaling in cancer. *Oncogene* **2017**, *36*, 1461–1473. [CrossRef] [PubMed]
4. Gong, X.; Carmon, K.S.; Lin, Q.; Thomas, A.; Yi, J.; Liu, Q. LGR6 is a high affinity receptor of R-spondins and potentially functions as a tumor suppressor. *PLoS ONE* **2012**, *7*, e34739. [CrossRef] [PubMed]
5. Chen, P.-H.; Chen, X.; Lin, Z.; Fang, D.; He, X. The structural basis of R-spondin recognition by LGR5 and RNF43. *Genes Dev.* **2013**, *27*, 1345–1350. [CrossRef] [PubMed]
6. Carmon, K.S.; Gong, X.; Lin, Q.; Thomas, A.; Liu, Q. R-spondins function as ligands of the orphan receptors LGR4 and LGR5 to regulate Wnt/beta-catenin signaling. *Proc. Natl. Acad. Sci. USA* **2011**, *108*, 11452–11457. [CrossRef]
7. De Lau, W.; Barker, N.; Low, T.Y.; Koo, B.-K.; Li, V.S.W.; Teunissen, H.; Kajula, P.; Haegebarth, A.; Peters, P.J.; van de Wetering, M.; et al. Lgr5 homologues associate with Wnt receptors and mediate R-spondin signaling. *Nature* **2011**, *476*, 293–297. [CrossRef]

8. Hao, H.X.; Xie, Y.; Zhang, Y.; Charlat, O.; Oster, E.; Avello, M.; Lei, H.; Mickanin, C.; Liu, D.; Ruffner, H.; et al. ZNRF3 promotes Wnt receptor turnover in an R-spondin-sensitive manner. *Nature* **2012**, *485*, 195–200. [CrossRef]
9. Kobayashi, M.; Honma, T.; Matsuda, Y.; Suzuki, Y.; Narisawa, R.; Ajioka, Y.; Asakura, H. Nuclear translocation of beta-catenin in colorectal cancer. *Br. J. Cancer* **2000**, *82*, 1689–1693.
10. Khramtsov, A.I.; Khramtsova, G.F.; Tretiakova, M.; Huo, D.; Olopade, O.I.; Goss, K.H. Wnt/beta-catenin pathway activation is enriched in basal-like breast cancers and predicts poor outcome. *Am. J. Pathol.* **2010**, *176*, 2911–2920. [CrossRef]
11. Damsky, W.E.; Curley, D.P.; Santhanakrishnan, M.; Rosenbaum, L.E.; Platt, J.T.; Gould Rothberg, B.E.; Taketo, M.M.; Dankort, D.; Rimm, D.L.; McMahon, M.; et al. beta-Catenin signaling controls metastasis in Braf-activated Pten-deficient melanomas. *Cancer Cell* **2011**, *20*, 741–754. [CrossRef] [PubMed]
12. Tao, J.; Calvisi, D.F.; Ranganathan, S.; Cigliano, A.; Zhou, L.; Singh, S.; Jiang, L.; Fan, B.; Terracciano, L.; Armeanu-Ebinger, S.; et al. Activation of beta-catenin and Yap1 in human hepatoblastoma and induction of hepatocarcinogenesis in mice. *Gastroenterology* **2014**, *147*, 690–701. [CrossRef] [PubMed]
13. Gekas, C.; D'Altri, T.; Aligué, R.; González, J.; Espinosa, L.; Bigas, A. beta-Catenin is required for T-cell leukemia initiation and MYC transcription downstream of Notch1. *Leukemia* **2016**, *30*, 2002–2010. [CrossRef] [PubMed]
14. Clevers, H.; Nusse, R. Wnt/beta-catenin signaling and disease. *Cell* **2012**, *149*, 1192–1205. [CrossRef]
15. Polakis, P. Wnt signaling in cancer. *Cold Spring Harb. Perspect. Biol.* **2012**, *4*, a008052. [CrossRef]
16. The Cancer Genome Atlas Network. Comprehensive molecular characterization of human colon and rectal cancer. *Nature* **2012**, *487*, 330–337. [CrossRef]
17. Seshagiri, S.; Stawiski, E.W.; Durinck, S.; Modrusan, Z.; Storm, E.E.; Conboy, C.B.; Chaudhuri, S.; Guan, Y.; Janakiraman, V.; Jaiswal, B.S.; et al. Recurrent R-spondin fusions in colon cancer. *Nature* **2012**, *488*, 660–664. [CrossRef]
18. Han, T.; Schatoff, E.M.; Murphy, C.; Zafra, M.P.; Wilkinson, J.E.; Elemento, O.; Dow, L.E. R-Spondin chromosome rearrangements drive Wnt-dependent tumour initiation and maintenance in the intestine. *Nat. Commun.* **2017**, *8*, 15945. [CrossRef]
19. Zucman-Rossi, J.; Jeannot, E.; Van Nhieu, J.T.; Scoazec, J.-Y.; Guettier, C.; Rebouissou, S.; Bacq, Y.; Leteurtre, E.; Paradis, V.; Michalak, S.; et al. Genotype-phenotype correlation in hepatocellular adenoma: New classification and relationship with HCC. *Hepatology* **2006**, *43*, 515–524. [CrossRef]
20. Austinat, M.; Dunsch, R.; Wittekind, C.; Tannapfel, A.; Gebhardt, R.; Gaunitz, F. Correlation between beta-catenin mutations and expression of Wnt-signaling target genes in hepatocellular carcinoma. *Mol. Cancer* **2008**, *7*, 21. [CrossRef]
21. White, B.D.; Chien, A.J.; Dawson, D.W. Dysregulation of Wnt/beta-catenin signaling in gastrointestinal cancers. *Gastroenterology* **2012**, *142*, 219–232. [CrossRef] [PubMed]
22. Howe, L.R.; Brown, A.M. Wnt signaling and breast cancer. *Cancer Biol. Ther.* **2004**, *3*, 36–41. [CrossRef] [PubMed]
23. Klarmann, G.J.; Decker, A.; Farrar, W. Epigenetic gene silencing in the Wnt pathway in breast cancer. *Epigenetics* **2008**, *3*, 59–63. [CrossRef] [PubMed]
24. Liu, C.C.; Prior, J.; Piwnica-Worms, D.; Bu, G. LRP6 overexpression defines a class of breast cancer subtype and is a target for therapy. *Proc. Natl. Acad. Sci. USA* **2010**, *107*, 5136–5141. [CrossRef]
25. Yang, L.; Wu, X.; Wang, Y.; Zhang, K.; Wu, J.; Yuan, Y.C.; Deng, X.; Chen, L.; Kim, C.C.; Lau, S.; et al. FZD7 has a critical role in cell proliferation in triple negative breast cancer. *Oncogene* **2011**, *30*, 4437–4446. [CrossRef] [PubMed]
26. Tammela, T.; Sanchez-Rivera, F.J.; Cetinbas, N.M.; Wu, K.; Joshi, N.S.; Helenius, K.; Park, Y.; Azimi, R.; Kerper, N.R.; Wesselhoeft, R.A.; et al. A Wnt-producing niche drives proliferative potential and progression in lung adenocarcinoma. *Nature* **2017**, *545*, 355–359. [CrossRef] [PubMed]
27. Van Schie, E.H.; van Amerongen, R. Aberrant WNT/CTNNB1 signaling as a therapeutic target in human breast cancer: Weighing the evidence. *Front. Cell Dev. Biol.* **2020**, *8*, 25. [CrossRef]
28. Holick, M.F.; Frommer, J.E.; McNeill, S.C.; Richtand, N.M.; Henley, J.W.; Potts, J.T., Jr. Photometabolism of 7-dehydrocholesterol to previtamin D3 in skin. *Biochem. Biophys. Res. Commun.* **1977**, *76*, 107–114. [CrossRef]
29. Christakos, S.; Dhawan, P.; Verstuyf, A.; Verlinden, L.; Carmeliet, G. Vitamin D: Metabolism, molecular mechanism of action, and pleiotropic effects. *Physiol. Rev.* **2016**, *96*, 365–408. [CrossRef]
30. Zerwekh, J.E. Blood biomarkers of vitamin D status. *Am. J. Clin. Nutr.* **2008**, *87*, 1087S–1091S. [CrossRef]

31. Carlberg, C.; Muñoz, A. An update on vitamin D signaling and cancer. *Semin. Cancer Biol.* **2020**. [CrossRef] [PubMed]
32. Haussler, M.R.; Jurutka, P.W.; Mizwicki, M.; Norman, A.W. Vitamin D receptor (VDR)-mediated actions of 1alpha,25(OH)2vitamin D3: Genomic and non-genomic mechanisms. *Best Pract. Res. Clin. Endocrinol. Metab.* **2011**, *25*, 543–559. [CrossRef] [PubMed]
33. Molnár, F.; Peräkylä, M.; Carlberg, C. Vitamin D receptor agonists specifically modulate the volume of the ligand-binding pocket. *J. Biol. Chem.* **2006**, *281*, 10516–10526. [CrossRef] [PubMed]
34. Ordóñez-Morán, P.; Larriba, M.J.; Pálmer, H.G.; Valero, R.A.; Barbáchano, A.; Dunach, M.; García de Herreros, A.; Villalobos, C.; Berciano, M.T.; Lafarga, M.; et al. RhoA—ROCK and p38MAPK-MSK1 mediate vitamin D effects on gene expression, phenotype, and Wnt pathway in colon cancer cells. *J. Cell Biol.* **2008**, *183*, 697–710. [CrossRef] [PubMed]
35. Hii, C.S.; Ferrante, A. The non-genomic actions of vitamin D. *Nutrients* **2016**, *8*, 135. [CrossRef] [PubMed]
36. Feldman, D.; Krishnan, A.V.; Swami, S.; Giovannucci, E.; Feldman, B.J. The role of vitamin D in reducing cancer risk and progression. *Nat. Rev. Cancer* **2014**, *14*, 342–357. [CrossRef]
37. Fernández-Barral, A.; Bustamante-Madrid, P.; Ferrer-Mayorga, G.; Barbáchano, A.; Larriba, M.J.; Muñoz, A. Vitamin D effects on cell differentiation and stemness in cancer. *Cancers* **2020**, *12*, 2413. [CrossRef]
38. Garland, C.F.; Garland, F.C. Do sunlight and vitamin D reduce the likelihood of colon cancer? *Int. J. Epidemiol.* **1980**, *9*, 65–71. [CrossRef]
39. Garland, C.F.; Garland, F.C.; Gorham, E.D.; Lipkin, M.; Newmark, H.; Mohr, S.B.; Holick, M.F. The role of vitamin D in cancer prevention. *Am. J. Public Health* **2006**, *96*, 252–261. [CrossRef]
40. Calderwood, A.H.; Baron, J.A.; Mott, L.A.; Ahnen, D.J.; Bostick, R.M.; Figueiredo, J.C.; Passarelli, M.N.; Rees, J.R.; Robertson, D.J.; Barry, E.L. No evidence for posttreatment effects of vitamin D and calcium supplementation on risk of colorectal adenomas in a randomized trial. *Cancer Prev. Res.* **2019**, *12*, 295–304. [CrossRef]
41. Markotic, A.; Langer, S.; Kelava, T.; Vucic, K.; Turcic, P.; Tokic, T.; Stefancic, L.; Radetic, E.; Farrington, S.; Timofeeva, M.; et al. Higher post-operative serum vitamin D level is associated with better survival outcome in colorectal cancer patients. *Nutr. Cancer* **2019**, *71*, 1078–1085. [CrossRef] [PubMed]
42. Ng, K.; Nimeiri, H.S.; McCleary, N.J.; Abrams, T.A.; Yurgelun, M.B.; Cleary, J.M.; Rubinson, D.A.; Schrag, D.; Miksad, R.; Bullock, A.J.; et al. Effect of high-dose vs standard-dose vitamin D3 supplementation on progression-free survival among patients with advanced or metastatic colorectal cancer: The SUNSHINE randomized clinical trial. *J. Am. Med. Assoc.* **2019**, *321*, 1370–1379. [CrossRef] [PubMed]
43. El-Sharkawy, A.; Malki, A. Vitamin D signaling in inflammation and cancer: Molecular mechanisms and therapeutic implications. *Molecules* **2020**, *25*, 3219. [CrossRef] [PubMed]
44. Negri, M.; Gentile, A.; de Angelis, C.; Montò, T.; Patalano, R.; Colao, A.; Pivonello, R.; Pivonello, C. Vitamin D-induced molecular mechanisms to potentiate cancer therapy and to reverse drug-resistance in cancer cells. *Nutrients* **2020**, *12*, 1798. [CrossRef] [PubMed]
45. Pálmer, H.G.; González-Sancho, J.M.; Espada, J.; Berciano, M.T.; Puig, I.; Baulida, J.; Quintanilla, M.; Cano, A.; García de Herreros, A.; Lafarga, M.; et al. Vitamin D3 promotes the differentiation of colon carcinoma cells by the induction of E-cadherin and the inhibition of beta-catenin signaling. *J. Cell Biol.* **2001**, *154*, 369–387. [CrossRef] [PubMed]
46. Easwaran, V.; Pishvaian, M.; Salimuddin; Byers, S. Cross-regulation of beta-catenin-LEF/TCF and retinoid signaling pathways. *Curr. Biol.* **1999**, *9*, 1415–1418. [CrossRef]
47. Truica, C.I.; Byers, S.; Gelmann, E.P. beta-Catenin affects androgen receptor transcriptional activity and ligand specificity. *Cancer Res.* **2000**, *60*, 4709–4713.
48. Shah, S.; Islam, M.N.; Dakshanamurthy, S.; Rizvi, I.; Rao, M.; Herrell, R.; Zinser, G.; Valrance, M.; Aranda, A.; Moras, D.; et al. The molecular basis of vitamin D receptor and beta-catenin crossregulation. *Mol. Cell* **2006**, *21*, 799–809. [CrossRef]
49. Egan, J.B.; Thompson, P.A.; Vitanov, M.V.; Bartik, L.; Jacobs, E.T.; Haussler, M.R.; Gerner, E.W.; Jurutka, P.W. Vitamin D receptor ligands, adenomatous polyposis coli, and the vitamin D receptor FokI polymorphism collectively modulate beta-catenin activity in colon cancer cells. *Mol. Carcinog.* **2010**, *49*, 337–352. [CrossRef]
50. Álvarez-Díaz, S.; Valle, N.; García, J.M.; Peña, C.; Freije, J.M.; Quesada, V.; Astudillo, A.; Bonilla, F.; López-Otín, C.; Muñoz, A. Cystatin D is a candidate tumor suppressor gene induced by vitamin D in human colon cancer cells. *J. Clin. Investig.* **2009**, *119*, 2343–2358. [CrossRef]

51. Barbáchano, A.; Ordóñez-Morán, P.; García, J.M.; Sánchez, A.; Pereira, F.; Larriba, M.J.; Martínez, N.; Hernández, J.; Landolfi, S.; Bonilla, F.; et al. SPROUTY-2 and E-cadherin regulate reciprocally and dictate colon cancer cell tumourigenicity. *Oncogene* **2010**, *29*, 4800–4813. [CrossRef] [PubMed]
52. Pereira, F.; Barbáchano, A.; Silva, J.; Bonilla, F.; Campbell, M.J.; Muñoz, A.; Larriba, M.J. KDM6B/JMJD3 histone demethylase is induced by vitamin D and modulates its effects in colon cancer cells. *Hum. Mol. Genet.* **2011**, *20*, 4655–4665. [CrossRef] [PubMed]
53. Xu, H.; McCann, M.; Zhang, Z.; Posner, G.H.; Bingham, V.; El-Tanani, M.; Campbell, F.C. Vitamin D receptor modulates the neoplastic phenotype through antagonistic growth regulatory signals. *Mol. Carcinog.* **2009**, *48*, 758–772. [CrossRef] [PubMed]
54. Aguilera, O.; Peña, C.; García, J.M.; Larriba, M.J.; Ordóñez-Morán, P.; Navarro, D.; Barbáchano, A.; López de Silanes, I.; Ballestar, E.; Fraga, M.F.; et al. The Wnt antagonist DICKKOPF-1 gene is induced by 1alpha,25-dihydroxyvitamin D3 associated to the differentiation of human colon cancer cells. *Carcinogenesis* **2007**, *28*, 1877–1884. [CrossRef]
55. Semenov, M.V.; Tamai, K.; Brott, B.K.; Kuhl, M.; Sokol, S.; He, X. Head inducer Dickkopf-1 is a ligand for Wnt coreceptor LRP6. *Curr. Biol.* **2001**, *11*, 951–961. [CrossRef]
56. Mao, B.; Wu, W.; Davidson, G.; Marhold, J.; Li, M.; Mechler, B.M.; Delius, H.; Hoppe, D.; Stannek, P.; Walter, C.; et al. Kremen proteins are Dickkopf receptors that regulate Wnt/beta-catenin signalling. *Nature* **2002**, *417*, 664–667. [CrossRef]
57. Niida, A.; Hiroko, T.; Kasai, M.; Furukawa, Y.; Nakamura, Y.; Suzuki, Y.; Sugano, S.; Akiyama, T. DKK1, a negative regulator of Wnt signaling, is a target of the beta-catenin/TCF pathway. *Oncogene* **2004**, *23*, 8520–8526. [CrossRef]
58. Chamorro, M.N.; Schwartz, D.R.; Vonica, A.; Brivanlou, A.H.; Cho, K.R.; Varmus, H.E. FGF-20 and DKK1 are transcriptional targets of beta-catenin and FGF-20 is implicated in cancer and development. *EMBO J.* **2005**, *24*, 73–84. [CrossRef]
59. González-Sancho, J.M.; Aguilera, O.; García, J.M.; Pendás-Franco, N.; Peña, C.; Cal, S.; García de Herreros, A.; Bonilla, F.; Muñoz, A. The Wnt antagonist DICKKOPF-1 gene is a downstream target of beta-catenin/TCF and is downregulated in human colon cancer. *Oncogene* **2005**, *24*, 1098–1103. [CrossRef]
60. Lee, A.Y.; He, B.; You, L.; Xu, Z.; Mazieres, J.; Reguart, N.; Mikami, I.; Batra, S.; Jablons, D.M. Dickkopf-1 antagonizes Wnt signaling independent of beta-catenin in human mesothelioma. *Biochem. Biophys. Res. Commun.* **2004**, *323*, 1246–1250. [CrossRef]
61. Mikheev, A.M.; Mikheeva, S.A.; Liu, B.; Cohen, P.; Zarbl, H. A functional genomics approach for the identification of putative tumor suppressor genes: Dickkopf-1 as suppressor of HeLa cell transformation. *Carcinogenesis* **2004**, *25*, 47–59. [CrossRef] [PubMed]
62. Aguilera, O.; Fraga, M.F.; Ballestar, E.; Paz, M.F.; Herranz, M.; Espada, J.; García, J.M.; Muñoz, A.; Esteller, M.; González-Sancho, J.M. Epigenetic inactivation of the Wnt antagonist DICKKOPF-1 (DKK-1) gene in human colorectal cancer. *Oncogene* **2006**, *25*, 4116–4121. [CrossRef] [PubMed]
63. Sato, H.; Suzuki, H.; Toyota, M.; Nojima, M.; Maruyama, R.; Sasaki, S.; Takagi, H.; Sogabe, Y.; Sasaki, Y.; Idogawa, M.; et al. Frequent epigenetic inactivation of DICKKOPF family genes in human gastrointestinal tumors. *Carcinogenesis* **2007**, *28*, 2459–2466. [CrossRef] [PubMed]
64. Rawson, J.B.; Manno, M.; Mrkonjic, M.; Daftary, D.; Dicks, E.; Buchanan, D.D.; Younghusband, H.B.; Parfrey, P.S.; Young, J.P.; Pollett, A.; et al. Promoter methylation of Wnt antagonists DKK1 and SFRP1 is associated with opposing tumor subtypes in two large populations of colorectal cancer patients. *Carcinogenesis* **2011**, *32*, 741–747. [CrossRef]
65. Rawson, J.B.; Sun, Z.; Dicks, E.; Daftary, D.; Parfrey, P.S.; Green, R.C.; Gallinger, S.; McLaughlin, J.R.; Wang, P.P.; Knight, J.A.; et al. Vitamin D intake is negatively associated with promoter methylation of the Wnt antagonist gene DKK1 in a large group of colorectal cancer patients. *Nutr. Cancer* **2012**, *64*, 919–928. [CrossRef] [PubMed]
66. Pendás-Franco, N.; García, J.M.; Peña, C.; Valle, N.; Pálmer, H.G.; Heinaniemi, M.; Carlberg, C.; Jiménez, B.; Bonilla, F.; Muñoz, A.; et al. DICKKOPF-4 is induced by TCF/beta-catenin and upregulated in human colon cancer, promotes tumour cell invasion and angiogenesis and is repressed by 1alpha,25-dihydroxyvitamin D3. *Oncogene* **2008**, *27*, 4467–4477. [CrossRef] [PubMed]
67. You, J.; Nguyen, A.V.; Albers, C.G.; Lin, F.; Holcombe, R.F. Wnt pathway-related gene expression in inflammatory bowel disease. *Dig. Dis. Sci.* **2008**, *53*, 1013–1019. [CrossRef] [PubMed]

68. Matsui, A.; Yamaguchi, T.; Maekawa, S.; Miyazaki, C.; Takano, S.; Uetake, T.; Inoue, T.; Otaka, M.; Otsuka, H.; Sato, T.; et al. DICKKOPF-4 and -2 genes are upregulated in human colorectal cancer. *Cancer Sci.* **2009**, *100*, 1923–1930. [CrossRef]
69. Hsieh, A.L.; Walton, Z.E.; Altman, B.J.; Stine, Z.E.; Dang, C.V. MYC and metabolism on the path to cancer. *Semin. Cell Dev. Biol.* **2015**, *43*, 11–21. [CrossRef]
70. Wolf, E.; Eilers, M. Targeting MYC proteins for tumor therapy. *Annu. Rev. Cancer Biol.* **2020**, *4*, 61–75. [CrossRef]
71. Meyer, M.B.; Goetsch, P.D.; Pike, J.W. VDR/RXR and TCF4/beta-catenin cistromes in colonic cells of colorectal tumor origin: Impact on c-FOS and c-MYC gene expression. *Mol. Endocrinol.* **2012**, *26*, 37–51. [CrossRef] [PubMed]
72. Toropainen, S.; Väisänen, S.; Heikkinen, S.; Carlberg, C. The down-regulation of the human MYC gene by the nuclear hormone 1alpha,25-dihydroxyvitamin D3 is associated with cycling of corepressors and histone deacetylases. *J. Mol. Biol.* **2010**, *400*, 284–294. [PubMed]
73. He, T.C.; Sparks, A.B.; Rago, C.; Hermeking, H.; Zawel, L.; da Costa, L.T.; Morin, P.J.; Vogelstein, B.; Kinzler, K.W. Identification of c-MYC as a target of the APC pathway. *Science* **1998**, *281*, 1509–1512. [CrossRef] [PubMed]
74. Beildeck, M.E.; Islam, M.; Shah, S.; Welsh, J.; Byers, S.W. Control of TCF-4 expression by VDR and vitamin D in the mouse mammary gland and colorectal cancer cell lines. *PLoS ONE* **2009**, *4*, e7872.
75. Tang, W.; Dodge, M.; Gundapaneni, D.; Michnoff, C.; Roth, M.; Lum, L. A genome-wide RNAi screen for Wnt/beta-catenin pathway components identifies unexpected roles for TCF transcription factors in cancer. *Proc. Natl. Acad. Sci. USA* **2008**, *105*, 9697–9702. [CrossRef] [PubMed]
76. Jin, D.; Zhang, Y.G.; Wu, S.; Lu, R.; Lin, Z.; Zheng, Y.; Chen, H.; Cs-Szabo, G.; Sun, J. Vitamin D receptor is a novel transcriptional regulator for Axin1. *J. Steroid Biochem. Mol. Biol.* **2017**, *165*, 430–437.
77. Groschel, C.; Aggarwal, A.; Tennakoon, S.; Hobaus, J.; Prinz-Wohlgenannt, M.; Marian, B.; Heffeter, P.; Berger, W.; Kallay, E. Effect of 1,25-dihydroxyvitamin D3 on the Wnt pathway in non-malignant colonic cells. *J. Steroid Biochem. Mol. Biol.* **2016**, *155*, 224–230. [CrossRef]
78. Kaler, P.; Augenlicht, L.; Klampfer, L. Macrophage-derived IL-1beta stimulates Wnt signaling and growth of colon cancer cells: A crosstalk interrupted by vitamin D3. *Oncogene* **2009**, *28*, 3892–3902. [CrossRef]
79. Ferrer-Mayorga, G.; Niell, N.; Cantero, R.; González-Sancho, J.M.; Del Peso, L.; Muñoz, A.; Larriba, M.J. Vitamin D and Wnt3A have additive and partially overlapping modulatory effects on gene expression and phenotype in human colon fibroblasts. *Sci. Rep.* **2019**, *9*, 8085.
80. Fernández-Barral, A.; Costales-Carrera, A.; Buira, S.P.; Jung, P.; Ferrer-Mayorga, G.; Larriba, M.J.; Bustamante-Madrid, P.; Domínguez, O.; Real, F.X.; Guerra-Pastrian, L.; et al. Vitamin D differentially regulates colon stem cells in patient-derived normal and tumor organoids. *FEBS J.* **2020**, *287*, 53–72. [CrossRef]
81. Larriba, M.J.; González-Sancho, J.M.; Barbáchano, A.; Niell, N.; Ferrer-Mayorga, G.; Muñoz, A. Vitamin D is a multilevel repressor of Wnt/beta-catenin signaling in cancer cells. *Cancers* **2013**, *5*, 1242–1260. [CrossRef] [PubMed]
82. Gómez-Oliva, R.; Geribaldi-Doldán, N.; Domínguez-García, S.; Carrascal, L.; Verástegui, C.; Nunez-Abades, P.; Castro, C. Vitamin D deficiency as a potential risk factor for accelerated aging, impaired hippocampal neurogenesis and cognitive decline: A role for Wnt/beta-catenin signaling. *Aging* **2020**, *12*, 13824–13844. [CrossRef] [PubMed]
83. Pálmer, H.G.; Larriba, M.J.; García, J.M.; Ordóñez-Morán, P.; Peña, C.; Peiró, S.; Puig, I.; Rodríguez, R.; de la Fuente, R.; Bernad, A.; et al. The transcription factor SNAIL represses vitamin D receptor expression and responsiveness in human colon cancer. *Nat. Med.* **2004**, *10*, 917–919. [CrossRef] [PubMed]
84. Larriba, M.J.; Valle, N.; Pálmer, H.G.; Ordóñez-Morán, P.; Alvarez-Díaz, S.; Becker, K.F.; Gamallo, C.; de García de Herreros, A.; González-Sancho, J.M.; Muñoz, A. The inhibition of Wnt/beta-catenin signalling by 1alpha,25-dihydroxyvitamin D3 is abrogated by Snail1 in human colon cancer cells. *Endocr. Relat. Cancer* **2007**, *14*, 141–151. [CrossRef] [PubMed]
85. Wali, R.K.; Khare, S.; Tretiakova, M.; Cohen, G.; Nguyen, L.; Hart, J.; Wang, J.; Wen, M.; Ramaswamy, A.; Joseph, L.; et al. Ursodeoxycholic acid and F_6-D_3 inhibit aberrant crypt proliferation in the rat azoxymethane model of colon cancer: Roles of cyclin D1 and E-cadherin. *Cancer Epidemiol. Biomark. Prev.* **2002**, *11*, 1653–1662.

86. Fichera, A.; Little, N.; Dougherty, U.; Mustafi, R.; Cerda, S.; Li, Y.C.; Delgado, J.; Arora, A.; Campbell, L.K.; Joseph, L.; et al. A vitamin D analogue inhibits colonic carcinogenesis in the AOM/DSS model. *J. Surg. Res.* **2007**, *142*, 239–245. [CrossRef]
87. Xu, H.; Posner, G.H.; Stevenson, M.; Campbell, F.C. Apc^{MIN} modulation of vitamin D secosteroid growth control. *Carcinogenesis* **2010**, *31*, 1434–1441. [CrossRef]
88. Yang, K.; Yang, W.; Mariadason, J.; Velcich, A.; Lipkin, M.; Augenlicht, L. Dietary components modify gene expression: Implications for carcinogenesis. *J. Nutr.* **2005**, *135*, 2710–2714. [CrossRef]
89. Yang, K.; Kurihara, N.; Fan, K.; Newmark, H.; Rigas, B.; Bancroft, L.; Corner, G.; Livote, E.; Lesser, M.; Edelmann, W.; et al. Dietary induction of colonic tumors in a mouse model of sporadic colon cancer. *Cancer Res.* **2008**, *68*, 7803–7810. [CrossRef]
90. Wang, D.; Peregrina, K.; Dhima, E.; Lin, E.Y.; Mariadason, J.M.; Augenlicht, L.H. Paneth cell marker expression in intestinal villi and colon crypts characterizes dietary induced risk for mouse sporadic intestinal cancer. *Proc. Natl. Acad. Sci. USA* **2011**, *108*, 10272–10277. [CrossRef]
91. Larriba, M.J.; Ordóñez-Morán, P.; Chicote, I.; Martín-Fernández, G.; Puig, I.; Muñoz, A.; Pálmer, H.G. Vitamin D receptor deficiency enhances Wnt/beta-catenin signaling and tumor burden in colon cancer. *PLoS ONE* **2011**, *6*, e23524. [CrossRef] [PubMed]
92. Zheng, W.; Wong, K.E.; Zhang, Z.; Dougherty, U.; Mustafi, R.; Kong, J.; Deb, D.K.; Zheng, H.; Bissonnette, M.; Li, Y.C. Inactivation of the vitamin D receptor in APCmin/+ mice reveals a critical role for the vitamin D receptor in intestinal tumor growth. *Int. J. Cancer* **2012**, *130*, 10–19. [CrossRef] [PubMed]
93. Fedirko, V.; Bostick, R.M.; Flanders, W.D.; Long, Q.; Sidelnikov, E.; Shaukat, A.; Daniel, C.R.; Rutherford, R.E.; Woodard, J.J. Effects of vitamin D and calcium on proliferation and differentiation in normal colon mucosa: A randomized clinical trial. *Cancer Epidemiol. Biomark. Prev.* **2009**, *18*, 2933–2941. [CrossRef] [PubMed]
94. Ahearn, T.U.; Shaukat, A.; Flanders, W.D.; Rutherford, R.E.; Bostick, R.M. A randomized clinical trial of the effects of supplemental calcium and vitamin D3 on the APC/beta-catenin pathway in the normal mucosa of colorectal adenoma patients. *Cancer Prev. Res.* **2012**, *5*, 1247–1256. [CrossRef] [PubMed]
95. Bostick, R.M. Effects of supplemental vitamin D and calcium on normal colon tissue and circulating biomarkers of risk for colorectal neoplasms. *J. Steroid Biochem. Mol. Biol.* **2015**, *148*, 86–95. [CrossRef] [PubMed]
96. Liu, S.; Barry, E.L.; Baron, J.A.; Rutherford, R.E.; Seabrook, M.E.; Bostick, R.M. Effects of supplemental calcium and vitamin D on the APC/beta-catenin pathway in the normal colorectal mucosa of colorectal adenoma patients. *Mol. Carcinog.* **2017**, *56*, 412–424. [CrossRef] [PubMed]
97. Boughanem, H.; Cabrera-Mulero, A.; Hernández-Alonso, P.; Clemente-Postigo, M.; Casanueva, F.F.; Tinahones, F.J.; Morcillo, S.; Crujeiras, A.B.; Macias-Gonzalez, M. Association between variation of circulating 25-OH vitamin D and methylation of secreted frizzled-related protein 2 in colorectal cancer. *Clin. Epigenetics* **2020**, *12*, 83. [CrossRef]
98. Nusse, R.; Varmus, H.E. Many tumors induced by the mouse mammary tumor virus contain a provirus integrated in the same region of the host genome. *Cell* **1982**, *31*, 99–109. [CrossRef]
99. Geyer, F.C.; Lacroix-Triki, M.; Savage, K.; Arnedos, M.; Lambros, M.B.; MacKay, A.; Natrajan, R.; Reis-Filho, J.S. beta-Catenin pathway activation in breast cancer is associated with triple-negative phenotype but not with CTNNB1 mutation. *Mod. Pathol.* **2011**, *24*, 209–231. [CrossRef]
100. Pendás-Franco, N.; González-Sancho, J.M.; Suarez, Y.; Aguilera, O.; Steinmeyer, A.; Gamallo, C.; Berciano, M.T.; Lafarga, M.; Muñoz, A. Vitamin D regulates the phenotype of human breast cancer cells. *Differentiation* **2007**, *75*, 193–207. [CrossRef]
101. Jeong, Y.; Swami, S.; Krishnan, A.V.; Williams, J.D.; Martin, S.; Horst, R.L.; Albertelli, M.A.; Feldman, B.J.; Feldman, D.; Diehn, M. Inhibition of Mouse Breast Tumor-Initiating Cells by Calcitriol and Dietary Vitamin D. *Mol. Cancer Ther.* **2015**, *14*, 1951–1961. [CrossRef] [PubMed]
102. Johnson, A.L.; Zinser, G.M.; Waltz, S.E. Vitamin D3-dependent VDR signaling delays ron-mediated breast tumorigenesis through suppression of beta-catenin activity. *Oncotarget* **2015**, *6*, 16304–16320. [CrossRef] [PubMed]
103. Zheng, W.; Duan, B.; Zhang, Q.; Ouyang, L.; Peng, W.; Qian, F.; Wang, Y.; Huang, S. Vitamin D-induced vitamin D receptor expression induces tamoxifen sensitivity in MCF-7 stem cells via suppression of Wnt/beta-catenin signaling. *Biosci. Rep.* **2018**, *38*, BSR20180595. [CrossRef] [PubMed]

104. Zheng, Y.; Trivedi, T.; Lin, R.C.; Fong-Yee, C.; Nolte, R.; Manibo, J.; Chen, Y.; Hossain, M.; Horas, K.; Dunstan, C.; et al. Loss of the vitamin D receptor in human breast and prostate cancers strongly induces cell apoptosis through downregulation of Wnt/beta-catenin signaling. *Bone Res.* **2017**, *5*, 17023. [CrossRef] [PubMed]
105. Wang, B.; Liu, M.; Zhuang, R.; Jiang, J.; Gao, J.; Wang, H.; Chen, H.; Zhang, Z.; Kuang, Y.; Li, P. Long non-coding RNA CCAT2 promotes epithelial-mesenchymal transition involving Wnt/beta-catenin pathway in epithelial ovarian carcinoma cells. *Oncol. Lett.* **2018**, *15*, 3369–3375. [PubMed]
106. Wang, L.; Zhou, S.; Guo, B. Vitamin D suppresses ovarian cancer growth and invasion by targeting long non-coding RNA CCAT2. *Int. J. Mol. Sci.* **2020**, *21*, 2334. [CrossRef] [PubMed]
107. Srivastava, A.K.; Rizvi, A.; Cui, T.; Han, C.; Banerjee, A.; Naseem, I.; Zheng, Y.; Wani, A.A.; Wang, Q.E. Depleting ovarian cancer stem cells with calcitriol. *Oncotarget* **2018**, *9*, 14481–14491. [CrossRef]
108. Corachán, A.; Ferrero, H.; Aguilar, A.; Garcia, N.; Monleon, J.; Faus, A.; Cervelló, I.; Pellicer, A. Inhibition of tumor cell proliferation in human uterine leiomyomas by vitamin D via Wnt/beta-catenin pathway. *Fertil. Steril.* **2019**, *111*, 397–407. [CrossRef]
109. Tapia, C.; Suares, A.; De Genaro, P.; Gonzalez-Pardo, V. In vitro studies revealed a downregulation of Wnt/beta-catenin cascade by active vitamin D and TX 527 analog in a Kaposi's sarcoma cellular model. *Toxicol. In Vitro* **2020**, *63*, 104748. [CrossRef]
110. Xu, S.; Zhang, Z.H.; Fu, L.; Song, J.; Xie, D.D.; Yu, D.X.; Xu, D.X.; Sun, G.P. Calcitriol inhibits migration and invasion of renal cell carcinoma cells by suppressing Smad2/3-, STAT3- and beta-catenin-mediated epithelial-mesenchymal transition. *Cancer Sci.* **2020**, *111*, 59–71. [CrossRef]
111. Arensman, M.D.; Nguyen, P.; Kershaw, K.M.; Lay, A.R.; Ostertag-Hill, C.A.; Sherman, M.H.; Downes, M.; Liddle, C.; Evans, R.M.; Dawson, D.W. Calcipotriol targets LRP6 to inhibit Wnt signaling in pancreatic cancer. *Mol. Cancer Res.* **2015**, *13*, 1509–1519. [CrossRef] [PubMed]
112. Zinser, G.M.; Sundberg, J.P.; Welsh, J. Vitamin D3 receptor ablation sensitizes skin to chemically induced tumorigenesis. *Carcinogenesis* **2002**, *23*, 2103–2109. [CrossRef] [PubMed]
113. Ellison, T.I.; Smith, M.K.; Gilliam, A.C.; MacDonald, P.N. Inactivation of the vitamin D receptor enhances susceptibility of murine skin to UV-induced tumorigenesis. *J. Investig. Dermatol.* **2008**, *128*, 2508–2517. [CrossRef] [PubMed]
114. Teichert, A.E.; Elalieh, H.; Elias, P.M.; Welsh, J.; Bikle, D.D. Overexpression of hedgehog signaling is associated with epidermal tumor formation in vitamin D receptor-null mice. *J. Investig. Dermatol.* **2011**, *131*, 2289–2297. [CrossRef]
115. Pálmer, H.G.; Anjos-Afonso, F.; Carmeliet, G.; Takeda, H.; Watt, F.M. The vitamin D receptor is a Wnt effector that controls hair follicle differentiation and specifies tumor type in adult epidermis. *PLoS ONE* **2008**, *3*, e1483. [CrossRef]
116. Jiang, Y.J.; Teichert, A.E.; Fong, F.; Oda, Y.; Bikle, D.D. 1alpha,25(OH)2-dihydroxyvitamin D3/VDR protects the skin from UVB-induced tumor formation by interacting with the beta-catenin pathway. *J. Steroid Biochem. Mol. Biol.* **2013**, *136*, 229–232. [CrossRef]
117. Bikle, D.D.; Oda, Y.; Tu, C.L.; Jiang, Y. Novel mechanisms for the vitamin D receptor (VDR) in the skin and in skin cancer. *J. Steroid Biochem. Mol. Biol.* **2015**, *148*, 47–51. [CrossRef]
118. Muralidhar, S.; Filia, A.; Nsengimana, J.; Poźniak, J.; O'Shea, S.J.; Diaz, J.M.; Harland, M.; Randerson-Moor, J.A.; Reichrath, J.; Laye, J.P.; et al. Vitamin D-VDR signaling inhibits Wnt/beta-catenin-mediated melanoma progression and promotes antitumor immunity. *Cancer Res.* **2019**, *79*, 5986–5998. [CrossRef]
119. Salehi-Tabar, R.; Nguyen-Yamamoto, L.; Tavera-Mendoza, L.E.; Quail, T.; Dimitrov, V.; An, B.S.; Glass, L.; Goltzman, D.; White, J.H. Vitamin D receptor as a master regulator of the c-MYC/MXD1 network. *Proc. Natl. Acad. Sci. USA* **2012**, *109*, 18827–18832. [CrossRef]
120. Oak, A.S.W.; Bocheva, G.; Kim, T.K.; Brożyna, A.A.; Janjetovic, Z.; Athar, M.; Tuckey, R.C.; Slominski, A.T. Noncalcemic vitamin D hydroxyderivatives inhibit human oral squamous cell carcinoma and down-regulate Hedgehog and WNT/beta-catenin pathways. *Anticancer Res.* **2020**, *40*, 2467–2474. [CrossRef]
121. Rubin, B.; Pilon, C.; Pezzani, R.; Rebellato, A.; Fallo, F. The effects of mitotane and 1alpha,25-dihydroxyvitamin D3 on Wnt/beta-catenin signaling in human adrenocortical carcinoma cells. *J. Endocrinol. Investig.* **2020**, *43*, 357–367. [CrossRef]

122. Chen, J.; Katz, L.H.; Muñoz, N.M.; Gu, S.; Shin, J.H.; Jogunoori, W.S.; Lee, M.H.; Belkin, M.D.; Kim, S.B.; White, J.C.; et al. Vitamin D deficiency promotes liver tumor growth in transforming growth factor-beta/smad3-deficient mice through Wnt and Toll-like receptor 7 pathway modulation. *Sci. Rep.* **2016**, *6*, 30217. [CrossRef]
123. Matsuda, A.; Ishiguro, K.; Yan, I.K.; Patel, T. Therapeutic efficacy of vitamin D in experimental c-MET-beta-catenin-driven hepatocellular cancer. *Gene Expr.* **2019**, *19*, 151–159. [CrossRef]
124. Rosen, C.J.; Adams, J.S.; Bikle, D.D.; Black, D.M.; Demay, M.B.; Manson, J.E.; Murad, M.H.; Kovacs, C.S. The nonskeletal effects of vitamin D: An Endocrine Society scientific statement. *Endocr. Rev.* **2012**, *33*, 456–492. [CrossRef] [PubMed]
125. Zenata, O.; Vrzal, R. Fine tuning of vitamin D receptor (VDR) activity by post-transcriptional and post-translational modifications. *Oncotarget* **2017**, *8*, 35390–35402. [CrossRef] [PubMed]
126. Anastas, J.N.; Moon, R.T. WNT signalling pathways as therapeutic targets in cancer. *Nat. Rev. Cancer* **2013**, *13*, 11–26. [CrossRef] [PubMed]
127. Dongre, A.; Weinberg, R.A. New insights into the mechanisms of epithelial-mesenchymal transition and implications for cancer. *Nat. Rev. Mol. Cell Biol.* **2019**, *20*, 69–84. [CrossRef]
128. Zhou, B.P.; Deng, J.; Xia, W.; Xu, J.; Li, Y.M.; Gunduz, M.; Hung, M.C. Dual regulation of Snail by GSK-3beta-mediated phosphorylation in control of epithelial-mesenchymal transition. *Nat. Cell Biol.* **2004**, *6*, 931–940. [CrossRef]
129. Yook, J.I.; Li, X.Y.; Ota, I.; Fearon, E.R.; Weiss, S.J. Wnt-dependent regulation of the E-cadherin repressor snail. *J. Biol. Chem.* **2005**, *280*, 11740–11748. [CrossRef]
130. Wu, Z.-Q.; Li, X.-Y.; Hu, C.Y.; Ford, M.; Kleer, C.G.; Weiss, S.J. Canonical Wnt signaling regulates Slug activity and links epithelial-mesenchymal transition with epigenetic Breast Cancer 1, Early Onset (BRCA1) repression. *Proc. Natl. Acad. Sci. USA* **2012**, *109*, 16654–16659. [CrossRef]
131. Bachelder, R.E.; Yoon, S.O.; Francí, C.; García de Herreros, A.; Mercurio, A.M. Glycogen synthase kinase-3 is an endogenous inhibitor of Snail transcription: Implications for the epithelial-mesenchymal transition. *J. Cell Biol.* **2005**, *168*, 29–33. [CrossRef] [PubMed]
132. Yook, J.I.; Li, X.Y.; Ota, I.; Hu, C.; Kim, H.S.; Kim, N.H.; Cha, S.Y.; Ryu, J.K.; Choi, Y.J.; Kim, J.; et al. A Wnt-Axin2-GSK3beta cascade regulates Snail1 activity in breast cancer cells. *Nat. Cell Biol.* **2006**, *8*, 1398–1406. [CrossRef] [PubMed]
133. Wu, Y.; Ginther, C.; Kim, J.; Mosher, N.; Chung, S.; Slamon, D.; Vadgama, J.V. Expression of Wnt3 activates Wnt/beta-catenin pathway and promotes EMT-like phenotype in trastuzumab-resistant HER2-overexpressing breast cancer cells. *Mol. Cancer Res.* **2012**, *10*, 1597–1606. [CrossRef] [PubMed]
134. Larriba, M.J.; Martín-Villar, E.; García, J.M.; Pereira, F.; Peña, C.; García de Herreros, A.; Bonilla, F.; Muñoz, A. Snail2 cooperates with Snail1 in the repression of vitamin D receptor in colon cancer. *Carcinogenesis* **2009**, *30*, 1459–1468. [CrossRef] [PubMed]
135. Peña, C.; García, J.M.; Silva, J.; García, V.; Rodríguez, R.; Alonso, I.; Millán, I.; Salas, C.; García de Herreros, A.; Muñoz, A.; et al. E-cadherin and vitamin D receptor regulation by SNAIL and ZEB1 in colon cancer: Clinicopathological correlations. *Hum. Mol. Genet.* **2005**, *14*, 3361–3370. [CrossRef]
136. Peña, C.; García, J.M.; García, V.; Silva, J.; Domínguez, G.; Rodríguez, R.; Maximiano, C.; García de Herreros, A.; Muñoz, A.; Bonilla, F. The expression levels of the transcriptional regulators p300 and CtBP modulate the correlations between SNAIL, ZEB1, E-cadherin and vitamin D receptor in human colon carcinomas. *Int. J. Cancer* **2006**, *119*, 2098–2104. [CrossRef]
137. Peña, C.; García, J.M.; Larriba, M.J.; Barderas, R.; Gómez, I.; Herrera, M.; García, V.; Silva, J.; Domínguez, G.; Rodríguez, R.; et al. SNAI1 expression in colon cancer related with CDH1 and VDR downregulation in normal adjacent tissue. *Oncogene* **2009**, *28*, 4375–4385. [CrossRef]
138. Mittal, M.K.; Myers, J.N.; Misra, S.; Bailey, C.K.; Chaudhuri, G. In vivo binding to and functional repression of the *VDR* gene promoter by SLUG in human breast cells. *Biochem. Biophys. Res. Commun.* **2008**, *372*, 30–34. [CrossRef]
139. Yang, H.; Zhang, Y.; Zhou, Z.; Jiang, X.; Shen, A. Snail-1 regulates VDR signaling and inhibits 1,25(OH)-D_3 action in osteosarcoma. *Eur. J. Pharmacol.* **2011**, *670*, 341–346. [CrossRef]
140. Knackstedt, R.W.; Moseley, V.R.; Sun, S.; Wargovich, M.J. Vitamin D receptor and retinoid X receptor α status and vitamin D insufficiency in models of murine colitis. *Cancer Prev. Res.* **2013**, *6*, 585–593. [CrossRef]

141. Zhou, A.D.; Diao, L.T.; Xu, H.; Xiao, Z.D.; Li, J.H.; Zhou, H.; Qu, L.H. beta-Catenin/LEF1 transactivates the microRNA-371-373 cluster that modulates the Wnt/beta-catenin-signaling pathway. *Oncogene* **2012**, *31*, 2968–2978. [CrossRef] [PubMed]
142. Loayza-Puch, F.; Yoshida, Y.; Matsuzaki, T.; Takahashi, C.; Kitayama, H.; Noda, M. Hypoxia and RAS-signaling pathways converge on, and cooperatively downregulate, the RECK tumor-suppressor protein through microRNAs. *Oncogene* **2010**, *29*, 2638–2648. [CrossRef] [PubMed]
143. Yamashita, S.; Yamamoto, H.; Mimori, K.; Nishida, N.; Takahashi, H.; Haraguchi, N.; Tanaka, F.; Shibata, K.; Sekimoto, M.; Ishii, H.; et al. MicroRNA-372 is associated with poor prognosis in colorectal cancer. *Oncology* **2012**, *82*, 205–212. [CrossRef] [PubMed]
144. Eyking, A.; Reis, H.; Frank, M.; Gerken, G.; Schmid, K.W.; Cario, E. MiR-205 and miR-373 are associated with aggressive human mucinous colorectal cancer. *PLoS ONE* **2016**, *11*, e0156871. [CrossRef] [PubMed]
145. Wang, L.Q.; Yu, P.; Li, B.; Guo, Y.H.; Liang, Z.R.; Zheng, L.L.; Yang, J.H.; Xu, H.; Liu, S.; Zheng, L.S.; et al. miR-372 and miR-373 enhance the stemness of colorectal cancer cells by repressing differentiation signaling pathways. *Mol. Oncol.* **2018**, *12*, 1949–1964. [CrossRef]

Publisher's Note: MDPI stays neutral with regard to jurisdictional claims in published maps and institutional affiliations.

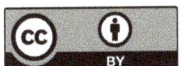

© 2020 by the authors. Licensee MDPI, Basel, Switzerland. This article is an open access article distributed under the terms and conditions of the Creative Commons Attribution (CC BY) license (http://creativecommons.org/licenses/by/4.0/).

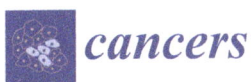

Review

Wnt/β-Catenin Target Genes in Colon Cancer Metastasis: The Special Case of L1CAM

Sanith Cheriyamundath and Avri Ben-Ze'ev *

Department of Molecular Cell Biology, Weizmann Institute of Science, Rehovot 76100, Israel; sanith.cheriyamundath@weizmann.ac.il
* Correspondence: avri.ben-zeev@weizmann.ac.il; Tel.: +972-8-934-2422

Received: 5 October 2020; Accepted: 17 November 2020; Published: 19 November 2020

Simple Summary: The Wnt/β-catenin cell–cell signaling pathway is one of the most basic and highly conserved pathways for intercellular communications regulating key steps during development, differentiation, and cancer. In colorectal cancer (CRC), in particular, aberrant activation of the Wnt/β-catenin pathway is believed to be responsible for perpetuating the disease from the very early stages of cancer development. A large number of downstream target genes of β-catenin-T-cell factor (TCF), including oncogenes, were detected as regulators of CRC development. In this review, we will summarize studies mainly on one such target gene, the L1CAM (L1) cell adhesion receptor, that is selectively induced in invasive and metastatic CRC cells and in regenerating cells of the intestine following injury. We will describe studies on the genes activated when the levels of L1 are increased in CRC cells and their effectiveness in propagating CRC development. These downstream targets of L1-signaling can serve in diagnosis and may provide additional targets for CRC therapy.

Abstract: Cell adhesion to neighboring cells is a fundamental biological process in multicellular organisms that is required for tissue morphogenesis. A tight coordination between cell–cell adhesion, signaling, and gene expression is a characteristic feature of normal tissues. Changes, and often disruption of this coordination, are common during invasive and metastatic cancer development. The Wnt/β-catenin signaling pathway is an excellent model for studying the role of adhesion-mediated signaling in colorectal cancer (CRC) invasion and metastasis, because β-catenin has a dual role in the cell; it is a major adhesion linker of cadherin transmembrane receptors to the cytoskeleton and, in addition, it is also a key transducer of Wnt signaling to the nucleus, where it acts as a co-transcriptional activator of Wnt target genes. Hyperactivation of Wnt/β-catenin signaling is a common feature in the majority of CRC patients. We found that the neural cell adhesion receptor L1CAM (L1) is a target gene of β-catenin signaling and is induced in carcinoma cells of CRC patients, where it plays an important role in CRC metastasis. In this review, we will discuss studies on β-catenin target genes activated during CRC development (in particular, L1), the signaling pathways affected by L1, and the role of downstream target genes activated by L1 overexpression, especially those that are also part of the intestinal stem cell gene signature. As intestinal stem cells are highly regulated by Wnt signaling and are believed to also play major roles in CRC progression, unravelling the mechanisms underlying the regulation of these genes will shed light on both normal intestinal homeostasis and the development of invasive and metastatic CRC.

Keywords: L1; Wnt target genes; β-catenin; cell adhesion; colon cancer; NF-κB; invasion and metastasis; cancer stem cells; EMT; Lgr5

1. Introduction

Cell–cell adhesion is a basic biological process in multicellular organisms that determines cellular and tissue morphogenesis, and its disruption is a hallmark of cancer development. Aberrant signaling mediated by changes in cell–cell adhesion is a characteristic feature of invasive and metastatic cancer cells. Wnt/β-catenin signaling is a key signaling pathway that is hyperactivated in the majority of inherited colorectal cancer (CRC) patients and serves as a very useful model for studying adhesion-mediated mechanisms underlying CRC development [1,2]. This notion is supported by findings demonstrating that β-catenin plays a dual role in the cell. It is a major linker of cell–cell adhesion receptors (of the cadherin type) to the actin-cytoskeleton and, in addition, β-catenin plays a critical role in transmitting the Wnt signal to the nucleus by being a co-transcriptional activator [together with T-cell factor (TCF)] of Wnt target genes in the nucleus [3,4]. These two seemingly unrelated roles of β-catenin and the characteristic hyperactivation of Wnt/β-catenin signaling in CRC can serve as a useful system for investigating the roles of adhesion-mediated and Wnt signaling in CRC invasion and metastasis.

Wnt signaling was discovered over 40 years ago [5,6] and was first shown to play a role in determining the segmentation pattern in *Drosophila* [7]. Following these original studies, in the coming years, a role for Wnt signaling in embryonic axis determination in vertebrates was reported [8], and the potential involvement of the Wnt pathway in cancer development in humans was suggested [9]. In parallel, numerous studies addressed the identification of downstream components in the Wnt signaling pathway and discovered that inactivating mutations in the adenomatous polyposis coli (APC) gene, which is involved in β-catenin degradation, is a key step in the activation of Wnt signaling during CRC development [10]. In addition, stabilizing mutations in β-catenin against degradation by the ubiquitin-proteasomal system were also identified in a minority of CRC cases [11,12]. At this stage, an important avenue of research consisted of unraveling the target genes of Wnt/β-catenin signaling that are responsible for human CRC development. As the early steps in tumorigenesis are driven by changes that lead to uncontrolled proliferation of cells, initial studies focused on asking whether key regulators of the cell cycle (especially those leading to increased cell proliferation) are target genes of Wnt signaling and contain β-catenin/TCF binding sites in their promoter region. These studies led to the discovery of c-myc [13] and cyclin D1 [14,15] as target genes of β-catenin/TCF transactivation. Since then, hundreds of additional β-catenin-TCF target genes were discovered; for most of these genes, their role in CRC development remains to be determined [16]. Initial immunohistochemical studies of human CRC tissue did not detect a significant accumulation of β-catenin in the nuclei of early-stage CRC tissue and β-catenin localization remained mostly at cell–cell junctions in both normal colonic epithelial cells and in differentiated areas of CRC tissue [17,18]. However, at the later stages of CRC development, especially during the invasive and metastatic stages of tumor progression, a vast accumulation of β-catenin could be demonstrated, mostly in the nuclei of cancer cells [17,18], in addition to a specific expression of β-catenin target genes at the invasive areas of the tumor [19].

In this review, we will describe studies mainly on one such β-catenin-TCF target gene, the neuronal cell adhesion receptor L1CAM (L1) and its downstream targets, and its role in CRC invasion and metastasis. We will also discuss studies suggesting that some genes induced by L1 overexpression are known genes of the colonic stem cell signature that control the homeostasis of the intestinal stem cell compartment. Because CRC is believed to originate from tumorigenic intestinal stem cells [20], we hope that studies on L1 and downstream Wnt/β-catenin target genes will provide novel insights into the control of normal intestinal homeostasis and will also provide new targets for CRC therapy.

2. Members of the L1 Family of Cell Adhesion Receptors Are β-Catenin-TCF Target Genes

Initial DNA microarray analyses of genes induced by activated β-catenin-TCF signaling in cancer cells identified two members of the L1 family of immunoglobulin-like cell adhesion receptors, NrCAM [21,22] and L1 [19]. These findings were unexpected because both L1 and NrCAM were known to be present mostly in nerve cells, playing key roles during brain development by regulating a number of dynamic cellular processes including axonal growth, fasciculation, and pathfinding [23,24]. In previous studies, numerous point mutations were discovered in the L1 molecule that have severe consequences on brain development, leading to mental retardation by a group of syndromes known as L1 syndrome, MASA syndrome, and X-linked hydrocephalus [25–29].

L1 is a cell adhesion transmembrane receptor, believed to act mostly by homophilic interactions with L1 on the surface of neighboring cells. L1 belongs to the superfamily of immunoglobulin-like cell adhesion receptors, containing six Ig-like domains and five fibronectin type III repeats; a transmembrane sequence; and a highly conserved (from *C. elegans* to man) cytoplasmic tail that has binding sites for ezrin, ankyrin, and other PDZ-containing proteins (Figure 1). In addition, L1 can be cleaved in the juxtamembrane region, outside the cell, by the metalloprotease ADAM10, and inside the cell, it has binding sites for the γ-secretase cleavage complex (Figure 1). Unlike cadherins that are characterized by strong homophilic interactions, L1 can interact via both homophilic and heterophilic binding to other neuronal cell adhesion molecules including neurocan, neuropilin1, axonin, and N-CAM [30]. In addition, L1 can associate with ECM components (fibronectin, laminin, tenascin) and ECM receptors (integrins) and can also bind to growth factor receptors, such as EGFR and basic FGFR [31]. Because of these numerous weak interactions of L1 with a variety of molecules, an increase in the expression of L1 in cancer cells could be advantageous for promoting the motile, invasive, and metastatic stages of tumorigenesis.

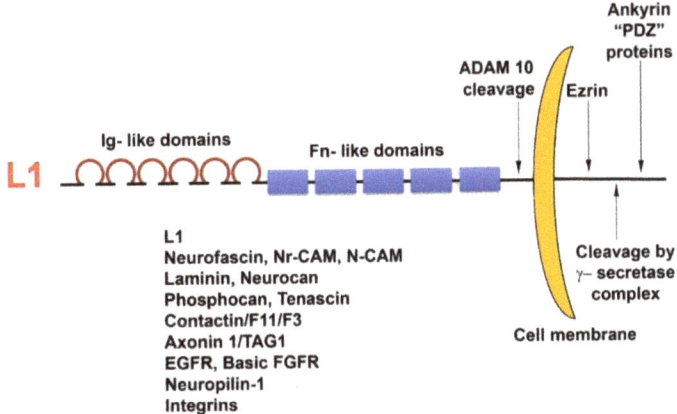

Figure 1. Domain structure and binding partners of L1. Note the numerous types of L1 ligands in the ectodomain as well as in the cytoplasmic tail domain of the molecule.

3. The Roles of L1 in Promoting CRC Cell Proliferation, Motility, Tumorigenesis, and Metastasis

Overexpression of L1 in 3T3 mouse fibroblasts and in human CRC cell lines results in elevated cell proliferation under stress (in the absence of serum); increased motility; invasion; tumorigenesis upon s.c injection into mice [19]; and, in the case of CRC cells, metastasis to the liver, a hallmark of human CRC progression [32]. The metalloprotease ADAM10, also a target gene of β-catenin-TCF transactivation, cleaves the ectodomain of L1 (Figure 1), thereby leading to its shedding, and promotes the rebinding of the shed L1 ectodomain to L1 molecules on the cell surface and enhances the metastatic potential of human CRC cells [32].

Immunohistochemical analysis of human CRC tissue revealed that the more differentiated areas of the tumor and the normal colonic epithelium do not express L1 [19]. L1 is exclusively expressed at the invading edge of human CRC tissue (Figure 2) in the membrane of cells that display strong nuclear β-catenin staining, indicative of a highly active β-catenin-TCF transactivation [19]. These results were recently confirmed and extended to show that, while L1 is not required for adenoma initiation, it plays multiple roles in cancer propagation, liver metastasis, and chemoresistance [33]. This study also demonstrated that L1 is not expressed in the homeostatic intestinal epithelium, but its expression is required for CRC organoid formation and metastasis initiation and growth. Finally, L1 expression was shown to be crucial for the regrowth occurring during wound healing in the intestine following injury [33]. Taken together, these results are reminiscent of the important roles played by L1 in the dynamic cellular processes occurring in nerve cells during brain development (i.e., axonal growth, pathfinding, and fasciculation) [34].

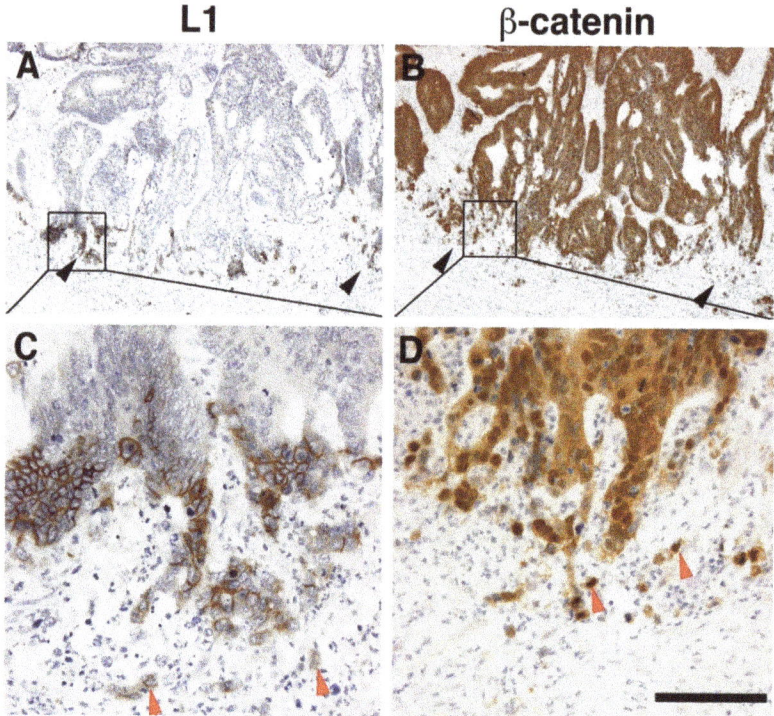

Figure 2. L1 is exclusively expressed at the invasive front of human colorectal cancer (CRC) tissue in cells expressing β-catenin in their nuclei. (**A**) Immunohistochemical staining of human CRC tissue for L1. Note the preferential localization of L1 in invasive areas of the tumor (black arrowheads), but not in the inner more differentiated areas of the tumor. (**B**) In contrast to L1 localization, a serial tissue section stained with anti β-catenin antibody displays a uniform staining of the same CRC tissue area. (**C**) Enlarged picture of the boxed area in (**A**) showing the membranal localization of L1. Single CRC cells invading into the stroma could also be seen (red arrowheads). (**D**) Magnified picture of the boxed area shown in (**B**) localizing β-catenin staining in both the cytoplasm and nuclei of CRC tissue cells and in the nuclei of single invasive cells (red arrowheads) at the tumor tissue edge [19]. Scale bar: (**A**,**B**) 375 µm, (**C**,**D**) 75 µm.

4. Mechanisms and Downstream Targets of L1 Signaling

Numerous studies have addressed the mechanisms underlying the downstream signaling of L1. In neuronal cells, neurite outgrowth was shown to involve the MAPK pathway by increasing the expression of MAP2 [35]. In addition, the involvement of PI3K, ERK, and Rac-1 was also implicated in L1 signaling [36–39]. More recent studies have shown that, in CRC cells [40] and in pancreatic cancer cells [41], the signaling downstream of L1 involves the NF-κB pathway. According to this model (Figure 3), the L1 signaling pathway includes the activation of the cytoskeletal protein ezrin by phosphorylation on Thr567 (by ROCK), which leads to the re-localization of ezrin from filopodia to L1 in the membrane domain (Figure 3) and requires Tyr1151 on the L1 cytodomain (Figure 3B). Point mutations in Tyr1151 abolish the tumorigenic and metastatic capacities conferred by L1 [40]. In the next step, the IκB–NFκB complex is recruited to this multimolecular assembly, which enhances IκB phosphorylation and its degradation by the proteasome, thereby releasing NF-κB from IκB, which enables the migration of NF-κB into the nucleus and the activation of NF-κB target genes (Figure 3C). In support of this model, the activated (phosphorylated) p65 NF-κB subunit was detected in the nuclei of CRC tissue cells in invasive areas of the tumor together with L1 and ezrin expression in the membrane and cytoplasm of the same cells [40]. In addition, blocking NF-κB signaling in CRC cells expressing elevated L1 expression abolishes the properties conferred by L1 including enhanced growth and motility, tumorigenesis, and metastasis [40].

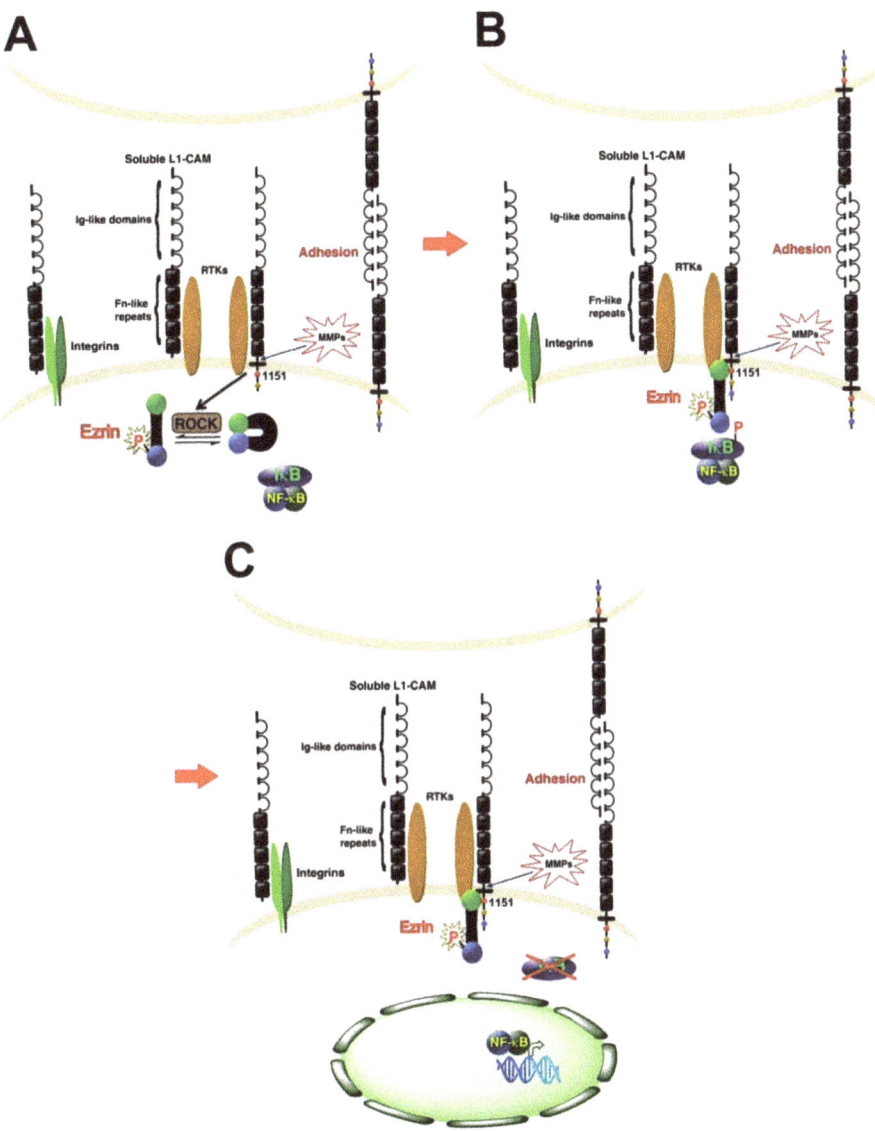

Figure 3. An NF-κB-ezrin signaling pathway is involved in L1 signaling in CRC cells. (**A**) The

cytoskeletal protein ezrin is recruited to the cytoplasmic tail of L1 after it is activated by ROCK phosphorylation. The binding of activated ezrin to L1 involves Tyr1151 on the L1 cytoplasmic tail. (**B**) The L1-activated ezrin complex recruits the cytoplasmic NF-κB–IκB complex and leads to increased phosphorylation of IκB. (**C**) Elevated IκB phosphorylation results in its increased degradation by the proteasome and the release of NF-κB from the complex followed by NF-κB migration into the nucleus and transcriptional activation of target genes [40].

5. Genes Induced or Suppressed by L1 That Affect CRC Progression

In the next step, we wished to determine the genes induced, or suppressed, by L1 in CRC cells via an NF-κB-dependent mechanism using cDNA microarrays and compared these gene expression patterns to those of a large set of human CRC tissue samples [42]. A rather unexpected result of these analyses was the finding that, among the genes whose expression was suppressed by L1 overexpression (and by NF-κB signaling), and was also suppressed in human CRC tissue samples, was the well-known oncogene c-KIT [42]. Reconstitution of c-KIT expression in human CRC cell lines overexpressing L1 resulted in the inhibition of the pro-metastatic properties promoted by L1 in these cells [42]. The mechanism underlying this anti-metastatic effect conferred by c-KIT also involves the NF-κB pathway, but in this case, NF-κB plays an inhibitory role by suppressing the expression of SP-1, a key transcription factor of the c-KIT gene. The inhibition of SP-1 expression resulted in decreased c-KIT levels. In addition, the reduction in c-KIT also promoted an elevation in E-cadherin levels, the growing of cells in flat epithelial-like colonies, and the inhibition of SLUG (a key transcription factor of the EMT process), suggesting a mesenchymal to epithelial conversion (MET) [42]. While these dramatic effects of c-KIT on metastasis and cell motility indicated a tumor suppressive effect played by c-KIT [42], the proliferation in vitro and in vivo (in mice) of c-KIT overexpressing CRC cells showed that c-KIT enhances tumorigenesis, thus pointing to distinct modes of action of c-KIT in early versus late phases of tumor progression. A similar result was also reported for the key oncogene c-myc [43], thus further arguing that separate pathways mediate the tumorigenic and metastatic processes by these oncogenic molecules.

Further insight into the nature of genes induced by L1 in CRC cells by the NF-κB-ezrin pathway and their role in CRC tumorigenesis was provided by the discovery of insulin like growth factor receptor 2 (IGFBP-2) among these genes [44]. IGFBP-2 overexpression mimics the effects conferred by L1 on cell proliferation, motility tumorigenesis and metastasis, and the suppression of IGFBP-2 levels in L1-overexpressing cells blocked these properties conferred by L1 in CRC cells [44]. Interestingly, IGFBP-2 forms a molecular complex with L1, further supporting the important role played by these molecules in CRC progression. A most significant finding regarding the possible role of IGFBP-2 in CRC was derived from immunohistochemical analyses of CRC tissue samples to detect the localization of IGFBP-2. We detected IGFBP-2 at increased levels throughout the human CRC tissue samples, co-localizing with the activated p65 NF-κB subunit [44]. Most importantly, in the adjacent normal colonic mucosa, IGFBP-2 was exclusively localized at the bottom of the colonic crypts (Figure 4A). Because cells in the colonic crypts, especially at the crypts bottom, contain the colonic stem cells [45], which are believed to also be progenitors of the developing human CRC [45], we have further investigated this relationship between L1-induced genes and the colonic stem cell signature genes.

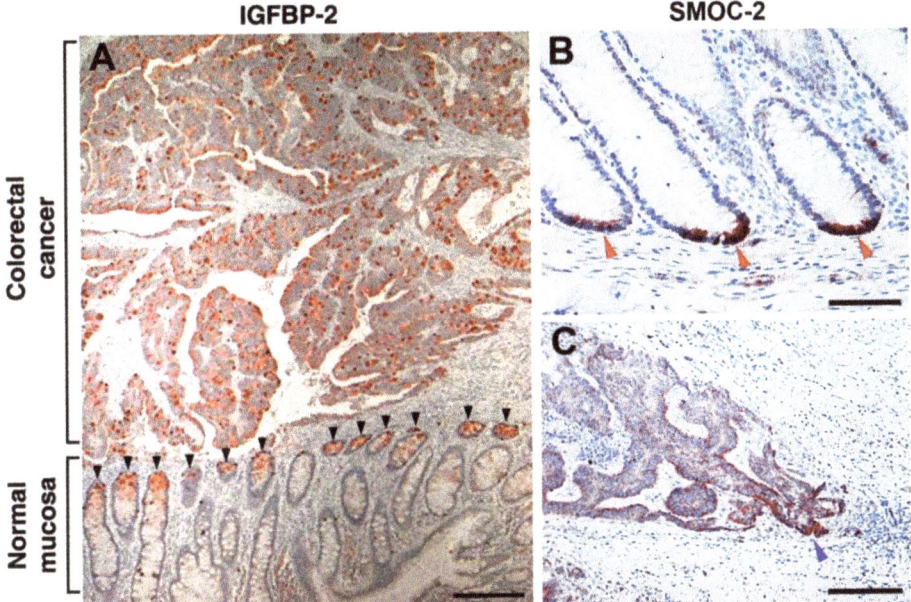

Figure 4. Genes induced by L1 in CRC cells include intestinal stem cell signature genes. (**A**) Insulin like growth factor receptor 2 (IGFBP-2) staining of CRC tissue revealed strong staining of the tumor tissue throughout the tissue, while in the adjacent normal mucosa, IGFBP-2 staining was exclusively confined to the bottom of colonic crypts (black arrowheads). (**B**) The intestinal stem cell signature gene secreted modular calcium-binding matricellular protein-2 (SMOC-2) was detected at the bottom of colonic crypts in normal colonic mucosa (red arrowheads). (**C**) In CRC tissue, SMOC-2 was localized in more differentiated areas of the tumor with stronger staining of invasive areas of the tumor (blue arrowhead) [44,46]. Scale bar: (**A**) 250 µm, (**B**) 50 µm, (**C**) 100 µm.

6. Colonic Stem Cell Signature Genes Induced by L1 in CRC Cells

The human intestinal epithelium contains invaginating crypts that harbor, at their base, the intestinal stem cells that express the Lgr5 molecular marker [20]. This epithelium is the most frequently regenerating tissue in the body and the lifetime of intestinal epithelial cells is less than a week. The stem cells fuel a continuous generation of all differentiated colonic cell types and are believed to be the progenitors of human CRC cells [47]. Among the genes induced by L1-ezrin-NF-κB signaling, we detected (in addition to IGFBP-2) the secreted modular calcium-binding matricellular protein-2 (SMOC-2). SMOC-2 is known as a representative of the group of Lgr5$^+$ intestinal stem cell signature genes in mice [48]. We found that the induction of SMOC-2 in human CRC cells was necessary for the pro-tumorigenic properties conferred by L1 [46]. SMOC-2 overexpression could mimic the increase in cell proliferation under stress, motility, tumorigenesis, and liver metastasis and confers a more mesenchymal phenotype characterized by suppression of E-cadherin levels and an increase in the EMT-promoting transcription factor SNAIL. These properties of SMOC-2 overexpressing in CRC cells involve signaling by integrin linked kinase (ILK) [46]. In addition, we found an increase in the intestinal stem cell signature gene Lgr5 in CRC cells overexpressing SMOC-2, L1, or the p65 subunit of NF-κB [46]. Most significantly, we detected SMOC-2 exclusively at the base of normal colonic epithelial crypts (Figure 4B) and a preferential increase in its expression at invasive areas of human CRC tissue (Figure 4C).

In the next step, we identified clusterin (CLU) as a gene induced by L1 that is also expressed at increased levels in Lgr5$^+$ intestinal stem cells of the mouse [49]. CLU is a secreted highly glycosylated protein that was implicated in playing a role in a variety of human tumors and is considered to be a marker for CRC development [50]. Similar to IGFBP-2 and SMOC-2, CLU overexpression induces CRC motility and tumorigenesis, but CLU does not promote experimental liver metastasis, implying the involvement of additional factors. However, the suppression of CLU in L1-overexpressing cells dramatically reduced their metastatic potential [49]. The mechanism of L1-mediated increase in CLU does not involve the NF-κB pathway, but rather a STAT-1-mediated elevation in the expression of the transcription factor SP-1 that activates the CLU gene promoter [49].

In the search for key intestinal/colonic stem cell compartment signature genes that could be activated by L1-mediated signaling in CRC, we turned to analyze the expression of ASCL2 in L1-overexpressing CRC cells. ASCL2 is a basic-helix-loop-helix transcription factor, a target gene of Wnt/β-catenin signaling and is restricted to Lgr5$^+$ basal crypt cells in both mice and humans [48]. A recent study identified ASCL2 as the key transcriptional regulator that is induced at a very early stage during regeneration of the intestinal stem cell compartment following injury [51]. We found that overexpression of L1 in CRC cells induces the expression and nuclear accumulation of ASCL2, a decrease in E-cadherin levels, and increased levels of β-catenin in the nucleus, together with elevated β-catenin-TCF transactivation of Wnt/β-catenin target genes [52]. This downregulation of E-cadherin expression, the increase in the accumulation of nuclear β-catenin, and the transactivation of Wnt/β-catenin-TCF target genes were also reported in breast cancer cells [53]. This suggests that the replacement of E-cadherin-mediated adhesions by L1 in CRC cells is a more general characteristic of cancer cells. In addition, we found that the overexpression of ASCL2 in CRC cells could mimic the effects conferred by L1 on cell proliferation, motility, tumorigenesis, and liver metastasis (including an elevation in the intestinal stem cell signature genes Lgr5, OLFM4, and SMOC-2), while ASCL2 suppression in L1-transfected CRC cells blocked these properties conferred by L1 [52]. We detected ASCL2 in invasive areas of human CRC tissue in cells expressing increased levels of L1 (but not in normal colon mucosa) [52], indicating that L1 and ASCL2 cooperate in promoting CRC progression.

7. Genes Affected by Point Mutations in the L1 Ectodomain That Regulate CRC Development

As inherited mutations in the L1 ectodomain were shown to affect the adhesive properties of L1 and are associated with severe human brain developmental diseases [25–29,54], we searched for genes induced by L1 that are affected by specific point mutations in the L1 ectodomain and examined their role in CRC development. All the known ectodomain point mutants of L1 that we analyzed lost their ability to confer the tumorigenic and metastatic properties in CRC cells [55]. Among the genes that are specifically affected by the L1/H210Q mutation, but not by other L1 mutations in the L1 ectodomain, we identified the membrane-associated neutral endopeptidase, neprilysin (CD10) [55]. We found that the induction of CD10 by L1 that is blocked by the L1/H210Q mutation is required for the pro-tumorigenic and metastatic capacities conferred by L1 [55]. As with several other L1-induced genes, CD10 expression was dependent on an NF-κB-ezrin signaling pathway and we identified L1 and CD10 in cells localized in invasive areas of CRC tissue, suggesting that the two molecules act together in promoting the invasive properties of CRC cells [55]. The identification of genes that are specifically affected by such L1 ectodomain point mutations could provide additional targets for CRC diagnosis and therapy.

8. Secreted Factors That Promote the Tumorigenesis Induced by L1 Overexpressing CRC Cells

Because a great number of genes that are induced by L1 overexpression in CRC cells are coding for either membrane bound proteins and are exposed to the extracellular milieu, or proteins secreted into the culture medium (see above, IGFBP-2, CLU, neprilysin, SMOC-2), we conducted a proteomic analysis of the secretome from L1 expressing CRC cells. Among the proteins whose levels were increased by L1 expression in CRC cells, we studied the role of the aspartate protease cathepsin D (CTSD), a lysosomal and secreted protein, because numerous studies reported on its association with the development of cancer in various tumors [56–61]. The levels of RNA, protein, and secreted CTSD protein were increased in response to L1 expression, and this induction of CTSD was necessary for L1-mediated CRC progression and liver metastasis [62]. The overexpression of CTSD in CRC cells, in the absence of L1, could confer increased proliferation, motility, tumorigenesis, and liver metastasis in these cells [62]. Enhancing Wnt/β-catenin signaling increased the levels of CTSD, suggesting its involvement in regulating CTSD expression. CTSD was detected in more invasive areas of the tumor in both epithelial cells and the adjacent stromal compartment, but not in normal mucosa, supporting a role for CTSD in L1-mediated CRC progression [62].

Another protein whose level is elevated in the secretome of CRC cells is the ubiquitin-like interferon induced gene 15 (ISG15), which operates much like ubiquitin by conjugating to target proteins (ISGylation) [63]. We found that increased ISG15 levels were required for L1-mediated CRC progression because suppression of ISG15 expression blocked the L1-mediated increase in CRC cell motility, tumorigenesis, and metastasis [63]. The induction of ISG15 was dependent on proper L1–L1 mediated adhesions, as point mutations in the L1 ectodomain abolished its ability to induce the expression of ISG15 [63]. The induction in ISG15 by L1 was dependent on the NF-κB pathway and ISG15 was detected in CRC tumor tissue and in the adjacent stroma, but not in normal colonic mucosa, suggesting that ISG15 could serve as a therapeutic target for CRC treatment [63].

9. Conclusions

L1, a cell adhesion receptor and a target gene of Wnt/β-catenin signaling, is a key perpetuator of CRC development and metastasis. L1 is not expressed in normal homeostatic colonic mucosa, but is induced at the invasive front of CRC tissue in cells expressing the Lgr5 intestinal stem cell marker as well as during regeneration of the intestinal/colonic tissue following injury. In addition, L1 was reported to contribute to the generation of an immunosuppressive tumor microenvironment [64] and promotes chemoresistance [33,65,66]. The studies summarized above point to the numerous genes that are induced (and suppressed) during CRC progression following L1 expression. Because the level of L1 expression was shown to be a powerful prognostic factor for indicating poor survival in a variety of cancer types, L1 is considered a promising target for cancer therapy that involves blocking L1 antibodies in combination with cytostatic drugs and/or radio-immunotherapy [67–70]. The downstream target genes of L1-mediated CRC progression described here could mimic the effects conferred by L1 on the motile, tumorigenic, and metastatic properties of CRC cells. Targeting these downstream effectors of L1-mediated signaling could provide additional approaches to CRC diagnosis and therapy.

Funding: This research received no external funding.

Conflicts of Interest: The authors declare no conflict of interest.

References

1. Valenta, T.; Hausmann, G.; Basler, K. The many faces and functions of β-catenin. *EMBO J.* **2012**, *31*, 2714–2736. [CrossRef] [PubMed]
2. Basu, S.; Cheriyamundath, S.; Ben-Ze'Ev, A. Cell–cell adhesion: Linking Wnt/β-catenin signaling with partial EMT and stemness traits in tumorigenesis. *F1000Research* **2018**, *7*, 1488. [CrossRef] [PubMed]
3. McCrea, P.D.; Gottardi, C.J. Beyond β-catenin: Prospects for a larger catenin network in the nucleus. *Nat. Rev. Mol. Cell Biol.* **2016**, *17*, 55–64. [CrossRef] [PubMed]
4. Gumbiner, B.M. Cell Adhesion: The Molecular Basis of Tissue Architecture and Morphogenesis. *Cell* **1996**, *84*, 345–357. [CrossRef]
5. Sharma, R. Wingless, a new mutant in *D. melanogaster*. *J. Dros. Inf. Service* **1973**, *50*, 134.
6. Sharma, R.; Chopra, V. Effect of the wingless (wg1) mutation on wing and haltere development in *Drosophila melanogaster*. *Dev. Biol.* **1976**, *48*, 461–465. [CrossRef]
7. Nüsslein-Volhard, C.; Wieschaus, E. Mutations affecting segment number and polarity in *Drosophila*. *Nat. Cell Biol.* **1980**, *287*, 795–801. [CrossRef]

8. McMahon, A.P.; Moon, R.T. Ectopic expression of the proto-oncogene int-1 in Xenopus embryos leads to duplication of the embryonic axis. *Cell* **1989**, *58*, 1075–1084. [CrossRef]
9. Nusse, R.; Varmus, H.E. Many tumors induced by the mouse mammary tumor virus contain a provirus integrated in the same region of the host genome. *Cell* **1982**, *31*, 99–109. [CrossRef]
10. Kinzler, K.W.; Vogelstein, B. Lessons from Hereditary Colorectal Cancer. *Cell* **1996**, *87*, 159–170. [CrossRef]
11. Korinek, V.; Barker, N.; Morin, P.J.; van Wichen, D.; de Weger, R.; Kinzler, K.W.; Vogelstein, B.; Clevers, H. Constitutive Transcriptional Activation by a beta -Catenin-Tcf Complex in APC-/- Colon Carcinoma. *Science* **1997**, *275*, 1784–1787. [CrossRef] [PubMed]
12. Morin, P.J.; Sparks, A.B.; Korinek, V.; Barker, N.; Clevers, H.; Vogelstein, B.; Kinzler, K.W. Activation of beta -Catenin-Tcf Signaling in Colon Cancer by Mutations in beta -Catenin or APC. *Science* **1997**, *275*, 1787–1790. [CrossRef] [PubMed]
13. He, T.-C.; Sparks, A.B.; Rago, C.; Hermeking, H.; Zawel, L.; da Costa, L.T.; Morin, P.J.; Vogelstein, B.; Kinzler, K.W. Identification of c-MYC as a Target of the APC Pathway. *Science* **1998**, *281*, 1509–1512. [CrossRef] [PubMed]
14. Shtutman, M.; Zhurinsky, J.; Simcha, I.; Albanese, C.; D'Amico, M.; Pestell, R.; Ben-Ze'Ev, A. The cyclin D1 gene is a target of the -catenin/LEF-1 pathway. *Proc. Natl. Acad. Sci. USA* **1999**, *96*, 5522–5527. [CrossRef] [PubMed]
15. Tetsu, O.; McCormick, F. β-Catenin regulates expression of cyclin D1 in colon carcinoma cells. *Nat. Cell Biol.* **1999**, *398*, 422–426. [CrossRef]
16. Herbst, A.; Jurinovic, V.; Krebs, S.; Thieme, S.E.; Blum, H.; Göke, B.; Kolligs, F.T. Comprehensive analysis of β-catenin target genes in colorectal carcinoma cell lines with deregulated Wnt/β-catenin signaling. *BMC Genom.* **2014**, *15*, 74. [CrossRef]
17. Brabletz, T.; Jung, A.; Hermann, K.; Günther, K.; Hohenberger, W.; Kirchner, T. Nuclear Overexpression of the Oncoprotein β-Catenin in Colorectal Cancer is Localized Predominantly at the Invasion Front. *Pathol.–Res. Pr.* **1998**, *194*, 701–704. [CrossRef]
18. Brabletz, T.; Jung, A.; Reu, S.; Porzner, M.; Hlubek, F.; Kunz-Schughart, L.A.; Knuechel, R.; Kirchner, T. Variable -catenin expression in colorectal cancers indicates tumor progression driven by the tumor environment. *Proc. Natl. Acad. Sci. USA* **2001**, *98*, 10356–10361. [CrossRef]
19. Gavert, N.; Conacci-Sorrell, M.; Gast, D.; Schneider, A.; Altevogt, P.; Brabletz, T.; Ben-Ze'Ev, A. L1, a novel target of β-catenin signaling, transforms cells and is expressed at the invasive front of colon cancers. *J. Cell Biol.* **2005**, *168*, 633–642. [CrossRef]
20. Barker, N.; van Es, J.H.; Kuipers, J.; Kujala, P.; Born, M.V.D.; Cozijnsen, M.; Haegebarth, A.; Korving, J.; Begthel, H.; Peters, P.J.; et al. Identification of stem cells in small intestine and colon by marker gene Lgr5. *Nat. Cell Biol.* **2007**, *449*, 1003–1007. [CrossRef]
21. Conacci-Sorrell, M.E.; Ben-Yedidia, T.; Shtutman, M.; Feinstein, E.; Einat, P.; Ben-Ze'Ev, A. Nr-CAM is a target gene of the beta -catenin/LEF-1 pathway in melanoma and colon cancer and its expression enhances motility and confers tumorigenesis. *Genes Dev.* **2002**, *16*, 2058–2072. [CrossRef]
22. Bottomly, D.; Kyler, S.L.; McWeeney, S.K.; Yochum, G.S. Identification of β-catenin binding regions in colon cancer cells using ChIP-Seq. *Nucleic Acids Res.* **2010**, *38*, 5735–5745. [CrossRef]
23. Zelina, P.; Avci, H.X.; Thelen, K.; Pollerberg, G.E. The cell adhesion molecule NrCAM is crucial for growth cone behaviour and pathfinding of retinal ganglion cell axons. *Development* **2005**, *132*, 3609–3618. [CrossRef]
24. Sakurai, T. The role of NrCAM in neural development and disorders—Beyond a simple glue in the brain. *Mol. Cell. Neurosci.* **2012**, *49*, 351–363. [CrossRef]
25. Jouet, M.; Rosenthal, A.; Armstrong, G.; MacFarlane, J.; Stevenson, R.; Paterson, J.; Metzenberg, A.; Ionasescu, V.; Temple, K.; Kenwrick, S. X–linked spastic paraplegia (SPG1), MASA syndrome and X–linked hydrocephalus result from mutations in the L1 gene. *Nat. Genet.* **1994**, *7*, 402–407. [CrossRef]
26. Wong, E.V.; Kenwrick, S.; Willems, P.; Lemmon, V.P. Mutations in the cell adhesion molecule LI cause mental retardation. *Trends Neurosci.* **1995**, *18*, 168–172. [CrossRef]
27. Fransen, E.; van Camp, G.; Vits, L.; Willems, P.J. L1-associated diseases: Clinical geneticists divide, molecular geneticists unite. *Hum. Mol. Genet.* **1997**, *6*, 1625–1632. [CrossRef]
28. Kamiguchi, H.; Hlavin, M.L.; Lemmon, V.P. Role of L1 in Neural Development: What the Knockouts Tell Us. *Mol. Cell. Neurosci.* **1998**, *12*, 48–55. [CrossRef]

29. Kenwrick, S.; Watkins, A.; de Angelis, E. Neural cell recognition molecule L1: Relating biological complexity to human disease mutations. *Hum. Mol. Genet.* **2000**, *9*, 879–886. [CrossRef]
30. Altevogt, P.; Doberstein, K.; Fogel, M. L1CAM in human cancer. *Int. J. Cancer* **2015**, *138*, 1565–1576. [CrossRef]
31. Schmid, R.S.; Maness, P.F. L1 and NCAM adhesion molecules as signaling coreceptors in neuronal migration and process outgrowth. *Curr. Opin. Neurobiol.* **2008**, *18*, 245–250. [CrossRef]
32. Gavert, N.; Sheffer, M.; Raveh, S.; Spaderna, S.; Shtutman, M.S.; Brabletz, T.; Barany, F.; Paty, P.; Notterman, D.; Domany, E.; et al. Expression of L1-CAM and ADAM10 in Human Colon Cancer Cells Induces Metastasis. *Cancer Res.* **2007**, *67*, 7703–7712. [CrossRef]
33. Ganesh, K.; Basnet, H.; Kaygusuz, Y.; Laughney, A.M.; He, L.; Sharma, R.; O'Rourke, K.P.; Reuter, V.P.; Huang, Y.-H.; Turkekul, M.; et al. L1CAM defines the regenerative origin of metastasis-initiating cells in colorectal cancer. *Nat. Rev. Cancer* **2020**, *1*, 28–45. [CrossRef]
34. Wiencken-Barger, A.; Mavity-Hudson, J.; Bartsch, U.; Schachner, M.; Casagrande, V.A. The Role of L1 in Axon Pathfinding and Fasciculation. *Cereb. Cortex* **2004**, *14*, 121–131. [CrossRef]
35. Schaefer, A.W.; Kamiguchi, H.; Wong, E.V.; Beach, C.M.; Landreth, G.; Lemmon, V.P. Activation of the MAPK Signal Cascade by the Neural Cell Adhesion Molecule L1 Requires L1 Internalization. *J. Biol. Chem.* **1999**, *274*, 37965–37973. [CrossRef]
36. Silletti, S.; Yebra, M.; Perez, B.; Cirulli, V.; McMahon, M.; Montgomery, A.M.P. Extracellular Signal-regulated Kinase (ERK)-dependent Gene Expression Contributes to L1 Cell Adhesion Molecule-dependent Motility and Invasion. *J. Biol. Chem.* **2004**, *279*, 28880–28888. [CrossRef]
37. Cheng, L.; Lemmon, S.; Lemmon, V.P. RanBPM is an L1-interacting protein that regulates L1-mediated mitogen-activated protein kinase activation. *J. Neurochem.* **2005**, *94*, 1102–1110. [CrossRef]
38. Schmid, R.S.; Pruitt, W.M.; Maness, P.F. A MAP Kinase-Signaling Pathway Mediates Neurite Outgrowth on L1 and Requires Src-Dependent Endocytosis. *J. Neurosci.* **2000**, *20*, 4177–4188. [CrossRef]
39. Kiefel, H.; Bondong, S.; Hazin, J.; Ridinger, J.; Schirmer, U.; Riedle, S.; Altevogt, P. L1CAM. *Cell Adhes. Migr.* **2012**, *6*, 374–384. [CrossRef]
40. Gavert, N.; Ben-Shmuel, A.; Lemmon, V.; Brabletz, T.; Ben-Ze'Ev, A. Nuclear factor- B signaling and ezrin are essential for L1-mediated metastasis of colon cancer cells. *J. Cell Sci.* **2010**, *123*, 2135–2143. [CrossRef]
41. Kiefel, H.; Bondong, S.; Erbe-Hoffmann, N.; Hazin, J.; Riedle, S.; Wolf, J.; Pfeifer, M.; Arlt, A.; Schäfer, H.; Müerköster, S.S.; et al. L1CAM-integrin interaction induces constitutive NF-κB activation in pancreatic adenocarcinoma cells by enhancing IL-1β expression. *Oncogene* **2010**, *29*, 4766–4778. [CrossRef]
42. Gavert, N.; Shvab, A.; Sheffer, M.; Ben-Shmuel, A.; Haase, G.; Bakos, E.; Domany, E.; Ben-Ze'Ev, A. c-Kit Is Suppressed in Human Colon Cancer Tissue and Contributes to L1-Mediated Metastasis. *Cancer Res.* **2013**, *73*, 5754–5763. [CrossRef]
43. Liu, H.; Radisky, D.C.; Yang, D.; Xu, R.; Radisky, E.S.; Bissell, M.J.; Bishop, J.M. MYC suppresses cancer metastasis by direct transcriptional silencing of αv and β3 integrin subunits. *Nat. Cell Biol.* **2012**, *14*, 567–574. [CrossRef]
44. Ben-Shmuel, A.; Shvab, A.; Gavert, N.; Brabletz, T.; Ben-Ze'Ev, A. Global analysis of L1-transcriptomes identified IGFBP-2 as a target of ezrin and NF-κB signaling that promotes colon cancer progression. *Oncogene* **2012**, *32*, 3220–3230. [CrossRef]
45. Humphries, A.; Wright, N.A. Colonic crypt organization and tumorigenesis. *Nat. Rev. Cancer* **2008**, *8*, 415–424. [CrossRef]
46. Shvab, A.; Haase, G.M.; Benshmuel, A.; Gavert, N.; Brabletz, T.; Dedhar, S.; BenZeev, A. Induction of the intestinal stem cell signature gene SMOC-2 is required for L1-mediated colon cancer progression. *Oncogene* **2016**, *35*, 549–557. [CrossRef]
47. Zeuner, A.; Todaro, M.; Stassi, G.; de Maria, R. Colorectal Cancer Stem Cells: From the Crypt to the Clinic. *Cell Stem Cell* **2014**, *15*, 692–705. [CrossRef]
48. Muñoz, J.; Stange, D.E.; Schepers, A.G.; van de Wetering, M.; Koo, B.-K.; Itzkovitz, S.; Volckmann, R.; Kung, K.S.; Koster, J.; Radulescu, S.; et al. The Lgr5 intestinal stem cell signature: Robust expression of proposed quiescent '+4' cell markers. *EMBO J.* **2012**, *31*, 3079–3091. [CrossRef]
49. Shapiro, B.; Tocci, P.; Haase, G.; Gavert, N.; Ben-Ze'Ev, A. Clusterin, a gene enriched in intestinal stem cells, is required for L1-mediated colon cancer metastasis. *Oncotarget* **2015**, *6*, 34389–34401. [CrossRef]

50. Rodriguez-Pineiro, A.M.; García-Lorenzo, A.; Blanco-Prieto, S.; Álvarez-Chaver, P.; Rodríguez-Berrocal, F.J.; de la Cadena, M.P.; Martinez-Zorzano, V.S. Secreted Clusterin in Colon Tumor Cell Models and Its Potentialas Diagnostic Marker for Colorectal Cancer. *Cancer Investig.* **2012**, *30*, 72–78. [CrossRef]
51. Murata, K.; Jadhav, U.; Madha, S.; van Es, J.; Dean, J.; Cavazza, A.; Wucherpfennig, K.; Michor, F.; Clevers, H.; Shivdasani, R.A. Ascl2-Dependent Cell Dedifferentiation Drives Regeneration of Ablated Intestinal Stem Cells. *Cell Stem Cell* **2020**, *26*, 377–390. [CrossRef]
52. Basu, S.; Gavert, N.; Brabletz, T.; Ben-Ze'Ev, A. The intestinal stem cell regulating gene ASCL2 is required for L1-mediated colon cancer progression. *Cancer Lett.* **2018**, *424*, 9–18. [CrossRef]
53. Shtutman, M.S.; Levina, E.; Ohouo, P.; Baig, M.; Roninson, I.B. Cell Adhesion Molecule L1 Disrupts E-Cadherin-Containing Adherens Junctions and Increases Scattering and Motility of MCF7 Breast Carcinoma Cells. *Cancer Res.* **2006**, *66*, 11370–11380. [CrossRef]
54. Kong, W.; Wang, X.; Zhao, J.; Kang, M.; Xi, N.; Li, S. A new frameshift mutation in L1CAM producing X-linked hydrocephalus. *Mol. Genet. Genom. Med.* **2019**, *8*, e1031. [CrossRef]
55. Haase, G.; Gavert, N.; Brabletz, T.; Ben-Ze'Ev, A. A point mutation in the extracellular domain of L1 blocks its capacity to confer metastasis in colon cancer cells via CD10. *Oncogene* **2017**, *36*, 1597–1606. [CrossRef]
56. Zhang, C.; Zhang, M.; Song, S. Cathepsin D enhances breast cancer invasion and metastasis through promoting hepsin ubiquitin-proteasome degradation. *Cancer Lett.* **2018**, *438*, 105–115. [CrossRef]
57. Vetvicka, V.; Vetvickova, J.; Fusek, M. Role of procathepsin D activation peptide in prostate cancer growth. *Prostate* **2000**, *44*, 1–7. [CrossRef]
58. Yang, L.; Cui, M.; Zhang, L.; Song, L. FOXM1 facilitates gastric cancer cell migration and invasion by inducing Cathepsin D. *Oncotarget* **2017**, *8*, 68180–68190. [CrossRef]
59. Gemoll, T.; Epping, F.; Heinrich, L.; Fritzsche, B.; Roblick, U.J.; Szymczak, S.; Hartwig, S.; Depping, R.; Bruch, H.-P.; Thorns, C.; et al. Increased cathepsin D protein expression is a biomarker for osteosarcomas, pulmonary metastases and other bone malignancies. *Oncotarget* **2015**, *6*, 16517–16526. [CrossRef]
60. Pranjol, Z.I.; Gutowski, N.J.; Hannemann, M.M.; Whatmore, J.L. The Potential Role of the Proteases Cathepsin D and Cathepsin L in the Progression and Metastasis of Epithelial Ovarian Cancer. *Biomolecules* **2015**, *5*, 3260–3279. [CrossRef]
61. Oh-E, H.; Tanaka, S.; Kitadai, Y.; Shimamoto, F.; Yoshihara, M.; Haruma, K. Cathepsin D expression as a possible predictor of lymph node metastasis in submucosal colorectal cancer. *Eur. J. Cancer* **2001**, *37*, 180–188. [CrossRef]
62. Basu, S.; Cheriyamundath, S.; Gavert, N.; Brabletz, T.; Haase, G.; Ben-Ze'Ev, A. Increased expression of cathepsin D is required for L1-mediated colon cancer progression. *Oncotarget* **2019**, *10*, 5217–5228. [CrossRef] [PubMed]
63. Cheriyamundath, S.; Basu, S.; Haase, G.; Doernberg, H.; Gavert, N.; Brabletz, T.; Ben-Ze'Ev, A. ISG15 induction is required during L1-mediated colon cancer progression and metastasis. *Oncotarget* **2019**, *10*, 7122–7131. [CrossRef] [PubMed]
64. Grage-Griebenow, E.; Jerg, E.; Gorys, A.; Wicklein, D.; Wesch, D.; Freitag-Wolf, S.; Goebel, L.; Vogel, I.; Becker, T.; Ebsen, M.; et al. L1CAM promotes enrichment of immunosuppressive T cells in human pancreatic cancer correlating with malignant progression. *Mol. Oncol.* **2014**, *8*, 982–997. [CrossRef]
65. Müerköster, S.S.; Kötteritzsch, J.; Geismann, C.; Gast, D.; Kruse, M.-L.; Altevogt, P.; Fölsch, U.R.; Schäfer, H. α5-integrin is crucial for L1CAM-mediated chemoresistance in pancreatic adenocarcinoma. *Int. J. Oncol.* **1992**, *34*, 243–253. [CrossRef]
66. Müerköster, S.S.; Werbing, V.; Sipos, B.; Debus, M.A.; Witt, M.; Großmann, M.; Leisner, D.; Kötteritzsch, J.; Kappes, H.; Klöppel, G.; et al. Drug-induced expression of the cellular adhesion molecule L1CAM confers anti-apoptotic protection and chemoresistance in pancreatic ductal adenocarcinoma cells. *Oncogene* **2006**, *26*, 2759–2768. [CrossRef]
67. Cho, S.; Lee, T.S.; Song, I.H.; Kim, A.-R.; Lee, Y.-J.; Kim, H.; Hwang, H.; Jeong, M.S.; Kang, S.G.; Hong, H.J. Combination of anti-L1 cell adhesion molecule antibody and gemcitabine or cisplatin improves the therapeutic response of intrahepatic cholangiocarcinoma. *PLoS ONE* **2017**, *12*, e0170078. [CrossRef]
68. Schäfer, H.; Dieckmann, C.; Korniienko, O.; Moldenhauer, G.; Kiefel, H.; Salnikov, A.; Krüger, A.; Altevogt, P.; Sebens, S. Combined treatment of L1CAM antibodies and cytostatic drugs improve the therapeutic response of pancreatic and ovarian carcinoma. *Cancer Lett.* **2012**, *319*, 66–82. [CrossRef]

69. Grünberg, J.; Lindenblatt, D.; Dorrer, H.; Cohrs, S.; Zhernosekov, K.; Köster, U.; Türler, A.; Fischer, E.; Schibli, R. Anti-L1CAM radioimmunotherapy is more effective with the radiolanthanide terbium-161 compared to lutetium-177 in an ovarian cancer model. *Eur. J. Nucl. Med. Mol. Imaging* **2014**, *41*, 1907–1915. [CrossRef]
70. Lindenblatt, D.; Fischer, E.; Cohrs, S.; Schibli, R.; Grünberg, J. Paclitaxel improved anti-L1CAM lutetium-177 radioimmunotherapy in an ovarian cancer xenograft model. *EJNMMI Res.* **2014**, *4*, 1–10. [CrossRef]

Publisher's Note: MDPI stays neutral with regard to jurisdictional claims in published maps and institutional affiliations.

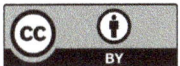 © 2020 by the authors. Licensee MDPI, Basel, Switzerland. This article is an open access article distributed under the terms and conditions of the Creative Commons Attribution (CC BY) license (http://creativecommons.org/licenses/by/4.0/).

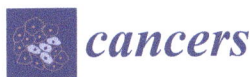

Review

Angiogenesis-Related Functions of Wnt Signaling in Colorectal Carcinogenesis

Aldona Kasprzak

Department of Histology and Embryology, Poznan University of Medical Sciences, Swiecicki Street 6, 60-781 Poznań, Poland; akasprza@ump.edu.pl; Tel.: +48-61-8546441; Fax: +48-61-8546440

Received: 28 October 2020; Accepted: 1 December 2020; Published: 2 December 2020

Simple Summary: Angiogenesis belongs to the most clinical characteristics of colorectal cancer (CRC) and is strongly linked to the activation of Wnt/β-catenin signaling. The most prominent factors stimulating constitutive activation of this pathway, and in consequence angiogenesis, are genetic alterations (mainly mutations) concerning *APC* and the β-catenin encoding gene (*CTNNB1*), detected in a large majority of CRC patients. Wnt/β-catenin signaling is involved in the basic types of vascularization (sprouting and nonsprouting angiogenesis), vasculogenic mimicry as well as the formation of mosaic vessels. The number of known Wnt/β-catenin signaling components and other pathways interacting with Wnt signaling, regulating angiogenesis, and enabling CRC progression continuously increases. This review summarizes the current knowledge about the role of the Wnt/Fzd/β-catenin signaling pathway in the process of CRC angiogenesis, aiming to improve the understanding of the mechanisms of metastasis as well as improvements in the management of this cancer.

Abstract: Aberrant activation of the Wnt/Fzd/β-catenin signaling pathway is one of the major molecular mechanisms of colorectal cancer (CRC) development and progression. On the other hand, one of the most common clinical CRC characteristics include high levels of angiogenesis, which is a key event in cancer cell dissemination and distant metastasis. The canonical Wnt/β-catenin downstream signaling regulates the most important pro-angiogenic molecules including vascular endothelial growth factor (VEGF) family members, matrix metalloproteinases (MMPs), and chemokines. Furthermore, mutations of the β-catenin gene associated with nuclear localization of the protein have been mainly detected in microsatellite unstable CRC. Elevated nuclear β-catenin increases the expression of many genes involved in tumor angiogenesis. Factors regulating angiogenesis with the participation of Wnt/β-catenin signaling include different groups of biologically active molecules including Wnt pathway components (e.g., Wnt2, DKK, BCL9 proteins), and non-Wnt pathway factors (e.g., chemoattractant cytokines, enzymatic proteins, and bioactive compounds of plants). Several lines of evidence argue for the use of angiogenesis inhibition in the treatment of CRC. In the context of this paper, components of the Wnt pathway are among the most promising targets for CRC therapy. This review summarizes the current knowledge about the role of the Wnt/Fzd/β-catenin signaling pathway in the process of CRC angiogenesis, aiming to improve the understanding of the mechanisms of metastasis as well as improvements in the management of this cancer.

Keywords: colorectal cancer; Wnt/beta-catenin signaling; angiogenesis; anti-angiogenic therapy

1. Introduction

The Wnt/Frizzled (Fzd)/β-catenin signaling pathway plays a significant role in physiology and pathology (including carcinogenesis) [1–4]. Since the pioneering mouse model genetic studies and *Drosophila* as well as the discovery of the first mammalian Wnt gene (1982), the role of Wnt signaling was mostly implied in cell growth regulation during embryonic development and maintenance of adult tissue structure [5–7]. Aberrant activation of the Wnt/β-catenin signaling pathway as well as its interactions with other pathways is characteristic for various types of carcinogenesis [6,8,9].

The elements of canonical Wnt signaling include both a range of extracellular factors (e.g., Wnts) and cytoplasmic proteins (e.g., β-catenin). Wnt ligands, which consist of more than 19 cysteine-rich secreted glycoproteins, mediate cell–cell communication and adhesion, while β-catenin acts as the main downstream effector of the pathway in a target cell [4,9–12]. The Wnt protein binding cell surface receptor complex is composed of two molecules, the Fzd protein and the single-pass transmembrane molecule, low-density lipoprotein-related protein 5/6 (LPR5/6). There are also several other transmembrane molecules that function as alternative Wnt receptors (e.g., the retinoic acid receptor (RAR)-related orphan receptor (ROR) and related to receptor tyrosine kinase (RYK)) [9]. In turn, there are also Wnt isoforms with the ability to activate the Wnt/β-catenin-independent signaling (e.g., Wnt/calcium and the Wnt/planar cell polarity pathways). Moreover, a number of secreted proteins regulating Wnt signaling have been identified (e.g., Dickkopf (DKK) family proteins, Fzd-related Proteins (FRPs), and Wnt Inhibitory Factor-1 (WIF-1)) [6,9].

It was long suggested that the Wnt/Fzd/β-catenin signaling pathway regulates the development of blood vessels in physiological and pathological conditions due to the presence of Wnt ligands (e.g., Wnt-2, -5a, -7a, and -10b), Wnt receptors (e.g., Fzd-1, -2, -3, and -5), and Wnt inhibitors (e.g., FRP-1 and -3) in vascular cells [13]. Descriptions of the biological activity of several identified human Wnt isoforms are already the subject of a number of excellent reviews [1,4,6,9,14].

Wnt/β-catenin signaling plays an especially important role in the carcinogenesis of the organs of the gastrointestinal tract in which this pathway takes part in the regulation of embryonic development as well as the homeostasis of adult tissues [1,8,15–17]. This group includes colorectal cancer (CRC), the third most commonly diagnosed tumor as well as the second leading cause of cancer-related deaths worldwide [18].

The most common clinical CRC characteristics include high levels of angiogenesis, metastasis, and chemoresistance [19]. In CRC etiology, the decisive role is attributed to the genetic changes (especially mutations of tumor suppressor genes and/or proto-oncogenes) occurring in different stages of carcinogenesis (e.g., mutation of the Adenomatous Polyposis Coli (APC) gene during the initiation, and Kirsten Rat Sarcoma Virus (KRAS, K-Ras) gene mutation during the progression of the tumorigenesis) [20]. Currently (2020), a classical *APC-KRAS-TP53* progression model, described by Fearon and Vogelstein in the 1990s [21], has been confirmed, proving that APC mutations have the highest odds of occurring early, followed by *KRAS*, loss of 17p and Tumor Protein 53 (TP53), and SMAD family member 4 (SMAD4) gene mutations [22]. Inactivating mutations of *APC* leads to constitutive activation of Wnt/β-catenin signaling and tumor development. The CRC is therefore considered a prototype example of an oncogenic function of the Wnt/β-catenin signaling [6,8,20].

The key component of the Wnt signaling is the cytoplasmic protein β-catenin, serving two important cellular functions. In the cytoplasm, it participates in a so-called destruction complex (DC), together with Axin, APC, and a two serine-threonine kinases: glycogen synthase kinase 3α/β (GSK3α/β) and casein kinase 1 α/δ (CK1 α/δ). Phosphorylation of the β-catenin N terminus represents a pre-requirement for recognition by E3-ubiquitin ligase β-TrCP, with its subsequent degradation in proteasomes. The second important cellular function of β-catenin in epithelial cells is the formation of intercellular junctions of *zonulae adherens* type, together with other catenins (α and γ) and E-cadherin. Activation of the canonical Wnt signaling inhibits β-catenin phosphorylation and protein degradation. Stabilization and cytoplasmic accumulation of β-catenin leads to its transport to the cell nucleus, resulting in the indirect regulation of transcription by the binding of sequence-specific Lymphoid Enhancer Factor/T cell Factor (LEF/TCF) DNA binding factors that upregulate target genes [9,23]. A recent meta-analysis of transcriptomic studies suggests that LEF/TCF-specific transcriptional regulation of Wnt target genes in CRC is relevant for tumor progression and metastasis [24]. It is worth noting that a subset of β-catenin transcriptional targets is LEF/TCF-independent [25].

Hence, particular actions of Wnt/β-catenin signaling can be regulated through interactions with various molecular partners including the molecules of adherent junction (E-cadherin), DC elements (axin/conductin, APC, GSK3α/β, CK1 α/δ, and β-TrCP) as well as LEF/TCF family transcription factors [9].

The *APC* and catenin β1 (β-catenin) encoding gene (*CTNNB1*) mutations are observed in familial adenomatosis polyposis and 60–90% of sporadic CRC [8,26]. Recently, splice alterations in intronic regions of *APC* and large-frame deletions in *CTNNB1* have been described, increasing Wnt/β-catenin signaling oncogenic alterations to 96% of CRC [27]. Mutations of *APC* encompassing at least two β-catenin downregulating motifs are significantly more frequent in microsatellite unstable (MSI-H) than in microsatellite stable (MSS) CRC [28]. However, the functional effects of *APC* and *CTNNB1* mutations might differ, sparking the search for other factors influencing the action of the Wnt/β-catenin signaling pathway, especially in the context of CRC treatment.

Several lines of evidence argue for the use of angiogenesis inhibition in the treatment of CRC. In the context of this paper, components of the Wnt pathway with anti-angiogenic activity are among the most promising targets for CRC therapy [6,8,20].

This review summarizes the current knowledge about the role of the Wnt/Fzd/β-catenin signaling pathway in the process of CRC angiogenesis for a better understanding of the mechanisms of metastasis as well as improvements in the management of this cancer.

2. Wnt/β-Catenin Signaling and Colorectal Cancer–General Comments

The link between hyperactivation of the Wnt/Fzd/β-catenin signaling and the development of colorectal cancer has been long recognized [2,19,20,29,30]. The activated Wnt/β-catenin signaling promotes CRC cell invasion and migration in vitro, subcutaneous tumor growth, angiogenesis, and liver metastases in vivo [31].

The activation of the Wnt canonical pathway causes inhibition of β-catenin phosphorylation as well as the absence of its degradation. Its stabilization and accumulation in the cytoplasm facilitate the transport of β-catenin to the cell nucleus. In the cell nucleus, β-catenin forms a complex with LEF/TCF and intensifies the expression of various target genes associated with proliferation, differentiation, migration, and angiogenesis [2,15,17,30]. In CRC progression and angiogenesis, simultaneous hyperactivation of Wnt/β-catenin signaling and inhibition of the phosphatidylinositol 3′ kinase (PI3K)/Akt pathway promote nuclear accumulation of β-catenin and the Forkhead box 03 protein (FOXO3a), respectively, promoting metastasis by regulating a panel of target genes [2]. Recently, a total of 13 target genes, highly functionally correlated with β-catenin, were identified to be significantly altered in CRC [30].

Evaluation of Wnt signaling activity in CRC became a basis to indicate molecular subtypes of this cancer. Hence, based on different responses to epidermal growth factor receptor (EGFR)-targeted therapy (cetuximab), six CRC subtypes were characterized and associated with distinctive anatomical regions of the colon crypts (phenotype), with location-dependent differentiation states and Wnt signaling activity [32]. In another molecular characterization of CRC, four consensus molecular subtypes (CMSs) were indicated including CMS2 ("canonical" subtype) (37%), which is characterized as epithelial and chromosomally unstable with marked Wnt and Myc signaling activation [33]. The most recent classification, among CRC intrinsic subtypes (CRIS), indicates CRIS-D, and to a lesser extent, CRIS-E as subtypes with high Wnt activity and a bottom crypt phenotype [34].

3. Typical Features of Angiogenesis in Solid Tumors (Including Colorectal Cancer (CRC))

Angiogenesis is one of the key mechanisms of tumor development and is critical for invasive tumor growth and metastasis [31,35–37]. The notion that "sustained angiogenesis" is one of the six key processes enabling malignant growth [38], tumor progression, and is one of the commonly accepted indicators of prognosis, is still valid [39]. This process (interchangeably called neoangiogenesis) enables new blood vessel formation through sprouting and splitting from the pre-existing ones.

Hence, cancer-focused research currently indicates two major types of angiogenesis: sprouting and nonsprouting (intussusceptive), dependent or independent of endothelial cell (EC) proliferation, respectively [40]. Other authors have reported six mechanisms of vascularization observed in solid tumors. These include, apart from the above-mentioned, recruitment of endothelial progenitor cells (EPCs), vessel co-option, vasculogenic mimicry (VM), and lymphangiogenesis [41]. In CRC, the two main types of angiogenesis (sprouting and nonsprouting) are most commonly described, with the addition of VM [42–44]. The "mosaic" vessels have also been reported in the xenograft of human colon adenocarcinoma cells (LS174T) and in human CRC tissues in which both ECs and tumor cells form the lumen. Potential mechanisms of mosaic vessel formation are discussed [45].

Among the cells participating in neoangiogenesis/neovascularization in CRC, EPCs, and ECs co-opted from surrounding vessels [41,46,47] as well as cancer stem cells (CSCs) are all indicated [40].

The process known as VM is based on the formation of vascular channels without ECs. It is carried out through transdifferentiation of colorectal CSCs (CRCSCs) to form vascular-tube structures (mimic the function of vessels) that facilitate tumor perfusion independently of tumor angiogenesis [40,43,44]. VM formation in CRC is promoted by the Zinc Finger E-box Binding Homeobox 1 (ZEB1) protein. Its silencing resulted in VM inhibition and vascular endothelial (VE)-cadherin downregulation in colon cancer cells (HCT116) [48]. Canonical Wnt signaling also participates in VM. It was demonstrated that in VM-positive CRC samples, the expression of Wnt3a and nuclear expression of β-catenin is increased compared to VM-negative samples. In in vitro (HT29 cells) studies as well as in the mouse xenograft model, the tube-like structure formation was confirmed with the mechanism of overregulated Wnt3a participation in this process explained (through increased expression of vascular endothelial growth factor receptor type 2 (VEGFR-2) and VE-cadherin) [11].

The best-known molecular pathway driving tumor vascularization (including CRC) is the hypoxia-adaptation mechanism. When the tumors grow to 0.2–2.0 mm in diameter, they become hypoxic and hindered in growth in the absence of angiogenesis. During the angiogenic switch, pro-angiogenic factors predominate and result in a transition from a vascularized hyperplasia to vascularized tumor, and eventually, to malignant tumor progression [46,49–51]. Pro-angiogenic proteins are produced by the tumor and stromal cells and include (i.e., VEGF, transforming growth factor (TGF), basic fibroblast growth factor (bFGF), and platelet-derived growth factor (PDGF)) [35,52,53]. The two latter growth factors are indispensable in the maintenance of the angiogenic process [35].

The best-studied pro-angiogenic factor in solid tumors is VEGF, which is important for sprouting angiogenesis as well as the recruitment of circulating EPCs to tumor vasculature [46,47,54]. Several members of the VEGF family have been described, namely the VEGF-A, B, C, D, E and placental growth factor (PlGF, PGF) [50]. These factors bind specific receptors present on the EC surface (VEGFR-1, VEGFR-2, VEGFR-3, neuropilin-1 and -2), which dimerize and activate the intracellular tyrosine kinases (TKs), conducting the angiogenesis promoting signals [41]. VEGF-dependent tumor angiogenesis appears to activate inverse and reciprocal regulation of both VEGFR-1 and VEGFR-2. The VEGFR-1 signaling is required for EC survival, while VEGFR-2 regulates capillary tube formation [55].

Increased production of VEGF follows for upregulation of the hypoxia-inducible transcription factor 1 (HIF-1) complex [56,57]. In turn, other factors regulate the HIF-1 complex. An increase in HIF1α expression was reported to be invoked by overexpression of Sine Oculis Homeobox Homolog 4 (SIX4) via Akt signaling. SIX4 also intensified VEGF-A expression by coordinating with HIF-1α in CRC, promoting angiogenesis and tumor growth both in vivo and in vitro [57]. Other pro-angiogenic genes, activated through HIF-1 binding to hypoxia response sequence element (5'-CGTG-3') in their promoters, are PDGF and TGF-α, activation of which results in blood vessel remodeling and angiogenesis [53,58]. Other HIF-1 target genes with proven roles in colon carcinoma cell invasion include vimentin, keratins 14, -18, -19, fibronectin 1, matrix metalloproteinase 2 (MMP-2), urokinase-type plasminogen activator receptor (uPAR), cathepsin D, and autocrine motility factor (AMF) [58]. In turn, HIF-1α and HIF-2α were proven to play different, or even opposing, roles in canonical Wnt signaling in colon cancer cells. Hence, while HIF-1α silencing negatively affected the stability and transcriptional activity of β-catenin,

HIF-2α knockdown did not affect β-catenin level, increasing the transcriptional activity of this protein by inducing its nuclear transport.

Participation of the Wnt/β-catenin axis in CRC angiogenesis is a complex process. It was proven that β-catenin induces VEGF-A expression (mRNA and protein) in human colon cancer cells, underlining the importance of this protein in early and stepwise events of CRC neoangiogenesis [59,60]. Furthermore, VEGF expression positively correlates with cytoplasmic β-catenin expression in tumor cells as well as with tumor progression in vivo [61]. In turn, while VEGFR-1 (Flt-1) is considered specific for ECs, it is also present and functional in different CRC cell lines [62]. Moreover, the study of Ahluwalia et al. reported strong expression of not only VEGF but also VEGFR-1 and VEGFR-2 in human CRC specimens as well as in in vitro studies (HCT116 and HT29 cells). This indicates an autocrine mechanism of action of cancer cell produced VEGF, independent of its primary function in the induction of angiogenesis [63]. Other studies indicate that in CRC, VEGF is secreted through a K-ras/PI3K/Rho/ROCK/c-Myc axis [64]. There are also reports of Wnt signaling promotion by K-ras activation as well as the cooperation of these signaling pathways in the CRC angiogenesis process [59].

In CRC cells, non-endothelial interactions between both VEGF receptor type 1 and 2 (VEGFR-1, VEGFR-2) and the Wnt/β-catenin pathway have also been reported [10,65]. Naik et al. showed that VEGFR-1 is a positive regulator of the Wnt/β-catenin pathway, functioning in a GSK3β-independent manner [65]. Inhibition of VEGFR-1 action by RNA interference (RNAi) or TK inhibitors (TKIs) in Wnt-addicted CRC cells leads to cell death via direct disruption of the Wnt/β-catenin "survival" signaling [10,65].

An interesting model of the regulating influence of Wnt signaling on cancer metabolism and angiogenesis through pyruvate dehydrogenase kinase 1 (PDK1), as a direct Wnt target gene, was demonstrated by Pate et al. They reported that Wnt/β-catenin signaling directs a metabolic program of glycolysis in colon cancer cells (as a common cancer phenotype called the Warburg effect) and affects the tumor microenvironment through increased vessel development [66].

When it comes to mechanisms of CRC angiogenesis regulated through Wnt/β-catenin signaling, a growing number of factors promoting or inhibiting this process are described [67–69].

4. Factors Promoting CRC Angiogenesis via Wnt/β-Catenin Signaling

Many described factors promote angiogenesis through Wnt/β-catenin signaling pathway regulation. These include Wnt pathway components and non-Wnt signaling biologically active molecules such as chemoattractant cytokines (chemokines) [70] and various enzymatic proteins including transcription factors [71–78]. The components of the Wnt pathway include agonists (e.g., B cell Lymphoma 9 protein (BCL9)) [67,79,80] as well as antagonists such as the DKK-4 (also called the Dickkopf Wnt signaling pathway inhibitor 4) [81]. An increase in DKK-4 mRNA production was observed in CRC tissues, with elevated ectopic expression of the DKK-4 protein intensifying cell migration and invasion. Moreover, conditioned media from DKK-4 expressing cells also promoted the migrative abilities of CRC as well as the formation of capillary-like tubules of human primary microvascular ECs [81].

It needs to be noted that the activity of many classical pro-angiogenic factors (e.g., VEGF-A, MMPs, inducible nitric oxide synthase (iNOS), and chemokines) is usually regulated by at least two signaling pathways (e.g., PI3K/Phosphatase and the Tensin Homolog Deleted on Chromosome Ten (PTEN)/Akt pathway and canonical Wnt/β-catenin downstream signaling). Hence, aberrant Wnt/β-catenin signaling, along with the production of nitric oxide (NO), can positively regulate tumor angiogenesis [68].

The BCL9 protein, a transcriptional Wnt/β-catenin cofactor, is the angiogenesis promoting element of the Wnt pathway in CRC [80]. An β-catenin independent function of the BCL9 was also proven, correlating with poor prognosis subtype of the CRC [82]. In the past, it has been underlined that BCL9 intensifies β-catenin-mediated transcriptional activity, independently of Wnt signaling component mutations. BCL9 knockdown enhanced the survival of the xenograft mouse model of CRC and attenuated the expression of pro-angiogenic factors (e.g., CD44, and VEGF), which resulted in a reduction of tumor metastasis and angiogenesis [67]. Hence, BCL9 is a coactivator of the β-catenin-mediated transcription that is highly expressed in tumors, but not in the physiological cells of their origin. The mechanism of BCL9 action in Wnt signaling is based on its direct binding to a unique BCL9-β-catenin binding domain [79], corresponding to its Homology Domain 2 (HD2), which contains a single amphipathic α-helix [83].

(C-X-C motif) ligand 8 (CXCL8) (also known as interleukin (IL)-8) is one of the proinflammatory chemokines produced by CRC cells at the tumor invasion front. It promotes angiogenesis through VEGF-A upregulation and cell invasion via the Akt/GSK3β/β-catenin/MMP-7 pathway, by upregulating the anti-apoptotic B-cell lymphoma protein 2 (Bcl-2) [70]. Participation of stromal cell-derived factor 1 (SDF-1) and its receptor (C-X-C chemokine receptor type 4 (CXCR4, fusin, CD184)) was also proven in the mechanisms of CRC progression. In vitro studies confirmed that stromal cell-derived factor 1 (SDF-1) induced CXCR4-positive CRC cell invasion and epithelial-mesenchymal transition (EMT) via activation of the Wnt/β-catenin signaling [84].

DEAH box protein 32 (DHX32), one of the RNA helicases, also belongs to the group of angiogenesis promoting enzymes. This transcriptional regulator enhanced the expression of VEGF-A in CRC cells, interacting and stabilizing β-catenin. Thus, the study showed that DHX32 overexpression was associated with angiogenesis in CRC as well as poor outcomes of human CRC patients [72]. Another factor, overexpression of which influences the aggressive phenotype, angiogenesis, chemoresistance, and metastasis of CRC cells, is gankyrin (PSMD10). It is a regulatory subunit of the 26S proteasome complex. A unique pathway participates in the regulation of the above-mentioned processes by gankyrin, namely the PI3K/GSK3β/β-catenin (a cross-talk between the PI3K/Akt and Wnt/β-catenin canonical signaling pathways) [19]. In turn, Cheng et al. proved the stimulating influence on CRC progression and metastasis exhibited by Uba2, a vital component of small ubiquitin-like protein SUMO-activating enzyme, occurring through the regulation of Wnt signaling and EMT enhancement [85].

A positive influence on CRC angiogenesis is also attributed to tissue transglutaminase 2 (TGM2). It was reported that silencing of TGM2 inhibited angiogenesis and suppressed the expression of MMP-2, MMP-9, Wnt3a, β-catenin, and cyclin D1 [75]. Similar results were obtained by other authors, describing a decrease in both stemness and angiogenesis through TGM2 inhibition [86]. Similarly, in the case of the Casitas B-lineage lymphoma (c-Cbl) gene encoding CBL protein, which plays a role as an E3 ubiquitin-protein ligase, it was proven that mutant *C-Cbl-Y371H* resulted in augmented Wnt/β-catenin signaling, increasing Wnt gene expression, angiogenesis, and CRC growth. Furthermore, for the regulation of nuclear β-catenin and angiogenesis, phosphorylation of c-Cbl Tyr^{371} is also required [73].

High aggressiveness and intense angiogenesis were also attributed to the HCT-116 CRC cells stably overexpressing Akt. In these cells, an increased expression of EMT-related transcription factors was noted including β-catenin. Akt/HCT-116 xenografts were highly aggressive and angiogenic (with high microvessel formation and increased expression of Factor VIII) compared to the pCMV/HCT-116 xenografts. Additionally, the tumors were characterized by the nuclear localization of β-catenin and lower expression of E-cadherin [71].

Among the transcription factors, interesting correlations can be observed between Wnt/β-catenin signaling and Zink Finger Transcription Factor Spalt (Sall)-like Protein 4 (SALL4). In a study of the SALL4 gene promoter, a consensus TCF/LEF-binding site within a region of 31 bp was described, possibly playing a role in the stimulation of Wnt/β-catenin signaling in various cancers (including CRC) through direct β-catenin biding and oncogene action [76,78]. In CRC cells, co-expression and correlation between SALL4 and β-catenin expression was described, promoting lymph node metastasis and advanced CRC clinical stage [78]. Recently, it was also demonstrated that SALL4 participates in the process of human umbilical vein ECs (HUVECs) angiogenesis, modulating VEGF-A expression [87].

When it comes to other transcription factors, it was demonstrated that the Forkhead Box Q1 protein (FOXQ1) protein is overexpressed in CRC and correlates with stage of tumor and lymph node metastasis. Small iRNA knockdown experiments on the SW480 cell line weakened the aggressive potential of cancer, downregulating angiogenesis, invasion, EMT, and resistance to drug-induced apoptosis through the inhibition of nuclear translocation of β-catenin. It was also demonstrated that the expression and action of FOXQ1 were promoted by TGF-β1. Hence, CRC progression via angiogenesis was enabled by the co-operation of two signaling pathways: Wnt and TGF-β1 [77].

The influence of several plant-based compounds on CRC angiogenesis [88] as well as the connection between the activity of such compounds and Wnt/β-catenin signaling in CRC, were also investigated [89]. These compounds include the water solutions of *Aloe vera* extracts (with two active components: aloin and aloesin). It seems that the action of active *Aloe Vera* components on angiogenesis and tumor growth depends on the activity of more than one signaling pathway. It was proven that aloin promotes activation of the Wnt/β-catenin signaling as well as inhibits the Notch signaling pathway in CRC cells only in the presence of Wnt3a. In turn, aloesin directly activates Wnt signaling and inhibits the Notch pathway in a Wnt3a independent manner [89]. These results are contradictory to previous reports describing the inhibiting influence of aloin on CRC angiogenesis via signal transducer and activator of transcription protein 3 (STAT3) activation [88].

5. Factors Inhibiting CRC Angiogenesis via Wnt/β-Catenin Signaling

Furthermore, various factors inhibiting angiogenesis CRC via Wnt/β-catenin signaling were also described. These include antagonists of Wnt (e.g., DKK-1 genes) [90]. DKK-1 protein expression in CRC tissues was downregulated during the CRC adenoma-carcinoma sequence, correlating with the downregulation of VEGF expression and decreased microvessel density. Overexpression of DKK-1 in CRC cells in vitro (HCT116) inhibited the formation of tube-like structures and downregulated VEGF expression in HUVECs. Xenografts of DKK-1 overexpressing CRC cells have decreased microvessel density (MVD) and VEGF expression vs. the control cells [90].

Angiogenesis inhibiting factors also include tumor suppressors (e.g., tumor necrosis factor α (TNFα)-induced protein 8 like 2 (TIPE2, TNFAIP8L2)) [91]. TIPE2 plays a role in immune homeostasis and is associated with carcinogenesis on many tumors [92]. The study by Wu et al. on human rectal adenocarcinoma demonstrated that the expression of this protein was higher in tumor tissues compared to the control. However, TIPE2 overexpression increased cell apoptosis through downregulation of Wnt3a, phospho-β-catenin, and GSK3β expression in rectal adenocarcinoma cells. It was proven that TIPE2 knockdown promoted the growth of this tumor through angiogenesis modulation. The participation of TIPE2 in the regulation of proliferation, migration, invasion, and, consequently, angiogenesis involves the Wnt/β-catenin and TGF-β/Smad2/3 signaling pathways [91].

A relation between re-expression of type 1 cyclic guanosine monophosphate (cGMP)-dependent protein kinase (PKG) in metastatic colon carcinoma and reduced tumor angiogenesis was also described. In vivo studies confirmed reduced levels of VEGF in PKG-expressed tumors compared with tumors that were derived from parental SW620 cells. Moreover, PKG expression was associated with reduced levels of β-catenin in comparison with the parental cells. Administration of exogenous PKG in SW620 cells also inhibited the expression of β-catenin and resulted in a decrease of TCF-dependent transcription [93].

Another molecule inhibiting β-catenin mRNA production and promoter activity is the scaffold/matrix attachment region binding protein 1 (SMAR1). Effects inhibiting the Wnt/β-catenin signaling activity were obtained by recruiting histone deacetylase-5 to the β-catenin promoter, resulting in decreased CRC cell migration and invasion as well as indirectly inhibiting cancer progression and angiogenesis. Moreover, smaller tumor size in in vivo NOD-SCID mice correlated with the suppression of β-catenin [94].

Protein kinase C-α (PKCα) can also function as a Wnt/β-catenin inhibitor, participating in RORα phosphorylation, hence inhibiting transcriptional activity of β-catenin. The key mechanism of that Wnt/β-catenin signaling inhibition is Wnt5a/PKCα-dependent phosphorylation on SER^{35} of RORα. Reduction of RORα phosphorylation in >70% of CRC cases appears clinically important, together with a significant correlation of this reduction and PKCα phosphorylation in tumor samples compared to normal tissue specimens [95]. It was also proven that PKCα also phosphorylates β-catenin itself, leading to its physiological degradation in proteasomes [96]. Recent in vitro (DLD-1 cells incubated with PKCα activators) and in vivo (C57BL/6J mice) studies with knocked-out *PRKCA* (gene encoding mouse PKCα) confirmed that this kinase exerts an anti-tumor (anti-growth, stimulating cell death) effect on cancer cells [97].

Similarly, an inhibitory influence of certain plant-based compounds (known and used in traditional Chinese medicine) on angiogenesis is described. The research indicates the inhibiting function of sporamin (a Kunitz-type trypsin inhibitor, found in sweet potato (*Ipomea batatas*)) on the number and mass of tumor nodules formed in the abdominal cavity via reduction of β-catenin (mRNA and protein) and VEGF concentration in the liver of mouse xenografted with LoVo CRC cells [97]. Another such compound is Tanshinone IIA (Tan IIA, TSA), the active lipophilic component of a Chinese *Salvia miltiorrhiza Bunge* plant. The mechanism of its action in normoxic and hypoxic microenvironment conditions is based on the inhibition of TGF-β secretion via inhibition of HIF-1α, which drives angiogenesis by promoting β-catenin nuclear translocation and TCF/LEF activation [98].

A significant influence on Wnt/β-catenin signaling and downregulation of the key genes: TCF4 (transcription factor 7-like 2, TCF7L2), cyclin D1, and c-Myc in CRC are also exerted by emodin (the anthraquinone-active substance) [99,100]. This active component of the roots and bark of several plants regulates the expression of key components of Wnt signaling, namely β-catenin and TCF7L2 as well as several downstream targets of this pathway. Additionally, two new targets of emodin action, the p300 Wnt co-activator (downregulated), and the HMG-box transcription factor 1 (HBP1) repressor (upregulated) were indicated in CRC cell lines [99]. Recent research confirmed these observations through the demonstration of EMT and tumor growth inhibition. After emodin administration, a decrease in the expression of MMPs (MMP-7 and MMP-9), VEGF, N-cadherin, Snail, and β-catenin was observed together with an increase in E-cadherin mRNA expression [100].

A recent study (2020) indicated the inhibitory influence of 6-Gingerol (6-G) on mouse CRC tumorigenesis and angiogenesis, with the participation of the Wnt/β-catenin signaling [101]. The use of ginger (*Zingiber officinale*) extract and 6-G in therapy against cancers (including CRC) is very well known in medicine (reviewed in [102]). After 6-G exposition, downregulation of various oncogenic proteins' expression was demonstrated, including Wnt3a and β-catenin. Inhibition of angiogenesis occurred through the downregulation of the concentration of VEGF, Angiopoietin-1 (ANG-1), FGF, and growth differentiation factor 15 (GDF-15) in the colon of benzo[a]pyrene and dextran sulfate sodium (DSS)-exposed mouse [101].

Furthermore, the inhibitory action of Raddeanin A (RA), an active oleanane type triterpenoid saponin and a major compound isolated from *Anemone raddeana Regel* was also described in CRC, influencing invasion and metastasis of this cancer's cells. This process occurred via nuclear-factor kappa B (NF-κB) and STAT3 signaling pathways. However, the main signaling pathway associated with RA action seems to be the PI3K/Akt (reviewed in [103]). Inhibition of cell proliferation and tumor growth occurs through the downregulation of canonical Wnt/β-catenin and NF-κB signaling pathways. In the mechanism of Wnt pathway downregulation, suppression of phosphorylated lipoprotein-related protein 6 (p-LPR6), Akt inactivation, the release of GSK3β inhibition, and attenuation of β-catenin expression were noted [104]. It was proven that RA inhibits HUVEC proliferation, motility, migration, and tube formation as well as reduces angiogenesis in the chick embryo chorioallantoic membrane. As an anti-tumor plant-based compound, RA also inhibits angiogenesis in vitro (HCT-15 cell line) as well as in preclinical models in vivo. Mechanism of its action in CRC is based on the modulation of VEGF-mediated phosphorylation of VEGFR-2 as well as downstream focal adhesion kinase (FAK), phospholipase C γ1 (PLCγ1), Src, and Akt kinases [105].

Pan et al. demonstrated the inhibitory action of aloin (derived from *Aloe barbadensis Miller* (*Aloe vera*) leaves) on angiogenesis, mainly occurring through the inhibition of the STAT3 signaling pathway. Aloin inhibited HUVEC proliferation, migration, and tube formation in vitro as well as activation of VEGFR-2 and STAT3 phosphorylation in ECs. After aloin administration in SW620 CRC cells, a downregulation of antiapoptotic (Bcl-xL), pro-proliferative (C-Myc), and angiogenic factors (e.g., VEGF) was also observed. Moreover, reduced tumor volumes and weight were noted in vivo (mice xenograft model) [88].

The activity of other plant-derived compounds as potential therapeutic targets will be discussed in further sections of this review.

In Table 1, a summary of pro- and anti-angiogenic activity of chosen factors influencing the Wnt/β-catenin signaling in CRC is presented.

Table 1. A list of known pro- and anti-angiogenetic factors and their influence on the regulation of the Wnt/β-catenin signaling pathway in colorectal cancer (CRC) angiogenesis.

Action	Family of Factors	Factor	Molecular Mechanisms/Effects on Angiogenesis	Ref.
Pro-angiogenic	Wnt pathway components	DKK-4	(i) ↑expression in CRC cells; (ii) ↑migration and formation of capillary-like tubules of human primary microvascular ECs	[81]
		BCL9	(i) directly binds to β-catenin; (ii)BCL9 knockdown attenuated the expression of pro-angiogenic factors (e.g., CD44, and VEGF), which resulted in a reduction of tumor metastasis and angiogenesis	[67,79,80]
		Wnt2	(i) ↑expression in CAFs, which correlates with clinical data; (ii) induces CRC cells and EC migration and invasion; (iii) ↑vessels density and tumor volume; (iv) activates Wnt signaling in autocrine and paracrine manner	[106–108]
		DHX32	(i) ↑VEGF-A and stabilization of β-catenin; (ii) ↑↑- is a poor prognostic factor	[72]
		gankyrin (PSMD10)	(i) coordinates cooperation between PI3K/Akt and canonical Wnt/β-catenin signaling pathways; (ii) overexpressing gankyrin promoted angiogenesis, chemoresistance and metastasis of CRC cells both in vitro and in vivo	[19]
	Non-Wnt pathway factors	Uba2	Regulates Wnt signaling and enhances EMT	[85]
		TGM2	↑expression of MMP-2, MMP-9, Wnt3a, β-catenin and cyclin D1	[75,86]
		c-Cbl gene	Mutant C-Cbl-Y371H shows ↑Wnt/β-catenin signaling, increased Wnt genes, angiogenesis, and CRC growth via phosphorylation of c-Cbl Tyr^{371}	[73]
		AKT	↑↑EMT-related transcription factors (including β-catenin)	[71]
		CXCL8	(i) ↑VEGF-A and Bcl2; (ii) ↑cell invasion via AKT/GSK3β/β-catenin/MMP7 pathway	[70]
		CXCR4	SDF-1 induces CXCR4-positive CRC cell invasion and EMT via activation of Wnt/β-catenin signaling	[84]
		SALL4	(i) directly binds to β-catenin; (ii) co-expression with β-catenin promoting lymph node metastasis and advanced stage; (iii) modulates VEGF-A expression in HUVECs	[76,78,87]
		FOXQ1	(i) ↑↑correlates with stage and lymph nodes metastasis; (ii) modulates cell invasion, EMT, and resistance to drug-induced apoptosis	[77]

Table 1. Cont.

Action	Family of Factors	Factor	Molecular Mechanisms/Effects on Angiogenesis	Ref.
Anti-angiogenic	Bioactive compound of plants	Aloin, aloesin	(i) aloin activates Wnt/β-catenin signaling in the presence of Wnt3a in CRC cells; (ii) aloesin directly activates Wnt signaling in Wnt3a independent manner	[89]
	Wnt pathway components	DKK-1	(i) ↓MVD and VEGF expression vs. control; (ii) inhibits tube-like structure formation and ↓VEGF expression in HUVECs	[90]
	Non-Wnt pathway factors	TIPE2 (TNFAIP8L2)	↓expression of Wnt3a, phospho-β-catenin, and GSK-3β in rectal adenocarcinoma cells; (ii) cooperates with Wnt/β-catenin and TGF-β/Smad2/3 signaling pathways	[91]
		SMAR1	Inhibits β-catenin mRNA production and promoter activity by recruiting Histone deacetylase-5 to β-catenin promoter	[94]
		PKG	↓VEGF and β-catenin expression in TCF-dependent transcription	[93]
		PKCα	(i) inhibits β-catenin transcriptional activity via Wnt5a/PKCα-dependent phosphorylation on SER35 of ROR α; (ii) phosphorylates of β-catenin	[95,96]
		Aloin	(i) inhibits HUVECs proliferation, migration and tube formation in vitro; (ii) inhibits VEGFR-2 and STAT3 phosphorylation in ECs; (iii) ↓VEGF antiapoptotic, pro-proliferative factors (C-Myc) in CRC cells	[88]
	Bioactive compound of plants	Sporamin	↓β-catenin and VEGF production	[97]
		Tan IIA (TSA)	(i) inhibits secretion of VEGF and bFGF; (ii) suppresses the proliferation, tube formation and metastasis of HUVECs; (iii) inhibits β-catenin/VEGF-mediated angiogenesis by decreasing TGF-β (via HIF-1α inhibition)	[98]

Table 1. Cont.

Action	Family of Factors	Factor	Molecular Mechanisms/Effects on Angiogenesis	Ref.
		Emodin	(i) ↓TCF/LEF transcriptional activity; (ii) inhibits EMT proteins, β-catenin and TCF7L2, VEGF production; (iii)↑cadherin E mRNA expression	[99,100]
		6-Gingerol	(i) inhibits Wnt3a and β-catenin expression; (ii) ↓VEGF, ANG-1, FGF, GDF-15 levels	[101]
		Raddeanin A	(i) modulates VEGF-mediated phosphorylation of VEGFR-2 and downstream kinases FAK, PLCγ1, Src, and Akt; (ii) inhibits p-LPR6, inactivates AKT, removes GSK-3β inhibition and attenuation of β-catenin; (iii) inhibits HUVECs proliferation, motility, migration, and tube formation	[104,105]

Abbreviations: ↑,↓—increase (upregulation)/decrease expression/level; ↑↑—overexpression; AKT (Akt)—Protein Kinase B; ANG-1—Angiopoietin-1; Bcl-2—B-cell lymphoma protein; BCL9—B cell lymphoma 9; CAFs—Cancer Associated Fibroblasts; c-Cbl—Casitas B-lineage lymphoma gene; CXCL8—the chemokine (C-C motif) ligand 8; CXCR4—C-X-C chemokine receptor type 4; DHX32—DEAH box protein 32; DKK—Dickkopf-related Protein; ECs—Endothelial Cells; EMT—Epithelial-Mesenchymal Transition; FAK—Focal Adhesion Kinase; FGF—Fibroblast Growth Factor; FOXQ1—Forkhead Box Q1 Protein; GDF-15—Growth Differentiation Factor 15; GSK-3β—Glycogen Synthase Kinase 3 β; HIF-1α—Hypoxia-inducible Factor 1 α; HUVECs—Human Umbilical Vein ECs; LEF—Lymphoid Enhancer Factor; MMP-2, -9—Matrix Metalloproteinase 2, -9; MVD—Microvessel Density; PI3K—Phosphatidylinositol 3′ Kinase; PKCα—Protein Kinase C α; PKG—type 1 cyclic guanosine monophosphate (cGMP)-dependent protein kinase; PLCγ1—Phospholipase C γ1; p-LPR6—phosphorylated Lipoprotein-related Protein 6; ROR α—RAR-related orphan receptor α; SALL4—Zink Finger Transcription Factor Spalt (Sall)-like Protein 4; SDF-1—Stromal Cell-derived Factor 1; SER—Serine; SMAR1—Scaffold/Matrix Attachment Region Binding protein 1; STAT3—Signal Transducer and Activator of Transcription Protein 3; Tan IIA/TSA—Tanshinone IIA; TCF—T cell Factor; TCF7L2—Transcription Factor 7-like 2; TGF-β—Tumor Growth Factor beta; TGM2—Tissue Transglutaminase 2; TIPE2 (TNFAIP8L2)—Tumor Necrosis Factor α (TNFα)-induced protein 8 like 2; VEGF (R)—Vascular Endothelial Growth Factor (Receptor).

6. Cellular Components of Tumors in Angiogenesis-Related Functions of Wnt/β-Catenin Signaling in CRC

Cells active in CRC angiogenesis mediated by Wnt/β-catenin signaling (interacting with vascular ECs) are tumor colorectal cells [109], CRC stem cells [40,64,110,111] and CRC-associated fibroblasts [35,64,106] (Figure 1). The group of cells crucial in the process of angiogenesis and metastasis promotion includes those directly associated with blood vessels, namely progenitor ECs (EPCs) [35,112], tumor-associated ECs (TECs) [37], pericytes [113], and platelets [35,53].

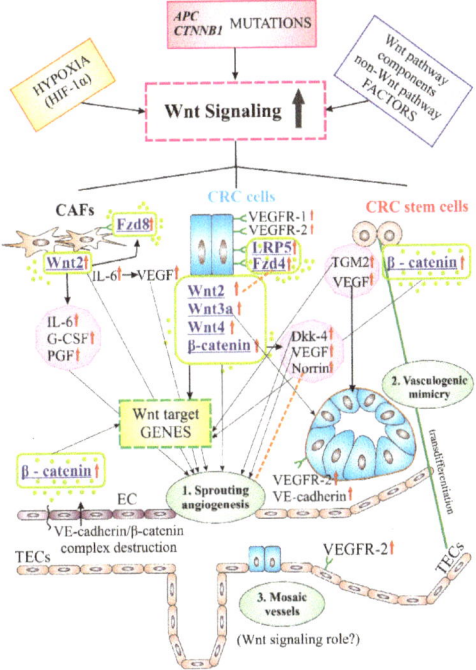

Figure 1. Angiogenesis-related functions of the Wnt/β-catenin signaling pathway in colorectal cancer (CRC). Schematic overview of the main components of the canonical and non-canonical Wnt signaling overexpressed (↑) in the main cells of the tumor (i.e., CRC cells, CRC stem cells, and cancer-associated fibroblasts (CAFs)). Various extracellular factors (e.g., Wnts) and cytoplasmic proteins (e.g., β-catenin) secreted by these cells play a stimulating (arrows) or regulating (dotted lines) role in angiogenesis. There are several other pro-angiogenic factors (e.g., VEGF, IL-6, Norrin) that interact with the Wnt pathway components to enhance angiogenesis in CRC. CRC stem cells can directly transdifferentiate into tumor endothelial cell (TECs) to form vascular-tube structures (vasculogenic mimicry). In the sprouting angiogenesis and vasculogenic mimicry, Wnt pathway-related mechanisms are well described. In turn, the role of Wnt signaling in mosaic vessel formation in CRC is poorly understood (for details see text). Abbreviations: APC—Adenomatous Polyposis Coli gene; CTNNB1—catenin β1 (β-catenin) gene; DKK—Dickkopf-related Protein; ECs—Endothelial Cells; Fzd4,8—Frizzleds 4,8 proteins; G-CSF—Granulocyte Colony-stimulating Factor; HIF-1α—Hypoxia-inducible Factor 1 α; IL-6—Interleukin 6; LRP5—Low-density Lipoprotein-related Protein 5; PGF—Placental Growth Factor; TGM2—Tissue Transglutaminase 2; VE-cadherin—Vascular Endothelial cadherin; VEGF (R)—Vascular Endothelial Growth Factor (Receptor).

6.1. Tumor Cells

β-catenin produced by the tumor directly induces VEGF production and an increase in vessel density, which was proved in the *Min/+* mouse model. Levels of VEGF-A (mRNA and protein) upregulated by 250–300% were observed in an in vitro model, using transfection of normal colon epithelial cell line NCM460 with activated β-catenin. The relation between β-catenin and regulation of VEGF-A expression was also proven on colon cancer cell lines (HCT116, SW620), which indicates the participation of β-catenin in angiogenesis initiation. A positive correlation was demonstrated between the upregulation of VEGF-A expression and *APC* mutational status [60].

Wnts are not the only ligands of the Fzd receptors. Norrin, a non-Wnt ligand, binds selectively to Fzd4 and stimulates Wnt signaling [9]. The norrin/Fzd4 interactions are modulated via the regulation of Fzd4 expression by Wnt2 [114]. Norrin produced by colon cancer cells increases EC growth and motility in a tumor microenvironment [114,115]. In turn, ECs in the microenvironment of colorectal tumor comprise all of the components of the Norrin signaling pathway. Hence, this signaling pathway has an important role in CRC tumor microenvironment angiogenesis [115].

In CRC cells, aberrant expression of E-cadherin/β-catenin complex can be observed as well as that of other angiogenesis markers such as Syndecan-1, platelet (Endothelial) cell adhesion molecule 1 [P(E)CAM-1, CD31], and endoglin (CD105), all involved in tumor progression and prognosis. Moreover, endoglin expression in tumor cells was positively correlated with E-cadherin, β-catenin, and Syndecan-1 [116].

It was demonstrated that exosomes derived from hypoxic CRC cells promote angiogenesis. These exosomes, enriched with Wnt4, promoted the proliferation and migration of ECs through Wnt4-induced β-catenin signaling. It was proved that Wnt4 increased nuclear translocation of β-catenin in ECs. Furthermore, an increase in tumor size and angiogenesis via CRC cell-derived exosomes was also confirmed in an animal in vivo model [109].

6.2. Colorectal Cancer Stem(-Like) Cells (CRCSCs)

CSCs of human CRC are unique cell types able to maintain tumor mass, modify the tumoral microenvironment by expressing angiogenic factors and enhanced neovascularization, and survive outside of the primary tumor at metastatic sites [40,64,110,111]. These cells play an important role in tumor vasculogenesis through their ability for transdifferentiation into human colorectal carcinoma ECs as well as to generate functional blood vessels [110]. Moreover, they also play a role in VM [40]. Surface markers of CSCs have been characterized, and their role in angiogenesis of all gastrointestinal cancers (including CRC) has been discussed in great detail in recent reviews [40,111]. Furthermore, it seems that CRCSCs cooperate with pericytes during angiogenesis initiation in CRC [113].

The mutual relations between CRCSCs and the canonical Wnt/β-catenin signaling pathway are also described in the case of CRC. This signaling pathway is a master regulator of a balance between stemness and differentiation in several adult stem cell niches including colon CSCs population in intestinal crypts of Lieberkühn. The colon-crypt base is characterized by high activity of Wnt signaling, especially in the bottom third of the crypts (where CSCs reside) due to signals from the stromal microenvironment cells [1,32]. In HCT116 and HT29 sphere models, Wei et al. demonstrated the promotion of proliferation, migration, and tube formation of EPCs via VEGF secretion by spheroid cells [112]. The malignancy in CRC spheroid cells (with high CSC characteristics) was associated with increased expression of TGM2 (TG2), β-catenin, VEGF, and EMT features [86]. Many new canonical Wnt signaling gene targets on CRCSCs were also identified as components of the stem-like subtype signature described by the authors [32].

6.3. Cancer-Associated Fibroblasts (CAFs)

Cancer-associated fibroblasts, as a major component of tumor stroma, play an underestimated role in the development and progression of various solid tumors (including CRC) [117,118]. Activated CAFs isolated from CRC produce IL-6, which induces angiogenesis mainly through intensification of VEGF-A expression in these cells [119]. Among the pro-angiogenic Wnt signaling components highly enriched in colorectal cancer CAFs is the Wnt2 protein [106–108,120]. Initially, overexpression of this protein was demonstrated in CRC cells, with a knockdown of Wnt2 downregulating Wnt/β-catenin target gene expression. Furthermore, the pro-proliferative properties of this protein were also observed [121]. The role of CAFs, as the main source of Wnt2 in CRC, was first demonstrated by Kramer et al. [107]. CAF-derived Wnt2 activates canonical signaling in APC/β-catenin wild-type colon cancer cells (but not in cells with APC/CTNNB1 mutations) in a paracrine manner. Fzd8, a putative Wnt2 receptor, was identified on CAFs. It was demonstrated that Wnt2 activates autocrine canonical Wnt signaling in primary fibroblasts, which was connected to the pro-migrative and pro-invasive phenotype. These studies indicate the major role of Wnt2 in the promotion of growth, invasion, and CRC metastasis in vivo [107]. Further research of this group demonstrated that Wnt2 intensifies EC migration and invasion. However, induction of the canonical Wnt pathway was only observed in a small number of cells. In turn, in the CRC xenograft model, Wnt2 overexpression led to enhanced vessel density and tumor volume. A correlation of Wnt2 levels was observed with the expression of vascular markers as well as an increase in pro-angiogenic functions of many proteins (e.g., ANG-2, IL-6, granulocyte colony-stimulating factor (G-CSF), and placental growth factor (PGF)). Three of them (IL-6, G-CSF, and PGF) have a major part in angiogenesis intensification via increased Wnt2. Hence, the authors proved the key role of Wnt2 in the formation of the active CAF phenotype in CRC, associated with the maintenance of pro-angiogenic secretome and extracellular matrix (ECM) remodeling signals [106]. The research of Aizawa et al. demonstrated that gene sets related to the Wnt signaling were highly expressed in CAFs (with Wnt2 specifically expressed). The authors observed Wnt2-induced cancer cell migration and invasion in CRC and confirmed the correlation between Wnt2 expression and clinicopathological data (including venous invasion) in CRC in vivo studies [108].

6.4. Tumor-Associated (Vascular) Endothelial Cells (TECs, TVECs)

In physiology, ECs are responsible for the formation of a semi-permeable barrier, a process enabled by the structure of intercellular connections as well as the presence of VE-cadherin (cadherin 5/CD144) and β-catenin, linking the VE-cadherin junction complex to the cytoskeleton [122,123]. The factors destroying intercellular connections in ECs also play a role in angiogenesis induction. Temporary and reversible damage of the VE-cadherin/β-catenin junctional complex was observed as a result of the activity of some inflammatory agents (e.g., histamine) [122]. A decrease in VE-cadherin expression, release of β-catenin from the complex, induction of nuclear accumulation of β-catenin, and an increase in MMP-7 mRNA expression in HUVECs were also observed after application of recombinant matrilysin (MMP-7) [124].

In tumor (including CRC) blood vessels, structural and functional changes can be observed, connected to alterations in leukocyte trafficking. It was demonstrated that VE-cadherin expression and downstream activation of the Akt/GSK3β/β-catenin signaling caused an increase in the expression of the chemokine (C-C motif) ligand 2 (CCL2) and CXCL10, which facilitate CD8+ T cell transmigration into tumor parenchyma. Restoration of proper EC junctions not only inhibits vascular leak, but also regulates immune cell infiltration into tumors [125]. The endothelial Wnt/β-catenin signaling also participates in angiogenesis through differentiation and sprouting of ECs, remodeling as well as arterio-venous specification [126,127].

The blood vessels produced within the tumor are lined by TECs, characterized by abnormal proliferation and apoptosis [35]. TECs exhibit many altered phenotypes compared with normal ECs and produce several "angiocrine factors", which promote tumor progression. One of these factors is biglycan, which is produced in highly metastatic tumors including CRC. Stages and mechanisms of tumor metastasis involving TECc as well as elements of the stromal microenvironment (cells, extracellular matrix) are well described in the literature [128]. In the case of diabetes-complicated CRC and liver metastasis, results of a recent study indicate that the expression of biglycan is particularly intense in the myxomatous stroma. Induction of its production in vitro (HT29 cells) is regulated by high sugar concentration, fatty acids, and insulin. In turn, the co-culture with mesenchymal stem cells (MSCs) resulted in enhanced stemness and EMT phenotype [129].

In the case of CRC, in contrast to normal ECs, TECs originate not only from EPCs but also from the differentiation of CSCs. It was shown that CRC cells (HCT116 line) can transform into TECs under hypoxia conditions via a VEGFR-2-dependent mechanism. These cells expressed EC markers and formed tube-like structures in vitro [130]. Characterization of CRC blood supply and the role of TECs in this type of cancer, depending on its stage and immune remodeling, can both be found in a recent review [37]. Recent studies on tumor vascular ECs (referred as TVECs) purified from CRC tissues using iTRAQ-based quantitative proteomics analysis, among several groups of differentially expressed proteins (DEPs) and signaling pathways, also indicated proteins important in angiogenesis (e.g., HIF1 and PI3K/Akt signaling pathway-related proteins) were upregulated in TVECs compared with the controls [131]. The role of EPCs in CRC angiogenesis was also emphasized, with these cells exhibiting the potential to increase the tumorigenic capacity of CRC spheroid cells through angiogenesis, making them responsible for CRC progression [112].

7. Tissue Expression and Serum Levels of Wnt/β-Catenin Signaling Molecules–Diagnostic and Prognostic Role in CRC

When it comes to the expression of Wnt signaling components in CRC tissues, nuclear localization of β-catenin is described in the invasive front, in close proximity of the tumor microenvironment cells (known as the β-catenin paradox) [17,26,132,133]. Such localization mostly concerns isolated, scattered tumor cells [26]. Moreover, a correlation is described between nuclear β-catenin at the invasive front of the primary tumor and liver metastases [132,133]. Nuclear accumulation of β-catenin in neoplastic cells and the blood vessels was even considered as the most powerful predictor of liver metastasis in CRC [133]. However, there are also studies of rectal cancer, which did not detect any correlation between the nuclear overexpression of β-catenin and distant metastases or disease-free survival (DFS) [29]. Apart from its localization in the invasive front, a more heterogenous distribution of β-catenin can be observed intracellularly, both in cell membranes and in the cytoplasm [15,17,26,133,134]. Serafino et al. used a multiparametric analysis of IHC expression and subcellular localization of Wnt/β-catenin upstream (e.g., β-catenin, E-cadherin) and downstream signaling components (e.g., C-Myc, cyclin D1) in an animal model (rats) of chemically-induced CRC and human samples obtained from patients with inflammatory bowel diseases (IBD) or at sequential stages of sporadic CRC. A similar trend of β-catenin expression was noted in human and rat samples, reaching maximal values of nuclear β-catenin upregulation or membranous β-catenin downregulation in high grade dysplasia vs. normal mucosa. In advanced CRC from humans, membranous β-catenin was predominant vs. nuclear β-catenin. In their conclusions, the authors state that the crucial components of the Wnt pathway could be important markers for diagnosis, prevention, and therapy in IBD and sporadic CRC, and also possess a predictive value for responsiveness to Wnt-targeting therapy [134].

It was also noted that the cytoplasmic levels of β-catenin increased in response to hypoxia [60]. Dilek et al. showed nuclear expression of β-catenin in only 26.1% of rectosigmoid tumors, also reporting positive correlation between cytoplasmic β-catenin expression and VEGF [61]. The presence of the high Wnt signaling activity observed in tumor cells localized in the closest proximity to stromal myofibroblasts suggests a significant influence of the tumor microenvironment in further promotion of the nuclear translocation of β-catenin [15,16]. However, the prognostic role of nuclear β-catenin for distant metastases in rectal cancers is still a matter of discussion [29]. Nuclear localization of β-catenin at the invasive front of CRC appears to be important in early stages of colorectal carcinogenesis. However, there is not yet a consensus on the prognostic significance of such an expression pattern. It was stated that mutations in *APC* and *CTNNB*, while crucial for constitutive Wnt pathway activation, are not sufficient for nuclear β-catenin accumulation and full action of this signaling pathway [15,16].

Another protein of the Wnt pathway, increased expression of which in tumor cells is important for the initiation of inhibition of CRC angiogenesis process, is Wnt2 [108,120,121]. Positive expression of this protein was mainly demonstrated in stromal cells (CAFs), with little presence in cancer cells themselves. In turn, expression in CAFs positively correlates with clinicopathological data (depth of tumor, lymph node metastasis, TNM stage, venous invasion, and recurrence) [108]. Zhang et al. showed a significant positive correlation between tissue expression of Wnt2, collagen type VIII (COL8A1) (i.e., produced in ECs) and worse survival outcomes in CRC patients. Hence, Wnt2 and COL8A1 were deemed as independent factors of poor CRC prognosis. Moreover, high levels of Wnt2 expression were connected to ECM receptor and focal adhesion pathways [120]. Apart from higher β-catenin (mRNA, protein) in CRC tissues compared to the control, a correlation with elevated expression of CXCR4 was observed. Furthermore, a correlation between CXCR4 expression and low E-cadherin, high N-cadherin, and high vimentin was also noted, suggesting links between the SDF-1/CXCR4 pathway and Wnt/β-catenin signaling [84].

When it comes to the role of serum concentration of Wnt signaling components, as markers of CRC angiogenesis, it was proven that serum VE-cadherin was about fourfold higher in CRC patients compared with the controls, but it was not correlated with the VEGF level and any clinicopathological data (sex, age, tumor site, lymph node metastasis, grade, the subtype of CRC). Hence, the authors suggest that these proteins can be considered as independent markers of CRC angiogenesis [135].

8. Wnt/β-Catenin Signaling and Other Signalizing Partners in CRC Angiogenesis

The number of known Wnt/β-catenin signaling components and other pathways interacting with Wnt signaling, regulating angiogenesis, and enabling CRC progression continuously increases [35,66,68,86,106,136,137]. The pro-angiogenic pathways include Akt [71], PI3K/GSK3β [19], RAS-extracellular signal-regulated kinase (ERK) [20,138], PI3K/Akt/I kappa B kinase (IKK), PI3K/Akt/FOXO3a [2,136], PI3K/PTEN/Akt [68], cAMP/protein kinase A [137], SDF-1/CXCR4 [84], Norrin [115], Notch and VEGF-A/VEGFR-2 [127], miR-27a-3p/RXRα [139], ECM receptor, and focal adhesion [120] signaling pathways.

In turn, anti-angiogenic signaling pathways interacting with Wnt signaling are TGF-β1 [77,98], HIF-1α/β-catenin/TCF3/LEF1 [98], and the protein kinase C-α (PKCα) signaling pathways [74,95,96,140].

9. The Role of Non-Coding RNAs in Angiogenesis via Wnt Signaling in CRC

MicroRNAs (miRNAs, MiRs) and long noncoding RNAs (lncRNAs) are two major families of non-protein-coding transcripts [141]. This group also includes circular RNAs (circRNAs), which are closed-loop RNAs formed by covalent bonds containing exons and introns [142]. The latter are generated via alternative back-splicing, which connects the terminal 5' and 3' ends of the single-stranded mRNA [143].

9.1. MicroRNAs (miRNAs, miRs)

MiRNAs are the most commonly studied form of non-coding RNAs, responsible for modulating up to 60% of protein-coding gene expression [144]. An increasing number of studies concerns the clarification of the role of micro-RNAs in CRC progression (including angiogenesis) via alteration of different signaling pathways including Wnt/β-catenin signaling (reviewed in [51,145]).

Notably, increased expression of β-catenin in CRC tissues of mice (C57BL/6Apc(min/+)) and human CRC cells positively correlated with significantly upregulated miR-574-5p. This miRNA changed the expression of β-catenin and p27 (Kip1 protein) as well as intensified the migration and invasion of cancer cells. Furthermore, in CRC tissues, miR-574-5p was negatively correlated with the expression of RNA binding protein Quaking (Qki) (associated with developmental defects in vascular tissues) [146].

Another study, among 26 deregulated miRNAs in an APC-inducible cell line, identified members of the miR-17-92 cluster that were inhibited by APC. In this process, the stabilized form of β-catenin (as a result of APC mutation) bound to and activated the miR-17-92 promoter. The main mechanism by which APC exerted its tumor suppressor activity was the reduction of miR-19a, the most important member of the miR-17-92 cluster. Therefore, the expression of miR-19a correlated with the level of β-catenin in the CRC samples, and was associated with an aggressive stage of cancer [147]. MiR-92a exhibits oncogene functions, being upregulated in chemoresistant CRC cells and tissues as well as intensifies Wnt/β-catenin signaling through Kruppel-like factor 4 (KLF4), GSK3β, and DKK-3. miR-92a expression was enhanced by IL-6/STAT, directly targeting its promoter. The authors also proved that increased miR-92a resulted in increased Wnt signaling and promotion of stem-like phenotypes of CRC cells [148].

Upregulation of miR-452 in ~70% CRC tissue samples vs. normal tissues was also reported, correlating with the clinical data. This MiR-452 promotes nuclear relocalization of β-catenin and the expression of target genes (e.g., C-Myc and cyclin D1). In turn, in vitro and xenograft mice models showed that MiR-452 can activate Wnt/β-catenin signaling and promotes an aggressive CRC phenotype through direct regulation of the 3′ untranslated region (3′UTR) of GSK3β. The miR-452 promoter is affected by the same transcription factors (TCF/LEF family of transcription factors). The authors conclude that a miR-452-GSK3β-TCF4/LEF1 positive feedback loop has an important role in CRC initiation and progression (including angiogenesis) [149].

Other MiRs promoting CRC proliferation, migration, invasion, and suppression of apoptosis in vitro, and in vivo include miR-27a-3p. This molecule acts through downregulation of nuclear receptor retinoid x receptor alpha (RXRα). On the tissue level, an increased expression of this MiR was demonstrated, correlating negatively with RXRα, and positively with various clinical (clinical-stage, distant metastasis, patients' survival) and histological data (tumor differentiation). The authors also noted that RXRα negatively regulates the expression of β-catenin by its ubiquitination in CRC [138]. This confirms earlier observations of the aberrant expression of β-catenin, upregulated by suppression of RXRα [150] as well as direct interactions between RXRα and β-catenin, which suppress β-catenin transcription and protein expression in CRC cells [151].

MiR-224 [152] or epigenetic silencing of miR-490-3p [153] also promotes the aggressive CRC phenotype through activation of Wnt/β-catenin signaling. Direct regulative effects of MiR-224 on the 3′UTR of GSK3β and secreted Frizzled-related protein 2 (SFRP2) genes was demonstrated, leading to the activation of Wnt signaling and nuclear localization of β-catenin. Furthermore, ectopic miR-224 expression enhanced CRC proliferation and invasion [152].

On the other hand, miR-490-3p inhibits β-catenin and suppresses cell proliferation as well as lowers cell invasiveness by repressing EMT. Its direct target was identified as the protooncogene frequently rearranged in advanced T-cell lymphoma 1 (FRAT1) protein, which is linked with nuclear accumulation of β-catenin. Furthermore, hypermethylation of the miR-490-3p promoter downregulated the expression of this miR in CRC cells. The authors conclude that alterations in the miR-490-3p/FRAT1/β-catenin pathway can play an important role in CRC progression (including angiogenesis) [153].

Antagonistic action in transactivation of Wnt signaling is also exhibited by ectopic miR-29b expression. This miR acts through downregulation of β-catenin coactivators (TCF7L2, Snail, BCL9L) in colon cancer cells (SW480). It binds the 3′UTR of BCL9L, lowering its expression and reducing nuclear translocation of β-catenin. As a consequence, MiR-29b inhibits anchorage-independent cell growth, promotes EMT reversal, and reduces the ability of CRC cell-conditioned medium to induce in vitro tube formation in ECs [154].

9.2. Long-Non Coding RNAs (lncRNAs)

Other commonly investigated molecules taking part in different stages of CRC progression (including angiogenesis) also include long non-coding RNAs [31,155–157]. These conserved, small non-coding RNAs, made up from 21–25 nucleotides, act as negative regulators of gene expression. In the context of angiogenesis, they are also known as "angiomiRs", directly or indirectly influencing this process (reviewed in [53]). Among this group of molecules, the Wnt/β-catenin signaling activating ability is attributed to lncRNA SLCO4A1-AS1. This molecule promotes β-catenin stabilization, impairing β-catenin-GSKβ interactions, and inhibiting its phosphorylation [156].

In turn, inhibition of tumorigenesis and progression (including angiogenesis and metastasis) in CRC is caused by lncRNA-CTD903 [155] and lncRNA-APC1 [158]. In CRC tissues, strong upregulation of CTD903 expression compared with adjacent normal tissues was observed. Furthermore, in the CTD903 knockdown model in CRC cell lines (RKO and SW480), both cell invasion and migration increased with EMT characteristics as well as reduced adherence ability. Downregulation of this lncRNA resulted in Wnt/β-catenin activation with increased transcription factors expression (e.g., Twist, Snail) [155], whereas overexpression of lncRNA-APC1 was sufficient to inhibit CRC cell growth, metastasis, and tumor angiogenesis by suppressing exosome production. Moreover, the results showed the oncogenic role of CRC-derived exosomal Wnt1, which acts in an autocrine manner through non-canonical Wnt signaling [158].

Inhibition of the Wnt signaling is also mediated by upregulation of lncRNA growth arrest specific 5 (lncRNA GAS5). This type of lncRNA plays a pivotal role in the prevention of angiogenesis, inhibiting invasion and CRC metastasis [31]. Other types of lncRNAs involved in Wnt signaling in CRC metastasis (e.g., colon cancer associated transcript 1/2 (CCAT-1/2), CASC11, PVT1, Wnt-regulated lincRNA-1 (WiNTRLINC1), PCAT1, and CCAL) are presented in recent reviews [157].

9.3. Circular RNAs (circRNAs)

One circRNA, namely circular decaprenyl-diphosphate synthase subunit 1 (PDSS1) was upregulated in CRC tissue compared to the control samples. All experiments showed that circPDSS1 is linked with local and distant metastasis as well as poor prognosis in CRC patients. Moreover, it was reported to stimulate angiogenesis in CRC via Wnt/β-catenin signaling. Knockdown experiments resulted in attenuated migratory ability and angiogenesis in CRC cells. The authors noted a downregulation of Wnt/β-catenin signaling proteins including β-catenin, GSK3β, C-Myc, MMP-9, and cyclin D1 protein levels in CRC transfected with sh-cicrPDSS1 [159].

The main types of non-coding RNAs in CRC angiogenesis regulated by Wnt/β-catenin signaling-mediated mechanisms are summarized in Table 2.

Table 2. The role of selected non-coding RNAs in colorectal cancer (CRC) angiogenesis regulated by Wnt/β-catenin signaling-mediated mechanisms.

Type of Non-Coding RNAs		Interacting Molecules	Molecular Mechanism of Angiogenesis	Effect on Wnt Pathway	Ref.
miRNAs	miR-574-5p	Qki	(i) ↑expression correlated with ↑expression of β-catenin and p27 (Kip1 protein), cell proliferation, invasion, and migration; (ii) ↑expression inversely correlated with Qkis isoforms	activates	[146]
	miR-17-92 cluster (including miR-19a)	β-catenin	(i) β-catenin binds to and activates the miR-17-92 promoter; (ii) miR-19a correlates with β-catenin level and aggressive stage of CRC	activates	[147]
	miR-92a	Wnt/β-catenin	(i) ↑expression in CRC cells; (ii) enhances Wnt/β-catenin signaling through KLF4, GSK3β and DKK-3; (iii) increased miR-92a promotes of stem-like phenotypes of CRC cells	activates	[148]
	miR-452	3′-UTR of GSK3β; β-catenin	(i) ↑expression in ~70% CRC tissue and CRC cell lines; (ii) promotes nuclear relocalization of β-catenin and the expression of the target genes; (iii) direct regulation on the 3′-UTR of the GSK3	activates	[149]
	miR-27a-3p	RXRα	(i) ↑expression in CRC tissue and positive correlation with clinical data; (ii) negative correlation with RXRα; (iii) downregulation of RXRα which prevents β-catenin degradation	activates	[139]
	miR-224	3′-UTR of GSK3β and SFRP2 genes	(i) leads to nuclear translocation of β-catenin; (ii) upregulated miR-224 inhibits the expression of GSK3β/SFRP2 and enhances CRC proliferation and invasion	activates	[152]
	miR-490-3p	FRAT1	(i) ↓expression in CRC cells via hypermethylation of the miR-490-3p promoter; (ii) suppresses CRC cells proliferation, inhibits invasion (via repressing EMT); (iii) inhibits β-catenin expression in nuclear fractions of CRC cells	inhibits	[153]
	miR-29b	3′UTR of BCL9L	(i) downregulates coactivators of β-catenin (TCF7L2, Snail, BCL9L); (ii) decreases nuclear translocation of β-catenin; (iii) ↓tube formation in ECs	inhibits	[154]
lncRNAs	lncRNA SLCO4A1-AS1	Wnt/β-catenin	(i) ↑expression in CRC tissues correlates with poor prognosis and metastasis; (ii) promotes cell proliferation, migration, and invasion (via EMT); (iii) enhances β-catenin stability	activates	[156]
	lncRNA-CTD903	Wnt/β-catenin	(i) ↑expression in CRC tissues vs. control; (ii) is independent factor of favorable prognosis; (iii) downregulated enhances Wnt/β-catenin activation and their downstream transcription factors	inhibits	[155]
	lncRNA GAS5	Wnt/β-catenin	(i) weak expression in CRC tissues and cells; (ii) upregulated inhibits CRC cells invasion and migration in vitro; (iii) inhibits of tumor growth, angiogenesis, and liver metastasis in vivo	inhibits	[31]
	lncRNA-APC1	APC	(i) ↑expression inhibits CRC cell growth, metastasis, and tumor angiogenesis by suppressing exosome production; (ii) inhibits MAPK pathway in ECs and suppress angiogenesis	inhibits	[158]
circRNAs	circPDSS1	Wnt/β-catenin	(i) ↑expression in CRC tissues vs. control; (ii) higher level predicts high rates of metastasis, and overall survival; (iii) knockdown of PDSS1 results in attenuation of migratory abilities and angiogenesis in CRC cells	activates	[159]

Abbreviations: ↑,↓—increase/decrease expression/level; APC—Adenomatous Polyposis Coli gene; BCL9L—B cell lymphoma 9-like protein; circ PDSS1—circular Decaprenyl-Diphosphate Synthase Subunit 1; circRNAs—circular RNAs; DKK—Dickkopf-related Protein; ECs—Endothelial Cells; EMT—Epithelial-Mesenchymal Transition; FRAT1—Frequently Rearranged in Advanced T-cell Lymphoma 1 Protein; GAS5—Growth Arrest Specific 5; GSK3β—Glycogen Synthase Kinase 3 β; KLF4—Kruppel-like Factor 4; lncRNA—long non-coding RNA; MAPK—A Mitogen-activated Protein Kinase; miR (miRNA)—microRNA; Qki—RNA family protein Quaking; RXRα—Nuclear Receptor Retinoid X Receptor alpha; SFRP2—Secreted Frizzled-related Protein 2; TCF7L2—Transcription Factor 7-like 2; 3′UTR—3′ Untranslated region of gene.

10. Anti-Angiogenic Therapy in CRC

Treatment of CRC patients, especially those affected by metastatic CRC (mCRC), still poses a major challenge and requires significant treatment personalization. Different forms of anti-angiogenic therapy have been attempted, taking into account the mechanisms of CRC angiogenesis, in which a major role is played by the VEGF pathway. There have been approaches based on the application of anti-angiogenic small-molecule TKIs (e.g., sorafenib, sunitinib, vatalanib, or tivozanib), with or without chemotherapy. Furthermore, monoclonal antibodies have also been used, both anti-VEGF pathway and EGFR targeting (cetuximab and panitumumab). The effectiveness of typical anti-VEGF-R TKIs (regorafenib, famitinib, axitinib, and apatinib) turned out to greatly vary in mCRC treatment. The first, most effective multikinase inhibitor of angiogenic (including VEGFR-1, -2, -3), stromal and oncogenic receptor TK, was regorafenib [160–162]. This drug evoked the most significant effects in cases of advanced, refractory disease [161], especially in anti-angiogenic-naïve patients with chemotherapy-refractory mCRC. The therapy with regorafenib showed antitumor activity in 59 CRC patients in a single-center, single-arm phase IIb study [162]. The most recent open-label, single center, single-arm, phase 3 study indicates clinical effectiveness of another multikinase inhibitor, lanvatinib, in the therapy of unresectable mCRC patients, especially refractory or intolerant to classical chemotherapy, anti-VEGF therapy, and anti-EGFR therapy (tumor with wt-*RAS* expression) [163]. Furthermore, promising results have also been reported for another highly-selective anti-VEGFR-1, -2, and -3 small molecule, fruquintinib, which improved both overall survival (OS), and progression-free survival (PFS) in mCRA patients compared with the placebo. This TKI was approved by the China Food and Drug Administration (CFDA) (2018) for mCRC patients after at least two standard anticancer therapies [164].

However, anti-angiogenic CRC therapies (also those combined with other forms of treatment) are not fully effective, being a matter of discussion in many excellent reviews [36,160,161,165]. Many individual variations have been observed in response to anti-angiogenic factor therapies, sparking the search for new compounds and/or identification of susceptibility markers [160,161,166]. An analysis of the profile of the expression of genes important for an effective response to cetuximab (anti-EGFR-targeted agent) therapy in 80 CRC tumors allowed for the identification of six clinically relevant CRC subtypes. Each of those subtypes showed differing degrees of "stemness" and Wnt signaling [32]. Furthermore, there has been a perspective for the improvement of efficacy and more targeted treatment in the form of studies on host genetic markers (reviewed in [166]).

There are currently a few anti-angiogenic agents approved by the U.S. FDA for mCRC treatment: anti-VEGF/VEGF-R agents (e.g., bevacizumab, ziv-aflibercept, regorafenib, ramucirumab), anti-EGFR agents (e.g., cetuximab, panitumubab), or immune-check-point inhibitors (e.g., pemprolizumab, nivolumab, ipilimubab). However, bevacizumab is the only anti-angiogenic compound for the first-line treatment of mCRC (from 2004) [36,165]. The subgroup analysis from the CONCUR trial suggests that regorafenib treatment prior to targeted therapy (including bevacizumab) may improve clinical outcomes [162].

Wnt/β-Catenin Signaling as a Potent Therapeutic Target in CRC-Associated Angiogenesis

Apart from anti-angiogenic therapy based on the VEGF pathway, Wnt/β-catenin signaling is among the pathways offering potential sites for targeting [140,165,167,168]. Most studies aiming to establish the most efficient anti-Wnt/β-catenin therapy concerned a better understanding of the mechanisms regulating APC signaling and/or factors downstream of APC that control β-catenin stability and/or co-transcriptional activity [74,140,168,169]. The confirmed factors inhibiting the Wnt/β-catenin signaling pathway include examples of potential CRC therapeutic factors, most of them exhibiting anti-tumor activity [83]. Their effects are mainly exerted through the inhibition of cell proliferation/migration/invasion, cancer progression delay as well as the prevention of CRC metastasis [83,140,165]. Furthermore, some drugs can be used to eliminate chemotherapy-resistance [167].

The most commonly mentioned existing anti-angiogenic drugs targeting the Wnt/β-catenin pathway in CRC include non-steroidal anti-inflammatory drugs (NSAIDs) (e.g., sulindac and celecoxib), which can "bypass" many carcinogenic effects, also regulating the increased expression of PTEN and GSK3β, inhibition of Akt (and β-catenin), and MMPs as well as iNOS activation, all of which induce cancer cell apoptosis [68,167]. Other anti-inflammatory drugs (e.g., artesunate and aspirin) caused a marked reduction in preneoplastic changes in a rat model. Both drugs also downregulated Wnt/β-catenin signaling and reduced the levels of angiogenic markers like VEGF and MMP-9. These drugs inhibited cellular proliferation and resulted in pro-apoptotic effects [170].

Apart from NSAIDs, vitamin A and D derivatives also showed efficacy in the disruption of a number of signaling pathways (e.g., Erk and PI3K/Akt) including Wnt. This fact, together with the introduction of new generations of their derivatives, creates a perspective for potential new interesting clinical trials [171–174]. Vitamin D3 metabolites, which generally inhibit growth and induce differentiation of cancer cells, have been found to also exert anti-proliferative effects on CRC cell lines (LoVo, HT29, and HCT116) and clinical samples [171]. There are reports stating that the active form of vitamin D3 and its analogs inhibit proliferation, angiogenesis, migration/invasion, and induce differentiation and apoptosis in malignant cell lines including CRC cells (reviewed in [175]). One of the newfound anti-tumor effects of $1,25(OH)_2D_3$ in human CRC occurs through the DKK-1 gene induction [176] and DKK-4 gene downregulation, both considered as novel mechanisms of Wnt signaling inhibition [81]. The use of protein-vitamin D-pectin nano-emulsion (NVD) induces cytotoxicity in CRC cells in a dose- and time-dependent manner. This compound inhibits the growth of CRC cells (HCT116 and HT29) through the regulation of proteins responsible for the G2 phase of the cell cycle (cyclins A, B1, E2, and decrease in Cdc25c) as well as encourages apoptosis. In the context of Wnt/β-catenin signaling, NVD causes a decrease in expression of β-catenin (mRNA, protein), Akt, and survivin genes in vitro as well as in vivo (mice xenograft model). NVD administration in CRC cells decreases PI3K and Akt phosphorylation as well as inhibits β-catenin production. Hence, the inhibitory effects of vitamin D derivatives on CRC cells also depend on blocking the Wnt/β-catenin signaling and its downstream targets (e.g., survivin) [173]. Therefore, NVD, as a Wnt/β-catenin inhibitor, has the potential to stop tumor invasion and metastasis processes (including angiogenesis). It was also proven that calcitriol (1α,25-dihydroxyvitamin D3), as an active vitamin D metabolite, inhibits the tumor-promoting properties of patient-derived CAFs, also modulating many types of immune cells expressing vitamin D receptor (VDR) [177]. Other mechanisms and factors increasing the anti-proliferative action of vitamin D derivatives in CRC cells (SW480) have also been examined. These include cytochrome P450 family 24 subfamily A member 1 (CYP24A1), overexpression of which can be observed in CRC. It was recently proven that CYP24A1 inhibition induces translocation of β-catenin from the nucleus to the cell membrane in SW480 cells, intensifying the inhibitory effect of $1,25(OH)_2D_3$ on C-Myc. Methylation of this factor increased the anti-tumor effects of vitamin D in CRC [172].

In turn, when it comes to vitamin A and its derivatives, it is worth noting that the pathways directing β-catenin for proteasome degradation (in addition to p53/Siah-1/APC and Wnt/GSK3β/APC) include the RXR-mediated pathway [178,179]. It was proven that retinol decreases the levels of β-catenin and increases ubiquitinated protein in three all-trans retinoic acid (ATRA)-resistant human CRC cells (HCT-116, WiDr, and SW620). Retinol treatment lowered the transcription of the TOPFlash reporter and mRNA levels of the endogenous β-catenin target genes (cyclin D1 and C-Myc). Hence, the potential influence of retinol on colon cancer cell growth inhibition occurs through an increase in β-catenin degradation in proteasomes with the use of the RXR-mediated pathway [180]. The research of the same group confirmed that retinol administration to ATRA-resistant human CRC cells increased β-catenin and RXRα protein interactions, inducing β-catenin transport to the degradation location in the cytoplasm [179].

A growing number of novel agents targeting the Wnt pathway are subjected to clinical trials including specific small molecules [165,168]. This group includes G007-LK and G244-LM, specific tankyrase inhibitor compounds, which reduce Wnt/β-catenin signaling through the prevention of Axin degradation, resulting in the promotion of β-catenin destabilization [169]. As β-catenin is considered the primary cause of dysregulated Wnt signaling, the action of a range of its direct inhibitors and knockdown strategies was examined. However, as of today, none of them have been introduced into oncological practice [74,140]. The usefulness of current approaches to target anti-Wnt therapy against CRC is the subject of recent reviews [181]. Furthermore, ongoing clinical trials 1-2 employ novel agents affecting this signaling pathway (with Wnt as targets), for example, Wnt-974, Foxy-5, and LGK-974 [165,167].

It was proven that aberrant activation of Wnt/β-catenin signaling mediates resistance of CRC cells to irradiation and 5-FU-based chemotherapy. Higher levels of active β-catenin and increased TCF/LEF reporter activity were observed in SW1463 cells that evolved radiation resistance. It was also demonstrated that inhibition of β-catenin (via siRNAs or small-molecule inhibitor of β-catenin transcription, XAV-939), sensitized CRC cells to chemoradiotherapy [182]. Other studies in in vitro and mice xenograft tumor models showed that PI3K/Akt signaling inhibition leads to nuclear β-catenin and FOXO3a accumulation (both promoting metastasis). It was proven that nuclear β-catenin confers resistance to the FOXO3a-mediated apoptosis induced by PI3K and Akt inhibitors (API-2), with this effect reversed by XAV-939 [2].

Recently, previous observations on some Wnt/β-catenin signaling inhibitors and downstream targets involving PKCα came back to light, indirectly related to the progression of CRC and angiogenesis. It was proven that PKCα is rarely mutated in CRC samples, hence its function might be activated with no side effects for the intestinal epithelium. Additionally, PKCα activation results in increased cell death and is drug-inducible. According to the authors of the study, there are ongoing phase II clinical trials on the application of natural PKCα activators (found in the Bryozoan species *Bugula neritina*) for CRC treatment [74]. The use of a stabilized form of BCL9 α-helix (SAH-BCL9) is also suggested in potential therapy, as its administration caused dissociation of the native β-catenin/BCL9 complex as well as suppressed tumor growth and angiogenesis in the mouse xenograft model of the Colo320 CRC cell [83].

Moreover, a growing number of publications have documented the action of anti-Wnt/β-catenin signaling plant based compounds (particularly those used in traditional Chinese medicine) However, anti-angiogenic actions linked to Wnt signaling are only attributed to some of them, for example, Raddeanin [103–105] and Tanshinone IIA [39,98,183] (Table 1). Other naturally occurring compounds that inhibit Wnt signaling include thymol, derived from *Thymus vulgaris L* [184,185]. One of the mechanisms of this factor's action in CRC in vitro (HCT116 and LoVo cells) as well as in vivo is the prevention of EMT, invasion, and metastasis through the inhibition of Wnt/β-catenin signaling [186]. In turn, in the case of Radix *Tetrastigma hemsleyani* flavone (RTHF), it was proven that this compound causes downregulation of β-catenin activation and downstream protein expression (Lgr5, C-Myc, and cyclin D1). It also decreased the size of tumors in vivo in mice through the inhibition of pro-proliferative properties of the Wnt pathway [187]. Another plant-based polyphenol compound extracted from the root of *Curcuma longa*, is curcumin. This phytochemical also shows an anti-inflammatory, anti-oxidant, and anti-cancer activity [188]. In studies of CRC cells (SW480) as well as in the xenograft tumor model, Dou et al. proved anti-tumor activity of curcumin via inhibition of cell proliferation by suppression of the Wnt/β-catenin pathway. It was also noted that overexpression of miR-130a could abolish the anti-tumor activity of curcumin [189]. Recently, a study of another CRC cell line (SW620 cells) reported an inhibitory influence of curcumin on cell viability as well as the promotion of apoptosis. At the same time, an increase in the expression of Caudal Type Homeobox-2 (CDX2) and decreased β-catenin nuclear translocation were observed. In turn, the expression of downstream proteins of Wnt/β-catenin signaling (Wnt3a, C-Myc, survivin, and cyclin D1) was reduced. Furthermore, it was reported that the inhibitory action of Wnt/β-catenin in these cells occurred due to CDX2 restoration [190]. The isobavachalcone, a flavonoid extracted from *Psoralea corylifolia*, also inhibits growth and colony formation of CRC tumor cells as well as the induction of apoptosis through the inhibition of the AKT/GSK3β/β-catenin pathway have been noted [191]. Promising study results in anti-Wnt/β-catenin signaling therapies also concern berberine (and its synthetic 13-arylalkyl derivatives) [192,193], an isoquinoline alkaloid present in several plants including *Coptis sp.* and *Berberis sp.* [194]. Special attention was given to its anti-tumor function, mediated by the inhibition of β-catenin transcriptional activity and weakening of anchorage-independent growth (decrease in E-cadherin expression) [192]. It was proven that berberine inhibits the function of β-catenin by direct binding to a unique RXRα region that contains the Gln^{275}, Arg^{316}, and Arg^{371} residues. As a result, a promotion of this receptor's interaction with nuclear β-catenin occurs, leading to c-Cbl mediated degradation of β-catenin, hence the inhibition of cell proliferation. Moreover, human CRC xenograft in nude mice also demonstrated the inhibition of tumor growth in an RXRα-dependent manner [193].

The basic drawbacks of anti-angiogenic and anti-Wnt signaling targeted therapies have been presented in several reviews [54,165]. These include the costs of treatment, extra adverse events, crossover, and bypass mechanisms between different signaling pathways and drug resistance as well as varying efficacy among patients [165]. The main challenges and complexities associated with creating the perfect therapeutic agents targeting the Wnt/β-catenin signaling pathway in CRC have been summarized by others [140].

Direct CRC angiogenesis inhibition mechanisms based on Wnt/β-catenin signaling are only described in a small number of existing or potential therapeutics. Nevertheless, previously mentioned results of studies (Sections 2–4) demonstrate a tight interaction of Wnt signaling with angiogenesis markers in CRC. It can therefore be assumed that the inhibition of upstream and/or downstream targets of Wnt signaling, apart from downregulating cell proliferation/migration/invasion, hence tumor growth and metastasis, is also a statement of angiogenesis inhibition in the tumor. More detailed information on the therapeutics targeting the Wnt/β-catenin signaling pathway in CRC can be found in existing works focused solely on this topic [140]. Table 3 summarizes the selected existing drugs and several agents under investigation for different Wnt/β-catenin targets in CRC with an indication of their influence on angiogenesis.

Table 3. Selected classes of existing/potential anti-Wnt/β-catenin signaling therapeutics with anti-angiogenic effects in colorectal cancer (CRC).

Class of Agents	Name of Targeted Agents	Target	Mechanism of Action and Effects in CRC Cells	Effect on Angiogenesis	Stage of Development	Ref.
NSAIDs	Sulindac (Clinoril)	β-catenin	(i) both drugs ↑ expression of PTEN and GSK3β, inhibit Akt (and β-catenin), MMPs, and iNOS activation; (ii) inhibit proliferation, have pro-apoptotic effects; (iii) ↓CD133 expression, a marker of cancer stem cells; (iv) inhibit COX-2 and progression of tumor	inhibits	clinical	[68,144,167,165]
	Celecoxib	TCF		inhibits	clinical	
Other anti-inflammatory drugs	Artesunate	β-catenin	(i) both drugs down-regulate β-catenin signaling and ↓levels of VEGF, and MMP-9; (ii) inhibit proliferation, and have pro-apoptotic effects	inhibits	clinical	[170]
	Aspirin	β-catenin		inhibits	clinical	
Vitamins and their derivatives	Vitamin D3 metabolites (Cholecalciferol)	Wnt/β-catenin with upstream and downstream targets	(i) anti-proliferative effects in vitro and in vivo; (ii) ↑DKK-1 gene and ↓DKK-4 gene	inhibits	Phase 1–3 *	[81,140,171–176]
	Vitamin A and its other forms (e.g., retinoic acid, retinol)	Wnt/β-catenin and downstream targets	(i) ↑β-catenin degradation in proteosomes via RXR-mediated pathway; (ii) ↓transcription of the TOPFlash reporter and mRNA levels of the cyclin D1 and C-Myc genes	nd	clinical	[178,180]
Specific small molecules	ETC-159	Wnt, PORCN	PORCN inhibitor; effective in treating RSPO-translocation bearing CRC patient-derived xenografts	nd	Phase 1	[196]
	Wnt-974	Wnt, PORCN	Inhibitory effects in metastatic CRC	nd	Phase 1/2	[165]
	LGK-974	Wnt, PORCN	Inhibitory effects in multiple tumor including CRC	nd	Phase 1	[144,165,167]
	Foxy-5	Wnt5 mimicking	Inhibitory effects in multiple tumors including CRC	nd	Phase 1	[165,167]
	G007-LK	Axin	Both are tankyrase inhibitors; both promote β-catenin destabilization; G007-LK inhibits tumor growth in vivo in a subset of APC-mutant CRC xenograft models	nd	preclinical	[169]
	G244-LM					
	LF3 (4-thioureido-benzenesulphonamide derivative)	β-catenin/TCF	(i) antagonises β-catenin/TCF4 interactions; (ii) suppresses cell motility, cell-cycle progression; (iii) ↓tumor growth and induces differentiation in a mouse xenografts of CRC	nd	discovery	[197]
	SAH-BCL9	Blockade of β-catenin protein-protein interactions	(i) dissociates native β-catenin/BCL9 complexes, selectively suppresses Wnt transcription, and exhibits antitumor effects; (ii) suppresses tumor growth and angiogenesis in mouse xenograft model of CRC	inhibits	preclinical	[83]
	XAV-939	β-catenin, Axin	Inhibits β-catenin which resulted in sensitization of CRC cells to chemotherapy	nd	discovery	[182]
Antibodies	Anti-RSPO3 mAb (Rosmantuzumab, OMP-131R10)	RSPO3 (Wnt agonist)	In PTPRK-RSPO3-fusion positive human colon tumors xenografts inhibits tumor growth and promotes differentiation	nd	Phase 1	[198]
	Berberine and synthetic 13-arylalkyl derivatives	β-catenin	(i) inhibits β-catenin transcriptional activity by binding to a unique RXRα region; (ii) weakening of anchorage-independent growth (↓E-cadherin expression)	nd	discovery	[192–194]
	Bryostatin 1	Wnt/β-catenin	(i) natural PKCα activator; (ii) PKCα triggers the death of CRC cells; (iii) PKCα activity is drug-inducible	nd	Phase 2	[74]
Plant-based agents	Curcumin (diferuloymethane)	Wnt/β-catenin and downstream proteins	anti-tumor activity via inhibition of cell proliferation, pro-apoptotic effects, decrease in CDX2 and expression of Wnt3α, c-Myc, survivin, and cyclin D1	nd	Phase 1–3 *	[140,188–190]
	Genistein	Wnt/β-catenin and downstream proteins	(i) ↓nuclear β-catenin and increases phospho-β-catenin accumulation; (ii) inhibits cell viability, cell invasion, cell migration by recovering WIF1, ↑apoptosis; (iii) ↑sFRP2 gene expression by demethylating its silenced promoter; (iv) ↓MMP-2 and MMP-9, but ↑E-cadherin	nd	Phase 1–2 *	[199,200]
	Isobavachalcone	AKT/GSK3β/β-catenin pathway	inhibits growth and colony formation of tumor cells, as well as induces apoptosis	nd	discovery	[191]
	Resveratrol (SRT501, grapes)	TCF4	(i) ↓cellular accumulation of endogenously-introduced TCF4 protein; (ii) represses the growth of CRC cells	nd	Phase 1	[140,201]
	RTHF	Wnt/β-catenin	↓β-catenin and downstream protein expression (Lgr5, c-Myc, and cyclin D1)	nd	discovery	[187]
	Thymol	Wnt/β-catenin	(i) prevents EMT, invasion, and CRC metastasis	nd	discovery	[186]

Abbreviations: ↑,↓—increase (up-regulation)/decrease expression/level; *—used also in combination with radiation therapy and chemotherapy; ANG—Angiopoietin; bFGF—(basic) Fibroblast Growth Factor; CDX2—Caudal Type Homeobox-2; COX-2—Cyclooxygenase-2; EMT—Epithelial-Mesenchymal Transition; GSK3β—Glycogen Synthase Kinase 3β; HUVECs—Human Umbilical Vein Endothelial Cells; nd—not determined; MMPs—Matrix Metalloproteinases; NSAIDs—non-steroidal anti-inflammatory drugs; PKCα—Protein Kinase C α; PORCN—Porcupine; PTPRK—Receptor-type Tyrosine-protein Phosphatase kappa; RSPO1-4—Wnt agonists of the R-spondin family; RTHF—Radix *Tetrastigma hemsleyani* flavone; RXR—retinoid X receptor; sFRP2—secreted Frizzled related protein 2; TCF4—Transcription Factor 4; TOPFlash—TCF Reporter Plasmid; WIF1—Wnt Inhibitory Factor 1.

11. Final Remarks and Future Perspectives

Angiogenesis belongs to the most clinical characteristics of CRC and is strongly linked to the activation of Wnt/β-catenin signaling. The most prominent factors stimulating constitutive activation of this pathway, and in consequence angiogenesis, are genetic alterations (mainly mutations) concerning *APC* and the β-catenin encoding gene (*CTNNB1*), detected in a large majority of CRC patients. These mutations lead to an intensification of CRC cell proliferation, migration, and invasion in vitro as well as tumor growth, angiogenesis, and distant metastases in vivo. In addition to the mutations mentioned, there are more and more genetic and epigenetic biomarkers used to determine CRC diagnosis, prognosis, and response to therapy, as summarized in excellent reviews [202]. There are also potential clinical applications of liquid biopsy biomarkers in CRC including circulating tumor cells, circulating tumor DNA, miRNAs, lncRNAs, and proteins from blood and body fluids, and their genomic and proteomic analyses (reviewed in [203]).

Wnt/β-catenin signaling is involved in the basic types of vascularization (sprouting and nonsprouting angiogenesis) and vasculogenic mimicry as well as the formation of mosaic vessels. In vascular cells, expression of Wnt ligands, Wnt receptors, and Wnt inhibitors has been reported. The main type of angiogenesis with the participation of Wnt signaling is currently assumed to occur through the hypoxia-adaptation mechanism mediated by VEGF-signaling and upregulation of the HIF-1 complex. β-catenin itself induces the expression of VEGF in colon cancer cells in the early steps of CRC neoangiogenesis. Furthermore, tissue VEGF expression positively correlates with the cytoplasmic expression of β-catenin in tumor cells and tumor progression in vivo. In turn, the influence of HIF-1α (increasing) and HIF-2α (decreasing) on β-catenin levels/transcriptional activity in CRC cells remains much more varied. Moreover, non-endothelial interactions between both VEGF receptor types (VEGFR-1, VEGFR-2) and Wnt/β-catenin signaling have also been reported. It was confirmed that VEGFR-1 positively regulates Wnt signaling in a GSK3β-independent manner. In contrary to the previous paradigm, the presence of both VEGF receptor types was also demonstrated on tumor CRC cells, suggesting the possibility of autocrine VEGF action.

Factors regulating angiogenesis with the participation of Wnt/β-catenin signaling include different groups of biologically active molecules, namely selected molecules belonging to Wnt family proteins (e.g., Wnt2, DKK, BCL9) as well as various factors outside the Wnt family (e.g., DHX32, gankyrin, Uba2, CXCL8, SALL4, FOXQ1, bioactive compounds of plants, etc.).

A direct influence of several pro-angiogenic factors (e.g., BCL9, SALL4) on Wnt signaling has been demonstrated (binding β-catenin) in the angiogenesis process. Other factors promoting angiogenesis (e.g., DHX32, gankyrin, Uba2, AKT) regulate Wnt signaling through β-catenin stabilization and increase Wnt gene expression as well as the intensification of EMT-related transcription factor expression (including β-catenin). This regulation results in EC migration and the formation of capillary-like tubules of human microvascular ECs. The opposite effects are evoked by the anti-angiogenic factors through the inhibition of production and transcriptional activity of β-catenin (e.g., TIPE2, SMAR1, PKG, PKCα, sporamin, emodin, 6-Gingerol, raddeanin A). Recently, an increasingly important role in Wnt signaling involving CRC angiogenesis is attributed to non-coding RNAs. A number of these molecules activate (e.g., miR-574-5p, miR-17-92, miR-92a, miR-452, miR-27a-3p, miR-224, lncRNA SLCO4A1-AS1, and circPDSS1), while other inhibit Wnt signaling (e.g., miR-490-3p, miR-29b, lncRNA-CTD903, lncRNA APC1, and lncRNAGAS5).

The active cellular components of CRC-related angiogenesis consist of tumor cells, CRC stem cells, and cancer-associated fibroblasts (CAFs) as well as cells directly linked to blood vessels (EPCs, TECs, pericytes). Moreover, complex intercellular interactions have been reported in tumors during angiogenesis. CRC cells produce β-catenin (mRNA and protein), which intensifies VEGF expression and increases vessel density. The norrin protein produced by cancer cells binds to Fzd4, regulating EC proliferation and motility. In turn, norrin/Fzd4 interactions are modulated via regulation of Fzd4 expression by Wnt2. Furthermore, exosomes enriched in Wnt4 produced by CRC cancer cells promote angiogenesis by increasing ECs proliferation and migration via Wnt signaling. Both tumor CRC cells and CAFs (main source) produce the Wnt2 protein, which plays a major role in the initiation and maintenance of the CRC angiogenesis process. Wnt2 expression in CAFs correlates with a number of clinicopathological data (including venous invasion) of CRC patients. Wnt2 intensifies EC migration and invasion, enhanced vessel density, and tumor volume. Wnt2 expression positively correlates with the expression of vascular markers and an increase in pro-angiogenic function of many proteins (e.g., IL-6, G-CSF, and PGF). When it comes to CRC stem cells, high Wnt activity is mostly present in the bottom third of the crypts (where CSCs reside). These cells have the ability of transdifferentiation into human TECs as well as the generation of functional blood vessels.

The list of Wnt/β-catenin signaling components and pathways interacting with Wnt signaling, regulating angiogenesis, and conditioning CRC progression, continuously increases.

As β-catenin is considered as a primary cause of dysregulated Wnt signaling in CRC as a consequence of APC/CTNNB1 mutations, there are ongoing studies on the action of a number of inhibitors of β-catenin itself as well as knockdown strategies. However, no results of such research have yet been introduced into CRC oncological practice, due to the relatively low effectiveness as well as significant intestinal toxicity. Small molecules blocking Wnt signaling in CRC also include tankyrase inhibitors (G007-LK and G244-LM). There are several clinical trials (phase 1/2, phase 1, and phase 2) on the use of novel Wnt targeting agents in CRC (e.g., Wnt-974, LGK-974, Foxy-5). Positive anti-angiogenic effects, disrupting Wnt/β-catenin signaling have been demonstrated for a number of NSAIDs (e.g., sulindac, celecoxib, artesunate, and aspirin) and vitamin A and D derivatives. Furthermore, many natural plant-derived compounds used in traditional Chinese medicine inhibits Wnt/β-catenin signaling and, directly or indirectly, CRC angiogenesis (e.g., RA, thymol, RTHF, curcumin, IBC, Tan IIA, and berberine). As for now, the available results mostly concern in vitro and mouse in vivo models.

12. Conclusions

As the reviewed literature shows, the role of aberrant Wnt/β-catenin signaling in CRC-related angiogenesis is undisputed. These activities mostly occur due to canonical APC/β-catenin pathway activation in tumor colorectal cells, CRC stem cells, cancer-associated fibroblasts and tumor ECs, intensification of β-catenin expression, and translocation to the nucleus as well as positive correlations with other typical pro-angiogenic factors (e.g., VEGF, VEGRs). Furthermore, the role of a number of active polypeptides, proteins, and non-coding RNAs is indicated in this process. However, when it comes to anti-angiogenic CRC treatments based on targeting the Wnt/β-catenin signaling, studied inhibitors of this pathway are still mostly in preclinical stages, with only a few compounds reaching phase 1 or 2 clinical trials. Individualized targeted CRC therapeutic strategies should take into account the newest findings of molecular biology, explaining the role of direct tumor cell interactions, and all pro- and anti-angiogenic factors acting on this type of signaling as well as other related pathways. An especially large number of publications in the last five years focusing on the role of Wnt/β-catenin signaling in cancer progression (including CRC) has certainly resulted in a better understanding of the mechanisms of metastasis as well as improvements in the management of this cancer.

Author Contributions: The author worked on the information compilation, analysis and manuscript writing. The author has read and agreed to the published version of the manuscript.

Funding: This research received no external funding.

Acknowledgments: My sincere apologies to researchers whose primary articles could not be cited due to length constraints of this review. I wish to thank Monika Świerczewska for her assistance in the artwork.

Conflicts of Interest: The author declares no conflict of interest.

Abbreviations

aa	Amino acids
Akt/AKT	Serine-threonine Protein Kinase (PKB, now called AKT1)
ANG-1, -2	Angiopoietin-1, -2
APC	Adenomatous Polyposis Coli
(b)FGF	(basic) Fibroblast Growth Factor
Bcl-2	B-cell lymphoma protein
BCL9	B cell CLL/lymphoma 9 protein
CDX	Caudal Type Homeobox-2 Protein
CD44, 184	Cluster of Differentiation 44, 184
COX-2	Cyclooxygenase-2
CRC	Colorectal Cancer
CXCL8	C-X-C motif ligand 8 (chemokine)
CXCR4	C-X-C chemokine receptor type 4
DKK-1, -4	Dickkopf-related protein 1;-4
ECs	Endothelial Cells
ECM	Extracellular Matrix
EMT	Epithelial-Mesenchymal Transition
ERK1/2	Extracellular Signal-regulated Kinase $\frac{1}{2}$
FAK	Focal Adhesion Kinase
FOXQ1	Forkhead Box Q1 Protein
FRAT1	Frequently Rearranged in Advanced T-cell Lymphoma 1 Protein
FRPs	Fzd-related Proteins
Fzd	Frizzleds proteins, a family of G protein-coupled receptor proteins
GDF-15	Growth Differentiation Factor 15
GSK3β	Glycogen Synthase Kinase 3 β
HIF-1α	Hypoxia-inducible Factor 1 α
HUVECs	Human Umbilical Vein ECs
IL	Interleukin
KRAS	Kirsten Rat Sarcoma Virus, proto-oncogene
LEF	Lymphoid Enhancer Factor
MAPK	A Mitogen-activated Protein Kinase
MMP-2, -9	Matrix Metalloproteinase 2, 9
MVD	Microvessel Density
PI3K	Phosphatidylinositol 3' Kinase
PKA, B (AKT), C α	Protein Kinase A, B (AKT), C α
PKG	Type 1 cyclic Guanosine Monophosphate (cGMP)-dependent Protein Kinase
PLCγ1	Phospholipase C γ1
p-LPR6	Phosphorylated Lipoprotein-related Protein 6
ROS	Reactive Oxygen Species
RAR	Retinoic Acid Receptor
RORα	RAR-related Orphan Receptor α;
RYK	Related to Receptor Tyrosine Kinase protein
SALL4	Zink Finger Transcription Factor Spalt (Sall)-like Protein 4
SFRP2	Secreted Frizzled-related Protein 2
SMAD4	SMAD family member 4, Mothers Against Decapentaplegic Homolog 4
SMAR1	Scaffold/Matrix Attachment Region Binding Protein 1

STAT3	Signal Transducer and Activator of Transcription Protein Activator of Transcription 3
Tan IIA, TSA	Tanshinone IIA
TCF	T cell Factor, Transcription Factor
TCF7L2	Transcription Factor 7-like 2
TGF-β	Tumor Growth Factor beta
TGM2	Tissue Transglutaminase 2
TIPE2 (TNFAIP8L2)	TNFα-induced protein 8 like 2
TNF-α	Tumor Necrosis Factor α
TNM	T—tumor; N—lymph nodes; M—metastasis
TOPFlash	TCF Reporter Plasmid
TP53	Tumor Protein 53
3'UTR	3' Untranslated Region
VEGF	Vascular Endothelial Growth Factor
VEGF (R)	Vascular Endothelial Growth Factor (Receptor)

References

1. Gregorieff, A.; Clevers, H. Wnt signaling in the intestinal epithelium: From endoderm to cancer. *Genes Dev.* **2005**, *19*, 877–890. [CrossRef]
2. Tenbaum, S.P.; Ordóñez-Morán, P.; Puig, I.; Chicote, I.; Arqués, O.; Landolfi, S.; Fernández, Y.; Herance, J.R.; Gispert, J.D.; Mendizabal, L.; et al. β-catenin confers resistance to PI3K and AKT inhibitors and subverts FOXO3a to promote metastasis in colon cancer. *Nat. Med.* **2012**, *18*, 892–901. [CrossRef]
3. Zhan, T.; Rindtorff, N.; Boutros, M. Wnt signaling in cancer. *Oncogene* **2017**, *36*, 1461–1473. [CrossRef]
4. Wiese, K.E.; Nusse, R.; van Amerongen, R. Wnt signalling: Conquering complexity. *Development* **2018**, *145*. [CrossRef]
5. Nusse, R.; Varmus, H.E. Many tumors induced by the mouse mammary tumor virus contain a provirus integrated in the same region of the host genome. *Cell* **1982**, *31*, 99–109. [CrossRef]
6. Chien, A.J.; Conrad, W.H.; Moon, R.T. A Wnt survival guide: From flies to human disease. *J. Investig. Dermatol.* **2009**, *129*, 1614–1627. [CrossRef]
7. Nusse, R.; Varmus, H. Three decades of Wnts: A personal perspective on how a scientific field developed. *EMBO J.* **2012**, *31*, 2670–2684. [CrossRef]
8. White, B.D.; Chien, A.J.; Dawson, D.W. Dysregulation of Wnt/β-catenin signaling in gastrointestinal cancers. *Gastroenterology* **2012**, *142*, 219–232. [CrossRef]
9. Nusse, R.; Clevers, H. Wnt/β-Catenin Signaling, Disease, and Emerging Therapeutic Modalities. *Cell* **2017**, *169*, 985–999. [CrossRef]
10. Zeitlin, B.D.; Ellis, L.M.; Nör, J.E. Inhibition of Vascular Endothelial Growth Factor Receptor-1/Wnt/{beta}-catenin Crosstalk Leads to Tumor Cell Death. *Clin. Cancer Res.* **2009**, *15*, 7453–7455. [CrossRef]
11. Qi, L.; Song, W.; Liu, Z.; Zhao, X.; Cao, W.; Sun, B. Wnt3a Promotes the Vasculogenic Mimicry Formation of Colon Cancer via Wnt/β-Catenin Signaling. *Int. J. Mol. Sci.* **2015**, *16*, 18564–18579. [CrossRef]
12. Olsen, J.J.; Pohl, S.Ö.; Deshmukh, A.; Visweswaran, M.; Ward, N.C.; Arfuso, F.; Agostino, M.; Dharmarajan, A. The Role of Wnt Signalling in Angiogenesis. *Clin. Biochem. Rev.* **2017**, *38*, 131–142. [PubMed]
13. Goodwin, A.M.; D'Amore, P.A. Wnt signaling in the vasculature. *Angiogenesis* **2002**, *5*, 1–9. [CrossRef]
14. Nie, X.; Liu, H.; Liu, L.; Wang, Y.D.; Chen, W.D. Emerging Roles of Wnt Ligands in Human Colorectal Cancer. *Front. Oncol.* **2020**, *10*. [CrossRef]
15. Fodde, R.; Brabletz, T. Wnt/beta-catenin signaling in cancer stemness and malignant behavior. *Curr. Opin. Cell Biol.* **2007**, *19*, 150–158. [CrossRef]
16. Vermeulen, L.; Felipe De Sousa, E.M.; Van Der Heijden, M.; Cameron, K.; De Jong, J.H.; Borovski, T.; Tuynman, J.B.; Todaro, M.; Merz, C.; Rodermond, H.; et al. Wnt activity defines colon cancer stem cells and is regulated by the microenvironment. *Nat. Cell Biol.* **2010**, *12*, 468–476. [CrossRef]
17. Teeuwssen, M.; Fodde, R. Cell Heterogeneity and Phenotypic Plasticity in Metastasis Formation: The Case of Colon Cancer. *Cancers* **2019**, *11*, 1368, Correction in *Cancers* **2020**, *12*, 1392. [CrossRef]

18. Keum, N.; Giovannucci, E. Global burden of colorectal cancer: Emerging trends, risk factors and prevention strategies. *Nat. Rev. Gastroenterol. Hepatol.* **2019**, *16*, 713–732. [CrossRef]
19. He, F.; Chen, H.; Yang, P.; Yin, H.; Zhang, X.; He, T.; Song, S.; Sun, S.; Wang, B.; Li, Z.; et al. Gankyrin sustains PI3K/GSK-3β/β-catenin signal activation and promotes colorectal cancer aggressiveness and progression. *Oncotarget* **2016**, *7*, 81156–81171. [CrossRef]
20. Lee, S.K.; Hwang, J.H.; Choi, K.Y. Interaction of the Wnt/β-catenin and RAS-ERK pathways involving co-stabilization of both β-catenin and RAS plays important roles in the colorectal tumorigenesis. *Adv. Biol. Regul.* **2018**, *68*, 46–54. [CrossRef]
21. Fearon, E.R.; Vogelstein, B. A genetic model for colorectal tumorigenesis. *Cell* **1990**, *61*, 759–767. [CrossRef]
22. Gerstung, M.; Jolly, C.; Leshchiner, I.; Dentro, S.C.; Gonzalez, S.; Rosebrock, D.; Mitchell, T.J.; Rubanova, Y.; Anur, P.; Yu, K.; et al. The evolutionary history of 2658 cancers. *Nature* **2020**, *578*, 122–128. [CrossRef] [PubMed]
23. Liu, C.; Li, Y.; Semenov, M.; Han, C.; Baeg, G.H.; Tan, Y.; Zhang, Z.; Lin, X.; He, X. Control of beta-catenin phosphorylation/degradation by a dual-kinase mechanism. *Cell* **2002**, *108*, 837–847. [CrossRef]
24. Mayer, C.D.; Giclais, S.M.; Alsehly, F.; Hoppler, S. Diverse LEF/TCF Expression in Human Colorectal Cancer Correlates with Altered Wnt-Regulated Transcriptome in a Meta-Analysis of Patient Biopsies. *Genes* **2020**, *11*, 538. [CrossRef]
25. Doumpas, N.; Lampart, F.; Robinson, M.D.; Lentini, A.; Nestor, C.E.; Cantù, C.; Basler, K. TCF/LEF dependent and independent transcriptional regulation of Wnt/β-catenin target genes. *EMBO J.* **2019**, *38*. [CrossRef]
26. Brabletz, T.; Jung, A.; Hermann, K.; Günther, K.; Hohenberger, W.; Kirchner, T. Nuclear overexpression of the oncoprotein beta-catenin in colorectal cancer is localized predominantly at the invasion front. *Pathol. Res. Pract.* **1998**, *194*, 701–704. [CrossRef]
27. Yaeger, R.; Chatila, W.K.; Lipsyc, M.D.; Hechtman, J.F.; Cercek, A.; Sanchez-Vega, F.; Jayakumaran, G.; Middha, S.; Zehir, A.; Donoghue, M.T.A.; et al. Clinical Sequencing Defines the Genomic Landscape of Metastatic Colorectal Cancer. *Cancer Cell* **2018**, *33*, 125–136. [CrossRef]
28. Albuquerque, C.; Baltazar, C.; Filipe, B.; Penha, F.; Pereira, T.; Smits, R.; Cravo, M.; Lage, P.; Fidalgo, P.; Claro, I.; et al. Colorectal cancers show distinct mutation spectra in members of the canonical WNT signaling pathway according to their anatomical location and type of genetic instability. *Genes Chromosomes Cancer* **2010**, *49*, 746–759. [CrossRef]
29. Günther, K.; Brabletz, T.; Kraus, C.; Dworak, O.; Reymond, M.A.; Jung, A.; Hohenberger, W.; Kirchner, T.; Köckerling, F.; Ballhausen, W.G. Predictive value of nuclear betacatenin expression for the occurrence of distant metastases in rectal cancer. *Dis. Colon Rectum* **1998**, *41*, 1256–1261. [CrossRef]
30. Zhao, H.; He, L.; Yin, D.; Song, B. Identification of β-catenin target genes in colorectal cancer by interrogating gene fitness screening data. *Oncol. Lett.* **2019**, *18*, 3769–3777. [CrossRef]
31. Song, J.; Shu, H.; Zhang, L.; Xiong, J. Long noncoding RNA GAS5 inhibits angiogenesis and metastasis of colorectal cancer through the Wnt/β-catenin signaling pathway. *J. Cell Biochem.* **2019**, *120*, 6937–6951. [CrossRef] [PubMed]
32. Sadanandam, A.; Lyssiotis, C.A.; Homicsko, K.; Collisson, E.A.; Gibb, W.J.; Wullschleger, S.; Ostos, L.C.; Lannon, W.A.; Grotzinger, C.; Del Rio, M.; et al. A colorectal cancer classification system that associates cellular phenotype and responses to therapy. *Nat. Med.* **2013**, *19*, 619–625. [CrossRef] [PubMed]
33. Guinney, J.; Dienstmann, R.; Wang, X.; de Reyniès, A.; Schlicker, A.; Soneson, C.; Marisa, L.; Roepman, P.; Nyamundanda, G.; Angelino, P.; et al. The consensus molecular subtypes of colorectal cancer. *Nat. Med.* **2015**, *21*, 1350–1356. [CrossRef]
34. Isella, C.; Brundu, F.; Bellomo, S.E.; Galimi, F.; Zanella, E.; Porporato, R.; Petti, C.; Fiori, A.; Orzan, F.; Senetta, R.; et al. Selective analysis of cancer-cell intrinsic transcriptional traits defines novel clinically relevant subtypes of colorectal cancer. *Nat. Commun.* **2017**, *8*, 1–16. [CrossRef] [PubMed]
35. Mathonnet, M.; Perraud, A.; Christou, N.; Akil, H.; Melin, C.; Battu, S.; Jauberteau, M.O.; Denizot, Y. Hallmarks in colorectal cancer: Angiogenesis and cancer stem-like cells. *World J. Gastroenterol.* **2014**, *20*, 4189–4196. [CrossRef]
36. Mody, K.; Baldeo, C.; Bekaii-Saab, T. Antiangiogenic Therapy in Colorectal Cancer. *Cancer J.* **2018**, *24*, 165–170. [CrossRef]
37. Chen, W.Z.; Jiang, J.X.; Yu, X.Y.; Xia, W.J.; Yu, P.X.; Wang, K.; Zhao, Z.Y.; Chen, Z.G. Endothelial cells in colorectal cancer. *World J. Gastrointest. Oncol.* **2019**, *11*, 946–956. [CrossRef]

38. Hanahan, D.; Weinberg, R.A. The hallmarks of cancer. *Cell* **2000**, *100*, 57–70. [CrossRef]
39. Xing, Y.; Tu, J.; Zheng, L.; Guo, L.; Xi, T. Anti-angiogenic effect of tanshinone IIA involves inhibition of the VEGF/VEGFR2 pathway in vascular endothelial cells. *Oncol. Rep.* **2015**, *33*, 163–170. [CrossRef]
40. Lizárraga-Verdugo, E.; Avendaño-Félix, M.; Bermúdez, M.; Ramos-Payán, R.; Pérez-Plasencia, C.; Aguilar-Medina, M. Cancer Stem Cells and Its Role in Angiogenesis and Vasculogenic Mimicry in Gastrointestinal Cancers. *Front. Oncol.* **2020**, *10*. [CrossRef]
41. Hillen, F.; Griffioen, A.W. Tumour vascularization: Sprouting angiogenesis and beyond. *Cancer Metastasis Rev.* **2007**, *26*, 489–502. [CrossRef]
42. Patan, S.; Munn, L.L.; Jain, R.K. Intussusceptive microvascular growth in a human colon adenocarcinoma xenograft: A novel mechanism of tumor angiogenesis. *Microvasc. Res.* **1996**, *51*, 260–272. [CrossRef] [PubMed]
43. Maniotis, A.J.; Folberg, R.; Hess, A.; Seftor, E.A.; Gardner, L.M.; Pe'er, J.; Trent, J.M.; Meltzer, P.S.; Hendrix, M.J. Vascular channel formation by human melanoma cells in vivo and in vitro: Vasculogenic mimicry. *Am. J. Pathol.* **1999**, *155*, 739–752. [CrossRef]
44. Folberg, R.; Hendrix, M.J.; Maniotis, A.J. Vasculogenic mimicry and tumor angiogenesis. *Am. J. Pathol.* **2000**, *156*, 361–381. [CrossRef]
45. Chang, Y.S.; di Tomaso, E.; McDonald, D.M.; Jones, R.; Jain, R.K.; Munn, L.L. Mosaic blood vessels in tumors: Frequency of cancer cells in contact with flowing blood. *Proc. Natl. Acad. Sci. USA* **2000**, *97*, 14608–14613. [CrossRef]
46. Folkman, J. Role of angiogenesis in tumor growth and metastasis. *Semin. Oncol.* **2002**, *29* (Suppl. S16), 15–18. [CrossRef]
47. Qian, C.N.; Tan, M.H.; Yang, J.P.; Cao, Y. Revisiting tumor angiogenesis: Vessel co-option, vessel remodeling, and cancer cell-derived vasculature formation. *Chin. J. Cancer.* **2016**, *35*, 10. [CrossRef]
48. Liu, Z.; Sun, B.; Qi, L.; Li, H.; Gao, J.; Leng, X. Zinc finger E-box binding homeobox 1 promotes vasculogenic mimicry in colorectal cancer through induction of epithelial-to-mesenchymal transition. *Cancer Sci.* **2012**, *103*, 813–820. [CrossRef]
49. Baeriswyl, V.; Christofori, G. The angiogenic switch in carcinogenesis. *Semin. Cancer Biol.* **2009**, *19*, 329–337. [CrossRef]
50. Shahneh, F.Z.; Baradaran, B.; Zamani, F.; Aghebati-Maleki, L. Tumor angiogenesis and anti-angiogenic therapies. *Hum. Antibodies* **2013**, *22*, 15–19. [CrossRef]
51. Soheilifar, M.; Grusch, M.; Neghab, H.K.; Amini, R.; Maadi, H.; Saidijam, M.; Wang, Z. Angioregulatory microRNAs in Colorectal Cancer. *Cancers* **2019**, *12*, 71. [CrossRef]
52. Folkman, J.; D'Amore, P.A. Blood vessel formation: What is its molecular basis? *Cell* **1996**, *87*, 1153–1155. [CrossRef]
53. Salinas-Vera, Y.M.; Marchat, L.A.; Gallardo-Rincón, D.; Ruiz-García, E.; Astudillo-De La Vega, H.; Echavarría-Zepeda, R.; López-Camarillo, C. AngiomiRs: MicroRNAs driving angiogenesis in cancer. *Int. J. Mol. Med.* **2019**, *43*, 657–670. [CrossRef]
54. Bridges, E.M.; Harris, A.L. The angiogenic process as a therapeutic target in cancer. *Biochem. Pharmacol.* **2011**, *81*, 1183–1191. [CrossRef]
55. Zhang, Z.; Neiva, K.G.; Lingen, M.W.; Ellis, L.M.; Nör, J.E. VEGF-dependent tumor angiogenesis requires inverse and reciprocal regulation of VEGFR1 and VEGFR2. *Cell Death Differ.* **2010**, *17*, 499–512. [CrossRef]
56. Carmeliet, P.; Dor, Y.; Herbert, J.M.; Fukumura, D.; Brusselmans, K.; Dewerchin, M.; Neeman, M.; Bono, F.; Abramovitch, R.; Maxwell, P.; et al. Role of HIF-1α in hypoxia-mediated apoptosis, cell proliferation and tumour angiogenesis. *Nature* **1998**, *394*, 485–490. [CrossRef]
57. Sun, X.; Hu, F.; Hou, Z.; Chen, Q.; Lan, J.; Luo, X.; Wang, G.; Hu, J.; Cao, Z. SIX4 activates Akt and promotes tumor angiogenesis. *Exp. Cell Res.* **2019**, *383*. [CrossRef]
58. Krishnamachary, B.; Berg-Dixon, S.; Kelly, B.; Agani, F.; Feldser, D.; Ferreira, G.; Iyer, N.; LaRusch, J.; Pak, B.; Taghavi, P.; et al. Regulation of colon carcinoma cell invasion by hypoxia-inducible factor 1. *Cancer Res.* **2003**, *63*, 1138–1143.
59. Zhang, X.; Gaspard, J.P.; Chung, D.C. Regulation of vascular endothelial growth factor by the Wnt and K-ras pathways in colonic neoplasia. *Cancer Res.* **2001**, *61*, 6050–6054.

60. Easwaran, V.; Lee, S.H.; Inge, L.; Guo, L.; Goldbeck, C.; Garrett, E.; Wiesmann, M.; Garcia, P.D.; Fuller, J.H.; Chan, V.; et al. β-Catenin regulates vascular endothelial growth factor expression in colon cancer. *Cancer Res.* **2003**, *63*, 3145–3153.
61. Dılek, F.H.; Topak, N.; Tokyol, Ç.; Akbulut, G.; Dılek, O.N. β-Catenin and its relation to VEGF and cyclin D1 expression in pT3 rectosigmoid cancers. *Turk. J. Gastroenterol.* **2010**, *21*, 365–371. [CrossRef]
62. Fan, F.; Wey, J.S.; McCarty, M.F.; Belcheva, A.; Liu, W.; Bauer, T.W.; Somcio, R.J.; Wu, Y.; Hooper, A.; Hicklin, D.J.; et al. Expression and function of vascular endothelial growth factor receptor-1 on human colorectal cancer cells. *Oncogene* **2005**, *24*, 2647–2653. [CrossRef]
63. Ahluwalia, A.; Jones, M.K.; Szabo, S.; Tarnawski, A.S. Aberrant, ectopic expression of VEGF and VEGF receptors 1 and 2 in malignant colonic epithelial cells. Implications for these cells growth via an autocrine mechanism. *Biochem. Biophys. Res. Commun.* **2013**, *437*, 515–520. [CrossRef]
64. Catalano, V.; Turdo, A.; Di Franco, S.; Dieli, F.; Todaro, M.; Stassi, G. Tumor and its microenvironment: A synergistic interplay. *Semin. Cancer Biol.* **2013**, *23*, 522–532. [CrossRef]
65. Naik, S.; Dothager, R.S.; Marasa, J.; Lewis, C.L.; Piwnica-Worms, D. Vascular Endothelial Growth Factor Receptor-1 Is Synthetic Lethal to Aberrant {beta}-Catenin Activation in Colon Cancer. *Clin. Cancer Res.* **2009**, *15*, 7529–7537. [CrossRef]
66. Pate, K.T.; Stringari, C.; Sprowl-Tanio, S.; Wang, K.; TeSlaa, T.; Hoverter, N.P.; McQuade, M.M.; Garner, C.; Digman, M.A.; Teitell, M.A.; et al. Wnt signaling directs a metabolic program of glycolysis and angiogenesis in colon cancer. *EMBO J.* **2014**, *33*, 1454–1473. [CrossRef] [PubMed]
67. Mani, M.; Carrasco, D.E.; Zhang, Y.; Takada, K.; Gatt, M.E.; Dutta-Simmons, J.; Ikeda, H.; Diaz-Griffero, F.; Pena-Cruz, V.; Bertagnolli, M.; et al. BCL9 promotes tumor progression by conferring enhanced proliferative, metastatic, and angiogenic properties to cancer cells. *Cancer Res.* **2009**, *69*, 7577–7586. [CrossRef]
68. Vaish, V.; Sanyal, S.N. Role of Sulindac and Celecoxib in the regulation of angiogenesis during the early neoplasm of colon: Exploring PI3-K/PTEN/Akt pathway to the canonical Wnt/β-catenin signaling. *Biomed. Pharmacother.* **2012**, *66*, 354–367. [CrossRef]
69. Santoyo-Ramos, P.; Likhatcheva, M.; García-Zepeda, E.A.; Castañeda-Patlán, M.C.; Robles-Flores, M. Hypoxia-inducible factors modulate the stemness and malignancy of colon cancer cells by playing opposite roles in canonical Wnt signaling. *PLoS ONE* **2014**, *9*. [CrossRef]
70. Kumar, A.; Cherukumilli, M.; Mahmoudpour, S.H.; Brand, K.; Bandapalli, O.R. ShRNA-mediated knock-down of CXCL8 inhibits tumor growth in colorectal liver metastasis. *Biochem. Biophys. Res. Commun.* **2018**, *500*, 731–737. [CrossRef]
71. Suman, S.; Kurisetty, V.; Das, T.P.; Vadodkar, A.; Ramos, G.; Lakshmanaswamy, R.; Damodaran, C. Activation of AKT signaling promotes epithelial-mesenchymal transition and tumor growth in colorectal cancer cells. *Mol. Carcinog.* **2014**, *53* (Suppl. 1), E151–E160. [CrossRef]
72. Lin, H.; Fang, Z.; Su, Y.; Li, P.; Wang, J.; Liao, H.; Hu, Q.; Ye, C.; Fang, Y.; Luo, Q.; et al. DHX32 Promotes Angiogenesis in Colorectal Cancer Through Augmenting β-catenin Signaling to Induce Expression of VEGFA. *EBioMedicine* **2017**, *18*, 62–72. [CrossRef]
73. Kumaradevan, S.; Lee, S.Y.; Richards, S.; Agani, F.; Feldser, D.; Ferreira, G.; Iyer, N.; LaRusch, J.; Pak, B.; Taghavi, P.; et al. c-Cbl Expression Correlates with Human Colorectal Cancer Survival and Its Wnt/β-Catenin Suppressor Function Is Regulated by Tyr371 Phosphorylation. *Am. J. Pathol.* **2018**, *188*, 1921–1933. [CrossRef]
74. Dupasquier, S.; Blache, P.; Picque Lasorsa, L.; Zhao, H.; Abraham, J.D.; Haigh, J.J.; Ychou, M.; Prévostel, C. Modulating PKCα Activity to Target Wnt/β-Catenin Signaling in Colon Cancer. *Cancers* **2019**, *11*, 693. [CrossRef]
75. Yang, P.; Yu, D.; Zhou, J.; Zhuang, S.; Jiang, T. TGM2 interference regulates the angiogenesis and apoptosis of colorectal cancer via Wnt/β-catenin pathway. *Cell Cycle* **2019**, *18*, 1122–1134. [CrossRef]
76. Böhm, J.; Sustmann, C.; Wilhelm, C.; Kohlhase, J. SALL4 is directly activated by TCF/LEF in the canonical Wnt signaling pathway. *Biochem. Biophys. Res. Commun.* **2006**, *348*, 898–907. [CrossRef]
77. Peng, X.; Luo, Z.; Kang, Q.; Deng, D.; Wang, Q.; Peng, H.; Wang, S.; Wei, Z. FOXQ1 mediates the crosstalk between TGF-β and Wnt signaling pathways in the progression of colorectal cancer. *Cancer Biol. Ther.* **2015**, *16*, 1099–1109. [CrossRef]
78. Hao, L.; Zhao, Y.; Wang, Z.; Yin, H.; Zhang, X.; He, T.; Song, S.; Sun, S.; Wang, B.; Li, Z.; et al. Expression and clinical significance of SALL4 and β-catenin in colorectal cancer. *J. Mol. Histol.* **2016**, *47*, 117–128. [CrossRef]

79. Sampietro, J.; Dahlberg, C.L.; Cho, U.S.; Hinds, T.R.; Kimelman, D.; Xu, W. Crystal structure of a β-catenin/BCL9/Tcf4 complex. *Mol. Cell.* **2006**, *24*, 293–300. [CrossRef]
80. Mosimann, C.; Hausmann, G.; Basler, K. β-catenin hits chromatin: Regulation of Wnt target gene activation. *Nat. Rev. Mol. Cell Biol.* **2009**, *10*, 276–286. [CrossRef]
81. Pendás-Franco, N.; García, J.M.; Peña, C.; Valle, N.; Pálmer, H.G.; Heinäniemi, M.; Carlberg, C.; Jiménez, B.; Bonilla, F.; Muñoz, A.; et al. DICKKOPF-4 is induced by TCF/β-catenin and upregulated in human colon cancer, promotes tumour cell invasion and angiogenesis and is repressed by 1α,25-dihydroxyvitamin D3. *Oncogene* **2008**, *27*, 4467–4477. [CrossRef]
82. Jiang, M.; Kang, Y.; Sewastianik, T.; Wang, J.; Tanton, H.; Alder, K.; Dennis, P.; Xin, Y.; Wang, Z.; Liu, R.; et al. BCL9 provides multi-cellular communication properties in colorectal cancer by interacting with paraspeckle proteins. *Nat. Commun.* **2020**, *11*. [CrossRef]
83. Takada, K.; Zhu, D.; Bird, G.H.; Sukhdeo, K.; Zhao, J.J.; Mani, M.; Lemieux, M.; Carrasco, D.E.; Ryan, J.; Horst, D.; et al. Targeted disruption of the BCL9/β-catenin complex inhibits oncogenic Wnt signaling. *Sci. Transl. Med.* **2012**, *4*. [CrossRef]
84. Hu, T.H.; Yao, Y.; Yu, S.; Han, L.L.; Wang, W.J.; Guo, H.; Tian, T.; Ruan, Z.P.; Kang, X.M.; Wang, J.; et al. SDF-1/CXCR4 promotes epithelial-mesenchymal transition and progression of colorectal cancer by activation of the Wnt/β-catenin signaling pathway. *Cancer Lett.* **2014**, *354*, 417–426. [CrossRef]
85. Cheng, H.; Sun, X.; Li, J.; He, P.; Liu, W.; Meng, X. Knockdown of Uba2 inhibits colorectal cancer cell invasion and migration through downregulation of the Wnt/β-catenin signaling pathway. *J. Cell Biochem.* **2018**, *119*, 6914–6925. [CrossRef]
86. Ayinde, O.; Wang, Z.; Pinton, G.; Moro, L.; Griffin, M. Transglutaminase 2 maintains a colorectal cancer stem phenotype by regulating epithelial-mesenchymal transition. *Oncotarget* **2019**, *10*, 4556–4569. [CrossRef]
87. Sun, J.; Zhao, Z.; Zhang, W.; Tang, Q.; Yang, F.; Hu, X.; Liu, C.; Song, B.; Zhang, B.; Wang, H. Spalt-Like Protein 4 (SALL4) Promotes Angiogenesis by Activating Vascular Endothelial Growth Factor A (VEGFA) Signaling. *Med. Sci. Monit.* **2020**, *26*. [CrossRef]
88. Pan, Q.; Pan, H.; Lou, H.; Xu, Y.; Tian, L. Inhibition of the angiogenesis and growth of Aloin in human colorectal cancer in vitro and in vivo. *Cancer Cell Int.* **2013**, *13*. [CrossRef]
89. Peng, C.; Zhang, W.; Dai, C.; Li, W.; Shen, X.; Yuan, Y.; Yan, L.; Zhang, W.; Yao, M. Study of the aqueous extract of Aloe vera and its two active components on the Wnt/β-catenin and Notch signaling pathways in colorectal cancer cells. *J. Ethnopharmacol.* **2019**, *243*. [CrossRef]
90. Liu, Z.; Sun, B.; Qi, L.; Li, Y.; Zhao, X.; Zhang, D.; Zhang, Y. Dickkopf-1 expression is down-regulated during the colorectal adenoma-carcinoma sequence and correlates with reduced microvessel density and VEGF expression. *Histopathology* **2015**, *67*, 158–166. [CrossRef]
91. Wu, D.D.; Liu, S.Y.; Gao, Y.R.; Lu, D.; Hong, Y.; Chen, Y.G.; Dong, P.Z.; Wang, D.Y.; Li, T.; Li, H.M.; et al. Tumour necrosis factor-α-induced protein 8-like 2 is a novel regulator of proliferation, migration, and invasion in human rectal adenocarcinoma cells. *J. Cell Mol. Med.* **2019**, *23*, 1698–1713. [CrossRef]
92. Lou, Y.; Liu, S. The TIPE (TNFAIP8) family in inflammation, immunity, and cancer. *Mol. Immunol.* **2011**, *49*, 4–7. [CrossRef]
93. Kwon, I.K.; Schoenlein, P.V.; Delk, J.; Liu, K.; Thangaraju, M.; Dulin, N.O.; Ganapathy, V.; Berger, F.G.; Browning, D.D. Expression of cyclic guanosine monophosphate-dependent protein kinase in metastatic colon carcinoma cells blocks tumor angiogenesis. *Cancer* **2008**, *112*, 1462–1470. [CrossRef]
94. Taye, N.; Alam, A.; Ghorai, S.; Chatterji, D.G.; Parulekar, A.; Mogare, D.; Singh, S.; Sengupta, P.; Chatterjee, S.; Bhat, M.K.; et al. SMAR1 inhibits Wnt/β-catenin signaling and prevents colorectal cancer progression. *Oncotarget* **2018**, *9*, 21322–21336. [CrossRef]
95. Lee, J.M.; Kim, I.S.; Kim, H.; Lee, J.S.; Kim, K.; Yim, H.Y.; Jeong, J.; Kim, J.H.; Kim, J.Y.; Lee, H.; et al. RORalpha attenuates Wnt/beta-catenin signaling by PKCalpha-dependent phosphorylation in colon cancer. *Mol. Cell* **2010**, *37*, 183–195. [CrossRef]
96. Gwak, J.; Cho, M.; Gong, S.J.; Won, J.; Kim, D.E.; Kim, E.Y.; Lee, S.S.; Kim, M.; Kim, T.K.; Shin, J.G.; et al. Protein-kinase-C-mediated β-catenin phosphorylation negatively regulates the Wnt/β-catenin pathway. *J. Cell Sci.* **2006**, *119*, 4702–4709. [CrossRef]
97. Yang, C.; Zhang, J.J.; Zhang, X.P.; Xiao, R.; Li, P.G. Sporamin suppresses growth of xenografted colorectal carcinoma in athymic BALB/c mice by inhibiting liver β-catenin and vascular endothelial growth factor expression. *World J. Gastroenterol.* **2019**, *25*, 3196–3206. [CrossRef]

98. Sui, H.; Zhao, J.; Zhou, L.; Wen, H.; Deng, W.; Li, C.; Ji, Q.; Liu, X.; Feng, Y.; Chai, N.; et al. Tanshinone IIA inhibits β-catenin/VEGF-mediated angiogenesis by targeting TGF-β1 in normoxic and HIF-1α in hypoxic microenvironments in human colorectal cancer. *Cancer Lett.* **2017**, *403*, 86–97. [CrossRef]
99. Pooja, T.; Karunagaran, D. Emodin suppresses Wnt signaling in human colorectal cancer cells SW480 and SW620. *Eur. J. Pharmacol.* **2014**, *742*, 55–64. [CrossRef]
100. Gu, J.; Cui, C.F.; Yang, L.; Wang, L.; Jiang, X.H. Emodin Inhibits Colon Cancer Cell Invasion and Migration by Suppressing Epithelial-Mesenchymal Transition via the Wnt/β-Catenin Pathway. *Oncol. Res.* **2019**, *27*, 193–202. [CrossRef]
101. Farombi, E.O.; Ajayi, B.O.; Adedara, I.A. 6-Gingerol delays tumorigenesis in benzo [a] pyrene and dextran sulphate sodium-induced colorectal cancer in mice. *Food Chem. Toxicol.* **2020**, *142*. [CrossRef]
102. de Lima, R.M.T.; Dos Reis, A.C.; de Menezes, A.P.M.; Santos, J.V.O.; Filho, J.W.G.O.; Ferreira, J.R.O.; de Alencar, M.V.O.B.; da Mata, A.M.O.F.; Khan, I.N.; Islam, A.; et al. Protective and therapeutic potential of ginger (*Zingiber officinale*) extract and [6]-gingerol in cancer: A comprehensive review. *Phytother. Res.* **2018**, *32*, 1885–1907. [CrossRef] [PubMed]
103. Naz, I.; Ramchandani, S.; Khan, M.R.; Yang, M.H.; Ahn, K.S. Anticancer Potential of Raddeanin A, a Natural Triterpenoid Isolated from *Anemone raddeana Regel*. *Molecules* **2020**, *25*, 1035. [CrossRef]
104. Wang, Y.; Bao, X.; Zhao, A.; Zhang, J.; Zhang, M.; Zhang, Q.; Ma, B. Raddeanin A inhibits growth and induces apoptosis in human colorectal cancer through downregulating the Wnt/β-catenin and NF-κB signaling pathway. *Life Sci.* **2018**, *207*, 532–549. [CrossRef]
105. Guan, Y.Y.; Liu, H.J.; Luan, X.; Xu, J.R.; Lu, Q.; Liu, Y.R.; Gao, Y.G.; Zhao, M.; Chen, H.Z.; Fang, C. Raddeanin A, a triterpenoid saponin isolated from *Anemone raddeana*, suppresses the angiogenesis and growth of human colorectal tumor by inhibiting VEGFR2 signaling. *Phytomedicine* **2015**, *22*, 103–110. [CrossRef]
106. Unterleuthner, D.; Neuhold, P.; Schwarz, K.; Janker, L.; Neuditschko, B.; Nivarthi, H.; Crncec, I.; Kramer, N.; Unger, C.; Hengstschläger, M.; et al. Cancer-associated fibroblast-derived WNT2 increases tumor angiogenesis in colon cancer. *Angiogenesis* **2020**, *23*, 159–177. [CrossRef]
107. Kramer, N.; Schmöllerl, J.; Unger, C.; Nivarthi, H.; Rudisch, A.; Unterleuthner, D.; Scherzer, M.; Riedl, A.; Artaker, M.; Crncec, I.; et al. Autocrine WNT2 signaling in fibroblasts promotes colorectal cancer progression. *Oncogene* **2017**, *36*, 5460–5472. [CrossRef]
108. Aizawa, T.; Karasawa, H.; Funayama, R.; Shirota, M.; Suzuki, T.; Maeda, S.; Suzuki, H.; Yamamura, A.; Naitoh, T.; Nakayama, K.; et al. Cancer-associated fibroblasts secrete Wnt2 to promote cancer progression in colorectal cancer. *Cancer Med.* **2019**, *8*, 6370–6382. [CrossRef]
109. Huang, Z.; Feng, Y. Exosomes derived from hypoxic colorectal cancer cells promote angiogenesis through Wnt4-induced β-catenin signaling in endothelial cells. *Oncol. Res. Featur. Preclin. Clin. Cancer Ther.* **2017**, *25*, 651–661. [CrossRef]
110. Shangguan, W.; Fan, C.; Chen, X.; Lu, R.; Liu, Y.; Li, Y.; Shang, Y.; Yin, D.; Zhang, S.; Huang, Q.; et al. Endothelium originated from colorectal cancer stem cells constitute cancer blood vessels. *Cancer Sci.* **2017**, *108*, 1357–1367. [CrossRef]
111. Munro, M.J.; Wickremesekera, S.K.; Peng, L.; Tan, S.T.; Itinteang, T. Cancer stem cells in colorectal cancer: A review. *J. Clin. Pathol.* **2018**, *71*, 110–116. [CrossRef]
112. Wei, B.; Han, X.Y.; Qi, C.L.; Zhang, S.; Zheng, Z.H.; Huang, Y.; Chen, T.F.; Wei, H.B. Coaction of spheroid-derived stem-like cells and endothelial progenitor cells promotes development of colon cancer. *PLoS ONE* **2012**, *7*. [CrossRef]
113. Garza Treviño, E.N.; González, P.D.; Valencia Salgado, C.I.; Martinez Garza, A. Effects of pericytes and colon cancer stem cells in the tumor microenvironment. *Cancer Cell. Int.* **2019**, *19*, 173. [CrossRef]
114. Planutis, K.; Planutiene, M.; Moyer, M.P.; Nguyen, A.V.; Pérez, C.A.; Holcombe, R.F. Regulation of norrin receptor frizzled-4 by Wnt2 in colon-derived cells. *BMC Mol. Cell Biol.* **2007**, *8*. [CrossRef]
115. Planutis, K.; Planutiene, M.; Holcombe, R.F. A novel signaling pathway regulates colon cancer angiogenesis through Norrin. *Sci. Rep.* **2014**, *4*, 1–5. [CrossRef]
116. Mitselou, A.; Galani, V.; Skoufi, U.; Arvanitis, D.L.; Lampri, E.; Ioachim, E. Syndecan-1, Epithelial-Mesenchymal Transition Markers (E-cadherin/β-catenin) and Neoangiogenesis-related Proteins (PCAM-1 and Endoglin) in Colorectal Cancer. *Anticancer Res.* **2016**, *36*, 2271–2280.
117. Bhowmick, N.A.; Neilson, E.G.; Moses, H.L. Stromal fibroblasts in cancer initiation and progression. *Nature* **2004**, *432*, 332–337. [CrossRef]

118. Wang, F.T.; Sun, W.; Zhang, J.T.; Fan, Y.Z. Cancer-associated fibroblast regulation of tumor neo-angiogenesis as a therapeutic target in cancer. *Oncol. Lett.* **2019**, *17*, 3055–3065. [CrossRef]
119. Nagasaki, T.; Hara, M.; Nakanishi, H.; Takahashi, H.; Sato, M.; Takeyama, H. Interleukin-6 released by colon cancer-associated fibroblasts is critical for tumour angiogenesis: Anti-interleukin-6 receptor antibody suppressed angiogenesis and inhibited tumour-stroma interaction. *Br. J. Cancer.* **2014**, *110*, 469–478. [CrossRef]
120. Zhang, L.; Jiang, X.; Li, Y.; Fan, Q.; Li, H.; Jin, L.; Li, L.; Jin, Y.; Zhang, T.; Mao, Y.; et al. Clinical correlation of Wnt2 and COL8A1 with colon adenocarcinoma prognosis. *Front. Oncol.* **2020**, *10*. [CrossRef]
121. Jung, Y.S.; Jun, S.; Lee, S.H.; Sharma, A.; Park, J.I. Wnt2 complements Wnt/β-catenin signaling in colorectal cancer. *Oncotarget* **2015**, *6*, 37257–37268. [CrossRef]
122. Guo, M.; Breslin, J.W.; Wu, M.H.; Gottardi, C.J.; Yuan, S.Y. VE-cadherin and beta-catenin binding dynamics during histamine-induced endothelial hyperpermeability. *Am. J. Physiol. Cell Physiol.* **2008**, *294*, 977–984. [CrossRef] [PubMed]
123. Gavard, J. Endothelial permeability and VE-cadherin: A wacky comradeship. *Cell Adhes. Migr.* **2013**, *7*, 455–461. [CrossRef]
124. Ichikawa, Y.; Ishikawa, T.; Momiyama, N.; Kamiyama, M.; Sakurada, H.; Matsuyama, R.; Hasegawa, S.; Chishima, T.; Hamaguchi, Y.; Fujii, S.; et al. Matrilysin (MMP-7) degrades VE-cadherin and accelerates accumulation of beta-catenin in the nucleus of human umbilical vein endothelial cells. *Oncol. Rep.* **2006**, *15*, 311–315. [CrossRef]
125. Zhao, Y.; Li, J.; Ting, K.K.; Chen, J.; Coleman, P.; Liu, K.; Wan, L.; Moller, T.; Vadas, M.A.; Gamble, J.R. The VE-Cadherin/β-catenin signalling axis regulates immune cell infiltration into tumours. *Cancer Lett.* **2020**, *496*, 1–15. [CrossRef]
126. Reis, M.; Liebner, S. Wnt signaling in the vasculature. *Exp. Cell Res.* **2013**, *319*, 1317–1323. [CrossRef]
127. Martowicz, A.; Trusohamn, M.; Jensen, N.; Wisniewska-Kruk, J.; Corada, M.; Ning, F.C.; Kele, J.; Dejana, E.; Nyqvist, D. Endothelial β-Catenin Signaling Supports Postnatal Brain and Retinal Angiogenesis by Promoting Sprouting, Tip Cell Formation, and VEGFR (Vascular Endothelial Growth Factor Receptor) 2 Expression. *Arterioscler. Thromb. Vasc. Biol.* **2019**, *39*, 2273–2288. [CrossRef]
128. Maishi, N.; Hida, K. Tumor endothelial cells accelerate tumor metastasis. *Cancer Sci.* **2017**, *108*, 1921–1926. [CrossRef]
129. Fujiwara-Tani, R.; Sasaki, T.; Fujii, K.; Luo, Y.; Mori, T.; Kishi, S.; Mori, S.; Matsushima-Otsuka, S.; Nishiguchi, Y.; Goto, K.; et al. Diabetes mellitus is associated with liver metastasis of colorectal cancer through production of biglycan-rich cancer stroma. *Oncotarget* **2020**, *11*, 2982–2994. [CrossRef]
130. Liu, Z.; Qi, L.; Li, Y.; Zhao, X.; Sun, B. VEGFR2 regulates endothelial differentiation of colon cancer cells. *BMC Cancer* **2017**, *17*, 593. [CrossRef]
131. Wang, G.; Yang, Q.; Li, M.; Zhang, Y.; Cai, Y.; Liang, X.; Fu, Y.; Xiao, Z.; Zhou, M.; Xie, Z.; et al. Quantitative proteomic profiling of tumor-associated vascular endothelial cells in colorectal cancer. *Biol. Open* **2019**, *8*. [CrossRef]
132. Suzuki, H.; Masuda, N.; Shimura, T.; Araki, K.; Kobayashi, T.; Tsutsumi, S.; Asao, T.; Kuwano, H. Nuclear β-catenin expression at the invasive front and in the vessels predicts liver metastasis in colorectal carcinoma. *Anticancer Res.* **2008**, *28*, 1821–1830.
133. Wang, L.; Cheng, H.; Liu, Y.; Wang, L.; Yu, W.; Zhang, G.; Chen, B.; Yu, Z.; Hu, S. Prognostic value of nuclear β-catenin overexpression at invasive front in colorectal cancer for synchronous liver metastasis. *Ann. Surg. Oncol.* **2011**, *18*, 1553–1559. [CrossRef]
134. Serafino, A.; Moroni, N.; Zonfrillo, M.; Andreola, F.; Mercuri, L.; Nicotera, G.; Nunziata, J.; Ricci, R.; Antinori, A.; Rasi, G.; et al. WNT-pathway components as predictive markers useful for diagnosis, prevention and therapy in inflammatory bowel disease and sporadic colorectal cancer. *Oncotarget* **2014**, *5*, 978–992. [CrossRef]
135. Sulkowska, M.; Famulski, W.; Wincewicz, A.; Moniuszko, T.; Kedra, B.; Koda, M.; Zalewski, B.; Baltaziak, M.; Sulkowski, S. Levels of VE-cadherin increase independently of VEGF in preoperative sera of patients with colorectal cancer. *Tumori J.* **2006**, *92*, 67–71. [CrossRef]
136. Agarwal, A.; Das, K.; Lerner, N.; Sathe, S.; Cicek, M.; Casey, G.; Sizemore, N. The AKT/I κB kinase pathway promotes angiogenic/metastatic gene expression in colorectal cancer by actiating nuclear factor-κB and β-catenin. *Oncogene* **2005**, *24*, 1021–1031. [CrossRef]

137. Shao, J.; Jung, C.; Liu, C.; Sheng, H. Prostaglandin E2 Stimulates the β-catenin/T cell factor-dependent transcription in colon cancer. *J. Biol. Chem.* **2005**, *280*, 26565–26572. [CrossRef]
138. Jeong, W.J.; Ro, E.J.; Choi, K.Y. Interaction between Wnt/β-catenin and RAS-ERK pathways and an anti-cancer strategy via degradations of β-catenin and RAS by targeting the Wnt/β-catenin pathway. *NPJ Precis. Oncol.* **2018**, *2*, 5. [CrossRef]
139. Liang, J.; Tang, J.; Shi, H.; Li, H.; Zhen, T.; Duan, J.; Kang, L.; Zhang, F.; Dong, Y.; Han, A. miR-27a-3p targeting RXRα promotes colorectal cancer progression by activating Wnt/β-catenin pathway. *Oncotarget* **2017**, *8*, 82991–83008. [CrossRef]
140. Cheng, X.; Xu, X.; Chen, D.; Zhao, F.; Wang, W. Therapeutic potential of targeting the Wnt/β-catenin signaling pathway in colorectal cancer. *Biomed. Pharmacother.* **2019**, *110*, 473–481. [CrossRef]
141. Xue, M.; Zhuo, Y.; Shan, B. MicroRNAs, Long Noncoding RNAs, and Their Functions in Human Disease. *Methods Mol. Biol.* **2017**, *1617*, 1–25. [CrossRef] [PubMed]
142. Patop, I.L.; Kadener, S. circRNAs in Cancer. *Curr. Opin. Genet. Dev.* **2018**, *48*, 121–127. [CrossRef]
143. Zhao, W.; Dong, M.; Pan, J.; Wang, Y.; Zhou, J.; Ma, J.; Liu, S. Circular RNAs: A novel target among non-coding RNAs with potential roles in malignant tumors. *Mol. Med. Rep.* **2019**, *20*, 3463–3474. [CrossRef]
144. Lewis, B.P.; Burge, C.B.; Bartel, D.P. Conserved seed pairing, often flanked by adenosines, indicates that thousands of human genes are microRNA targets. *Cell* **2005**, *120*, 15–20. [CrossRef]
145. Balacescu, O.; Sur, D.; Cainap, C.; Visan, S.; Cruceriu, D.; Manzat-Saplacan, R.; Muresan, M.S.; Balacescu, L.; Lisencu, C.; Irimie, A. The Impact of miRNA in Colorectal Cancer Progression and Its Liver Metastases. *Int. J. Mol. Sci.* **2018**, *19*, 3711. [CrossRef] [PubMed]
146. Ji, S.; Ye, G.; Zhang, J.; Wang, L.; Wang, T.; Wang, Z.; Zhang, T.; Wang, G.; Guo, Z.; Luo, Y.; et al. miR-574-5p negatively regulates Qki6/7 to impact β-catenin/Wnt signalling and the development of colorectal cancer. *Gut* **2013**, *62*, 716–726. [CrossRef]
147. Li, Y.; Lauriola, M.; Kim, D.; Francesconi, M.; D'Uva, G.; Shibata, D.; Malafa, M.P.; Yeatman, T.J.; Coppola, D.; Solmi, R.; et al. Adenomatous polyposis coli (APC) regulates miR17-92 cluster through β-catenin pathway in colorectal cancer. *Oncogene* **2016**, *35*, 4558–4568. [CrossRef]
148. Zhang, G.J.; Li, L.F.; Yang, G.D.; Xia, S.S.; Wang, R.; Leng, Z.W.; Liu, Z.L.; Tian, H.P.; He, Y.; Meng, C.Y.; et al. MiR-92a promotes stem cell-like properties by activating Wnt/β-catenin signaling in colorectal cancer. *Oncotarget* **2017**, *8*, 101760–101770. [CrossRef]
149. Li, T.; Jian, X.; He, H.; Lai, Q.; Li, X.; Deng, D.; Liu, T.; Zhu, J.; Jiao, H.; Ye, Y.; et al. MiR-452 promotes an aggressive colorectal cancer phenotype by regulating a Wnt/β-catenin positive feedback loop. *J. Exp. Clin. Cancer Res.* **2018**, *37*, 238. [CrossRef]
150. Zhang, F.; Meng, F.; Li, H.; Dong, Y.; Yang, W.; Han, A. Suppression of retinoid X receptor alpha and aberrant β-catenin expression significantly associates with progression of colorectal carcinoma. *Eur. J. Cancer* **2011**, *47*, 2060–2067. [CrossRef]
151. Han, A.; Tong, C.; Hu, D.; Bi, X.; Yang, W. A direct protein-protein interaction is involved in the suppression of beta-catenin transcription by retinoid X receptor alpha in colorectal cancer cells. *Cancer Biol. Ther.* **2008**, *7*, 454–459. [CrossRef]
152. Li, T.; Lai, Q.; Wang, S.; Cai, J.; Xiao, Z.; Deng, D.; He, L.; Jiao, H.; Ye, Y.; Liang, L.; et al. MicroRNA-224 sustains Wnt/β-catenin signaling and promotes aggressive phenotype of colorectal cancer. *J. Exp. Clin. Cancer Res.* **2016**, *35*, 21. [CrossRef]
153. Zheng, K.; Zhou, X.; Yu, J.; Li, Q.; Wang, H.; Li, M.; Shao, Z.; Zhang, F.; Luo, Y.; Shen, Z.; et al. Epigenetic silencing of miR-490-3p promotes development of an aggressive colorectal cancer phenotype through activation of the Wnt/β-catenin signaling pathway. *Cancer Lett.* **2016**, *376*, 178–187. [CrossRef] [PubMed]
154. Subramanian, M.; Rao, S.R.; Thacker, P.; Chatterjee, S.; Karunagaran, D. MiR-29b downregulates canonical Wnt signaling by suppressing coactivators of β-catenin in human colorectal cancer cells. *J. Cell Biochem.* **2014**, *115*, 1974–1984. [CrossRef]
155. Yuan, Z.; Yu, X.; Ni, B.; Chen, D.; Yang, Z.; Huang, J.; Wang, J.; Chen, D.; Wang, L. Overexpression of long non-coding RNA-CTD903 inhibits colorectal cancer invasion and migration by repressing Wnt/β-catenin signaling and predicts favorable prognosis. *Int. J. Oncol.* **2016**, *48*, 2675–2685. [CrossRef]
156. Yu, J.; Han, Z.; Sun, Z.; Wang, Y.; Zheng, M.; Song, C. LncRNA SLCO4A1-AS1 facilitates growth and metastasis of colorectal cancer through β-catenin-dependent Wnt pathway. *J. Exp. Clin. Cancer Res.* **2018**, *37*, 222. [CrossRef]

157. Javed, Z.; Khan, K.; Sadia, H.; Raza, S.; Salehi, B.; Sharifi-Rad, J.; Cho, W.C. LncRNA & Wnt signaling in colorectal cancer. *Cancer Cell Int.* **2020**, *20*, 326. [CrossRef]
158. Wang, F.W.; Cao, C.H.; Han, K.; Zhao, Y.X.; Cai, M.Y.; Xiang, Z.C.; Zhang, J.X.; Chen, J.W.; Zhong, L.P.; Huang, Y.; et al. APC-activated long noncoding RNA inhibits colorectal carcinoma pathogenesis through reduction of exosome production. *J. Clin. Investig.* **2019**, *129*, 727–743. [CrossRef]
159. Fang, Q.; Yang, A.; Dong, A.; Zhao, L. circPDSS1 Stimulates the Development of Colorectal Cancer via Activating the Wnt/β-Catenin Signaling. *Onco Targets Ther.* **2020**, *13*, 6329–6337. [CrossRef]
160. Kircher, S.M.; Nimeiri, H.S.; Benson, A.B., III. Targeting Angiogenesis in Colorectal Cancer: Tyrosine Kinase Inhibitors. *Cancer J.* **2016**, *22*, 182–189. [CrossRef]
161. Karasic, T.B.; Rosen, M.A.; O'Dwyer, P.J. Antiangiogenic tyrosine kinase inhibitors in colorectal cancer: Is there a path to making them more effective? *Cancer Chemother. Pharmacol.* **2017**, *80*, 661–671. [CrossRef]
162. Riechelmann, R.P.; Leite, L.S.; Bariani, G.M.; Glasberg, J.; Rivelli, T.G.; da Fonseca, L.G.; Nebuloni, D.R.; Braghiroli, M.I.; Queiroz, M.A.; Isejima, A.M.; et al. Regorafenib in Patients with Antiangiogenic-Naïve and Chemotherapy-Refractory Advanced Colorectal Cancer: Results from a Phase IIb Trial. *Oncologist* **2019**, *24*, 1180–1187. [CrossRef]
163. Iwasa, S.; Okita, N.; Kuchiba, A.; Ogawa, G.; Kawasaki, M.; Nakamura, K.; Shoji, H.; Honma, Y.; Takashima, A.; Kato, K.; et al. Phase II study of lenvatinib for metastatic colorectal cancer refractory to standard chemotherapy: The LEMON study (NCCH1503). *ESMO Open* **2020**, *5*. [CrossRef]
164. Zhang, Y.; Zou, J.Y.; Wang, Z.; Wang, Y. Fruquintinib: A novel antivascular endothelial growth factor receptor tyrosine kinase inhibitor for the treatment of metastatic colorectal cancer. *Cancer Manag. Res.* **2019**, *11*, 7787–7803. [CrossRef]
165. Xie, Y.H.; Chen, Y.X.; Fang, J.Y. Comprehensive review of targeted therapy for colorectal cancer. *Signal. Transduct. Target. Ther.* **2020**, *5*, 22. [CrossRef]
166. De Mattia, E.; Bignucolo, A.; Toffoli, G.; Cecchin, E. Genetic Markers of the Host to Predict the Efficacy of Colorectal Cancer Targeted Therapy. *Curr. Med. Chem.* **2020**, *27*, 4249–4273. [CrossRef]
167. Sebio, A.; Kahn, M.; Lenz, H.J. The potential of targeting Wnt/β-catenin in colon cancer. *Expert Opin. Ther. Targets* **2014**, *18*, 611–615. [CrossRef]
168. Katoh, M.; Katoh, M. Molecular genetics and targeted therapy of WNT-related human diseases. *Int. J. Mol. Med.* **2017**, *40*, 587–606. [CrossRef]
169. Lau, T.; Chan, E.; Callow, M.; Waaler, J.; Boggs, J.; Blake, R.A.; Magnuson, S.; Sambrone, A.; Schutten, M.; Firestein, R.; et al. A novel tankyrase small-molecule inhibitor suppresses APC mutation-driven colorectal tumor growth. *Cancer Res.* **2013**, *73*, 3132–3144. [CrossRef]
170. Verma, S.; Das, P.; Kumar, V.L. Chemoprevention by artesunate in a preclinical model of colorectal cancer involves down regulation of β-catenin, suppression of angiogenesis, cellular proliferation and induction of apoptosis. *Chem. Biol. Interact.* **2017**, *278*, 84–91. [CrossRef]
171. Wierzbicka, J.M.; Binek, A.; Ahrends, T.; Nowacka, J.D.; Szydłowska, A.; Turczyk, Ł.; Wąsiewicz, T.; Wierzbicki, P.M.; Sądej, R.; Tuckey, R.C.; et al. Differential antitumor effects of vitamin D analogues on colorectal carcinoma in culture. *Int. J. Oncol.* **2015**, *47*, 1084–1096. [CrossRef]
172. Sun, H.; Jiang, C.; Cong, L.; Wu, N.; Wang, X.; Hao, M.; Liu, T.; Wang, L.; Liu, Y.; Cong, X. CYP24A1 Inhibition Facilitates the Antiproliferative Effect of 1,25(OH)$_2$D$_3$ Through Downregulation of the WNT/β-Catenin Pathway and Methylation-Mediated Regulation of CYP24A1 in Colorectal Cancer Cells. *DNA Cell Biol.* **2018**, *37*, 742–749. [CrossRef]
173. Razak, S.; Afsar, T.; Almajwal, A.; Alam, I.; Jahan, S. Growth inhibition and apoptosis in colorectal cancer cells induced by Vitamin D-Nanoemulsion (NVD): Involvement of Wnt/β-catenin and other signal transduction pathways. *Cell Biosci.* **2019**, *9*, 15. [CrossRef]
174. Ferrer-Mayorga, G.; Larriba, M.J.; Crespo, P.; Muñoz, A. Mechanisms of action of vitamin D in colon cancer. *J. Steroid Biochem. Mol. Biol.* **2019**, *185*, 1–6. [CrossRef]
175. Leyssens, C.; Verlinden, L.; Verstuyf, A. Antineoplastic effects of 1,25(OH)$_2$D$_3$ and its analogs in breast, prostate and colorectal cancer. *Endocr. Relat. Cancer* **2013**, *20*, 31–47. [CrossRef]
176. Aguilera, O.; Peña, C.; García, J.M.; Larriba, M.J.; Ordóñez-Morán, P.; Navarro, D.; Barbáchano, A.; López de Silanes, I.; Ballestar, E.; Fraga, M.F.; et al. The Wnt antagonist DICKKOPF-1 gene is induced by 1alpha,25-dihydroxyvitamin D$_3$ associated to the differentiation of human colon cancer cells. *Carcinogenesis* **2007**, *28*, 1877–1884. [CrossRef]

177. Ferrer-Mayorga, G.; Gómez-López, G.; Barbáchano, A.; Fernández-Barral, A.; Peña, C.; Pisano, D.G.; Cantero, R.; Rojo, F.; Muñoz, A.; Larriba, M.J. Vitamin D receptor expression and associated gene signature in tumour stromal fibroblasts predict clinical outcome in colorectal cancer. *Gut* **2017**, *66*, 1449–1462. [CrossRef]

178. Xiao, J.H.; Ghosn, C.; Hinchman, C.; Forbes, C.; Wang, J.; Snider, N.; Cordrey, A.; Zhao, Y.; Chandraratna, R.A. Adenomatous polyposis coli (APC)-independent regulation of beta-catenin degradation via a retinoid X receptor-mediated pathway. *J. Biol. Chem.* **2003**, *278*, 29954–29962. [CrossRef]

179. Dillard, A.C.; Lane, M.A. Retinol Increases beta-catenin-RXRα binding leading to the increased proteasomal degradation of β-catenin and RXRα. *Nutr. Cancer* **2008**, *60*, 97–108. [CrossRef]

180. Dillard, A.C.; Lane, M.A. Retinol decreases β-catenin protein levels in retinoic acid-resistant colon cancer cell lines. *Mol. Carcinog.* **2007**, *46*, 315–329. [CrossRef]

181. Ghosh, N.; Hossain, U.; Mandal, A.; Sil, P.C. The Wnt signaling pathway: A potential therapeutic target against cancer. *Ann. N. Y. Acad. Sci.* **2019**, *1443*, 54–74. [CrossRef]

182. Emons, G.; Spitzner, M.; Reineke, S.; Möller, J.; Auslander, N.; Kramer, F.; Hu, Y.; Beissbarth, T.; Wolff, H.A.; Rave-Fränk, M.; et al. Chemoradiotherapy Resistance in Colorectal Cancer Cells is Mediated by Wnt/β-catenin Signaling. *Mol. Cancer Res.* **2017**, *15*, 1481–1490. [CrossRef] [PubMed]

183. Zhou, L.H.; Hu, Q.; Sui, H.; Ci, S.J.; Wang, Y.; Liu, X.; Liu, N.N.; Yin, P.H.; Qin, J.M.; Li, Q. Tanshinone II-a inhibits angiogenesis through down regulation of COX-2 in human colorectal cancer. *Asian Pac. J. Cancer Prev.* **2012**, *13*, 4453–4458. [CrossRef]

184. Nagoor Meeran, M.F.; Javed, H.; Al Taee, H.; Azimullah, S.; Ojha, S.K. Pharmacological Properties and Molecular Mechanisms of Thymol: Prospects for Its Therapeutic Potential and Pharmaceutical Development. *Front. Pharmacol.* **2017**, *8*. [CrossRef]

185. Chauhan, A.K.; Bahuguna, A.; Paul, S.; Kang, S.C. Thymol Elicits HCT-116 Colorectal Carcinoma Cell Death Through Induction of Oxidative Stress. *Anticancer Agents Med. Chem.* **2018**, *17*, 1942–1950. [CrossRef]

186. Zeng, Q.; Che, Y.; Zhang, Y.; Chen, M.; Guo, Q.; Zhang, W. Thymol Isolated from *Thymus vulgaris* L. Inhibits Colorectal Cancer Cell Growth and Metastasis by Suppressing the Wnt/β-Catenin Pathway. *Drug Des. Dev. Ther.* **2020**, *14*, 2535–2547. [CrossRef]

187. Wu, X.; Yu, N.; Zhang, Y.; Ye, Y.; Sun, W.; Ye, L.; Wu, H.; Yang, Z.; Wu, L.; Wang, F. Radix *Tetrastigma hemsleyani* flavone exhibits antitumor activity in colorectal cancer via Wnt/β-catenin signaling pathway. *Onco Targets Ther.* **2018**, *11*, 6437–6446. [CrossRef]

188. Deguchi, A. Curcumin targets in inflammation and cancer. *Endocr. Metab. Immune Disord. Drug Targets* **2015**, *15*, 88–96. [CrossRef]

189. Dou, H.; Shen, R.; Tao, J.; Huang, L.; Shi, H.; Chen, H.; Wang, Y.; Wang, T. Curcumin Suppresses the Colon Cancer Proliferation by Inhibiting Wnt/β-Catenin Pathways via miR-130a. *Front. Pharmacol.* **2017**, *8*. [CrossRef]

190. Jiang, X.; Li, S.; Qiu, X.; Cong, J.; Zhou, J.; Miu, W. Curcumin Inhibits Cell Viability and Increases Apoptosis of SW620 Human Colon Adenocarcinoma Cells via the Caudal Type Homeobox-2 (CDX2)/Wnt/β-Catenin Pathway. *Med. Sci Monit.* **2019**, *25*, 7451–7458. [CrossRef]

191. Li, Y.; Qin, X.; Li, P.; Zhang, H.; Lin, T.; Miao, Z.; Ma, S. Isobavachalcone isolated from *Psoralea corylifolia* inhibits cell proliferation and induces apoptosis via inhibiting the AKT/GSK-3β/β-catenin pathway in colorectal cancer cells. *Drug Des. Dev. Ther.* **2019**, *13*, 1449–1460. [CrossRef]

192. Albring, K.F.; Weidemüller, J.; Mittag, S.; Weiske, J.; Friedrich, K.; Geroni, M.C.; Lombardi, P.; Huber, O. Berberine acts as a natural inhibitor of Wnt/β-catenin signaling—Identification of more active 13-arylalkyl derivatives. *Biofactors* **2013**, *39*, 652–662. [CrossRef]

193. Ruan, H.; Zhan, Y.Y.; Hou, J.; Xu, B.; Chen, B.; Tian, Y.; Wu, D.; Zhao, Y.; Zhang, Y.; Chen, X.; et al. Berberine binds RXRα to suppress β-catenin signaling in colon cancer cells. *Oncogene* **2017**, *36*, 6906–6918. [CrossRef]

194. Ortiz, L.M.; Lombardi, P.; Tillhon, M.; Scovassi, A.I. Berberine, an epiphany against cancer. *Molecules* **2014**, *19*, 12349–12367. [CrossRef]

195. Gungor, H.; Ilhan, N.; Eroksuz, H. The effectiveness of cyclooxygenase-2 inhibitors and evaluation of angiogenesis in the model of experimental colorectal cancer. *Biomed. Pharmacother.* **2018**, *102*, 221–229. [CrossRef]

196. Madan, B.; Ke, Z.; Harmston, N.; Ho, S.Y.; Frois, A.O.; Alam, J.; Jeyaraj, D.A.; Pendharkar, V.; Ghosh, K.; Virshup, I.H.; et al. Wnt addiction of genetically defined cancers reversed by PORCN inhibition. *Oncogene* **2016**, *35*, 2197–2207. [CrossRef]

197. Fang, L.; Zhu, Q.; Neuenschwander, M.; Specker, E.; Wulf-Goldenberg, A.; Weis, W.I.; von Kries, J.P.; Birchmeier, W. A Small-Molecule Antagonist of the β-Catenin/TCF4 Interaction Blocks the Self-Renewal of Cancer Stem Cells and Suppresses Tumorigenesis. *Cancer Res.* **2016**, *76*, 891–901. [CrossRef]
198. Storm, E.E.; Durinck, S.; de Sousa e Melo, F.; Tremayne, J.; Kljavin, N.; Tan, C.; Ye, X.; Chiu, C.; Pham, T.; Hongo, J.A.; et al. Targeting PTPRK-RSPO3 colon tumours promotes differentiation and loss of stem-cell function. *Nature* **2016**, *529*, 97–100. [CrossRef]
199. Zhang, Y.; Chen, H. Genistein attenuates WNT signaling by up-regulating sFRP2 in a human colon cancer cell line. *Exp. Biol. Med.* **2011**, *236*, 714–722. [CrossRef]
200. Zhu, J.; Ren, J.; Tang, L. Genistein inhibits invasion and migration of colon cancer cells by recovering WIF1 expression. *Mol. Med. Rep.* **2018**, *17*, 7265–7273. [CrossRef]
201. Jeong, J.B.; Lee, J.; Lee, S.H. TCF4 Is a Molecular Target of Resveratrol in the Prevention of Colorectal Cancer. *Int. J. Mol. Sci.* **2015**, *16*, 10411–10425. [CrossRef]
202. Vacante, M.; Borzì, A.M.; Basile, F.; Biondi, A. Biomarkers in colorectal cancer: Current clinical utility and future perspectives. *World J. Clin. Cases* **2018**, *6*, 869–881. [CrossRef]
203. Vacante, M.; Ciuni, R.; Basile, F.; Biondi, A. The Liquid Biopsy in the Management of Colorectal Cancer: An Overview. *Biomedicines* **2020**, *8*, 308. [CrossRef]

Publisher's Note: MDPI stays neutral with regard to jurisdictional claims in published maps and institutional affiliations.

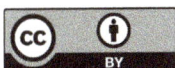

© 2020 by the author. Licensee MDPI, Basel, Switzerland. This article is an open access article distributed under the terms and conditions of the Creative Commons Attribution (CC BY) license (http://creativecommons.org/licenses/by/4.0/).

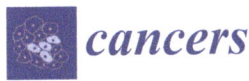

Review

Targeting Wnt Signaling for Gastrointestinal Cancer Therapy: Present and Evolving Views

Moon Jong Kim [1,†], **Yuanjian Huang** [1,†] **and Jae-Il Park** [1,2,3,*]

1. Department of Experimental Radiation Oncology, The University of Texas MD Anderson Cancer Center, Houston, TX 77030, USA; mkim312@mdanderson.org (M.J.K.); yhuang14@mdanderson.org (Y.H.)
2. Graduate School of Biomedical Sciences, The University of Texas MD Anderson Cancer Center and Health Science Center, Houston, TX 77030, USA
3. Program in Genetics and Epigenetics, The University of Texas MD Anderson Cancer Center, Houston, TX 77030, USA
* Correspondence: jaeil@mdanderson.org
† These authors contributed equally.

Received: 27 October 2020; Accepted: 1 December 2020; Published: 4 December 2020

Simple Summary: Therapeutic targeting of Wnt has long been suggested for gastrointestinal (GI) cancer treatment because deregulation of Wnt signaling is associated with GI cancers. However, therapeutic targeting of Wnt is still challenging because of the pleiotropic roles of Wnt signaling in the human body. Thus, targeting strategies of Wnt signaling are continuously evolving. The current flows of targeting Wnt signaling for cancer treatment are focused on increasing the specificity of drugs and combinatory treatment with other cancer drugs that minimize side effects and increase efficacy. Additionally, increased knowledge about the β-catenin paradox has expanded the cases that can be treated with Wnt targeting therapy, not strictly considering Wnt upstream and downstream mutations. Here, we discuss these evolving views of targeting Wnt signaling and describe examples of current clinical trials.

Abstract: Wnt signaling governs tissue development, homeostasis, and regeneration. However, aberrant activation of Wnt promotes tumorigenesis. Despite the ongoing efforts to manipulate Wnt signaling, therapeutic targeting of Wnt signaling remains challenging. In this review, we provide an overview of current clinical trials to target Wnt signaling, with a major focus on gastrointestinal cancers. In addition, we discuss the caveats and alternative strategies for therapeutically targeting Wnt signaling for cancer treatment.

Keywords: Wnt signaling; β-catenin; cancer; gastrointestinal cancers; therapeutic targeting of Wnt signaling; β-catenin paradox; molecular targeting

1. Introduction

Evolutionarily conserved Wnt signaling was initially identified in *Drosophila* (Wingless) and the mammalian system (Int-1) [1,2]. Wnt signaling has been extensively studied, revealing its pivotal roles in orchestrating embryonic development, tissue homeostasis, and regeneration [3–5]. Notably, the deregulation of Wnt signaling is associated with many human diseases, including cancers [6]. Therefore, the manipulation of Wnt signaling has gained attention as a means of disease treatment and prevention [7,8].

Although it has been confirmed in in vitro and in vivo cancer studies that targeting Wnt signaling has drastic tumor-suppressing effects, no targeted drugs have been successively advanced to clinical applications to date [7–9]. This is mainly because Wnt signaling plays essential roles in maintaining a broad range of physiological events [3–5]. Therefore, blocking Wnt signaling has detrimental impacts on tissue homeostasis and regeneration. In this review, we discuss current views on therapeutically targeting Wnt signaling and describe related clinical trials in gastrointestinal (GI) cancer.

2. Wnt Signaling

Wnt signaling is an autocrine and paracrine signal-transducing module that is activated by lipid-modified WNT ligands and their receptors [10,11]. In humans, 19 WNT ligands and 18 receptors and coreceptors have been identified [10,12]. The Wnt ligand–receptor interaction activates a downstream cascade in a β-catenin-dependent or -independent manner [13] (Figure 1).

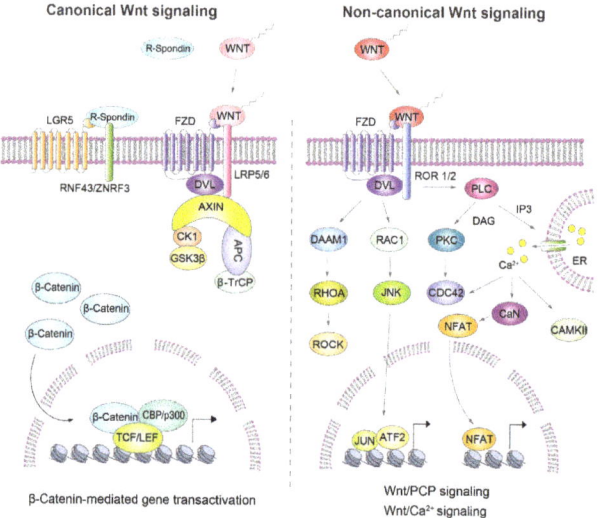

Figure 1. General view of canonical and non-canonical Wnt signaling. The switch of the canonical Wnt/β-catenin signaling pathway depends on the subcellular location of β-catenin. The stability of β-catenin is controlled by the destruction complex, consisting of AXIN, APC, CK1, and GSK3. In the absence of WNT ligands, cytoplasmic β-catenin is first phosphorylated by CK1 at Ser45 residue, followed by GSK3 phosphorylation at the Thr41, Ser37, and Ser33 residues. Next, the phosphorylated motif of β-catenin acts as a docking site for βTrCP, which induces the final ubiquitin-mediated degradation of β-catenin (Wnt off). When WNT ligands bind to Frizzled receptors (FZDs) and low density lipoprotein receptor-related protein co-receptor 5/6 (LRP 5/6), the destruction complex is recruited to the plasma membrane, triggering the translocation of β-catenin into the nucleus and activating its downstream target genes via binding directly to the TCF/LEF transcription factor family (Wnt on). Wnt/PCP signaling involves the triggering of a cascade that contains small GTPases RHOA (transforming protein RhoA) and Ras-related C3 botulinum toxin substrate 1 (RAC1), activating Rho-associated protein kinases (ROCKs) and JUN N-terminal kinases, respectively. Wnt/Ca^{2+} signaling involves the activation of phospholipase C, which in turn triggers the release of Ca^{2+} from intracellular stores and the activation of effectors such as calcium- or calmodulin-dependent protein kinase II, protein kinase C, and calcineurin (CaN). Next, CaN activates the nuclear factor of activated T cells, activating the transcription of downstream target genes.

β-catenin is an Armadillo repeat protein that is mainly associated with E-cadherin at the inner plasma membrane. The β-catenin level is tightly regulated by the protein destruction complex, which is composed of the axis inhibitor (AXIN1), adenomatous polyposis coli (APC), casein kinase 1 (CK1), glycogen synthase kinase 3 (GSK3), and β-transducin repeat-containing protein (βTrCP) and induces β-catenin degradation through phosphorylation-mediated ubiquitination [11,14–17]. In β-catenin-dependent Wnt signaling (canonical Wnt signaling), the destruction complex is sequestered upon WNT ligand stimulation and disrupted by the formation of the WNT-receptor-disheveled (DVL) complex [18], resulting in the stabilization and nuclear translocation of β-catenin [19]. Next, nuclear β-catenin interacts with the TCF/LEF transcription factor family (TCF7, LEF1, TCF7L1, and TCF7L2), which recruits coactivators to transactivate downstream target genes [20–23]. β-catenin-independent Wnt signaling (also referred to as non-canonical Wnt signaling) activates downstream modules through the planar cell polarity (Wnt/PCP) pathway or Wnt/Ca^{2+} signaling pathway [10] (Figure 1).

In the Wnt/PCP pathway, the binding of WNT-FZDs triggers a cascade involving small GTPases RHOA (transforming protein RhoA) and RAC1 (Ras-related C3 botulinum toxin substrate 1), which in turn activates ROCKs (Rho-associated protein kinases) and JUN-N-terminal kinases, respectively [10,24,25]. It mainly regulates cell polarity, cell motility, and morphogenetic movements [10,24,25]. In the Wnt/Ca^{2+} signaling pathway, the binding of WNT-FZDs activates phospholipase C (PLC), which in turn triggers the release of Ca^{2+} from intracellular stores and the activation of effectors such as calcium- and calmodulin-dependent protein kinase II (CAMKII), protein kinase C (PKC), and calcineurin (CaN) [10,26]. CaN activates the nuclear factor of activated T cells, which regulates the transcription of the genes that control cell fate and cell migration [10,26]. Although both β-catenin-dependent and -independent Wnt signaling are involved in tumorigenesis, β-catenin-dependent Wnt signaling is relatively well defined in various cancer models. In line with this, current pharmacological trials targeting Wnt signaling have mainly focused on β-catenin-dependent Wnt signaling.

3. Wnt Signaling Alteration in GI Cancers

Hyperactivation of Wnt signaling is frequently observed in GI cancers, including colorectal cancer (CRC), hepatocellular carcinoma, gastric cancer, and pancreatic cancer. Approximately 90% of CRC demonstrates Wnt signaling-related gene alterations [27]. More than 70% of the genetic alterations in CRC are *APC* mutations [27,28]. Unlike CRC, *APC* mutations are rare in hepatocellular carcinoma. Hepatocellular carcinoma mainly displays *CTNNB1* mutations (20–35%) [29], *AXIN1* mutations (8–15%) [30], and Frizzled-7 (*FZD7*) overexpression (90%) [31]. In addition to mutations in the negative feedback regulator of the FZD receptor, the E3 ubiquitin-protein ligases *ZNRF3* and *RNF43* and their ligands, R-spondins (RSPOs), are frequently observed in pancreatic and gastric cancers [32,33].

4. Therapeutically Targeting Wnt Signaling in GI Cancer

Targeting Wnt signaling for cancer treatment normalizes the hyperactivated Wnt signaling that promotes cancer progression. For this purpose, many targeting strategies have been evaluated, including the inhibition of Wnt ligands and receptors or coreceptors, restoration of the destructive complex, and inhibition of β-catenin/β-catenin-dependent transcriptional machinery. Although these approaches have not been studied in phase III clinical trials or used clinically, dozens of Wnt-targeting agents are currently being evaluated in phase II clinical trials (Table 1). These important phase II clinical trials include LGK974, genistein, Foxy-5, DKN-01, niclosamide, PRI-724, and chloroquine/hydroxychloroquine.

In the next section, we provide an overview of the known and potential agents that target Wnt signaling, especially for GI cancers; we also describe their mechanisms of action and related clinical trials (Table 2). All potential agents that inhibit Wnt signaling are listed in Table 3. In addition, the molecular targets of representative Wnt inhibitors on WNT signaling are illustrated in Figure 2.

Table 1. Agents inhibiting Wnt signaling for GI cancers in phase II clinical trials.

Agent	Mechanism	Trial	Cancer
LGK974	PORCN inhibitor	NCT02278133	BRAF V600-mutated metastatic colorectal cancer
Genistein	*SFRP2* silencer inhibitor	NCT01985763	Metastatic colorectal cancer
Foxy-5	WNT5A mimic	Vermorken 2019	WNT5A-negative colon cancer

Table 1. *Cont.*

Agent	Mechanism	Trial	Cancer
DKN-01	Monoclonal antibody against DKK1	NCT03645980; NCT04166721	Advanced hepatocellular carcinoma; Advanced gastroesophageal adenocarcinoma
Niclosamide	FZD1 inhibitor, LRP6 inhibitor	NCT02519582	Progressed colorectal cancer
PRI-724	β-catenin/CREBBP inhibitor	NCT02413853	Metastatic colorectal adenocarcinoma
Chloroquine	v-ATPase inhibitor	NCT02496741	Advanced solid malignancies, including intrahepatic cholangiocarcinoma
Hydroxy-chloroquine	v-ATPase inhibitor	NCT01006369, etc. (total 13 trials)	Advanced colorectal carcinoma; Advanced hepatocellular carcinoma; Advanced cholangiocarcinoma; Pancreatic adenocarcinoma

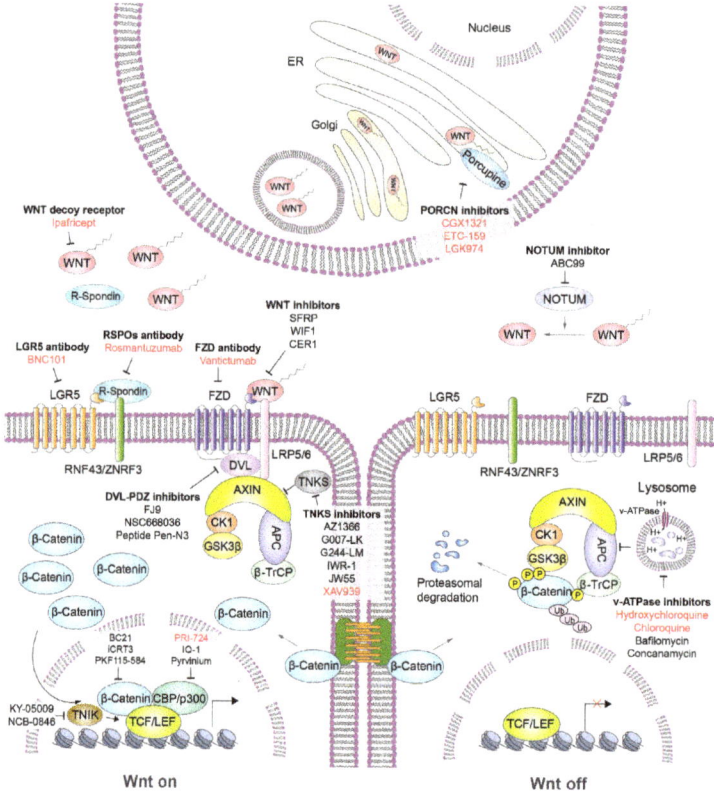

Figure 2. Wnt targeting agents for the Wnt/β-catenin signaling pathway. Wnt targeting agents for GI cancers mainly focus on the inhibition of the key molecules in Wnt/β-catenin signaling, such as inhibiting WNT ligands (ipafricept, LGK794), inhibiting Wnt receptors/coreceptors (vanticumab, rosmantuzumab), stabilizing the destruction complex (AZ1366, hydroxychloroquine), and inhibiting β-catenin-dependent transcriptional machinery (MSAB, PRI-724).

Table 2. Agents inhibiting Wnt signaling for GI cancers in clinical trials.

Trial	Agent	Mechanism	Design	Cancer	Interventions	Status
NCT02675946	CGX1321	Porcupine inhibitor	Phase I; Single group	Advanced GI cancers	CGX1321; CGX1321 + pembrolizumab	Recruiting
NCT03507998	CGX1321	Porcupine inhibitor	Phase I; Single group	Advanced GI cancers	CGX1321	Recruiting
Ng 2017 (NCT02521844) [34]	ETC-159	Porcupine inhibitor	Phase I; Single group	Advanced solid malignancies, including colorectal cancer, etc.	ETC-159; ETC-159 + pembrolizumab	Ongoing
NCT01351103	LGK974	Porcupine inhibitor	Phase I; Single group	Solid malignancies, including esophageal squamous-cell carcinoma, pancreatic adenocarcinoma, BRAF-mutated colorectal cancer, etc.	LGK974; LGK974 + spartalizumab	Recruiting
NCT02278133	LGK974	Porcupine inhibitor	Phase II; Single group	BRAF V600-mutated metastatic colorectal cancer with RNF43 mutations and/or R-spondin fusions	LGK974 + LGX818 + cetuximab	Completed
Pintova 2019 (NCT01985763) [35]	Genistein	SFRP2 silencer inhibitor	Phase II; Single group	Metastatic colorectal cancer	Genistein + FOLFOX; Genistein + FOLFOX + bevacizumab	Completed
Jimeno 2017 (NCT01608867) [36]	Ipafricept (OMP-54F28)	WNT decoy receptor	Phase I; Single group	Solid malignancies, including pancreatic cancer, colorectal cancer, etc.	Ipafricept	Completed
Dotan 2019 (NCT02050178) [37]	Ipafricept (OMP-54F28)	WNT decoy receptor	Phase I; Single group	Metastatic pancreatic ductal adenocarcinoma	Ipafricept + nab-paclitaxel + gemcitabine	Completed
NCT02069145	Ipafricept (OMP-54F28)	WNT decoy receptor	Phase I; Single group	Advanced hepatocellular carcinoma	Ipafricept + sorafenib	Completed
NCT02020291	Foxy-5	WNT5A mimic	Phase I; Single group	Metastatic breast, colon, prostate cancer	Foxy-5	Completed
NCT02655952	Foxy-5	WNT5A mimic	Phase I; Single group	Metastatic breast, colon, prostate cancer	Foxy-5	Completed

Table 2. Cont.

Trial	Agent	Mechanism	Design	Cancer	Interventions	Status
Vermorken 2019 [38]	Foxy-5	WNT5A mimic	Phase II; Randomized; Parallel	WNT5A-negative colon cancer	Foxy-5 vs placebo	Recruiting
Davis 2019 (NCT02005315) [39]	Vantictumab (OMP-18R5)	Monoclonal antibody against FZDs	Phase I; Single group	Metastatic pancreatic ductal adenocarcinoma	Vantictumab + nab-paclitaxel + gemcitabine	Terminated
Ryan 2016 (NCT02013154) [40]	DKN-01	Monoclonal antibody against DKK1	Phase I; Non-randomized; Parallel	Recurrent or metastatic esophageal cancer, gastro-esophageal junction cancer	DKN-01; DKN-01 vs paclitaxel; DKN-01 vs pembrolizumab	Ongoing
Eads 2016 (NCT02375880) [41]	DKN-01	Monoclonal antibody against DKK1	Phase I; Single group	Advanced cholangiocarcinoma	DKN-01 + gemcitabine + cisplatin	Ongoing
NCT03645980	DKN-01	Monoclonal antibody against DKK1	Phase II; Non-randomized; Sequential	Advanced hepatocellular carcinoma	DKN-01 vs sequential DKN-01 + sorafenib	Recruiting
NCT04166721	DKN-01	Monoclonal antibody against DKK1	Phase II; Single group	Advanced gastroesophageal adenocarcinoma	DKN-01 + atezolizumab	Recruiting
Bendell 2016 (NCT02482441) [42]	Rosmantuzumab (OMP-131R10)	Monoclonal antibody against RSPO3	Phase I; Single group	Advanced solid malignancies, including metastatic colorectal cancer, etc.	OMP-131R10	Completed
NIKOLO trial (NCT02519582) [43]	Niclosamide	FZD1 inhibitor, LRP6 inhibitor	Phase II; Single group	Progressed colorectal cancer	Niclosamide	Recruiting
NCT02687009	Niclosamide	FZD1 inhibitor, LRP6 inhibitor	Phase I; Single group	Colorectal adenocarcinoma	Niclosamide	Terminated
NCT02726334	BNC101	Monoclonal antibody against LGR5	Phase I; Single group	Metastatic colorectal cancer	BNC101; BNC101+ FOLFIRI	Terminated
NCT01777477	Chloroquine	v-ATPase inhibitor	Phase I; Single group	Advanced pancreatic adenocarcinoma	Chloroquine + gemcitabine	Completed
Molenaar 2017 (NCT02496741) [44]	Chloroquine	v-ATPase inhibitor	Phase II; Single group	Advanced solid malignancies, including intrahepatic cholangiocarcinoma	Chloroquine + metformin	Completed

Table 2. Cont.

Trial	Agent	Mechanism	Design	Cancer	Interventions	Status
NCT01006369	Hydroxy-chloroquine	v-ATPase inhibitor	Phase II; Non-randomized; Parallel	Metastatic colorectal carcinoma	Hydroxychloroquine + FOLFOX6 + bevacizumab vs Hydroxychloroquine + XELOX + bevacizumab	Completed
Mahalingam 2014 (NCT01023737) [45]	Hydroxy-chloroquine	v-ATPase inhibitor	Phase I; Single group	Advanced solid malignancies, including colorectal cancer, etc.	Hydroxychloroquine + vorinostat	Completed
Boone 2015 (NCT01128296) [46]	Hydroxy-chloroquine	v-ATPase inhibitor	Phase II; Single group	Unresectable pancreatic ductal adenocarcinoma	Hydroxychloroquine + gemcitabine	Completed
Loaiza-Bonilla 2015 (NCT01206530) [47]	Hydroxy-chloroquine	v-ATPase inhibitor	Phase I; Single group	Advanced colorectal adenocarcinoma	Hydroxychloroquine + FOLFOX + bevacizumab	Completed
Wolpin 2014 (NCT01273805) [48]	Hydroxy-chloroquine	v-ATPase inhibitor	Phase I; Single group	Metastatic pancreatic cancer	Hydroxychloroquine	Completed
Hong 2017 (NCT01494155) [49]	Hydroxy-chloroquine	v-ATPase inhibitor	Phase II; Single group	Early pancreatic ductal carcinoma	Short course radiation therapy preoperatively. Hydroxychloroquine + capecitabine postoperatively	Ongoing
Karasic 2019 (NCT01506973) [50]	Hydroxy-chloroquine	v-ATPase inhibitor	Phase II; Randomized; Parallel	Advanced pancreatic adenocarcinoma	Hydroxychloroquine + nab-paclitacel + gemcitabine vs nab-paclitacel + gemcitabine	Ongoing
NCT01978184	Hydroxy-chloroquine	v-ATPase inhibitor	Phase II; Randomized; Parallel	Resectable pancreatic adenocarcinoma	Hydroxychloroquine + nab-paclitacel + gemcitabine vs nab-paclitacel + gemcitabine	Completed
NCT02013778	Hydroxy-chloroquine	v-ATPase inhibitor	Phase II; Single group	Unresectable hepatocellular carcinoma	Hydroxychloroquine + transarterial chemoembolization	Terminated

Table 2. Cont.

Trial	Agent	Mechanism	Design	Cancer	Interventions	Status
Arora 2019 (NCT02316340) [51]	Hydroxy-chloroquine	v-ATPase inhibitor	Phase II; Randomized; Crossover	Metastatic colorectal cancer	Hydroxychloroquine + vorinostat vs regorafenib	Completed
NCT03037437	Hydroxy-chloroquine	v-ATPase inhibitor	Phase II; Non-randomized; Parallel	Advanced hepatocellular cancer	Hydroxychloroquine + sorafenib vs sorafenib	Ongoing
NCT03215264	Hydroxy-chloroquine	v-ATPase inhibitor	Phase II; Single group	Metastatic colorectal cancer	Hydroxychloroquine + entinostat + regorafenib	Suspended
NCT03344172	Hydroxy-chloroquine	v-ATPase inhibitor	Phase II; Randomized; Parallel	Resectable pancreatic adenocarcinoma	Hydroxychloroquine + gemcitabine + nab-paclitaxel + avelumab vs hydroxychloroquine + gemcitabine + nab-paclitaxel	Suspended
NCT03377179	Hydroxy-chloroquine	v-ATPase inhibitor	Phase II; Single group	Advanced cholangiocarcinoma	ABC294640; Hydroxychloroquine + ABC294640	Ongoing
NCT03825289	Hydroxy-chloroquine	v-ATPase inhibitor	Phase I; Single group	Advanced pancreatic cancer	Hydroxychloroquine + trametinib	Ongoing
NCT04132505	Hydroxy-chloroquine	v-ATPase inhibitor	Phase I; Single group	KRAS-mutated metastatic pancreatic adenocarcinoma	Hydroxychloroquine + binimetinib	Ongoing
NCT04145297	Hydroxy-chloroquine	v-ATPase inhibitor	Phase I; Single group	MAPK-mutated GI cancers	Hydroxychloroquine + ulixertinib	Ongoing
NCT04214418	Hydroxy-chloroquine	v-ATPase inhibitor	Phase II; Non-randomized; Sequential	KRAS-mutated advanced solid malignancies, including pancreatic adenocarcinoma, colorectal adenocarcinoma, etc.	Hydroxychloroquine + atezolizumab + cobimetinib	Ongoing
El-Khoueiry 2013 (NCT01302405) [52]	PRI-724	β-catenin/CREBBP inhibitor	Phase I; Single group	Advanced solid malignancies, including colorectal cancer, etc.	PRI-724	Terminated

Table 2. *Cont.*

Trial	Agent	Mechanism	Design	Cancer	Interventions	Status
Ko 2016 (NCT01764477) [53]	PRI-724	β-catenin/CREBBP inhibitor	Phase I; Single group	Recurrent or advanced pancreatic adenocarcinoma	PRI-724 + gemcitabine	Completed
NCT02413853	PRI-724	β-catenin/CREBBP inhibitor	Phase II; Randomized; Parallel	Metastatic colorectal adenocarcinoma	mFOLFOX6/Bevacizumab + PRI-724 vs mFOLFOX6/Bevacizumab	Withdrawn
NCT03355066	SM08502	CLK inhibitor	Phase I; Single group	Advanced solid malignancies, including pancreatic cancer, colorectal cancer, etc.	SM08502	Recruiting

Table 3. All potential agents inhibiting Wnt signaling.

Mechanism	Agents
PORCN inhibitor	CGX1321, ETC-159, LGK974, GNF-6231, IWP-2, IWP-3, IWP-4, IWP-12, IWP-L6, IWP-O1, RXC004, WNT-C59
SFRP1 inhibitor	WAY-316606
SFRP2 silencer inhibitor	Genistein
WNT5A mimic	Foxy-5
WNT inhibitor	Ant1.4Br/Ant1.4Cl, wogonin
WNT decoy receptor	Ipafricept
WNT3A-LRP5 complex inhibitor	APCDD1
FZD inhibitor	Vantictumab
FZD1&LRP6 inhibitor	Niclosamide
FZD4 inhibitor	FzM1
FZD7 inhibitor	Fz7-21
FZD10 inhibitor	OTSA101, OTSA101-DTPA-90Y
LGR5 inhibitor	BNC101
LRP6 inhibitor	Gigantol, salinomycin
FZD8-LRP6 heterodimer inhibitor	IGFBP-4

Table 3. Cont.

Mechanism	Agents
DKK1 inhibitor	DKN-01
DVL-PDZ domain inhibitor	Compound 3289-8625, FJ9, NSC668036, peptide Pen-N3
RSPO3 inhibitor	Rosmantuzumab
TNKS inhibitor	2X-121, AZ1366, AZ-6102, G007-LK, G244-LM, IWR-1, JW55, JW67, JW74, K-756, MN-64, MSC2504877, NVP-TNKS656, RK-287107, TC-E5001, WIKI4, XAV939
v-ATPase inhibitor	Apicularen, archazolid, bafilomycin, chloroquine, chondropsine, concanamycin, cruentaren, disulfiramthe, FR167356, FR177995, FR202126, hydroxychloroquine, indolyl, KM91104, lobatamide, NiK12192, oximidine, salicylihamide, SB 242784, tributyltin chloride
CK1 activator	Pyrvinium
GSK3β fragment mimic	TCS 183
β-catenin inhibitor	21H7, isoquercitrin, KY1220, KYA1797K, triptonide (NSC 165677, PG 492)
β-catenin degrader	MSAB, NRX-252114
β-catenin/TCF inhibitor	BC21, BC2059, CCT031374, CCT036477, CGP049090, CWP232228, ethacrynic acid, FH535, iCRT3, iCRT5, iCRT14, LF3, NLS-StAx-h, PKF115-584, PKF118-310, PKF118-744, PNU-74654, quercetin, ZTM000990
TNIK inhibitor	KY-05009, NCB-0846
β-catenin/EP300 inhibitor	IQ-1, windorphen, YH249/250
β-catenin/CREBBP&EP300 inhibitor	C-82, ICG-001, PRI-724, retinoids, vitamin D3
β-catenin/PYGO inhibitor	Pyrvinium
β-catenin/BCL9 inhibitor	Compound 22, carnosic acid, SAH-BCL9
CLK inhibitor	SM08502
Wnt/β-catenin signaling inhibitor	Adavivint (SM04690, lorecivivint), artesunate, cardamonin, cardionogen, CCT031374, diethyl benzylphosphonate, echinacoside, KY02111, pamidronic acid, specnuezhemide

5. Targeting WNT Ligands

5.1. Inhibiting WNT Ligands

Ipafricept (OMP-54F28) is a recombinant receptor that is comprised of the cysteine-rich domain of FZD8 fused to the human IgG1 Fc domain; it inhibits Wnt signaling by neutralizing WNT ligands [54]. Three trials evaluated ipafricept and its combination therapies (Table 2). A phase I trial evaluated the best dosage of ipafricept and revealed grade 1–2 adverse events (AEs), including dysgeusia, decreased appetite, fatigue, and muscle spasms [36]. Another phase I trial evaluated ipafricept combined with nab-paclitaxel and gemcitabine in metastatic pancreatic cancer and revealed grade ≥ 3 AEs, including increased aspartate aminotransferase, nausea, maculopapular rash, vomiting, and decreased white blood cells [37].

Secreted frizzled-related proteins (SFRPs) bound directly to WNTs via the cysteine-rich domain, preventing the WNT–FZD interaction [55–57]. SFRPs also form dimers with FZDs via the respective cysteine-rich domain to activate or inhibit WNT3A/β-catenin signaling, depending on their concentration [58]. In the nucleus, SFRPs act as biphasic modulators of β-catenin-mediated transcription, which promotes TCF7L2 recruitment and transactivation of cancer stem cell-related genes by binding to the β-catenin's C-terminus; however, they suppress transcriptional activities by binding to the N-terminus [59]. The phase II trial evaluated genistein, an *SFRP2* silencer inhibitor, in combination with FOLFOX and bevacizumab in metastatic CRC; the study revealed mild AEs, including headaches, nausea, and hot flashes (Table 2) [35]. In addition, Wnt inhibitory factor 1 directly binds to WNTs through the Wnt inhibitory factor domain and prevents WNTs from transducing Wnt signaling [60]. Cerberus also binds to and inhibits WNT8, inhibiting Wnt signaling [61]. However, no agents mimicking Wnt inhibitory factor 1 and Cerberus have been identified.

5.2. Targeting Lipid Modification of WNT Ligands

The palmitoylation of WNT ligands by the protein-serine O-palmitoleoyltransferase porcupine in the endoplasmic reticulum [62] is essential for the maturation and extracellular secretion of WNT ligands. The palmitoylated WNT ligands bind to Wntless homolog in the Golgi and are ferried to the plasma membrane via secretory exosomes [63]. Porcupine inhibitors (CGX1321, ETC-159, and LGK974 [WNT794]), which suppress Wnt signaling by blocking the secretion of WNT ligands, are currently being evaluated in clinical trials (Table 2). A phase I trial evaluated the best dosage of ETC-159 and revealed well-tolerated AEs, including vomiting, anorexia and fatigue, dysgeusia, and constipation [34]. The lipid modification of WNTs can be enzymatically removed by the palmitoleoyl-protein carboxylesterase NOTUM, thereby inhibiting Wnt signaling [64]. The NOTUM inhibitor, ABC99, is effective in the treatment of benefiting osteopenia and osteoporosis by enhancing Wnt signaling (Table 3) [64,65]. However, no agents have been identified that mimic NOTUM to inhibit GI cancers. Alternatively, metalloprotease TIKI1 (Trabd2a) acts as a protease to cleave eight amino acid residues of WNTs, resulting in oxidized WNT oligomers with minimized receptor binding capability in frogs [66,67]. However, no agents have been identified that mimic the impact of TRABD on Wnt signaling in humans.

6. Targeting Wnt Receptors and Co-Receptors

6.1. Antibodies against FZDs

Vantictumab (OMP-18R5) is a monoclonal antibody that binds to FZD 1, 2, 5, 7, and 8 and inhibits Wnt signal transduction [54]. A phase I trial evaluating the best dosage of vantictumab combined with nab-paclitaxel and gemcitabine in metastatic pancreatic cancer was terminated because of the increased risk of bone fracture [39]. Moreover, FZD5 has been identified as a dominant FZD receptor in RNF43-mutant pancreatic cancer cells and may be a therapeutic index [68]. However, no agents targeting FZD5 have been introduced.

6.2. Mimetic Agents Binding to FZDs

Initially, WNT5A was classified as a non-canonical Wnt family member. It activates Wnt/Ca^{2+} signaling by stimulating intracellular Ca^{2+} flux in zebrafish and frogs [69–72]. In 2006, Mikels et al. found that WNT5A also activates canonical Wnt signaling via FZD4 and LRP5 [73]. Intriguingly, WNT5A additionally inhibits WNT3A-induced canonical Wnt signaling via FZD2 and tyrosine-protein kinase transmembrane receptor ROR2 [73,74]. Therefore, the function of WNT5A is considered not limited to the field of Wnt signaling and is more dependent on the context of receptors. Foxy-5, a WNT5A peptide mimic, reduces the metastatic capacity of invasive breast cancer via epithelial discoidin domain-containing receptor 1 (DDR1), which decreases the motility and the invasive potential of breast epithelial cells [75–77]. However, whether these mechanisms are also true in GI cancers remains unknown. Foxy-5 is being evaluated in phase I-II clinical trials of metastatic CRC, but no results have been published [38] (Table 2).

6.3. Inhibiting LRP5/6

Given that dickkopf-related protein 1 (DKK1) inhibits Wnt signaling through its direct binding to LRP5/6 [78,79], DKK1 was initially considered a tumor suppressor in the β-catenin-dependent context. Conversely, several studies have shown that DKK1 promotes tumor cell proliferation, metastasis, and angiogenesis, which might be mediated by β-catenin-independent signaling [80–86]. One available explanation is that DKK1 interacts with both glypican4 (GPC4) and the LRP/KREMEN complex to induce the endocytosis of LRP5/6, transforming the biochemical properties of FZDs and their cytoplasmic components from the Wnt/β-catenin pathway to the Wnt/PCP signaling axis [87,88]. This mechanism activating β-catenin-independent signaling and inhibiting β-catenin-dependent signaling was validated in zebrafish and frogs [87,88].

On the basis of the tumorigenic role of DKK1, DKN-01, a DKK1 monoclonal antibody, was developed for cancer therapy. Four trials evaluating DKN-01 and its combination therapies are ongoing (Table 2). A phase I trial assessing DKN-01 combined with paclitaxel in advanced esophageal and gastroesophageal junction cancer revealed that 35% of patients experienced a partial response [40,89]. Another phase I trial of the best dosage of DKN-01 combined with gemcitabine and cisplatin in advanced biliary cancer revealed that 33.3% of patients experienced a partial response [41]. Sclerostin domain-containing protein 1 can activate or inhibit Wnt signaling by mimicking WNT ligands or by competing with WNT8 for binding to LRP6, respectively [90,91]. However, no agents simulating sclerostin domain-containing protein 1 have been identified.

6.4. Accelerating the Degradation of FZD/LRP Receptors

Secreted RSPOs (RSPO1-3) and their receptors, RNF43/ZNRF3, are required to potentiate Wnt signaling in various development and tissue homeostasis contexts [92–94]. In addition, leucine-rich repeat-containing G-protein-coupled receptors (LGRs, LGR4-6) are required for the interaction between RSPOs and their receptors [92]. Without RSPOs and LGRs, RNF43/ZNRF3 induces the internalization and degradation of FZD receptors and negatively regulates Wnt signaling [92,95,96].

A phase I trial evaluated the best dosage of rosmantuzumab (OMP-131R10), a monoclonal antibody against RSPO3, for metastatic CRC; no results have been published (Table 2). BNC101, a monoclonal antibody against LGR5, demonstrated antitumor activity in multiple CRC patient-derived xenografts, but the clinical trial was terminated (Table 2) [97]. Niclosamide, a teniacide in the anthelmintic family, promotes FZD1 endocytosis, inhibiting WNT3A/β-catenin signaling in CRC and osteosarcoma and inducing LRP6 degradation in prostate and breast cancer [98–100]. The NIKOLO trial and NCT02687009 have been evaluating niclosamide in CRC (Table 2). The NIKOLO trial has revealed no drug-related AEs [43].

7. Targeting the Destruction Complex

7.1. Inhibiting the DVL–FZD Interaction

In the presence of WNT ligands, DVLs bind to the cytoplasmic domain of FZDs via the PDZ (PSD95, DLG1, and ZO1) domain, which provides a platform for the interaction between the LRP's tail and AXIN to recruit the destruction complex onto the cytoplasmic membrane [101,102]. This process inhibits destruction complex-mediated β-catenin protein degradation [93]. Several inhibitors (compound 3289-8625, FJ9, NSC668036, and peptide Pen-N3) that directly inhibit DVL binding with FZDs are currently being evaluated in preclinical studies (Table 3) [103–106].

7.2. Stabilizing AXIN

Tankyrase is a member of the poly ADP-ribose polymerase superfamily of proteins which mediates the PARsylation and proteasomal degradation of AXIN [107,108]. Tankyrase inhibitors (AZ1366, G007-LK, G244-LM, IWR-1, JW55, and XAV939) that stabilize AXIN and activate the destruction complex are being evaluated in preclinical studies (Table 3) [109–113]. The E3 ubiquitin-protein ligase SIAH, a potent activator of Wnt signaling, promotes the ubiquitination and proteasomal degradation of AXIN by interacting with a VxP motif in the GSK3-binding domain of AXIN [114]. Ubiquitin carboxyl-terminal hydrolase 7 (USP7), a potent negative regulator of Wnt/β-catenin signaling, promotes the deubiquitination and stabilization of AXIN by interacting with AXIN through its TRAF domain [115]. However, no agents that inhibit SIAH or mimic USP7 have been identified.

7.3. Stabilizing APC

Transmembrane protein 9 (TMEM9) binds to and facilitates the assembly of vacuolar-type H^+-ATPase (v-ATPase), resulting in enhanced vesicular acidification and trafficking for subsequent lysosomal degradation of APC and hyperactivation of Wnt/β-catenin signaling [116]. Conversely, pharmacological targeting of v-ATPase using bafilomycin, concanamycin, hydroxychloroquine, or KM91104 inhibits Wnt/β-catenin signaling and suppresses intestinal tumorigenesis (Table 3) [116]. Twenty trials are currently evaluating v-ATPase inhibitors (Table 2). A phase II trial assessing hydroxychloroquine combined with gemcitabine in unresectable pancreatic cancer revealed no dose-limiting AEs [46]. Another phase II trial revealed an increased overall response rate (38.2 vs. 21.1%; $P = 0.047$) but no survival benefits (hazard ratio, 1.14; 95% CI, 0.76–1.69; $P = 0.53$) when adding hydroxychloroquine to combination therapy with nab-paclitaxel and gemcitabine for advanced pancreatic cancer [50].

7.4. Activating CK1 and GSK3

CK1 and GSK3 sequentially phosphorylate β-catenin to induce the ubiquitination and proteasomal degradation of β-catenin [16]. Therefore, CK1 and GSK3 activators likely reduce the level of β-catenin that translocates into the nucleus, consequently inactivating Wnt signaling. pyrvinium, a CK1 activator that binds to the C-terminal regulatory domain of its isoform CK1A1, has been introduced, but it has not been evaluated in clinical trials (Table 3) [117]. In addition, no GSK3 activators have been introduced.

8. Targeting β-Catenin and β-Catenin-Dependent Transcriptional Machinery

8.1. Promoting β-Catenin Degradation

Methyl 3-[[(4-methylphenyl)sulfonyl]amino] benzoate (MSAB) [12] binds to the Armadillo repeat domain of β-catenin and promotes its degradation [118]. NRX-252114, a protein–protein interaction enhancer, enhances the interaction between β-catenin and its cognate E3 ligase, potentiating the ubiquitination-mediated degradation of β-catenin [119]. No clinical trials have evaluated MSAB and NRX-252114.

8.2. Inhibiting the β-Catenin–TCF/LEF Complex

With its increased fold change, nuclear β-catenin replaces the transducin-like enhancer protein corepressor with coactivators by forming the β-catenin–TCF/LEF complex [93,120]. This complex transactivates Wnt target genes through its sequence-specific DNA binding and context-dependent interaction [121]. β-catenin-TCF/LEF complex inhibitors (BC21, iCRT3, and PKF115-584) were introduced in preclinical studies (Table 3) [122–124].

8.3. Manipulating TCF/LEF Phosphatases

TRAF2 and NCK-interacting protein kinase (TNIK) phosphorylates the serine 169 residue of TCF7L1 and the serine 154 residue of TCF7L2, acting as an activating kinase of the β-catenin-TCF/LEF transcriptional complex [125–127]. TNIK inhibitors (KY-05009 and NCB-0846) are being evaluated in preclinical studies [126,128] (Table 3). Serine/threonine-protein kinase NLK phosphorylates the threonine 155 and serine 166 residues of LEF1 and the threonine 178, 189 residues of TCF7L2, triggering their dissociation from DNA and inhibiting Wnt target gene transactivation [129,130]. Homeodomain-interacting protein kinase 2 (HIPK2) phosphorylates LEF1, TCF7L1, and TCF7L2 to dissociate them from DNA, which positively or negatively modulates Wnt/β-catenin signaling [131,132]. However, no agents targeting NLK and HIPK2 have been identified.

8.4. Inhibiting Coactivators

CREB-binding protein (CREBBP), histone acetyltransferase EP300, pygopus homolog (PYGO), and B-cell CLL/lymphoma 9 protein (BCL9) are coactivators that interact with the β-catenin–TCF/LEF complex [10]. PRI-724 competes with β-catenin to bind with CREBBP, suppressing the transcriptional activation of β-catenin target genes [133]. Three trials have been evaluating PRI-724, two of which were terminated or withdrawn because of low enrollment or a drug supply issue (Table 2). A phase I trial evaluating the best dosage of PRI-724 revealed grade 2 AEs, including diarrhea, bilirubin elevation, hypophosphatemia, nausea, fatigue, anorexia, thrombocytopenia, and alkaline phosphatase elevation [52]. Another phase I trial evaluating the best dosage of PRI-724 combined with gemcitabine as second-line therapy for advanced pancreatic cancer revealed grade ≥ 3 AEs, including abdominal pain, neutropenia, anemia, fatigue, and alkaline phosphatase elevation [53]. The inhibitors of EP300, PYGO, and BCL9 (IQ-1, pyrvinium, and carnosic acid, respectively) have been evaluated in preclinical studies (Table 3) [117,134,135]. In addition, SM08502, a CDC-like kinase (CLK) inhibitor that blocks the phosphorylation of serine/arginine-rich splicing factors and consequently disrupts spliceosome activity, has been shown to inhibit Wnt signaling in preclinical models [136–138]. A phase I trial evaluating SM08502 for advanced GI cancers is ongoing (Table 2).

9. Caveats in Targeting Wnt Signaling

9.1. Targeting Core Components of Wnt Signaling

The major caveat in Wnt targeting strategies is their detrimental side effects on normal cells in which Wnt signaling plays pivotal roles in tissue homeostasis and regeneration [3–5]. For example, intestinal stem cells replenish the intestinal epithelium every 3 to 4 days; this is tightly regulated by constitutively active Wnt signaling in the crypt bottom [139,140]. Inhibiting Wnt signaling disrupts intestinal homeostasis and induces the severe loss of the crypt-villi structure. Similarly, upon Wnt blockade, tissue homeostasis disruption also takes place in hair follicles, the stomach, and the hematopoietic system, where Wnt signaling is indispensable for the maintenance of stem cells and their niches [141–143]. Indeed, the treatment of the FZD inhibitor (vanctumab) and antagonist (ipafricept) leads to side effects, including tiredness, diarrhea, vomiting, constipation, bone metabolism disorders, and abdominal pain [36,54]. Wnt signaling is also required for tissue homeostasis and regeneration in the lungs, liver, skin, and pancreas [3–5]. Therefore, Wnt signaling targeting strategies need to be meticulously designed and evaluated on the basis of their specificity and efficacy, which is discussed in the next section.

9.2. Targeting Upstream vs. Downstream

Targeting the downstream effectors of Wnt signaling, e.g., β-catenin and TCF/LEF, might maximize Wnt signaling inhibition on the basis of signaling convergence into downstream gene regulation. However, targeting downstream Wnt signaling might also generate severe side effects by disrupting Wnt signaling in normal tissues. Conversely, targeting the upstream molecules of Wnt signaling, e.g., ligands and receptors, was initially considered ineffectual in cancer cells carrying mutations in Wnt signaling downstream (i.e., *APC* and β-catenin/*CTNNB1*) [93]. Intriguingly, accumulating evidence suggests that targeting Wnt signaling upstream is also effective independent of Wnt signaling downstream mutations. This evolving concept, the "β-catenin paradox", is discussed below.

10. Evolving Views in Targeting Wnt Signaling

10.1. Cancer- and Tissue-Specific Wnt Signaling Targeting

Targeting cancer type- or tissue-specific Wnt signaling components or modulators may overcome the side effects of Wnt signaling blockade on normal tissues. For instance, specifically targeting the constitutively active form of β-catenin mutants may be ideal. A recent study found that small-molecule enhancers of mutant β-catenin and its E3 ligase (β-TrCP) interaction potentiate the ubiquitination-mediated degradation of mutant β-catenin [119], suggesting one possible approach to targeting the mutant form of β-catenin.

There are also several promising preclinical and clinical studies evaluating antibodies against RSPOs and LGRs, Wnt signaling amplifiers [42]. Since RSPOs and LGRs are differently expressed in different tissues and cancers [144,145], targeting them might diminish normal tissue damage. LGR5 has been suggested as a cancer stem cell marker [146,147], and targeting LGR5+ cells with anti-LGR5 antibody–drug conjugates suppressed tumor growth and metastasis in a preclinical model [145,148]. Anti-LGR5 therapy and anti-RSPO3 (rosmantuzumab) are currently being evaluated in phase I trials for the treatment of metastatic CRC (NCT02726334 and NCT02005315) (Table 2). RSPO3-LGR4-maintained Wnt signaling is essential for the stemness of acute myeloid leukemia, and the clinical-grade anti-RSPO3 antibody eradicated leukemia stem cells [149], which might be effective in GI cancer. The results of these studies indicate that blockage of cancer- or tissue-specific Wnt signaling components or regulators are viable options for GI cancer treatment.

10.2. Efficacy and Combination Therapy

An alternative method of overcoming limitations in Wnt signaling targeting strategies is to identify a safe dose that is highly effective but does not disrupt normal physiologic processes. A specific dose of LGK794 had lower severity of side effects with effective pharmacologic outcomes in a phase I clinical trial [7]. It is also noteworthy that different tissues showed different levels of Wnt signaling threshold in vivo [150], supporting the theory that localizing treatment is an alternative strategy to avoid toxicity and side effects.

In general, combination therapy is considered to result in more AEs. However, it does not always induce more AEs than does monotherapy. The incidences and degrees of AEs depend on various factors, such as the doses of single drugs, the timing of administration, the period of treatment, the supportive treatment, and the heterogeneity of the patients themselves. Thus, certain drug dose combinations may be more effective, with fewer AEs. Furthermore, monotherapy targeting one pathway does not guarantee complete anticancer activity because of multiple crosstalks and compensations by other signaling pathways. Although its efficacy may be counterbalanced by correspondingly increased toxicity, combination therapy that simultaneously targets several pathways might be more efficient.

In addition, combination therapy is the most common approach to achieving survival benefits in clinical practice, and most promising phase III Wnt targeting trials use combination therapy.

ICG-001 and PRI-724 inhibit Wnt target gene expression by antagonizing CBP, a β-catenin coactivator [133,151]. PRI-724 was effective in a phase I clinical trial of PDAC when used in combination with gemcitabine (NCT01764477). Other cases include the combination of anti-FZD antibody with chemotherapy. Vantictumab (OMP-18R5) resulted in promising outcomes in the preclinical setting [152,153] and is currently being evaluated in phase I clinical trials for multiple cancers in combination with paclitaxel [154]. Ipafricept (OMP-54F28/FZD8-Fc) is being evaluated in a phase I clinical trial to treat advanced pancreatic cancer in combination with nab-paclitaxel and gemcitabine [36]. Although antibodies against pan-Wnts or pan-FZD were not tissue-specific, their combination in advanced solid tumors had promising effects [36,154]. In addition, as a neoadjuvant therapy, Foxy-5 is currently being evaluated in phase II trials for colon cancer, as described above (NCT03883802).

10.3. β-Catenin Paradox

The β-catenin paradox was introduced on the basis of heterogeneous Wnt signaling activity in CRC cells, carrying homogenous genetic alterations in *APC* or β-catenin/*CTNNB1* [155]. This observation was followed by discoveries of several Wnt signaling regulators and multiple crosstalks of Wnt/β-catenin signaling with MAPK and PI3K pathways [156–165]. Additionally, accumulating evidence suggests that the blockade of Wnt signaling upstream molecules suppresses tumor growth despite the presence of oncogenic mutations in Wnt signaling components [96,108,116,152,166,167], demonstrating the existence of additional regulatory modules in Wnt signaling, independent of genetic alterations. Additionally, truncated mutant APC remains partially functional to induce β-catenin protein degradation [116,167]. Moreover, the blockade of WNTs/RSPOs inhibits the growth of tumor cells that harbor *APC* mutations [96,116]. In line with this, Tankyrase inhibitor-stabilized AXIN protein suppresses the proliferation of CRC cells that carry constitutively active mutations in β-catenin or *APC* [108,110]. A recent gastric cancer mouse model study also revealed that vantictumab, the pan-FZD inhibitor, inhibits gastric adenoma growth independently of *APC* mutations [152]. Therefore, molecular targeting of the upstream molecules of APC and β-catenin might be promising in Wnt/β-catenin signaling-associated cancer.

10.4. Generalization of Wnt Targeting Therapy

Aberrant Wnt signaling is crucial for the potential clonal source of tumor cells and is considered an environmental and metastatic niche for tumor progression. Indeed, LGR5+ colon cancer cells are required for the formation of metastatic colonization in the liver [146]. A study using patient-derived pancreatic organoids revealed differing Wnt-niche dependency among organoids [168]. Furthermore, in a recent study of lung cancers that barely harbor Wnt mutations, Wnt signaling was shown to be required for lung cancer progression as a niche factor in a mouse lung adenocarcinoma model [169]. In that context, Wnt targeting by porcupine inhibitor, WNT794 (LGK794), revealed the suppression of lung tumor progression [169]. These results suggest that Wnt targeting therapy can be generalized to various types of non-Wnt-mutated cancers in which Wnt signaling has tumor-promoting or metastatic roles.

11. New Candidates for Targeting Wnt Signaling in GI Cancers

Several cancer-specific Wnt signaling regulators were identified in GI cancers. Amplification of USP21 deubiquitinase promotes pancreatic cancer cell growth and stemness via Wnt/β-catenin signaling [170]. RNF6, a CRC-upregulated E3 ligase, promotes CRC cell growth through the degradation of Tele3, a transcriptional repressor of the β-catenin/TCF4 complex [171]. Another deubiquitinase USP7 serves as a tumor-specific Wnt activator in *APC*-mutated CRC by promoting β-catenin deubiquitination [172]. Transcriptional coactivators of β-catenin, BCL9 and BCL9l, redundantly demonstrated CRC-specific upregulation, and their loss suppressed intestinal tumorigenesis in a mouse model [173]. BCL9 and BCL9l inhibitors were recently developed [135,174,175]. Targeting BCL9 and BCL9l has been suggested as a therapeutic approach to CRC-specific treatment. FZD5 mainly expressed in RNF43 mutated tumor cells was proposed as a molecular target for pancreatic cancer treatment [68]. Given that gut-specific knockout of *FZD5* is feasible in the mouse models [176,177], it is likely that targeting of FZD5 can be used in RNF43 mutated intestinal or gastric tumors. In addition, CRC-upregulated PAF/KIAA0101 hyperactivates Wnt/β-catenin signaling and accelerates tumorigenesis in vitro and in vivo [178,179]. As an amplifier of Wnt signaling, TMEM9 hyperactivates β-catenin via APC degradation to promote intestinal and hepatic tumorigenesis [116,166]. Of note, germline deletion of *Tmem9* or *Paf* did not display any discernible phenotypes, suggests that blockade of cancer-related Wnt signaling activators or amplifiers minimizes side effects in Wnt signaling targeting approaches.

Additionally, recent technological advances in organoids made it feasible to perform high-throughput chemical screening (clinical drugs or drug library) and genetic screening (gene knock-out or knock-down) of tumor organoids [180–182]. Moreover, patient-derived organoids become valuable resources to identify most effective drug(s) for precision medicine including pharmacogenomics [183–185]. Therefore, with the emergence of such new technology, it is anticipated that novel tumor-specific and druggable vulnerabilities related to Wnt signaling hyperactivation will be identified.

12. Conclusions

To date, many studies have reported the marked impact of molecular targeting of Wnt signaling on tumor suppression in preclinical settings. Despite the ongoing clinical trials, it is still imperative to overcome recurring pitfalls—catastrophic adverse effects on tissue homeostasis and regeneration. Like the sword of Damocles, targeting Wnt signaling poses a high risk but has significant potential in cancer therapy. With evolving concepts in Wnt signaling deregulation and manipulation, new and improved approaches, including molecular targeting of upstream signaling modules or cancer-specific regulators and combination therapy, are expected to open a new window of opportunity in the treatment of Wnt signaling-associated cancer.

Author Contributions: M.J.K., Y.H., and J.-I.P. wrote the manuscript. All authors have read and agreed to the published version of the manuscript.

Funding: This work was supported by grants to the Cancer Prevention and Research Institute of Texas (RP140563 and RP200315 to J.-I.P.), the National Institutes of Health (2R01 CA193297 to J.-I.P.), the Department of Defense Peer Reviewed Cancer Research Program (CA140572 to J.-I.P.), an Institutional Research Grant (MD Anderson to J.-I.P.), a Specialized Program of Research Excellence (SPORE) grant in endometrial cancer (P50 CA83639), and an ROSI Seed Award (00057597 to M.J.K.).

Acknowledgments: We apologize for all of the studies we were not able to cite because of space limitations.

Conflicts of Interest: The authors declare no conflict of interest.

References

1. Nusse, R.; Varmus, H.E. Many tumors induced by the mouse mammary tumor virus contain a provirus integrated in the same region of the host genome. *Cell* **1982**, *31*, 99–109. [CrossRef]
2. Nusslein-Volhard, C.; Wieschaus, E. Mutations affecting segment number and polarity in Drosophila. *Nature* **1980**, *287*, 795–801. [CrossRef] [PubMed]
3. Steinhart, Z.; Angers, S. Wnt signaling in development and tissue homeostasis. *Development* **2018**, *145*, dev146589. [CrossRef] [PubMed]
4. Clevers, H.; Loh, K.M.; Nusse, R. Stem cell signaling. An integral program for tissue renewal and regeneration: Wnt signaling and stem cell control. *Science* **2014**, *346*, 1248012. [CrossRef]
5. Logan, C.Y.; Nusse, R. The Wnt signaling pathway in development and disease. *Annu. Rev. Cell Dev. Biol.* **2004**, *20*, 781–810. [CrossRef]
6. Nusse, R. Wnt signaling in disease and in development. *Cell Res.* **2005**, *15*, 28–32. [CrossRef]

7. Kahn, M. Can we safely target the WNT pathway? *Nat. Rev. Drug Discov.* **2014**, *13*, 513–532. [CrossRef]
8. Anastas, J.N.; Moon, R.T. WNT signalling pathways as therapeutic targets in cancer. *Nat. Rev. Cancer* **2013**, *13*, 11–26. [CrossRef]
9. Jung, Y.S.; Park, J.I. Wnt signaling in cancer: Therapeutic targeting of Wnt signaling beyond beta-catenin and the destruction complex. *Exp. Mol. Med.* **2020**, *52*, 183–191. [CrossRef]
10. Niehrs, C. The complex world of WNT receptor signalling. *Nat. Rev. Mol. Cell Biol.* **2012**, *13*, 767–779. [CrossRef]
11. Li, V.S.; Ng, S.S.; Boersema, P.J.; Low, T.Y.; Karthaus, W.R.; Gerlach, J.P.; Mohammed, S.; Heck, A.J.; Maurice, M.M.; Mahmoudi, T.; et al. Wnt signaling through inhibition of beta-catenin degradation in an intact Axin1 complex. *Cell* **2012**, *149*, 1245–1256. [CrossRef] [PubMed]
12. Papkoff, J.; Brown, A.M.; Varmus, H.E. The int-1 proto-oncogene products are glycoproteins that appear to enter the secretory pathway. *Mol. Cell Biol.* **1987**, *7*, 3978–3984. [CrossRef] [PubMed]
13. Grumolato, L.; Liu, G.; Mong, P.; Mudbhary, R.; Biswas, R.; Arroyave, R.; Vijayakumar, S.; Economides, A.N.; Aaronson, S.A. Canonical and noncanonical Wnts use a common mechanism to activate completely unrelated coreceptors. *Genes Dev.* **2010**, *24*, 2517–2530. [CrossRef] [PubMed]
14. Gao, Z.H.; Seeling, J.M.; Hill, V.; Yochum, A.; Virshup, D.M. Casein kinase I phosphorylates and destabilizes the beta-catenin degradation complex. *Proc. Natl. Acad. Sci. USA* **2002**, *99*, 1182–1187. [CrossRef] [PubMed]
15. Ha, N.C.; Tonozuka, T.; Stamos, J.L.; Choi, H.J.; Weis, W.I. Mechanism of phosphorylation-dependent binding of APC to beta-catenin and its role in beta-catenin degradation. *Mol. Cell* **2004**, *15*, 511–521. [CrossRef]
16. Liu, C.; Li, Y.; Semenov, M.; Han, C.; Baeg, G.-H.; Tan, Y.; Zhang, Z.; Lin, X.; He, X. Control of beta-catenin phosphorylation/degradation by a dual-kinase mechanism. *Cell* **2002**, *108*, 837–847. [CrossRef]
17. Stamos, J.L.; Weis, W.I. The beta-catenin destruction complex. *Cold Spring Harb. Perspect. Biol.* **2013**, *5*, a007898. [CrossRef]
18. He, X.; Semenov, M.; Tamai, K.; Zeng, X. LDL receptor-related proteins 5 and 6 in Wnt/beta-catenin signaling: Arrows point the way. *Development* **2004**, *131*, 1663–1677. [CrossRef]
19. Kishida, S.; Yamamoto, H.; Hino, S.; Ikeda, S.; Kishida, M.; Kikuchi, A. DIX domains of Dvl and axin are necessary for protein interactions and their ability to regulate beta-catenin stability. *Mol. Cell Biol.* **1999**, *19*, 4414–4422. [CrossRef]
20. Brunner, E.; Peter, O.; Schweizer, L.; Basler, K. Pangolin encodes a Lef-1 homologue that acts downstream of Armadillo to transduce the Wingless signal in Drosophila. *Nature* **1997**, *385*, 829–833. [CrossRef]
21. van de Wetering, M.; Cavallo, R.; Dooijes, D.; van Beest, M.; van Es, J.; Loureiro, J.; Ypma, A.; Hursh, D.; Jones, T.; Bejsovec, A.; et al. Armadillo coactivates transcription driven by the product of the Drosophila segment polarity gene dTCF. *Cell* **1997**, *88*, 789–799. [CrossRef]
22. Takemaru, K.I.; Moon, R.T. The transcriptional coactivator CBP interacts with beta-catenin to activate gene expression. *J. Cell Biol.* **2000**, *149*, 249–254. [CrossRef]
23. Hecht, A.; Vleminckx, K.; Stemmler, M.P.; van Roy, F.; Kemler, R. The p300/CBP acetyltransferases function as transcriptional coactivators of beta-catenin in vertebrates. *EMBO J.* **2000**, *19*, 1839–1850. [CrossRef] [PubMed]
24. Kikuchi, A.; Yamamoto, H.; Sato, A.; Matsumoto, S. New insights into the mechanism of Wnt signaling pathway activation. *Int. Rev. Cell Mol. Biol.* **2011**, *291*, 21–71. [PubMed]
25. Simons, M.; Mlodzik, M. Planar cell polarity signaling: From fly development to human disease. *Annu. Rev. Genet.* **2008**, *42*, 517–540. [CrossRef] [PubMed]
26. De, A. Wnt/Ca^{2+} signaling pathway: A brief overview. *Acta Biochim. Biophys. Sin.* **2011**, *43*, 745–756. [CrossRef] [PubMed]
27. Cancer Genome Atlas Network. Comprehensive molecular characterization of human colon and rectal cancer. *Nature* **2012**, *487*, 330–337. [CrossRef]
28. Rowan, A.J.; Lamlum, H.; Ilyas, M.; Wheeler, J.; Straub, J.; Papadopoulou, A.; Bicknell, D.; Bodmer, W.F.; Tomlinson, I.P. APC mutations in sporadic colorectal tumors: A mutational "hotspot" and interdependence of the "two hits". *Proc. Natl. Acad. Sci. USA* **2000**, *97*, 3352–3357. [CrossRef]
29. Russell, J.O.; Monga, S.P. Wnt/beta-catenin signaling in liver development, homeostasis, and pathobiology. *Annu. Rev. Pathol.* **2018**, *13*, 351–378. [CrossRef]
30. Khalaf, A.M.; Fuentes, D.; Morshid, A.I.; Burke, M.R.; Kaseb, A.O.; Hassan, M.; Hazle, J.D.; Elsayes, K.M. Role of Wnt/beta-catenin signaling in hepatocellular carcinoma, pathogenesis, and clinical significance. *J. Hepatocell. Carcinoma* **2018**, *5*, 61–73. [CrossRef]

31. Merle, P.; de la Monte, S.; Kim, M.; Herrmann, M.; Tanaka, S.; Von Dem Bussche, A.; Kew, M.C.; Trepo, C.; Wands, J.R. Functional consequences of frizzled-7 receptor overexpression in human hepatocellular carcinoma. *Gastroenterology* **2004**, *127*, 1110–1122. [CrossRef]
32. Waddell, N.; Pajic, M.; Patch, A.M.; Chang, D.K.; Kassahn, K.S.; Bailey, P.; Johns, A.L.; Miller, D.; Nones, K.; Quek, K.; et al. Whole genomes redefine the mutational landscape of pancreatic cancer. *Nature* **2015**, *518*, 495–501. [CrossRef]
33. Cancer Genome Atlas Research Network. Comprehensive molecular characterization of gastric adenocarcinoma. *Nature* **2014**, *513*, 202–209. [CrossRef] [PubMed]
34. Ng, M.; Tan, D.S.; Subbiah, V.; Weekes, C.D.; Teneggi, V.; Diermayr, V.; Ethirajulu, K.; Yeo, P.; Chen, D.; Blanchard, S. First-in-human phase 1 study of ETC-159 an oral PORCN inhbitor in patients with advanced solid tumours. *Am. Soc. Clin. Oncol.* **2017**, *35*. [CrossRef]
35. Pintova, S.; Dharmupari, S.; Moshier, E.; Zubizarreta, N.; Ang, C.; Holcombe, R.F. Genistein combined with FOLFOX or FOLFOX-Bevacizumab for the treatment of metastatic colorectal cancer: Phase I/II pilot study. *Cancer Chemother. Pharmacol.* **2019**, *84*, 591–598. [CrossRef] [PubMed]
36. Jimeno, A.; Gordon, M.; Chugh, R.; Messersmith, W.; Mendelson, D.; Dupont, J.; Stagg, R.; Kapoun, A.M.; Xu, L.; Uttamsingh, S.; et al. A first-in-human phase I study of the anticancer stem cell agent ipafricept (OMP-54F28), a decoy receptor for Wnt ligands, in patients with advanced solid tumors. *Clin. Cancer Res. Off. J. Am. Assoc. Cancer Res.* **2017**, *23*, 7490–7497. [CrossRef] [PubMed]
37. Dotan, E.; Cardin, D.B.; Lenz, H.-J.; Messersmith, W.A.; O'Neil, B.; Cohen, S.J.; Denlinger, C.S.; Shahda, S.; Kapoun, A.M.; Brachmann, R.K.; et al. Phase Ib study of WNT inhibitor ipafricept (IPA) with nab-paclitaxel (Nab-P) and gemcitabine (G) in patients (pts) with previously untreated stage IV pancreatic cancer (mPC). *Am. Soc. Clin. Oncol.* **2019**, *37*. [CrossRef]
38. Vermorken, J.; Cervantes, A.; Morsing, P.; Johansson, K.; Andersson, T.; Roest, N.L.; Gullbo, J.; Salazar, R. P-133 A randomized, multicenter, open-label controlled phase 2 trial of Foxy-5 as neoadjuvant therapy in patients with WNT5A negative colon cancer. *Ann. Oncol.* **2019**, *30* (Suppl. S4). [CrossRef]
39. Davis, S.L.; Cardin, D.B.; Shahda, S.; Lenz, H.J.; Dotan, E.; O'Neil, B.H.; Kapoun, A.M.; Stagg, R.J.; Berlin, J.; Messersmith, W.A.; et al. A phase 1b dose escalation study of Wnt pathway inhibitor vantictumab in combination with nab-paclitaxel and gemcitabine in patients with previously untreated metastatic pancreatic cancer. *Investig. New Drugs* **2019**, *38*, 821–830. [CrossRef]
40. Ryan, D.; Murphy, J.; Mahalingam, D.; Strickler, J.; Stein, S.; Sirard, C.; Landau, S.; Bendell, J. PD-016 Current results of a phase I study of DKN-01 in combination with paclitaxel (P) in patients (pts) with advanced DKK1+ esophageal cancer (EC) or gastro-esophageal junction tumors (GEJ). *Ann. Oncol.* **2016**, *27* (Suppl. S2), ii108. [CrossRef]
41. Eads, J.R.; Goyal, L.; Stein, S.; El-Khoueiry, A.B.; Manji, G.A.; Abrams, T.A.; Landau, S.B.; Sirard, C.A. Phase I study of DKN-01, an anti-DKK1 antibody, in combination with gemcitabine (G) and cisplatin (C) in patients (pts) with advanced biliary cancer. *J. Clin. Oncol.* **2016**, *34* (Suppl. S15), e15603. [CrossRef]
42. Bendell, J.; Eckhardt, G.; Hochster, H.; Morris, V.; Strickler, J.; Kapoun, A.; Wang, M.; Xu, L.; McGuire, K.; Dupont, J. Initial results from a phase 1a/b study of OMP-131R10, a first-in-class anti-RSPO3 antibody, in advanced solid tumors and previously treated metastatic colorectal cancer (CRC). *Eur. J. Cancer* **2016**, *69* (Suppl. 1), S29–S30. [CrossRef]
43. Burock, S.; Daum, S.; Tröger, H.; Kim, T.D.; Krüger, S.; Rieke, D.T.; Ochsenreither, S.; Welter, K.; Herrmann, P.; Sleegers, A. Niclosamide a new chemotherapy agent? Pharmacokinetics of the potential anticancer drug in a patient cohort of the NIKOLO trial. *Am. Soc. Clin. Oncol.* **2018**, *36*, e14536. [CrossRef]
44. Molenaar, R.J.; Coelen, R.J.S.; Khurshed, M.; Roos, E.; Caan, M.W.A.; van Linde, M.E.; Kouwenhoven, M.; Bramer, J.A.M.; Bovee, J.; Mathot, R.A.; et al. Study protocol of a phase IB/II clinical trial of metformin and chloroquine in patients with IDH1-mutated or IDH2-mutated solid tumours. *BMJ Open* **2017**, *7*, e014961. [CrossRef] [PubMed]
45. Mahalingam, D.; Mita, M.; Sarantopoulos, J.; Wood, L.; Amaravadi, R.K.; Davis, L.E.; Mita, A.C.; Curiel, T.J.; Espitia, C.M.; Nawrocki, S.T.; et al. Combined autophagy and HDAC inhibition: A phase I safety, tolerability, pharmacokinetic, and pharmacodynamic analysis of hydroxychloroquine in combination with the HDAC inhibitor vorinostat in patients with advanced solid tumors. *Autophagy* **2014**, *10*, 1403–1414. [CrossRef]

46. Boone, B.A.; Bahary, N.; Zureikat, A.H.; Moser, A.J.; Normolle, D.P.; Wu, W.C.; Singhi, A.D.; Bao, P.; Bartlett, D.L.; Liotta, L.A.; et al. Safety and biologic response of pre-operative autophagy inhibition in combination with gemcitabine in patients with pancreatic adenocarcinoma. *Ann. Surg. Oncol.* **2015**, *22*, 4402–4410. [CrossRef]
47. Loaiza-Bonilla, A.; O'Hara, M.H.; Redlinger, M.; Damjanov, N.; Teitelbaum, U.R.; Vasilevskaya, I.; Rosen, M.A.; Heitjan, D.F.; Amaravadi, R.K.; O'Dwyer, P.J. Phase II trial of autophagy inhibition using hydroxychloroquine (HCQ) with FOLFOX/bevacizumab in the first-line treatment of advanced colorectal cancer. *J. Clin. Oncol.* **2015**, *33*, 3614. [CrossRef]
48. Wolpin, B.M.; Rubinson, D.A.; Wang, X.; Chan, J.A.; Cleary, J.M.; Enzinger, P.C.; Fuchs, C.S.; McCleary, N.J.; Meyerhardt, J.A.; Ng, K.; et al. Phase II and pharmacodynamic study of autophagy inhibition using hydroxychloroquine in patients with metastatic pancreatic adenocarcinoma. *Oncologist* **2014**, *19*, 637–648. [CrossRef]
49. Hong, T.S.; Wo, J.Y.-L.; Jiang, W.; Yeap, B.Y.; Clark, J.W.; Ryan, D.P.; Blaszkowsky, L.S.; Drapek, L.C.; Mamon, H.J.; Murphy, J.E.; et al. Phase II study of autophagy inhibition with hydroxychloroquine (HCQ) and preoperative (preop) short course chemoradiation (SCRT) followed by early surgery for resectable ductal adenocarcinoma of the head of pancreas (PDAC). *J. Clin. Oncol.* **2017**, *35*, 4118. [CrossRef]
50. Karasic, T.B.; O'Hara, M.H.; Loaiza-Bonilla, A.; Reiss, K.A.; Teitelbaum, U.R.; Borazanci, E.; De Jesus-Acosta, A.; Redlinger, C.; Burrell, J.A.; Laheru, D.A.; et al. Effect of gemcitabine and nab-paclitaxel with or without hydroxychloroquine on patients with advanced pancreatic cancer: A phase 2 randomized clinical trial. *JAMA Oncol.* **2019**, *5*, 993–998. [CrossRef]
51. Arora, S.P.; Tenner, L.L.; Sarantopoulos, J.; Morris, J.L.; Longoria, L.; Liu, Q.; Michalek, J.; Mahalingam, D. Modulation of autophagy: A phase II study of vorinostat (VOR) plus hydroxychloroquine (HCQ) vs regorafenib (RGF) in chemo-refractory metastatic colorectal cancer (mCRC). *J. Clin. Oncol.* **2019**, *37*, 3551. [CrossRef]
52. El-Khoueiry, A.B.; Ning, Y.; Yang, D.; Cole, S.; Kahn, M.; Zoghbi, M.; Berg, J.; Fujimori, M.; Inada, T.; Kouji, H. A phase I first-in-human study of PRI-724 in patients (pts) with advanced solid tumors. *Am. Soc. Clin. Oncol.* **2013**, *31*, 2501. [CrossRef]
53. Ko, A.H.; Chiorean, E.G.; Kwak, E.L.; Lenz, H.-J.; Nadler, P.I.; Wood, D.L.; Fujimori, M.; Inada, T.; Kouji, H.; McWilliams, R.R. Final results of a phase Ib dose-escalation study of PRI-724, a CBP/beta-catenin modulator, plus gemcitabine (GEM) in patients with advanced pancreatic adenocarcinoma (APC) as second-line therapy after FOLFIRINOX or FOLFOX. *Am. Soc. Clin. Oncol.* **2016**, *34*, e15721. [CrossRef]
54. Fischer, M.M.; Cancilla, B.; Yeung, V.P.; Cattaruzza, F.; Chartier, C.; Murriel, C.L.; Cain, J.; Tam, R.; Cheng, C.Y.; Evans, J.W.; et al. WNT antagonists exhibit unique combinatorial antitumor activity with taxanes by potentiating mitotic cell death. *Sci. Adv.* **2017**, *3*, e1700090. [CrossRef]
55. Lopez-Rios, J.; Esteve, P.; Ruiz, J.M.; Bovolenta, P. The Netrin-related domain of Sfrp1 interacts with Wnt ligands and antagonizes their activity in the anterior neural plate. *Neural Dev.* **2008**, *3*, 19. [CrossRef]
56. Bu, Q.; Li, Z.; Zhang, J.; Xu, F.; Liu, J.; Liu, H. The crystal structure of full-length Sizzled from Xenopus laevis yields insights into Wnt-antagonistic function of secreted Frizzled-related proteins. *J. Biol. Chem.* **2017**, *292*, 16055–16069. [CrossRef]
57. Agostino, M.; Pohl, S.O.; Dharmarajan, A. Structure-based prediction of Wnt binding affinities for Frizzled-type cysteine-rich domains. *J. Biol. Chem.* **2017**, *292*, 11218–11229. [CrossRef]
58. Xavier, C.P.; Melikova, M.; Chuman, Y.; Uren, A.; Baljinnyam, B.; Rubin, J.S. Secreted Frizzled-related protein potentiation versus inhibition of Wnt3a/beta-catenin signaling. *Cell. Signal.* **2014**, *26*, 94–101. [CrossRef]
59. Liang, C.J.; Wang, Z.W.; Chang, Y.W.; Lee, K.C.; Lin, W.H.; Lee, J.L. SFRPs are biphasic modulators of Wnt-signaling-elicited cancer stem cell properties beyond extracellular control. *Cell Rep.* **2019**, *28*, 1511–1525.e5. [CrossRef]
60. Malinauskas, T.; Aricescu, A.R.; Lu, W.; Siebold, C.; Jones, E.Y. Modular mechanism of Wnt signaling inhibition by Wnt inhibitory factor 1. *Nat. Struct. Mol. Biol.* **2011**, *18*, 886–893. [CrossRef]
61. Piccolo, S.; Agius, E.; Leyns, L.; Bhattacharyya, S.; Grunz, H.; Bouwmeester, T.; De Robertis, E.M. The head inducer Cerberus is a multifunctional antagonist of Nodal, BMP and Wnt signals. *Nature* **1999**, *397*, 707–710. [CrossRef] [PubMed]
62. Rios-Esteves, J.; Haugen, B.; Resh, M.D. Identification of key residues and regions important for porcupine-mediated Wnt acylation. *J. Biol. Chem.* **2014**, *289*, 17009–17019. [CrossRef] [PubMed]

63. Yu, J.; Chia, J.; Canning, C.A.; Jones, C.M.; Bard, F.A.; Virshup, D.M. WLS retrograde transport to the endoplasmic reticulum during Wnt secretion. *Dev. Cell* **2014**, *29*, 277–291. [CrossRef] [PubMed]
64. Suciu, R.M.; Cognetta, A.B., 3rd; Potter, Z.E.; Cravatt, B.F. Selective irreversible inhibitors of the Wnt-deacylating enzyme NOTUM developed by activity-based protein profiling. *ACS Med. Chem. Lett.* **2018**, *9*, 563–568. [CrossRef]
65. Moverare-Skrtic, S.; Nilsson, K.H.; Henning, P.; Funck-Brentano, T.; Nethander, M.; Rivadeneira, F.; Nunes, G.C.; Koskela, A.; Tuukkanen, J.; Tuckermann, J.; et al. Osteoblast-derived NOTUM reduces cortical bone mass in mice and the NOTUM locus is associated with bone mineral density in humans. *FASEB J. Off. Publ. Fed. Am. Soc. Exp. Biol.* **2019**, *33*, 11163–11179. [CrossRef]
66. Zhang, X.; Abreu, J.G.; Yokota, C.; MacDonald, B.T.; Singh, S.; Coburn, K.L.; Cheong, S.M.; Zhang, M.M.; Ye, Q.Z.; Hang, H.C.; et al. Tiki1 is required for head formation via Wnt cleavage-oxidation and inactivation. *Cell* **2012**, *149*, 1565–1577. [CrossRef]
67. Zhang, X.; MacDonald, B.T.; Gao, H.; Shamashkin, M.; Coyle, A.J.; Martinez, R.V.; He, X. Characterization of Tiki, a New Family of Wnt-specific Metalloproteases. *J. Biol. Chem.* **2016**, *291*, 2435–2443. [CrossRef]
68. Steinhart, Z.; Pavlovic, Z.; Chandrashekhar, M.; Hart, T.; Wang, X.; Zhang, X.; Robitaille, M.; Brown, K.R.; Jaksani, S.; Overmeer, R.; et al. Genome-wide CRISPR screens reveal a Wnt-FZD5 signaling circuit as a druggable vulnerability of RNF43-mutant pancreatic tumors. *Nat. Med.* **2017**, *23*, 60–68. [CrossRef]
69. Slusarski, D.C.; Yang-Snyder, J.; Busa, W.B.; Moon, R.T. Modulation of embryonic intracellular Ca^{2+} signaling by Wnt-5A. *Dev. Biol.* **1997**, *182*, 114–120. [CrossRef]
70. Murphy, L.L.; Hughes, C.C. Endothelial cells stimulate T cell NFAT nuclear translocation in the presence of cyclosporin A: Involvement of the wnt/glycogen synthase kinase-3 beta pathway. *J. Immunol.* **2002**, *169*, 3717–3725. [CrossRef]
71. Sheldahl, L.C.; Park, M.; Malbon, C.C.; Moon, R.T. Protein kinase C is differentially stimulated by Wnt and Frizzled homologs in a G-protein-dependent manner. *Curr. Biol. CB* **1999**, *9*, 695–698. [CrossRef]
72. Kühl, M.; Sheldahl, L.C.; Malbon, C.C.; Moon, R.T. Ca(2+)/calmodulin-dependent protein kinase II is stimulated by Wnt and Frizzled homologs and promotes ventral cell fates in Xenopus. *J. Biol. Chem.* **2000**, *275*, 12701–12711. [CrossRef] [PubMed]
73. Mikels, A.J.; Nusse, R. Purified Wnt5a protein activates or inhibits beta-catenin-TCF signaling depending on receptor context. *PLoS Biol.* **2006**, *4*, e115. [CrossRef] [PubMed]
74. Sato, A.; Yamamoto, H.; Sakane, H.; Koyama, H.; Kikuchi, A. Wnt5a regulates distinct signalling pathways by binding to Frizzled2. *EMBO J.* **2010**, *29*, 41–54. [CrossRef]
75. Safholm, A.; Tuomela, J.; Rosenkvist, J.; Dejmek, J.; Harkonen, P.; Andersson, T. The Wnt-5a-derived hexapeptide Foxy-5 inhibits breast cancer metastasis in vivo by targeting cell motility. *Clin. Cancer Res. Off. J. Am. Assoc. Cancer Res.* **2008**, *14*, 6556–6563. [CrossRef]
76. Safholm, A.; Leandersson, K.; Dejmek, J.; Nielsen, C.K.; Villoutreix, B.O.; Andersson, T. A formylated hexapeptide ligand mimics the ability of Wnt-5a to impair migration of human breast epithelial cells. *J. Biol. Chem.* **2006**, *281*, 2740–2749. [CrossRef]
77. Jönsson, M.; Andersson, T. Repression of Wnt-5a impairs DDR1 phosphorylation and modifies adhesion and migration of mammary cells. *J. Cell Sci.* **2001**, *114 Pt 11*, 2043–2053.
78. Glinka, A.; Wu, W.; Delius, H.; Monaghan, A.P.; Blumenstock, C.; Niehrs, C.J.N. Dickkopf-1 is a member of a new family of secreted proteins and functions in head induction. *Nature* **1998**, *391*, 357–362. [CrossRef]
79. Niehrs, C. Function and biological roles of the Dickkopf family of Wnt modulators. *Oncogene* **2006**, *25*, 7469–7481. [CrossRef]
80. Yu, B.; Yang, X.; Xu, Y.; Yao, G.; Shu, H.; Lin, B.; Hood, L.; Wang, H.; Yang, S.; Gu, J.; et al. Elevated expression of DKK1 is associated with cytoplasmic/nuclear beta-catenin accumulation and poor prognosis in hepatocellular carcinomas. *J. Hepatol.* **2009**, *50*, 948–957. [CrossRef]
81. Xu, W.H.; Liu, Z.B.; Yang, C.; Qin, W.; Shao, Z.M. Expression of dickkopf-1 and beta-catenin related to the prognosis of breast cancer patients with triple negative phenotype. *PLoS ONE* **2012**, *7*, e37624. [CrossRef] [PubMed]
82. Shi, R.Y.; Yang, X.R.; Shen, Q.J.; Yang, L.X.; Xu, Y.; Qiu, S.J.; Sun, Y.F.; Zhang, X.; Wang, Z.; Zhu, K.; et al. High expression of Dickkopf-related protein 1 is related to lymphatic metastasis and indicates poor prognosis in intrahepatic cholangiocarcinoma patients after surgery. *Cancer* **2013**, *119*, 993–1003. [CrossRef] [PubMed]

83. Chen, C.; Zhou, H.; Zhang, X.; Ma, X.; Liu, Z.; Liu, X. Elevated levels of Dickkopf-1 are associated with beta-catenin accumulation and poor prognosis in patients with chondrosarcoma. *PLoS ONE* **2014**, *9*, e105414.
84. Shi, Y.; Gong, H.L.; Zhou, L.; Tian, J.; Wang, Y. Dickkopf-1 is a novel prognostic biomarker for laryngeal squamous cell carcinoma. *Acta Otolaryngol.* **2014**, *134*, 753–759. [CrossRef]
85. Chen, W.; Zhang, Y.W.; Li, Y.; Zhang, J.W.; Zhang, T.; Fu, B.S.; Zhang, Q.; Jiang, N. Constitutive expression of Wnt/betacatenin target genes promotes proliferation and invasion of liver cancer stem cells. *Mol. Med. Rep.* **2016**, *13*, 3466–3474. [CrossRef]
86. Zhuang, X.; Zhang, H.; Li, X.; Li, X.; Cong, M.; Peng, F.; Yu, J.; Zhang, X.; Yang, Q.; Hu, G. Differential effects on lung and bone metastasis of breast cancer by Wnt signalling inhibitor DKK1. *Nat. Cell Biol.* **2017**, *19*, 1274–1285. [CrossRef]
87. Caneparo, L.; Huang, Y.L.; Staudt, N.; Tada, M.; Ahrendt, R.; Kazanskaya, O.; Niehrs, C.; Houart, C. Dickkopf-1 regulates gastrulation movements by coordinated modulation of Wnt/beta catenin and Wnt/PCP activities, through interaction with the Dally-like homolog Knypek. *Genes Dev.* **2007**, *21*, 465–480. [CrossRef]
88. Cha, S.W.; Tadjuidje, E.; Tao, Q.; Wylie, C.; Heasman, J. Wnt5a and Wnt11 interact in a maternal Dkk1-regulated fashion to activate both canonical and non-canonical signaling in Xenopus axis formation. *Development* **2008**, *135*, 3719–3729. [CrossRef]
89. Eisenhauer, E.A.; Therasse, P.; Bogaerts, J.; Schwartz, L.H.; Sargent, D.; Ford, R.; Dancey, J.; Arbuck, S.; Gwyther, S.; Mooney, M.; et al. New response evaluation criteria in solid tumours: Revised RECIST guideline (version 1.1). *Eur. J. Cancer* **2009**, *45*, 228–247. [CrossRef]
90. Yanagita, M.; Oka, M.; Watabe, T.; Iguchi, H.; Niida, A.; Takahashi, S.; Akiyama, T.; Miyazono, K.; Yanagisawa, M.; Sakurai, T. USAG-1: A bone morphogenetic protein antagonist abundantly expressed in the kidney. *Biochem. Biophys. Res. Commun.* **2004**, *316*, 490–500. [CrossRef]
91. Itasaki, N.; Jones, C.M.; Mercurio, S.; Rowe, A.; Domingos, P.M.; Smith, J.C.; Krumlauf, R. Wise, a context-dependent activator and inhibitor of Wnt signalling. *Development* **2003**, *130*, 4295–4305. [CrossRef] [PubMed]
92. de Lau, W.; Peng, W.C.; Gros, P.; Clevers, H. The R-spondin/Lgr5/Rnf43 module: Regulator of Wnt signal strength. *Genes Dev.* **2014**, *28*, 305–316. [CrossRef] [PubMed]
93. Nusse, R.; Clevers, H. Wnt/beta-catenin signaling, disease, and emerging therapeutic modalities. *Cell* **2017**, *169*, 985–999. [CrossRef] [PubMed]
94. Seshagiri, S.; Stawiski, E.W.; Durinck, S.; Modrusan, Z.; Storm, E.E.; Conboy, C.B.; Chaudhuri, S.; Guan, Y.; Janakiraman, V.; Jaiswal, B.S.; et al. Recurrent R-spondin fusions in colon cancer. *Nature* **2012**, *488*, 660–664. [CrossRef] [PubMed]
95. Koo, B.K.; Spit, M.; Jordens, I.; Low, T.Y.; Stange, D.E.; van de Wetering, M.; van Es, J.H.; Mohammed, S.; Heck, A.J.; Maurice, M.M.; et al. Tumour suppressor RNF43 is a stem-cell E3 ligase that induces endocytosis of Wnt receptors. *Nature* **2012**, *488*, 665–669. [CrossRef]
96. Hao, H.X.; Xie, Y.; Zhang, Y.; Charlat, O.; Oster, E.; Avello, M.; Lei, H.; Mickanin, C.; Liu, D.; Ruffner, H.; et al. ZNRF3 promotes Wnt receptor turnover in an R-spondin-sensitive manner. *Nature* **2012**, *485*, 195–200. [CrossRef] [PubMed]
97. Inglis, D.J.; Licari, J.; Georgiou, K.R.; Wittwer, N.L.; Hamilton, R.W.; Beaumont, D.M.; Scherer, M.A.; Lavranos, T.C. Abstract 3910: Characterization of BNC101 a human specific monoclonal antibody targeting the GPCR LGR5: First-in-human evidence of target engagement. *Cancer Res.* **2018**, *78* (Suppl. S13), 3910.
98. Osada, T.; Chen, M.; Yang, X.Y.; Spasojevic, I.; Vandeusen, J.B.; Hsu, D.; Clary, B.M.; Clay, T.M.; Chen, W.; Morse, M.A.; et al. Antihelminth compound niclosamide downregulates Wnt signaling and elicits antitumor responses in tumors with activating APC mutations. *Cancer Res.* **2011**, *71*, 4172–4182. [CrossRef]
99. Chen, M.; Wang, J.; Lu, J.; Bond, M.C.; Ren, X.R.; Lyerly, H.K.; Barak, L.S.; Chen, W. The anti-helminthic niclosamide inhibits Wnt/Frizzled1 signaling. *Biochemistry* **2009**, *48*, 10267–10274. [CrossRef]
100. Lu, W.; Lin, C.; Roberts, M.J.; Waud, W.R.; Piazza, G.A.; Li, Y. Niclosamide suppresses cancer cell growth by inducing Wnt co-receptor LRP6 degradation and inhibiting the Wnt/beta-catenin pathway. *PLoS ONE* **2011**, *6*, e29290. [CrossRef]
101. Wong, H.-C.; Bourdelas, A.; Krauss, A.; Lee, H.-J.; Shao, Y.; Wu, D.; Mlodzik, M.; Shi, D.-L.; Zheng, J. Direct binding of the PDZ domain of Dishevelled to a conserved internal sequence in the C-terminal region of Frizzled. *Mol. Cell* **2003**, *12*, 1251–1260. [CrossRef]

102. Fiedler, M.; Mendoza-Topaz, C.; Rutherford, T.J.; Mieszczanek, J.; Bienz, M. Dishevelled interacts with the DIX domain polymerization interface of Axin to interfere with its function in down-regulating beta-catenin. *Proc. Natl. Acad. Sci. USA* **2011**, *108*, 1937–1942. [CrossRef] [PubMed]
103. Grandy, D.; Shan, J.; Zhang, X.; Rao, S.; Akunuru, S.; Li, H.; Zhang, Y.; Alpatov, I.; Zhang, X.A.; Lang, R.A.; et al. Discovery and characterization of a small molecule inhibitor of the PDZ domain of dishevelled. *J. Biol. Chem.* **2009**, *284*, 16256–16263. [CrossRef] [PubMed]
104. Fujii, N.; You, L.; Xu, Z.; Uematsu, K.; Shan, J.; He, B.; Mikami, I.; Edmondson, L.R.; Neale, G.; Zheng, J.; et al. An antagonist of dishevelled protein-protein interaction suppresses beta-catenin-dependent tumor cell growth. *Cancer Res.* **2007**, *67*, 573–579. [CrossRef] [PubMed]
105. Shan, J.; Shi, D.L.; Wang, J.; Zheng, J. Identification of a specific inhibitor of the dishevelled PDZ domain. *Biochemistry* **2005**, *44*, 15495–15503. [CrossRef]
106. Zhang, Y.; Appleton, B.A.; Wiesmann, C.; Lau, T.; Costa, M.; Hannoush, R.N.; Sidhu, S.S. Inhibition of Wnt signaling by Dishevelled PDZ peptides. *Nat. Chem. Biol.* **2009**, *5*, 217–219. [CrossRef]
107. Riffell, J.L.; Lord, C.J.; Ashworth, A. Tankyrase-targeted therapeutics: Expanding opportunities in the PARP family. *Nat. Rev. Drug Discov.* **2012**, *11*, 923–936. [CrossRef]
108. Huang, S.M.; Mishina, Y.M.; Liu, S.; Cheung, A.; Stegmeier, F.; Michaud, G.A.; Charlat, O.; Wiellette, E.; Zhang, Y.; Wiessner, S.; et al. Tankyrase inhibition stabilizes axin and antagonizes Wnt signalling. *Nature* **2009**, *461*, 614–620. [CrossRef]
109. Huang, J.; Xiao, D.; Li, G.; Ma, J.; Chen, P.; Yuan, W.; Hou, F.; Ge, J.; Zhong, M.; Tang, Y.; et al. EphA2 promotes epithelial-mesenchymal transition through the Wnt/β-catenin pathway in gastric cancer cells. *Oncogene* **2014**, *33*, 2737–2747. [CrossRef]
110. Lau, T.; Chan, E.; Callow, M.; Waaler, J.; Boggs, J.; Blake, R.A.; Magnuson, S.; Sambrone, A.; Schutten, M.; Firestein, R.; et al. A novel tankyrase small-molecule inhibitor suppresses APC mutation-driven colorectal tumor growth. *Cancer Res.* **2013**, *73*, 3132–3144. [CrossRef]
111. Martins-Neves, S.R.; Paiva-Oliveira, D.I.; Fontes-Ribeiro, C.; Bovée, J.; Cleton-Jansen, A.M.; Gomes, C.M.F. IWR-1, a tankyrase inhibitor, attenuates Wnt/β-catenin signaling in cancer stem-like cells and inhibits in vivo the growth of a subcutaneous human osteosarcoma xenograft. *Cancer Lett.* **2018**, *414*, 1–15. [CrossRef] [PubMed]
112. Scarborough, H.A.; Helfrich, B.A.; Casás-Selves, M.; Schuller, A.G.; Grosskurth, S.E.; Kim, J.; Tan, A.C.; Chan, D.C.; Zhang, Z.; Zaberezhnyy, V.; et al. AZ1366: An inhibitor of tankyrase and the canonical Wnt pathway that limits the persistence of non-small cell lung cancer cells following EGFR inhibition. *Clin. Cancer Res. Off. J. Am. Assoc. Cancer Res.* **2017**, *23*, 1531–1541. [CrossRef] [PubMed]
113. Waaler, J.; Machon, O.; Tumova, L.; Dinh, H.; Korinek, V.; Wilson, S.R.; Paulsen, J.E.; Pedersen, N.M.; Eide, T.J.; Machonova, O.; et al. A novel tankyrase inhibitor decreases canonical Wnt signaling in colon carcinoma cells and reduces tumor growth in conditional APC mutant mice. *Cancer Res.* **2012**, *72*, 2822–2832. [CrossRef] [PubMed]
114. Ji, L.; Jiang, B.; Jiang, X.; Charlat, O.; Chen, A.; Mickanin, C.; Bauer, A.; Xu, W.; Yan, X.; Cong, F. The SIAH E3 ubiquitin ligases promote Wnt/beta-catenin signaling through mediating Wnt-induced Axin degradation. *Genes Dev.* **2017**, *31*, 904–915. [CrossRef]
115. Ji, L.; Lu, B.; Zamponi, R.; Charlat, O.; Aversa, R.; Yang, Z.; Sigoillot, F.; Zhu, X.; Hu, T.; Reece-Hoyes, J.S.; et al. USP7 inhibits Wnt/beta-catenin signaling through promoting stabilization of Axin. *Nat. Commun.* **2019**, *10*, 4184. [CrossRef]
116. Jung, Y.S.; Jun, S.; Kim, M.J.; Lee, S.H.; Suh, H.N.; Lien, E.M.; Jung, H.Y.; Lee, S.; Zhang, J.; Yang, J.I.; et al. TMEM9 promotes intestinal tumorigenesis through vacuolar-ATPase-activated Wnt/beta-catenin signalling. *Nat. Cell Biol.* **2018**, *20*, 1421–1433. [CrossRef]
117. Thorne, C.A.; Hanson, A.J.; Schneider, J.; Tahinci, E.; Orton, D.; Cselenyi, C.S.; Jernigan, K.K.; Meyers, K.C.; Hang, B.I.; Waterson, A.G.; et al. Small-molecule inhibition of Wnt signaling through activation of casein kinase 1alpha. *Nat. Chem. Biol.* **2010**, *6*, 829–836. [CrossRef]
118. Hwang, S.Y.; Deng, X.; Byun, S.; Lee, C.; Lee, S.J.; Suh, H.; Zhang, J.; Kang, Q.; Zhang, T.; Westover, K.D.; et al. Direct targeting of beta-catenin by a small molecule stimulates proteasomal degradation and suppresses oncogenic Wnt/beta-catenin signaling. *Cell Rep.* **2016**, *16*, 28–36. [CrossRef]

119. Simonetta, K.R.; Taygerly, J.; Boyle, K.; Basham, S.E.; Padovani, C.; Lou, Y.; Cummins, T.J.; Yung, S.L.; von Soly, S.K.; Kayser, F.; et al. Prospective discovery of small molecule enhancers of an E3 ligase-substrate interaction. *Nat. Commun.* **2019**, *10*, 1402. [CrossRef]
120. Goentoro, L.; Kirschner, M.W. Evidence that fold-change, and not absolute level, of beta-catenin dictates Wnt signaling. *Mol. Cell* **2009**, *36*, 872–884. [CrossRef]
121. Cadigan, K.M.; Waterman, M.L. TCF/LEFs and Wnt signaling in the nucleus. *Cold Spring Harb. Perspect. Biol.* **2012**, *4*, a007906. [CrossRef] [PubMed]
122. Gonsalves, F.C.; Klein, K.; Carson, B.B.; Katz, S.; Ekas, L.A.; Evans, S.; Nagourney, R.; Cardozo, T.; Brown, A.M.; DasGupta, R. An RNAi-based chemical genetic screen identifies three small-molecule inhibitors of the Wnt/wingless signaling pathway. *Proc. Natl. Acad. Sci. USA* **2011**, *108*, 5954–5963. [CrossRef] [PubMed]
123. Sukhdeo, K.; Mani, M.; Zhang, Y.; Dutta, J.; Yasui, H.; Rooney, M.D.; Carrasco, D.E.; Zheng, M.; He, H.; Tai, Y.T.; et al. Targeting the beta-catenin/TCF transcriptional complex in the treatment of multiple myeloma. *Proc. Natl. Acad. Sci. USA* **2007**, *104*, 7516–7521. [CrossRef] [PubMed]
124. Tian, W.; Han, X.; Yan, M.; Xu, Y.; Duggineni, S.; Lin, N.; Luo, G.; Li, Y.M.; Han, X.; Huang, Z.; et al. Structure-based discovery of a novel inhibitor targeting the beta-catenin/Tcf4 interaction. *Biochemistry* **2012**, *51*, 724–731. [CrossRef]
125. Mahmoudi, T.; Li, V.S.; Ng, S.S.; Taouatas, N.; Vries, R.G.; Mohammed, S.; Heck, A.J.; Clevers, H. The kinase TNIK is an essential activator of Wnt target genes. *EMBO J.* **2009**, *28*, 3329–3340. [CrossRef]
126. Masuda, M.; Uno, Y.; Ohbayashi, N.; Ohata, H.; Mimata, A.; Kukimoto-Niino, M.; Moriyama, H.; Kashimoto, S.; Inoue, T.; Goto, N.; et al. TNIK inhibition abrogates colorectal cancer stemness. *Nat. Commun.* **2016**, *7*, 12586. [CrossRef]
127. Shitashige, M.; Satow, R.; Jigami, T.; Aoki, K.; Honda, K.; Shibata, T.; Ono, M.; Hirohashi, S.; Yamada, T. Traf2- and Nck-interacting kinase is essential for Wnt signaling and colorectal cancer growth. *Cancer Res.* **2010**, *70*, 5024–5033. [CrossRef]
128. Lee, Y.; Jung, J.I.; Park, K.Y.; Kim, S.A.; Kim, J. Synergistic inhibition effect of TNIK inhibitor KY-05009 and receptor tyrosine kinase inhibitor dovitinib on IL-6-induced proliferation and Wnt signaling pathway in human multiple myeloma cells. *Oncotarget* **2017**, *8*, 41091–41101. [CrossRef]
129. Ishitani, T.; Ninomiya-Tsuji, J.; Nagai, S.; Nishita, M.; Meneghini, M.; Barker, N.; Waterman, M.; Bowerman, B.; Clevers, H.; Shibuya, H. The TAK1-NLK-MAPK-related pathway antagonizes signalling between beta-catenin and transcription factor TCF. *Nature* **1999**, *399*, 798–802. [CrossRef]
130. Ishitani, T.; Kishida, S.; Hyodo-Miura, J.; Ueno, N.; Yasuda, J.; Waterman, M.; Shibuya, H.; Moon, R.T.; Ninomiya-Tsuji, J.; Matsumoto, K. The TAK1-NLK mitogen-activated protein kinase cascade functions in the Wnt-5a/Ca^{2+} pathway to antagonize Wnt/beta-catenin signaling. *Mol. Cell Biol.* **2003**, *23*, 131–139. [CrossRef]
131. Hikasa, H.; Sokol, S.Y. Phosphorylation of TCF proteins by homeodomain-interacting protein kinase 2. *J. Biol. Chem.* **2011**, *286*, 12093–120100. [CrossRef] [PubMed]
132. Hikasa, H.; Ezan, J.; Itoh, K.; Li, X.; Klymkowsky, M.W.; Sokol, S.Y. Regulation of TCF3 by Wnt-dependent phosphorylation during vertebrate axis specification. *Dev. Cell* **2010**, *19*, 521–532. [CrossRef] [PubMed]
133. Emami, K.H.; Nguyen, C.; Ma, H.; Kim, D.H.; Jeong, K.W.; Eguchi, M.; Moon, R.T.; Teo, J.L.; Kim, H.Y.; Moon, S.H.; et al. A small molecule inhibitor of beta-catenin/CREB-binding protein transcription [corrected]. *Proc. Natl. Acad. Sci. USA* **2004**, *101*, 12682–12687. [CrossRef] [PubMed]
134. Miyabayashi, T.; Teo, J.L.; Yamamoto, M.; McMillan, M.; Nguyen, C.; Kahn, M. Wnt/beta-catenin/CBP signaling maintains long-term murine embryonic stem cell pluripotency. *Proc. Natl. Acad. Sci. USA* **2007**, *104*, 5668–5673. [CrossRef] [PubMed]
135. de la Roche, M.; Rutherford, T.J.; Gupta, D.; Veprintsev, D.B.; Saxty, B.; Freund, S.M.; Bienz, M. An intrinsically labile alpha-helix abutting the BCL9-binding site of beta-catenin is required for its inhibition by carnosic acid. *Nat. Commun.* **2012**, *3*, 680. [CrossRef] [PubMed]
136. Tam, B.Y.; Chiu, K.; Chung, H.; Bossard, C.; Nguyen, J.D.; Creger, E.; Eastman, B.W.; Mak, C.C.; Ibanez, M.; Ghias, A.; et al. The CLK inhibitor SM08502 induces anti-tumor activity and reduces Wnt pathway gene expression in gastrointestinal cancer models. *Cancer Lett.* **2020**, *473*, 186–197. [CrossRef]
137. Bossard, C.; Chiu, K.; Chung, H.; Nguyen, J.D.; Creger, E.; Eastman, B.; Mak, C.C.; Do, L.; Cho, S.; KC, S. Effects of SM08502, a novel, oral small-molecule inhibitor of Wnt pathway signaling, on gene expression and antitumor activity in colorectal cancer (CRC) models. *Am. Soc. Clin. Oncol.* **2019**, *37*, e15185. [CrossRef]

138. Bossard, C.; Cruz, N.; Eastman, B.; Mak, C.-C.; Sunil, K.; Tam, B.; Bucci, G.; Stewart, J.; Phalen, T.; Cha, S. Abstract A02: SM08502, a novel, small-molecule CDC-like kinase (CLK) inhibitor, downregulates the Wnt signaling pathway and demonstrates antitumor activity in pancreatic cancer cell lines and in vivo xenograft models. *AACR* **2019**. [CrossRef]

139. Pinto, D.; Gregorieff, A.; Begthel, H.; Clevers, H. Canonical Wnt signals are essential for homeostasis of the intestinal epithelium. *Genes Dev.* **2003**, *17*, 1709–1713. [CrossRef]

140. Fevr, T.; Robine, S.; Louvard, D.; Huelsken, J. Wnt/beta-catenin is essential for intestinal homeostasis and maintenance of intestinal stem cells. *Mol. Cell Biol.* **2007**, *27*, 7551–7559. [CrossRef]

141. Ito, M.; Yang, Z.; Andl, T.; Cui, C.; Kim, N.; Millar, S.E.; Cotsarelis, G. Wnt-dependent de novo hair follicle regeneration in adult mouse skin after wounding. *Nature* **2007**, *447*, 316–320. [CrossRef] [PubMed]

142. Duncan, A.W.; Rattis, F.M.; DiMascio, L.N.; Congdon, K.L.; Pazianos, G.; Zhao, C.; Yoon, K.; Cook, J.M.; Willert, K.; Gaiano, N.; et al. Integration of Notch and Wnt signaling in hematopoietic stem cell maintenance. *Nat. Immunol.* **2005**, *6*, 314–322. [CrossRef] [PubMed]

143. Schepers, A.; Clevers, H. Wnt signaling, stem cells, and cancer of the gastrointestinal tract. *Cold Spring Harb. Perspect. Biol.* **2012**, *4*, a007989. [CrossRef] [PubMed]

144. Barker, N.; Tan, S.; Clevers, H. Lgr proteins in epithelial stem cell biology. *Development* **2013**, *140*, 2484–2494. [CrossRef] [PubMed]

145. Junttila, M.R.; Mao, W.; Wang, X.; Wang, B.E.; Pham, T.; Flygare, J.; Yu, S.F.; Yee, S.; Goldenberg, D.; Fields, C.; et al. Targeting LGR5+ cells with an antibody-drug conjugate for the treatment of colon cancer. *Sci. Transl. Med.* **2015**, *7*, 314ra186. [CrossRef]

146. de Sousa e Melo, F.; Kurtova, A.V.; Harnoss, J.M.; Kljavin, N.; Hoeck, J.D.; Hung, J.; Anderson, J.E.; Storm, E.E.; Modrusan, Z.; Koeppen, H.; et al. A distinct role for Lgr5(+) stem cells in primary and metastatic colon cancer. *Nature* **2017**, *543*, 676–680. [CrossRef]

147. Shimokawa, M.; Ohta, Y.; Nishikori, S.; Matano, M.; Takano, A.; Fujii, M.; Date, S.; Sugimoto, S.; Kanai, T.; Sato, T. Visualization and targeting of LGR5(+) human colon cancer stem cells. *Nature* **2017**, *545*, 187–192. [CrossRef]

148. Gong, X.; Azhdarinia, A.; Ghosh, S.C.; Xiong, W.; An, Z.; Liu, Q.; Carmon, K.S. LGR5-targeted antibody-drug conjugate eradicates gastrointestinal tumors and prevents recurrence. *Mol. Cancer Ther.* **2016**, *15*, 1580–1590. [CrossRef]

149. Salik, B.; Yi, H.; Hassan, N.; Santiappillai, N.; Vick, B.; Connerty, P.; Duly, A.; Trahair, T.; Woo, A.J.; Beck, D.; et al. Targeting RSPO3-LGR4 signaling for leukemia stem cell eradication in acute myeloid leukemia. *Cancer Cell* **2020**, *38*, 263–278.e6. [CrossRef]

150. Buchert, M.; Athineos, D.; Abud, H.E.; Burke, Z.D.; Faux, M.C.; Samuel, M.S.; Jarnicki, A.G.; Winbanks, C.E.; Newton, I.P.; Meniel, V.S.; et al. Genetic dissection of differential signaling threshold requirements for the Wnt/beta-catenin pathway in vivo. *PLoS Genet.* **2010**, *6*, e1000816. [CrossRef]

151. Lenz, H.J.; Kahn, M. Safely targeting cancer stem cells via selective catenin coactivator antagonism. *Cancer Sci.* **2014**, *105*, 1087–1092. [CrossRef] [PubMed]

152. Flanagan, D.J.; Barker, N.; Costanzo, N.S.D.; Mason, E.A.; Gurney, A.; Meniel, V.S.; Koushyar, S.; Austin, C.R.; Ernst, M.; Pearson, H.B.; et al. Frizzled-7 is required for Wnt signaling in gastric tumors with and without Apc mutations. *Cancer Res.* **2019**, *79*, 970–981. [CrossRef] [PubMed]

153. Gurney, A.; Axelrod, F.; Bond, C.J.; Cain, J.; Chartier, C.; Donigan, L.; Fischer, M.; Chaudhari, A.; Ji, M.; Kapoun, A.M.; et al. Wnt pathway inhibition via the targeting of Frizzled receptors results in decreased growth and tumorigenicity of human tumors. *Proc. Natl. Acad. Sci. USA* **2012**, *109*, 11717–11722. [CrossRef] [PubMed]

154. Diamond, J.R.; Becerra, C.; Richards, D.; Mita, A.; Osborne, C.; O'Shaughnessy, J.; Zhang, C.; Henner, R.; Kapoun, A.M.; Xu, L.; et al. Phase Ib clinical trial of the anti-frizzled antibody vantictumab (OMP-18R5) plus paclitaxel in patients with locally advanced or metastatic HER2-negative breast cancer. *Breast Cancer Res. Treat.* **2020**, *184*, 53–62. [CrossRef]

155. Brabletz, T.; Jung, A.; Reu, S.; Porzner, M.; Hlubek, F.; Kunz-Schughart, L.A.; Knuechel, R.; Kirchner, T. Variable beta-catenin expression in colorectal cancers indicates tumor progression driven by the tumor environment. *Proc. Natl. Acad. Sci. USA* **2001**, *98*, 10356–10361. [CrossRef]

156. Fodde, R.; Tomlinson, I. Nuclear beta-catenin expression and Wnt signalling: In defence of the dogma. *J. Pathol.* **2010**, *221*, 239–241. [CrossRef]

157. Phelps, R.A.; Chidester, S.; Dehghanizadeh, S.; Phelps, J.; Sandoval, I.T.; Rai, K.; Broadbent, T.; Sarkar, S.; Burt, R.W.; Jones, D.A. A two-step model for colon adenoma initiation and progression caused by APC loss. *Cell* **2009**, *137*, 623–634. [CrossRef]
158. Janssen, K.P.; Alberici, P.; Fsihi, H.; Gaspar, C.; Breukel, C.; Franken, P.; Rosty, C.; Abal, M.; El Marjou, F.; Smits, R.; et al. APC and oncogenic KRAS are synergistic in enhancing Wnt signaling in intestinal tumor formation and progression. *Gastroenterology* **2006**, *131*, 1096–1109. [CrossRef]
159. Horst, D.; Chen, J.; Morikawa, T.; Ogino, S.; Kirchner, T.; Shivdasani, R.A. Differential WNT activity in colorectal cancer confers limited tumorigenic potential and is regulated by MAPK signaling. *Cancer Res.* **2012**, *72*, 1547–1556. [CrossRef]
160. Mzoughi, S.; Zhang, J.; Hequet, D.; Teo, S.X.; Fang, H.; Xing, Q.R.; Bezzi, M.; Seah, M.K.Y.; Ong, S.L.M.; Shin, E.M.; et al. PRDM15 safeguards naive pluripotency by transcriptionally regulating WNT and MAPK-ERK signaling. *Nat. Genet.* **2017**, *49*, 1354–1363. [CrossRef]
161. Jung, Y.S.; Jun, S.; Lee, S.H.; Sharma, A.; Park, J.I. Wnt2 complements Wnt/β-catenin signaling in colorectal cancer. *Oncotarget* **2015**, *6*, 37257–37268. [CrossRef] [PubMed]
162. Tomar, V.S.; Patil, V.; Somasundaram, K. Temozolomide induces activation of Wnt/beta-catenin signaling in glioma cells via PI3K/Akt pathway: Implications in glioma therapy. *Cell Biol. Toxicol.* **2020**, *36*, 273–278. [CrossRef] [PubMed]
163. Prossomariti, A.; Piazzi, G.; Alquati, C.; Ricciardiello, L. Are Wnt/beta-catenin and PI3K/AKT/mTORC1 distinct pathways in colorectal cancer? *Cell. Mol. Gastroenterol. Hepatol.* **2020**, *10*, 491–506. [CrossRef] [PubMed]
164. Shorning, B.Y.; Dass, M.S.; Smalley, M.J.; Pearson, H.B. The PI3K-AKT-mTOR pathway and prostate cancer: At the crossroads of AR, MAPK, and WNT signaling. *Int. J. Mol. Sci.* **2020**, *21*, 4507. [CrossRef]
165. Zhong, Z.; Sepramaniam, S.; Chew, X.H.; Wood, K.; Lee, M.A.; Madan, B.; Virshup, D.M. PORCN inhibition synergizes with PI3K/mTOR inhibition in Wnt-addicted cancers. *Oncogene* **2019**, *38*, 6662–6677. [CrossRef]
166. Jung, Y.S.; Stratton, S.A.; Lee, S.H.; Kim, M.J.; Jun, S.; Zhang, J.; Zheng, B.; Cervantes, C.L.; Cha, J.H.; Barton, M.C.; et al. TMEM9-v-ATPase activates Wnt/beta-catenin signaling via APC lysosomal degradation for liver regeneration and tumorigenesis. *Hepatology* **2020**. [CrossRef]
167. Voloshanenko, O.; Erdmann, G.; Dubash, T.D.; Augustin, I.; Metzig, M.; Moffa, G.; Hundsrucker, C.; Kerr, G.; Sandmann, T.; Anchang, B.; et al. Wnt secretion is required to maintain high levels of Wnt activity in colon cancer cells. *Nat. Commun.* **2013**, *4*, 2610. [CrossRef]
168. Seino, T.; Kawasaki, S.; Shimokawa, M.; Tamagawa, H.; Toshimitsu, K.; Fujii, M.; Ohta, Y.; Matano, M.; Nanki, K.; Kawasaki, K.; et al. Human pancreatic tumor organoids reveal loss of stem cell niche factor dependence during disease progression. *Cell Stem Cell* **2018**, *22*, 454–467.e6. [CrossRef]
169. Tammela, T.; Sanchez-Rivera, F.J.; Cetinbas, N.M.; Wu, K.; Joshi, N.S.; Helenius, K.; Park, Y.; Azimi, R.; Kerper, N.R.; Wesselhoeft, R.A.; et al. A Wnt-producing niche drives proliferative potential and progression in lung adenocarcinoma. *Nature* **2017**, *545*, 355–359. [CrossRef]
170. Hou, P.; Ma, X.; Zhang, Q.; Wu, C.J.; Liao, W.; Li, J.; Wang, H.; Zhao, J.; Zhou, X.; Guan, C.; et al. USP21 deubiquitinase promotes pancreas cancer cell stemness via Wnt pathway activation. *Genes Dev.* **2019**, *33*, 1361–1366. [CrossRef]
171. Liu, L.; Zhang, Y.; Wong, C.C.; Zhang, J.; Dong, Y.; Li, X.; Kang, W.; Chan, F.K.L.; Sung, J.J.Y.; Yu, J. RNF6 promotes colorectal cancer by activating the Wnt/beta-catenin pathway via ubiquitination of TLE3. *Cancer Res.* **2018**, *78*, 1958–1971. [CrossRef] [PubMed]
172. Novellasdemunt, L.; Foglizzo, V.; Cuadrado, L.; Antas, P.; Kucharska, A.; Encheva, V.; Snijders, A.P.; Li, V.S.W. USP7 is a tumor-specific WNT activator for APC-mutated colorectal cancer by mediating beta-catenin deubiquitination. *Cell Rep.* **2017**, *21*, 612–627. [CrossRef] [PubMed]
173. Gay, D.M.; Ridgway, R.A.; Muller, M.; Hodder, M.C.; Hedley, A.; Clark, W.; Leach, J.D.; Jackstadt, R.; Nixon, C.; Huels, D.J.; et al. Loss of BCL9/9l suppresses Wnt driven tumourigenesis in models that recapitulate human cancer. *Nat. Commun.* **2019**, *10*, 723. [CrossRef] [PubMed]
174. Deka, J.; Wiedemann, N.; Anderle, P.; Murphy-Seiler, F.; Bultinck, J.; Eyckerman, S.; Stehle, J.C.; Andre, S.; Vilain, N.; Zilian, O.; et al. Bcl9/Bcl9l are critical for Wnt-mediated regulation of stem cell traits in colon epithelium and adenocarcinomas. *Cancer Res.* **2010**, *70*, 6619–6628. [CrossRef]

175. Feng, M.; Jin, J.Q.; Xia, L.; Xiao, T.; Mei, S.; Wang, X.; Huang, X.; Chen, J.; Liu, M.; Chen, C.; et al. Pharmacological inhibition of β-catenin/BCL9 interaction overcomes resistance to immune checkpoint blockades by modulating T(reg) cells. *Sci. Adv.* **2019**, *5*, eaau5240. [CrossRef]
176. Flanagan, D.J.; Barker, N.; Nowell, C.; Clevers, H.; Ernst, M.; Phesse, T.J.; Vincan, E. Loss of the Wnt receptor frizzled 7 in the mouse gastric epithelium is deleterious and triggers rapid repopulation in vivo. *Dis. Models Mech.* **2017**, *10*, 971–980. [CrossRef]
177. Flanagan, D.J.; Phesse, T.J.; Barker, N.; Schwab, R.H.; Amin, N.; Malaterre, J.; Stange, D.E.; Nowell, C.J.; Currie, S.A.; Saw, J.T.; et al. Frizzled7 functions as a Wnt receptor in intestinal epithelial Lgr5(+) stem cells. *Stem Cell Rep.* **2015**, *4*, 759–767. [CrossRef]
178. Jung, H.Y.; Jun, S.; Lee, M.; Kim, H.C.; Wang, X.; Ji, H.; McCrea, P.D.; Park, J.I. PAF and EZH2 induce Wnt/beta-catenin signaling hyperactivation. *Mol. Cell* **2013**, *52*, 193–205. [CrossRef]
179. Kim, M.J.; Xia, B.; Suh, H.N.; Lee, S.H.; Jun, S.; Lien, E.M.; Zhang, J.; Chen, K.; Park, J.I. PAF-Myc-controlled cell stemness is required for intestinal regeneration and tumorigenesis. *Dev. Cell* **2018**, *44*, 582–596.e4. [CrossRef]
180. Schutgens, F.; Clevers, H. Human organoids: Tools for understanding biology and treating diseases. *Annu. Rev. Pathol.* **2020**, *15*, 211–234. [CrossRef]
181. Sato, T.; Vries, R.G.; Snippert, H.J.; van de Wetering, M.; Barker, N.; Stange, D.E.; van Es, J.H.; Abo, A.; Kujala, P.; Peters, P.J.; et al. Single Lgr5 stem cells build crypt-villus structures in vitro without a mesenchymal niche. *Nature* **2009**, *459*, 262–265. [CrossRef] [PubMed]
182. Clevers, H. Modeling development and disease with organoids. *Cell* **2016**, *165*, 1586–1597. [CrossRef] [PubMed]
183. Yao, Y.; Xu, X.; Yang, L.; Zhu, J.; Wan, J.; Shen, L.; Xia, F.; Fu, G.; Deng, Y.; Pan, M.; et al. Patient-derived organoids predict chemoradiation responses of locally advanced rectal cancer. *Cell Stem Cell* **2020**, *26*, 17–26.e6. [CrossRef] [PubMed]
184. Vlachogiannis, G.; Hedayat, S.; Vatsiou, A.; Jamin, Y.; Fernández-Mateos, J.; Khan, K.; Lampis, A.; Eason, K.; Huntingford, I.; Burke, R.; et al. Patient-derived organoids model treatment response of metastatic gastrointestinal cancers. *Science* **2018**, *359*, 920–926. [CrossRef]
185. Nagle, P.W.; Plukker, J.T.M.; Muijs, C.T.; van Luijk, P.; Coppes, R.P. Patient-derived tumor organoids for prediction of cancer treatment response. *Semin. Cancer Biol.* **2018**, *53*, 258–264. [CrossRef]

Publisher's Note: MDPI stays neutral with regard to jurisdictional claims in published maps and institutional affiliations.

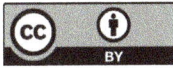

© 2020 by the authors. Licensee MDPI, Basel, Switzerland. This article is an open access article distributed under the terms and conditions of the Creative Commons Attribution (CC BY) license (http://creativecommons.org/licenses/by/4.0/).

Article

p300 Serine 89: A Critical Signaling Integrator and Its Effects on Intestinal Homeostasis and Repair

Keane K. Y. Lai [1,2,†], Xiaohui Hu [1,†], Keisuke Chosa [1,†], Cu Nguyen [1], David P. Lin [1], Keith K. Lai [3], Nobuo Kato [4], Yusuke Higuchi [1], Sarah K. Highlander [5], Elizabeth Melendez [1], Yoshihiro Eriguchi [6], Patrick T. Fueger [2,7], Andre J. Ouellette [6,8], Nyam-Osor Chimge [1], Masaya Ono [9] and Michael Kahn [1,2,8,10,*]

[1] Department of Molecular Medicine, Beckman Research Institute of City of Hope, Duarte, CA 91010, USA; klai@coh.org (K.K.Y.L.); huxiaohui@ahmu.edu.cn (X.H.); kchosa@coh.org (K.C.); cunguyen@coh.org (C.N.); dplin@hotmail.com (D.P.L.); yhiguchi@coh.org (Y.H.); emelendez@coh.org (E.M.); nchimge@coh.org (N.-O.C.)
[2] City of Hope Comprehensive Cancer Center, Duarte, CA 91010, USA; pfueger@coh.org
[3] Department of Anatomic Pathology, Cleveland Clinic, Cleveland, OH 44195, USA; LAIK2@ccf.org
[4] The Institute of Scientific and Industrial Research, Osaka University, Osaka 567-0047, Japan; kato-n@sanken.osaka-u.ac.jp
[5] Clinical Microbiome Service Center and Pathogen and Microbiome Division, Translational Genomics Research Institute, Flagstaff, AZ 86005, USA; shighlander@tgen.org
[6] Department of Pathology and Laboratory Medicine, Keck School of Medicine, University of Southern California, Los Angeles, CA 90033, USA; eriguchi@intmed1.med.kyushu-u.ac.jp (Y.E.); aouellet@med.usc.edu (A.J.O.)
[7] Department of Molecular and Cellular Endocrinology, Beckman Research Institute of City of Hope, Duarte, CA 91010, USA
[8] USC Norris Comprehensive Cancer Center, Keck School of Medicine, University of Southern California, Los Angeles, CA 90033, USA
[9] Department of Clinical Proteomics, National Cancer Center Research Institute, Tokyo 104-0045, Japan; masono@ncc.go.jp
[10] Department of Biochemistry and Molecular Biology, Keck School of Medicine, University of Southern California, Los Angeles, CA 90033, USA
* Correspondence: mkahn@coh.org
† These authors contributed equally to this work.

Simple Summary: Given their high degree of identity and even greater similarity at the amino acid level, Kat3 coactivators, CBP (Kat3A) and p300 (Kat3B), have long been considered redundant. We describe the generation of novel p300 S89A knock-in mice carrying a single site directed amino acid mutation in p300, changing the highly evolutionarily conserved serine 89 to alanine, thus enhancing Wnt/CBP/catenin signaling (at the expense of Wnt/p300/catenin signaling). p300 S89A knock-in mice exhibit multiple organ system, immunologic and metabolic differences, compared with their wild type counterparts. In particular, these p300 S89A knock-in mice are highly sensitive to intestinal injury resulting in colitis which is known to significantly predispose to colorectal cancer. Our results highlight the critical role of this region in p300 as a signaling nexus and provide further evidence that p300 and CBP are non-redundant, playing definite and distinctive roles in development and disease.

Abstract: Differential usage of Kat3 coactivators, CBP and p300, by β-catenin is a fundamental regulatory mechanism in stem cell maintenance and initiation of differentiation and repair. Based upon our earlier pharmacologic studies, p300 serine 89 (S89) is critical for controlling differential coactivator usage by β-catenin via post-translational phosphorylation in stem/progenitor populations, and appears to be a target for a number of kinase cascades. To further investigate mechanisms of signal integration effected by this domain, we generated p300 S89A knock-in mice. We show that S89A mice are extremely sensitive to intestinal insult resulting in colitis, which is known to significantly increase the risk of developing colorectal cancer. We demonstrate cell intrinsic differences, and microbiome compositional differences and differential immune responses, in intestine of S89A versus wild type mice. Genomic and proteomic analyses reveal pathway differences, including lipid metabolism, oxidative stress response, mitochondrial function and oxidative phosphorylation. The diverse effects on fundamental processes including epithelial differentiation, metabolism, immune response and microbiome colonization, all brought about by a single amino acid modification S89A, highlights the critical role of this region in p300 as a signaling nexus and the rationale for conservation of this residue and surrounding region for hundreds of million years of vertebrate evolution.

Keywords: CBP; p300; IBD; colitis; colorectal cancer; Wnt

1. Introduction

The vertebrate radiation, which was initiated approximately 450 million years ago, ushered in a major lifestyle change with a significant increase in adult lifespan [1,2] and with it, a requirement for high-fidelity, long-term homeostasis [2]. This change necessitated that somatic stem cells (SSC), in their respective niches, remain quiescent, in contrast to their differentiated daughter cells, which rapidly proliferate, in order to safeguard the integrity of the SSC's genetic material [1,3]. The gene duplication of the Kat3 coactivator family, which led to the evolution of Kat3A/CREBBP (cAMP response element binding protein (CREB)-binding protein) (CBP) and its closely related paralog Kat3B/E1A-binding protein, 300 kDa (p300), apparently occurred just prior to radiation of the vertebrate lineage [1]. The two Kat3 coactivators encode massive proteins of ~300 kDa over 33 and 31 exons, respectively [1]. CBP and p300 have maintained an extraordinarily high degree of identity—as high as 93%—and an even higher degree of similarity, particularly over an extensive central core region, which encompasses the CH1, KIX, bromodomain, CH2 and CH3 domains (Figure 1A) [1,2,4,5]. They both interact with a myriad of proteins, given their key roles in orchestrating transcription [1]. Due to their high degree of identity and even greater similarity at the amino acid level, CBP and p300 have long been considered redundant. However, mounting evidence clearly demonstrates that they are non-redundant, playing definite and distinctive roles in development and disease [1,6–10]. β-catenin, a key transcriptional component in Wnt signaling, must recruit CBP or p300 in addition to other components of the core transcriptional complex to initiate functional Wnt transcription [1,11,12]. The extreme N-terminal regions of CBP and p300, containing the lowest homology with approximately 66% identity, have been the focus of our interest. β-catenin and specific, direct small molecule CBP/catenin antagonists (ICG-001/PRI-724) [1,9,13,14] and direct small molecule p300/catenin antagonists (YH249/250) [15], competitively bind within this extreme N-terminal region (Figure 1A) [1]. This highly unstructured region of the Kat3 coactivators serves as a nexus for integrating the interactions of varied signal transduction pathways (e.g., nuclear receptor family, RAR/RXR, vitamin D, and Interferon STAT1/2) with the Wnt/catenin signaling cascade [1,9,16–19]. We originally identified p300 serine 89 as a critical residue (Figure 1B) controlling differential coactivator usage by β-catenin via post-translational phosphorylation in mouse embryonic stem cells [20]. p300 serine 89 appears to be a target for a number of kinase cascades including PKC [21,22], AMPK [23], and SIK2 [24], associated with an array of biological effects, including activation and inhibition of transcription [23,25], inhibition of histone acetyltransferase function [22], regulation of insulin/glucagon signaling [24], and differentiation of mES cells [20] and adult progenitor cells [26].

To further investigate the role that p300 serine 89 (S89) plays in vivo, we have generated p300 S89A knock-in mice. p300 S89A knock-in mice, albeit born at sub-Mendelian ratios, appear to be relatively normal. Nevertheless, these mice exhibit multiple organ system, immunologic and metabolic differences, compared with their wild type counterparts. We now initially report on the generation of these mice and their high sensitivity to intestinal injury, which is apparently related to a complex interplay between aberrant epithelial differentiation, gut immunity and changes in their intestinal microbiota and metabolites and which results in colitis, a significant risk factor predisposing to colorectal cancer [27,28].

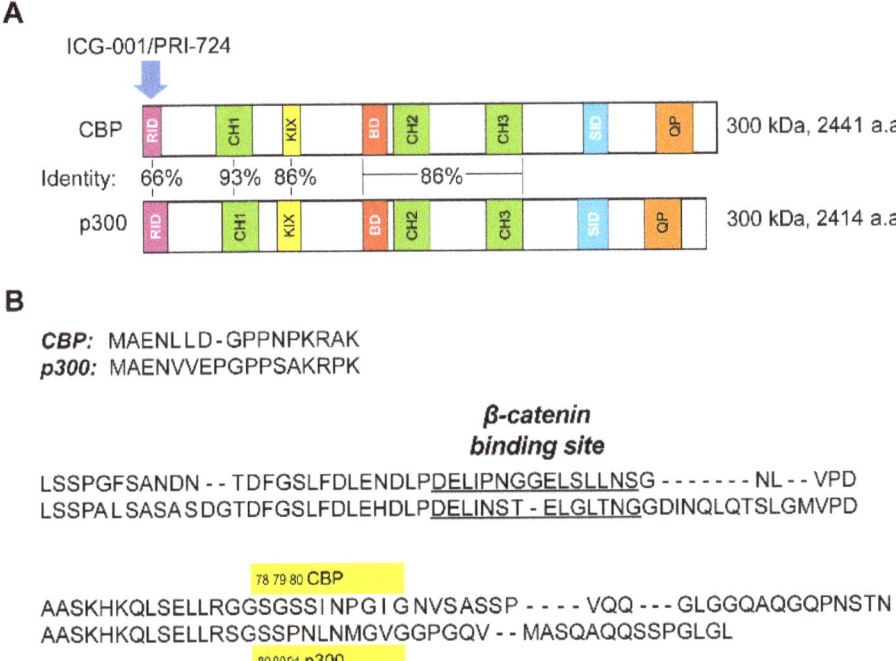

Figure 1. Differential usage of homologous Kat3 coactivators CBP and p300 by β-catenin. (**A**) Schematic representation displaying identity between CBP and p300. CBP and p300 have molecular weights of approximately 300 kDa and are encoded over 33 and 31 exons and consist of 2441 and 2414 amino acids (a.a.), respectively. β-catenin competes with direct small molecule CBP/catenin antagonists (PRI-724/ICG-001) for binding to CBP's (but not p300's) distal N-terminus, the least conserved region within these two Kat3 coactivators. CBP, cAMP response element binding protein (CREB)-binding protein; p300, E1A-binding protein, 300 kDa; RID, receptor-interacting domain; CH, cysteine/histidine region; KIX, kinase-inducible domain interacting domain; BD, bromodomain; SID, steroid receptor co-activator-1 interaction domain; QP, glutamine- and proline-rich domain. (**B**) Sequence alignment of the distal N-terminal regions of CBP and p300, showing conserved sites for binding of β-catenin (DELI motif). Note: p300 S89 is a critical residue controlling differential Kat3 coactivator usage by β-catenin. (Human CBP and p300 sequences are depicted.)

2. Materials and Methods

2.1. Mice

Animal studies were approved by the University of Southern California Institutional Animal Care and Use Committee (IACUC) as per protocol #11023. The S89A knock-in point mutation in exon 2 of the mouse p300 gene, via site-specific mutagenesis, was generated using the flip-excision (FLEx) switch construct. This mutation removes the highly conserved phosphorylation site at S89. The construct included five segments: the 5′ homology arm, a point-mutated exon 2 in inverted orientation, a PGK-Neo selection cassette, the wild type exon 2, and the 3′ homology arm. The design of the construct, cloning of the targeting vector, electroporation into mouse ES cells, screening of the 129 ES cells, injection into blastocysts, and screening of the chimeric mice were performed by Ozgene Pty Ltd. (Australia). In principle, transcription from the mutant exon 2 should have been activated via Cre recombinase in two steps. First, Cre recombinase would invert the mutated fragment flanked by the *loxP* site to correct the orientation to activate, and then excise the wild type fragment flanked by lox2272 to inactivate it. However, we found that mice homozygous for the knock-in construct displayed early embryonic stage lethality, similar to that of p300 knockout mice [29], suggesting that the wild type p300 protein was not being produced properly from the wild type fragment in vivo for unknown reasons. This malfunction of the wild type fragment caused us to revise our original plan of conditional mutagenesis, resulting in our decision to generate p300 S89A germ line mice. Mice were backcrossed onto C57BL/6 background (The Jackson Laboratory, Bar Harbor, ME, USA) for at least 10 generations before used for experiments. Hematology testing on mouse blood samples was performed on the Hemavet (Drew Scientific, Miami Lakes, FL, USA), and clinical chemistry testing was performed by Antech Diagnostics.

2.2. Isolation of Crypt Cells from Ileum

Crypt cells from ileum were isolated based on a previously described protocol [30] with minor modification. Ileum was dissected out, and lumen of the intestine was flushed with ice-cold PBS. Intestine was opened longitudinally and placed in tube containing ice-cold PBS. Tube was inverted 10–15 times, and then PBS removed and replaced with fresh ice-cold PBS. Washing with fresh ice-cold PBS was repeated until the supernatant no longer contained any visible debris. Intestine was cut into 5 mm pieces and placed into ice-cold 5 mM EDTA-PBS. Fragments of intestine were vigorously triturated by pipetting up and down 15 times, and then allowed to settle by gravity for 30 s. Supernatant was aspirated, and then 5 mM EDTA-PBS was added to the intestinal fragments and re-suspended intestinal fragments were placed at 4 °C on a benchtop roller for 10 min, after which supernatant was aspirated, and then intestinal fragments kept. 5 mM EDTA-PBS was added to the intestinal fragments and then placed at 4 °C on a benchtop roller for 30 min. Supernatant was aspirated and then ice-cold PBS was added to wash the crypts and then supernatant was aspirated. Ice-cold PBS was added, and the intestinal fragments were vigorously triturated 10 times. Supernatant fractions were collected and then mixed 1:1 with solution of basal media containing DNase I. (Final concentration of mixture: ~15 U/mL DNase I.) Mixture was first filtered through a 100 µm filter into a BSA (1%) coated conical tube, and then filtered through a 70 µm filter into a BSA (1%) coated tube, after which the filtrate was spun at $300\times g$ in a tabletop centrifuge for 5 min. Supernatant was aspirated, and the cell pellet was re-suspended in basal media containing 5% FBS and then centrifuged at $100\times g$ for 5 min, after which supernatant was removed and samples were frozen at −80 °C until further analysis.

2.3. Co-Immunoprecipitation

150–200 mg of intestinal crypt cells were re-suspended in CERI buffer (NE-PER, ThermoFisher, cat. #: 78833, Waltham, MA, USA) containing 5 mM DTT and 1X protease inhibitor cocktail, using a dounce homogenizer. After re-suspension in CERI buffer, the procedure for nuclear extraction was performed based on manufacturer protocol. Protein concentration of nuclear extract was performed using the Protein Assay Dye Reagent (Bio-Rad, cat. #: 500-0006, Hercules, CA, USA). 100–500 µg of nuclear protein was diluted in CoIP buffer (25 mM Tris-HCl, pH 8.0, 1% NP40, 5% glycerol, 150 mM NaCl, 1 mM EDTA, 5 mM DTT, 1X protease inhibitor cocktail (Calbiochem, cat. #: 539137, Burlington, MA, USA)) to a final volume of 1000 µL. 2 µg of CBP (Aviva Biosystems, cat. #: ARP43609_P050, San Diego, CA, USA), p300 (Aviva Biosystems, cat. #: OAAF01891-100UG, San Diego, CA, USA), 14-3-3-ε (Abcam, cat. #: ab43057, Cambridge, MA, USA), or normal IgG (Aviva Biosystems, cat. #: OAEF01185-1MG, San Diego, CA, USA) antibody was added and mixture incubated overnight at 4 °C on a tube shaker/rotator. 20 µL of Dynabeads Protein A (ThermoFisher, cat. #: 10001D, Waltham, MA, USA) was added and mixture incubated for 1 h at 4 °C on tube shaker/rotator. The magnetic beads were washed three times with 500 µL of CoIP Buffer each time, using the magnetic stand. 20 µL of 2× Laemmli buffer was added and mixture vortexed. Beads were boiled in 2× Laemmli buffer for 10 min. Supernatant containing proteins were separated from the magnetic beads, using the magnetic stand. Protein samples were subjected to electrophoresis on a 4–20% Teo-Tricine SDS-PAGE gel (VWR, cat. #: 71003-072, Radnor, PA, USA). Proteins were transferred onto PVDF membrane. Proteins of interest on the PVDF membrane were detected by incubating with β-catenin antibody (Santa Cruz Biotechnology, cat. #: sc-7199, Dallas, TX, USA) or p300 antibody (Aviva Biosystems, cat. #: OAAF01891-100UG, San Diego, CA, USA) as the primary antibody, and subsequent incubation with CleanBlot (ThermoFisher, cat. #: 21232, Waltham, MA, USA) as the secondary antibody, followed by application of chemiluminescent reagent ECL Plus (GE Healthcare, cat. #: RPN2132, Chicago, IL, USA) and imaging on the ChemiDoc Imaging System (Bio-Rad), after which relative protein concentration was determined by densitometry.

2.4. Western Blotting

Flash-frozen mouse ileum was resuspended in RIPA buffer (50 mM Tris-HCl, pH 7.5, 150 mM NaCl, 1% NP-40, 0.5% deoxycholate, 5 mM EDTA, 0.1% SDS), containing protease inhibitors (Roche, cat. #: 11836170001, South San Francisco, CA, USA). Tissue was homogenized and then centrifuged at $12,000\times g$ for 15 min, after which supernatants were collected. Protein concentration was determined using the Protein Assay Dye Reagent (Bio-Rad, cat. #: 500-0006, Hercules, CA, USA). 40 μg protein mixed with $4\times$ Laemmli sample buffer were incubated at 37 °C for 15 min and subjected to SDS-PAGE. After overnight transfer onto PVDF membrane (Bio-Rad, cat. #: 1620177, Hercules, CA, USA), membrane was incubated overnight with primary antibody at 4 °C. Membrane was washed and then incubated with secondary antibody for 1 h, followed by application of chemiluminescent reagent ECL (GE Healthcare, cat. #: RPN2232, Chicago, IL, USA) and imaging on the ChemiDoc Imaging System (Bio-Rad), after which relative protein concentration was determined by densitometry. The primary antibodies used were DUOX2 (Santa Cruz, cat. #: sc-398681, Dallas, TX, USA), GAPDH (Santa Cruz, cat. #: sc-32233, Dallas, TX, USA). The secondary antibody was mouse IgG kappa binding protein conjugated to horseradish peroxidase (Santa Cruz, cat. #: sc-516102, Dallas, TX, USA).

2.5. RT-qPCR and PCR

Total mRNA was extracted by TRIzol reagent (Invitrogen Carlsbad, CA, USA) according to the manufacturer's protocol. cDNA was synthesized using qScript cDNA Synthesis Kit (Quantabio, Beverly, MA, USA). cDNA template was used for qPCR with SYBR Green detection method utilizing the CFX Connect Real-Time PCR Detection System (Bio-Rad, Hercules, CA, USA). The PCR primer sequences used for mouse cells were as follows: Duox2 (F: 5′-CATTGCCACCTACCAGAACATTG-3′, R: 5′-AGATGCTGGGGTCCATG AAAG-3′); Duoxa2 (F: 5′-TAACATTACACTCCGAGGAACAC-3′, R: 5′-AGTCCCTTCTC CAAGGCATG-3′). Housekeeping gene PCR primer sequences for mouse Gusb were (F: 5′-TATGGAGCAGACGCAATCCC-3′, R: 5′-TTCGTCATGAAGTCGGCGAA-3′). Relative expression levels for genes of interest were calculated using the 2^{-ddCt} method. PCR primer sequences used for OTU217 were as follows: F: 5′-TACCGCATAAGCCTGCTGTG-3′, R: 5′-ATCGTTGTCTTGGTAGGCCG-3′. PCR products were resolved by agarose gel electrophoresis.

2.6. 16S rRNA Gene Sequencing of Microbiota

Stool samples from mice were collected and genomic DNA was extracted using the QIAAmp Fast Stool Mini Kit (Qiagen, Redwood City, CA, USA) as per manufacturer instructions. DNA samples were sent to Research and Testing Laboratory (currently RTL Genomics, Lubbock, TX, USA) for processing and analysis based on a previously described protocol [31,32]. 16S ribosomal RNA variable region was amplified and subjected to sequencing on an Illumina MiSeq as previously described [31]. Reads were processed and classified into operational taxonomic units (OTUs) as previously described [32]. Bacterial diversity between groups of mice were compared using the Shannon index (for alpha diversity) and the Bray–Curtis and Jaccard indices (for beta diversity).

2.7. Intestinal Organoids

Organoids were derived from mouse intestines and cultured based on a previously described protocol [33]. Briefly, mouse small intestine was isolated and opened longitudinally. After washing with ice-cold PBS, villi were scraped off using a coverslip. Intestine was then cut into fragments from which crypts were isolated. Crypts were resuspended with Matrigel, and cell suspension plated and cultured to form organoids.

2.8. Genomic Analysis

RNA-seq was performed on mouse intestine and intestinal organoids at the USC Core Lab, based on a previously described protocol [34]. Briefly, the Ovation RNA-Seq System V2 and Ovation Ultralow Library System V2 (NuGEN Technologies, Inc., San Carlos, CA, USA) were used for amplification of total RNA and library preparation. RNA-seq was performed on an Illumina HiSeq 2000 (Illumina, San Diego, CA, USA) using paired-end sequencing. Sequence data were analyzed using Partek Flow software (Partek Inc., Chesterfield, MO, USA). Differentially expressed gene lists were created, and differences were considered significant if false discovery rate (FDR) adjusted p-value, i.e., "q-value" < 0.05 or multimodel p-value < 0.05. Pathway analysis was performed using Ingenuity Pathway Analysis (IPA) (Qiagen).

2.9. Proteomic Analysis

Samples were prepared and subjected to proteomic analysis by 2DICAL as previously described [9]. Methanol solutions of whole cell extracts were dried and processed for trypsinization. After trypsinization, the obtained peptides were resolved and then quantified. Peptide solution was desalted, dried, and re-dissolved. The obtained peptide solution was subjected to nanoLC-Ultra 2D (AB SCIEX) coupled with to a TripleTOF5600 (AB SCIEX) mass spectrometer. The subjected peptides were directly injected onto a C18, non-end capping, ULTRON HF-ODS(N) (0.1mm I.D., 700 mm length, Shinwa Chemical Industries Ltd., Kyoto, Japan) and then separated by a binary gradient. The masses of the eluted peptides were determined using the TripleTOF5600. MS peaks were detected and quantified using 2DICAL. 2DICAL was developed as a shotgun proteomics analysis system. It analyzes the data of mass to charge ratio (m/z), retention time (RT) and peak intensity generated by liquid chromatography and mass spectrometer (LC/MS), and each sample as elemental data; it deploys various 2-dimensional images with different combinations of axes using these four elements. From the m/z–RT image, peaks derived from the same peptide in the direction of the acquiring time are integrated. By adding algorithms to ensure reproducibility of m/z and RT, the same peak can be compared precisely across different samples, and a statistical comparison of identical peaks in different samples leads to the discovery of specific differentially expressed peptide peaks. Specific peaks are designated by their m/z and RT coordinates, and further analysis is based on these identifiers. The peptide search engine used in 2DICAL is MASCOT software (version 2.5.1; Matrix Science) using the Swiss-Prot mouse database (SwissProt_2016_01.fasta). The mass spectrometry proteomics data have been deposited in the ProteomeXchange Consortium via the jPOST [35] partner repository with the data set identifier PXD021750. Statistical Analyses was performed with the open source statistical language R (version 3.3.0). The 2DICAL intensity data were converted to protein value averaging the intensity data of peptides derived from the protein.

2.10. Ingenuity Pathway Analysis of Proteomic Data

A total of 2836 proteins were detected in both wild type and p300 S89A mice. The proteomic data were quantile normalized and subjected to differential expression analysis. 93 proteins showed significant changes (fold change (FC) ≤ -1.2 or FC ≥ 1.2, and $p < 0.05$) and were subjected to Ingenuity Pathway Analysis (IPA) (Qiagen, Redwood City, CA, USA) to identify top canonical pathways associated with S89A mutation in mice.

2.11. DSS-induced Colitis Mouse Model

Mice were treated starting on day 1 for up to 5 days with low (2%) dose of dextran sodium sulfate (DSS) administered via the drinking water, based on a previously described protocol [36], after which treatment was discontinued for up to 7 days, and the effect of DSS on % original body weight, histology by hematoxylin and eosin (H&E) and Alcian blue staining, and colon length was assessed.

2.12. Data Analysis

Numerical data were expressed as the means ± standard deviation (s.d.) and Student's t-test was performed, unless otherwise noted. p-values < 0.05 were considered significant.

3. Results

3.1. Generation of p300 S89A Point Mutant Knock-in Mice

We previously utilized in vitro CRISPR/Cas9 editing of a highly conserved insertion in the N-terminus of p300 (aa 61–70) to demonstrate its importance in regulating Wnt/β-catenin/nuclear receptor interactions [9]. To further explore this critical signaling nexus within the N-terminal domain of the Kat3 coactivator p300, we generated an S89A knock-in point mutation in exon 2 of the mouse p300 gene via site-specific mutagenesis. This mutation removes the highly evolutionarily conserved phosphorylation site at S89 and consequently modulates the interaction of multiple proteins with the N-terminus of p300. The mutant fragment was cloned into a targeting vector for the murine p300 gene. The resultant flip-excision (FLEx) switch construct (Figure S1) was used to generate p300 S89A germ line mice. After crossing the mice with a CMV-Cre mouse line, we confirmed successful introduction of the point mutation and removal of the wild type fragment at both the genomic DNA and messenger RNA levels by PCR and DNA sequencing. The homozygous p300 S89A mice, although born at sub-Mendelian ratios (approximately 50% less than anticipated), did not demonstrate any obvious significant abnormalities (Figure S2 and Table S1) and were fertile, albeit both male and female S89A mice exhibited slightly decreased body weights (<10%) (Figure S2). The mice were subsequently backcrossed with C57BL/6 mice minimally for 10 generations before being used for further experiments.

3.2. p300 S89A Mice and Differential β-Catenin Kat3 Coactivator Usage

We previously reported that phosphorylation at S89 of p300 enhanced the association of β-catenin with p300 and mutation of serine 89 to alanine abrogated this phosphorylation dependent increase in vitro [20]. To confirm that this observation was also true in S89A knock-in mice, we performed a co-immunoprecipitation assay using tissue from intestinal crypts in which the Wnt signaling pathway is highly activated. As anticipated based on our previous in vitro studies, the association of β-catenin with p300 was significantly reduced in S89A mice compared with wild type (WT) mice (Figure 2).

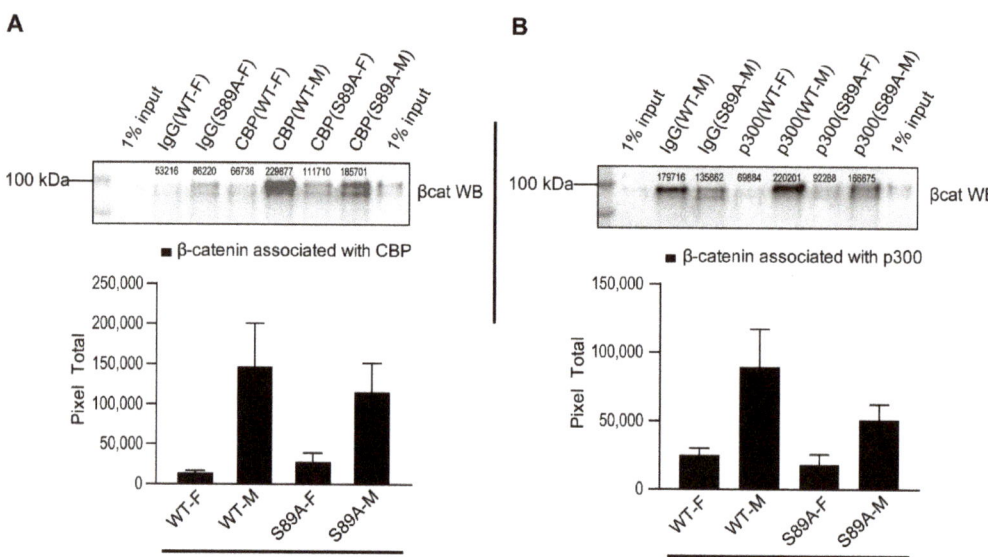

Figure 2. p300 S89A mice show differential usage of Kat3 coactivators CBP and p300 by β-catenin. Co-immunoprecipitation of β-catenin with CBP (**A**) or p300 (**B**) in S89A and WT mouse intestinal crypt cells. Control (IgG) antibody and anti-CBP antibody or anti-p300 antibody were used for immunoprecipitation followed by immunoblotting for β-catenin. Numerical values above protein bands indicate densitometric quantitation of β-catenin associated with CBP or p300. Bar graphs show densitometric quantitation normalized to respective control. Data in bar graphs (mean ± s.e.m.) representative of three independent experiments are shown. S89A, p300 S89A; WT, wild type; F, female; M, male; βcat, β-catenin; IP, immunoprecipitation. Whole immunoblots corresponding to immunoblot data are included in Figure S3.

3.3. p300 S89A Mice Are Extremely Sensitive to Intestinal Insult

Although p300 S89A mice did not exhibit obvious homeostatic defects under normal feeding and housing conditions, we decided to evaluate their response to insult. Inflammatory bowel disease (IBD), including Crohn's Disease and ulcerative colitis [36], may arise from infections caused by viruses or bacteria, damage due to ischemia, or disorders of autoimmunity in genetically predisposed individuals. One popular model of colitis utilizes dextran sodium sulfate (DSS) in the drinking water, which damages the intestinal epithelium and a vigorous inflammatory reaction within the intestine generally of several days duration [36]. One variation of this model involves repeated cycles of acute insult with subsequent repair via iterative cycles of DSS administration with intervening periods of recovery, thereby simulating chronic IBD [36]. We chose a relatively low (2%) dose of DSS and proceeded to administer it to seven-week-old female mice, both S89A and wild type C57BL/6 (WT), in their drinking water. After only one round of DSS, effects on control WT mice were minor, with only slight body weight reduction at day eight/nine (~2–3 days after withdrawal of DSS), whereas in sharp contrast, there was a dramatic (~20%) body weight reduction in the mutant mice and two S89A mice died at day 12 (Figure 3A, left panel). A similar trend was observed with male mice (Figure 3A, right panel).

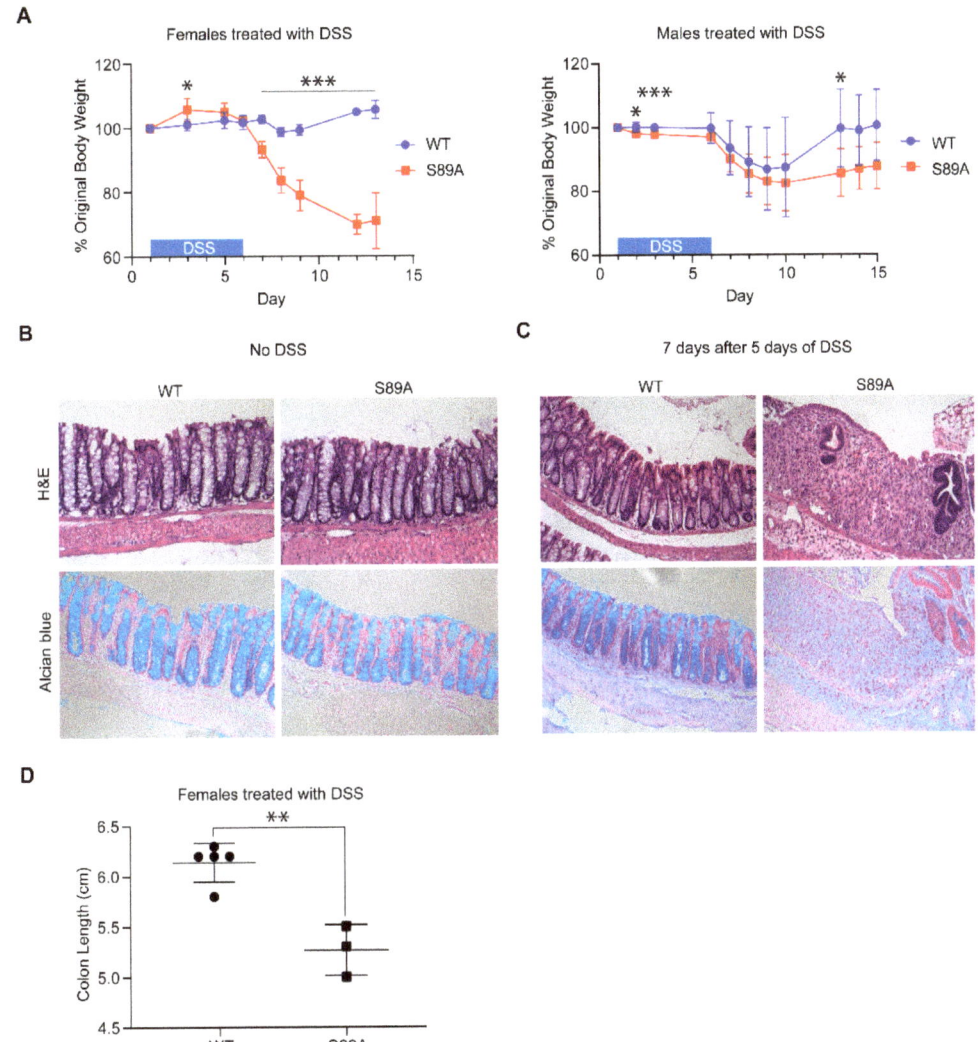

Figure 3. p300 S89A mice are extremely sensitive to intestinal insult. S89A and WT mice were treated starting on day 1 for ~5 days with low (2%) dose of dextran sodium sulfate (DSS) (or vehicle (**B**) after which treatment was discontinued for ~7 days and the effect of DSS on % original body weight (**A**), histology (**B**,**C**), and colon length (**D**) was assessed. Data are mean ± s.d. (n = 3–9 per group). * $p < 0.05$, ** $p < 0.01$, *** $p < 0.001$. (**B**) For both WT and S89A mice without DSS treatment: H&E staining shows normal colonic mucosa. The crypt architecture is preserved and there is no evidence of acute, neutrophil-mediated epithelial injury or histologic features suggestive of ongoing, chronic mucosal injury. Alcian blue staining highlights intact goblet cells. (**C**) With DSS treatment: For WT mice: H&E staining shows normal colonic mucosa. The crypt architecture is preserved and there is no evidence of acute, neutrophil-mediated epithelial injury or histologic features suggestive of ongoing, chronic mucosal injury. Alcian blue staining highlights intact goblet cells. For S89A mice: H&E staining shows colonic mucosa with lamina propria replacement by granulation tissue and fibrinopurulent exudate, consistent with ulcer. The few remaining crypts exhibit architectural distortion, indicative of chronic mucosal injury. Alcian blue staining highlights mucin loss and decreased goblet cells, consistent with epithelial injury.

Prior to DSS treatment, the colonic epithelium of S89A mice was normal, essentially the same as WT mice. Prior to treatment, in both S89A and WT mice, crypt architecture was intact and there was no evidence of neutrophil mediated epithelial injury or histological features suggestive of ongoing chronic mucosal injury. Alcian blue staining demonstrated the presence of intact goblet cells (Figure 3B). Histological examination of control and mutant mouse colons at day 12 after DSS treatment (five days treatment, seven days off) showed that S89A mice were nearly devoid of normal colonic epithelium. Hematoxylin and eosin staining showed colonic mucosa with lamina propria replacement by granulated tissue and fibrinopurulent exudate, consistent with ulceration. The few remaining crypts exhibited architectural distortion, indicative of chronic mucosal injury. Alcian blue staining highlighted mucin loss and decreased goblet cells consistent with epithelial injury (Figure 3C), whereas the tissue from WT mice was normal. The colon length of S89A female mice compared to WT controls, one week after 5 days of DSS administration, was somewhat shorter (5.3 versus 6.1 cm) (Figure 3D).

Perturbations of host–microbiota homeostasis induced by the host genetics and/or environmental factors can fuel inflammation at mucosal surfaces [37,38]. S89A mice were initially housed separately from control mice. We therefore decided to examine whether cohousing and thereby intermixing of the microbiota of S89A and WT mice would affect sensitivity to DSS induced colitis. Although separately housed S89A mice were dramatically more sensitive to 2% DSS treatment (Figure 4A), S89A mice were protected against the effects of the 2% DSS treatment when co-housed with WT mice (Figure 4A, left panel and Figure 4B). Interestingly, if mice subsequently were separated again for four weeks after four weeks of co-housing, both WT and S89A mice had intermediate sensitivity to DSS treatment (Figure 4C). 16S rRNA gene sequencing of stool samples from the separately housed WT and S89A mice demonstrated large taxonomic differences in the microbiota as depicted in a barplot of the top ~20 taxa in each sample (Figure 4D, upper panel). The Shannon (alpha) diversity of the two groups was not significantly different, indicating that the communities had about the same evenness and similar numbers of organisms and similar distribution. On the other hand, the Bray–Curtis and Jaccard (beta) diversity (Figures S5 and S6) was different between the two groups, indicating that the two groups were significantly different in their composition (that is members of the communities). Interestingly, at least one particular bacterial species, OTU-217, which we identified as Kineothrix alysoides and was present in S89A mice yet absent or at very low levels in WT mice housed separately, was transferred effectively during cohousing, and may contribute to enhancing the sensitivity of WT mice to DSS induced colitis (Figure 4D, lower panel).

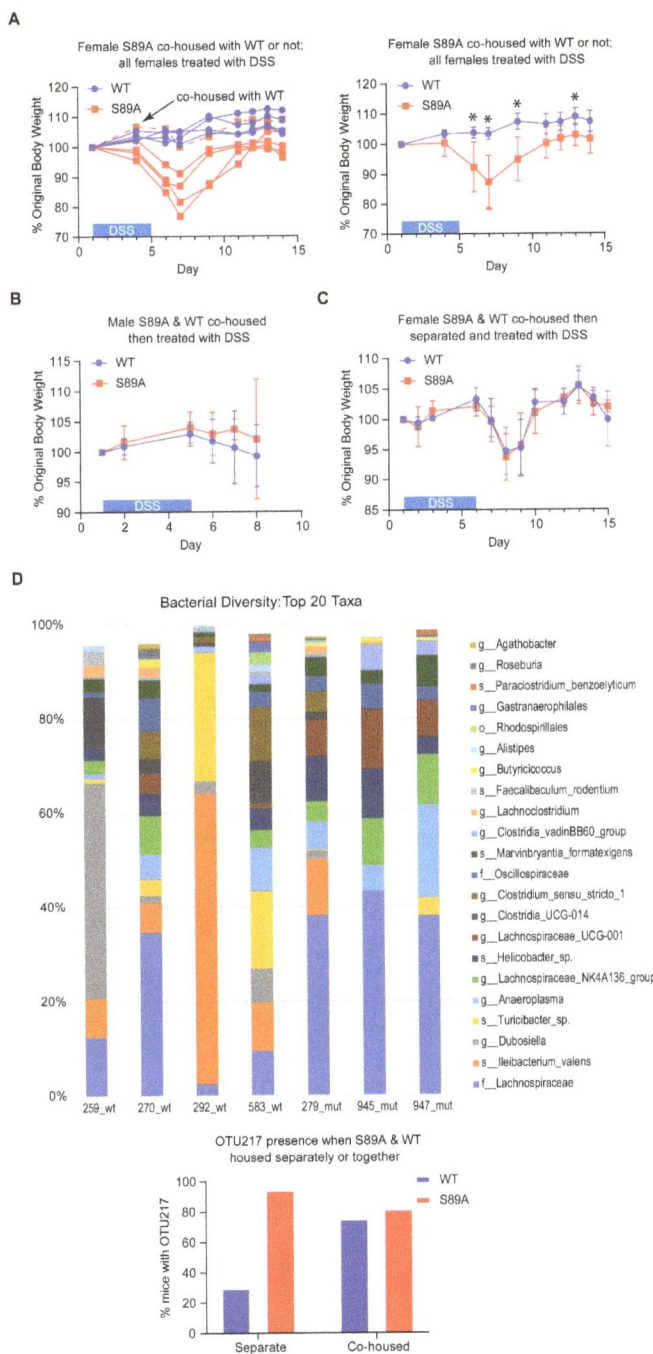

Figure 4. Co-housing of p300 S89A mice with wild type mice modulates severity of intestinal injury potentially via intermixing of microbiota. S89A and WT mice were treated on day 1 for ~4–5 days with low (2%) dose of dextran sodium sulfate (DSS) after which treatment was discontinued for ~7 days (**A**, **C**) or ~2 days (**B**), and the effect of DSS on % original body weight was assessed. A single

S89A mouse (dashed red line arrow) which was co-housed with WT mice, from ~4 weeks prior to the start of DSS treatment, was protected from intestinal injury similar to WT mice (**A**, left panel: individual mouse data), while the other S89A mice (not co-housed with WT mice) remained extremely sensitive to intestinal injury (**A**, right panel: aggregate mouse data according to genotype). S89A mice co-housed with WT mice, from ~4 weeks prior to the start of DSS treatment, were protected from intestinal injury (**B**). S89A and wild type mice co-housed ~4 weeks and then separated for ~4 weeks prior to the start of DSS treatment demonstrated an intermediate sensitivity to DSS treatment (**C**). Data are mean ± s.d. (n = 4–5 per group) unless otherwise indicated. * p < 0.05. (**D**) 16S rRNA gene sequencing of stool samples from separately housed WT and S89A mice demonstrated large taxonomic differences in the microbiota (**D**, top). (n = 3–4 per group.) Bacterial species, OTU-217, was detected by PCR in most of the S89A mice and largely absent in the separately housed WT mice, whereas OTU-217 was detected in most of the co-housed WT and S89A mice (**D**, bottom). (n = 12–20 per group.) OTU, operational taxonomic unit.

3.4. Genomic Analysis

To further explore the impact of the knock-in point mutation on gene expression, we performed RNA-seq on tissue from the intestines from separately housed untreated p300 S89A and WT mice. To examine epithelium-specific gene expression, intestinal organoids were also grown from both p300 S89A and WT mice and analyzed by RNA-seq. Interestingly, between the organoids and whole ileum RNA-seq (Tables S2 and S3, respectively), there was limited overlap within the statistically significantly regulated genes (400 genes, 2.18% in organoids and 785, 2.86% in ileum q < 0.05), with only nine genes (*DUOX2*, *ERO1l*, *GSR* and *MPTX2* up-regulated and *BCMO1*, *PMP22*, *PRELP*, *SLC13A1* and *SST* down-regulated) (Figure 5A) being common to both. Ingenuity Pathway Analysis (IPA) showed that in the organoids, the top affected network functions were: (1) Embryonic Development, Organismal Development and Function; (2) Cell-To-Cell Signaling and Interaction; (3) Cellular Assembly and Organization, Cell-To-Cell Signaling and Interaction; and (4) Lipid Metabolism, Molecular Transport, Small Molecule Biochemistry. The NRF2-mediated Oxidative Stress Response pathway was also strongly affected. DUOX2 and DUOXA2 members of the NADPH oxidase family, serve as the first line of defense against enteric pathogens by producing microbicidal reactive oxygen species and are the predominant H_2O_2-producing system in human colorectal mucosa [39,40].

Duox2 expression was significantly increased in both ileum (2.6-fold $p = 5.00 \times 10^{-5}$) and intestinal organoids (1.5-fold $p = 7.99 \times 10^{-6}$). We further confirmed increased expression of Duox2 and Duoxa2 at both the message (Figure 5B) and increased expression of Duox2 (~3-fold) at the protein level (Figure 5C) in S89A mice. The transcription factor *GATA4*, which has been demonstrated to play a crucial role in patterning the intestinal epithelium and acts as a critical determinant of enterocyte identity in the jejunum [41] was up-regulated 3.6-fold ($p = 1.08 \times 10^{-32}$) in intestinal organoids. Among the significantly down-regulated genes in the ileum was *REG3A* (~50% $p = 5.00 \times 10^{-5}$), an antibacterial C-type lectin, which is constitutively generated in the intestine and displays anti-Gram-positive bactericidal activity [42]. There was also a significant almost 50% reduction in the expression of the interferon-induced transmembrane protein 3, *IFITM3* (p = 0.047) in intestinal organoids. Differential expression of *IFITM3* has been found in endoscopic biopsies from Crohn's Disease patients [43]. In addition, the sulfate transporter *SLC13A1*, an FXR transcriptional target was down-regulated 2.5-fold ($p = 4.67 \times 10^{-8}$) in organoids with an approximately 50% reduction in ileum ($p = 5.00 \times 10^{-5}$), consistent with the importance of p300 Ser89 phosphorylation on p300/nuclear receptor interactions [44,45]. Additionally, members of the HOXB cluster, which is critical for specification of the digestive tract [46], including *HOXB3* and *HOXB5-9* were all down-regulated more than 2-fold in intestinal organoids ($p = 7.97 \times 10^{-7}$ to 4.49×10^{-5}). Among the top canonical pathways affected in the IPA analysis of the ileum RNA-seq were, interferon signaling, LPS/IL1 mediated inhibition of RXR function, estrogen biosynthesis and fatty acid and xenobiotic metabolism. 1.4-fold increases in Stat1 ($p = 5.00 \times 10^{-5}$) and Irf8 ($p = 5.00 \times 10^{-5}$), 2-fold ($p = 5.00 \times 10^{-5}$)

increases in granzyme b (*Gzmb*) and immunity-related GTPase family M member 1 (*Irgm1*) and a 1.6-fold ($p = 5.00 \times 10^{-5}$) up-regulation of the Interferon Inducible Protein 47 gene (*IFI47*) were observed in S89A mice consistent with the known IFN/STAT1 pathway dysregulation in IBD [47]. Serum Amyloid A1 (*SAA1*), which demonstrates bactericidal action in vitro, may provide a feedback protective mechanism in S89A mice and was increased 5.3-fold ($p = 5.00 \times 10^{-5}$) [48].

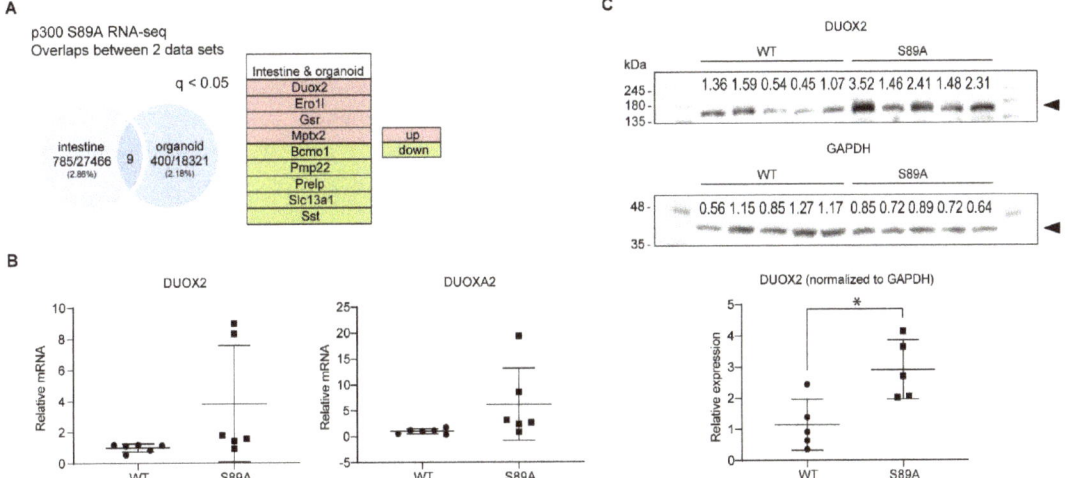

Figure 5. Genomic analysis of p300 S89A mice intestinal tissue. (**A**) RNA-seq analysis identifies 9 genes significantly differentially expressed in intestinal tissue and intestinal organoids derived from S89A mice versus those derived from WT mice. up, up-regulated; down, down-regulated. (*n* = 3 per group.) (**B**) RT-qPCR analysis of Duox2 and Duoxa2 mRNA levels in intestine of S89A and WT mice. (**C**) Immunoblot analysis of Duox2 protein levels in intestinal tissue of S89A and WT mice. Numerical values above protein bands indicate densitometric quantitation. Data in graphs are mean ± s.d. (*n* = 5–6 per group). * $p < 0.05$. Whole immunoblots corresponding to immunoblot data are included in Figure S4.

3.5. Proteomic Analysis

We performed a targeted proteomic analysis of intestinal proteins associated with CBP and/or p300 in wild type versus p300 S89A mice. Interestingly, the aryl hydrocarbon receptor nuclear translocator-like protein 2 (Bmal2) demonstrated increased association with CBP versus p300 in both wild type and p300 S89A mice under both fed or fasted conditions, and although the ratio of CBP to p300 binding did not change significantly in the male mice, fed female p300 S89A mice showed a somewhat decreased Bmal2/CBP versus Bmal2/p300 interaction (Table S4). *BMAL2*, similar to its paralog *BMAL1*, forms a dimer with *CLOCK*, to activate E-box-dependent transcription thereby playing an active role in circadian-regulated transcription [49]. Bmal1 regulates Bmal2, therefore Bmal1 deletion by itself effects combined Bmal1/Bmal2 deletion [50]. Clock/Bmal1-mediated transcription is associated with rhythmic recruitment of Clock to p300 by Bmal1 [51] and differential avidity and timing of binding to CBP versus p300, may affect circadian regulation in S89A mice. Differential association of the N6 methyl adenosine 70 kDa subunit Mettl3 with enhanced p300 association in the female p300 S89A mice was also demonstrated. These results are interesting given the recent report of circadian clock regulation of lipid metabolism and in particular PPARα-mediated transcription being modulated by m6A mRNA methylation [52] and the role of p300 Ser89 in PPAR transcriptional regulation [23]. The effect of the p300 S89A mutation on circadian regulation was not investigated in this study, however given the effect of this mutation on nuclear receptor signaling in both the intestine and in the liver (to be reported separately), and the crosstalk between nuclear receptors and core circadian transcriptional regulators [53], this area will be the focus of future investigations.

We next undertook global proteomic analysis of intestinal tissue from wild type and p300 S89A mice (Table S5), which revealed that 93 of the 2836 proteins detected in both WT and S89 mice proteins were significantly differentially expressed (with fold change ≤ -1.2 or fold change ≥ 1.2 and $p < 0.05$) (Table S6). IPA analysis of the 93 proteins showed that Mitochondrial Dysfunction, Oxidative Phosphorylation and Virus Entry via Endocytic Pathway were the top canonical pathways associated with S89A mutation (Figure 6). Interestingly, we have identified similar effects on mitochondrial dysfunction and oxidative phosphorylation in other organ systems in S89A mice (e.g., brain, liver, adipose tissue, to be reported separately) as well as cell-based model systems that affect differential Kat3 coactivator usage (i.e., P19 p300 N-terminally edited cells Ono et al. [9]). Metabolic dysfunction appears to be a fundamental feature associated with aberrant differential Kat3/β-catenin coactivator usage (Kahn lab manuscript in preparation). Further, the protein expression level of the bile acid transporter protein FABP6, the 2nd most down-regulated protein found in S89A mice, was approximately 10% of that in their wild type counterparts. This result is consistent with FABP6, which is required for efficient absorption and transport of bile acids in the distal intestine, being a PPAR target gene [54] that is repressed by GATA4 in the small intestine. *FABP6* message was also significantly decreased in S89A mice ($p = 0.00035$). Bile acids and their FXR nuclear receptors play important roles in inflammatory response and intestinal barrier function and are involved in IBD pathophysiology [55]. Calreticulin (CALR), which appears to play a role in leukocyte infiltration in mouse models of colitis via its interaction with alpha integrins, was down-regulated in S89A mice (~30%) [56]. Calreticulin, also is secreted by macrophages and binds to target cells marking them for removal by programmed cell phagocytosis [57] and believed to function as an "eat me" signal. Viable cells also can expose calreticulin on their surfaces, apparently protected from engulfment via concurrently expressed so called "don't eat me" signals, e.g., CD200 and CD47 [57]. Interestingly, the expression of the OX-2 membrane glycoprotein (CD200) is increased 1.5-fold in S89A intestines. The role of these differentially expressed proteins in innate immunity and the intestinal phenotype displayed in S89A mice will require further investigation.

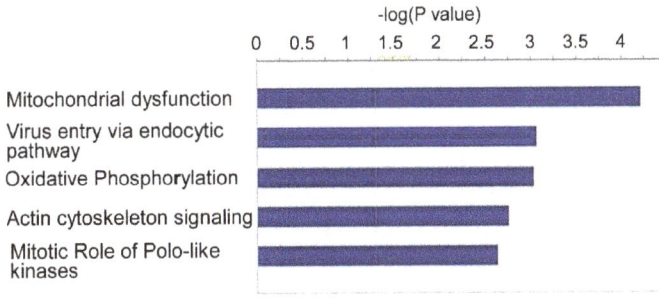

Mitochondrial dysfunction

Symbol	Protein	P value	FC S89A vs WT
COX7C	cytochrome c oxidase subunit 7C	0.0207	−1.75
NDUFA3	NADH:ubiquinone oxidoreductase subunit A3	0.0234	−1.70
NDUFA5	NADH:ubiquinone oxidoreductase subunit A5	0.0362	−1.39
NDUFB6	NADH:ubiquinone oxidoreductase subunit B6	0.0487	−1.39
PRDX3	peroxiredoxin 3	0.0295	−1.35
PRDX5	peroxiredoxin 5	0.0147	1.51

Virus entry

Symbol	Protein	P value	FC S89A vs WT
AP2M1	adaptor related protein complex 2 subunit mu 1	0.029	−1.50
CAV1	caveolin 1	0.0118	−2.44
FLNC	filamin C	0.00966	−1.73
NRAS	NRAS proto-oncogene, GTPase	0.037	1.24

Figure 6. Bioinformatic analysis of proteins differentially expressed in p300 S89A mice intestinal tissue. IPA bioinformatic analysis of the 93 genes identified by proteomic analysis to be significantly differentially expressed in intestinal tissues of S89A versus WT mice (with fold change ≤ -1.2 or fold change ≥ 1.2 and $p < 0.05$) revealed the Mitochondrial dysfunction and Virus entry via endocytic pathway as top canonical pathways associated with S89A mutation (top). Differentially expressed proteins comprising the Mitochondrial dysfunction and Virus entry via endocytic pathways and associated fold change (FC) in intestinal tissues of S89A versus WT mice (bottom). ($n = 3$–4 per group).

3.6. p300 S89A Is a Part of a 14-3-3 Binding Motif

The 14-3-3 protein family of scaffolding chaperones regulates diverse intracellular signaling pathways [58]. We observed that the p300 sequence LLRSGSSP (aa 84–91) is a member of the consensus 14-3-3 binding site sequence (LX(R/K)SX(pS/pT)XP) [59]. It is unique to p300 and not conserved in CBP. We therefore anticipated that mutation of serine 89 to alanine would disrupt the binding of 14-3-3 proteins to p300. Immunoprecipitation of 14-3-3 epsilon (14-3-3ε) was performed using protein from intestines of WT and S89A mice and subsequently immunoblotted with an antibody specific for p300. As shown (Figure 7) a substantial decrease in the association of 14-3-3ε with p300 was demonstrated in intestinal tissue from S89A mutant mice. To confirm these findings, we carried out the reverse experiment, i.e., anti-p300 antibody was used for immunoprecipitation followed by immunoblotting for 14-3-3ε. Again, we found a substantial decrease in the association of 14-3-3ε with p300 in S89A mutant mouse intestinal tissue (Figure S7). Further studies are needed to address the importance of this interaction, however differential subcellular localization of p300 regulated by its interaction with 14-3-3 proteins could potentially affect its role as a nuclear transcriptional coactivator.

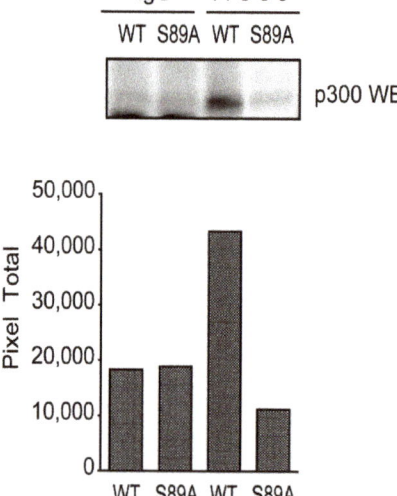

Figure 7. Association of 14-3-3ε with p300 is decreased in intestinal tissue from p300 S89A mice. Co-immunoprecipitation of p300 with 14-3-3ε in S89A and WT mouse intestinal crypt cells. Control (IgG) antibody and anti-14-3-3ε antibody were used for immunoprecipitation followed by immunoblot for p300. Bar graphs show densitometric quantitation of p300 associated with 14-3-3ε versus control IgG in intestinal tissues of S89A versus WT mice.

4. Discussion

Differential Kat3 coactivator usage by β-catenin is a fundamental regulatory mechanism in stem cell maintenance and the initiation of differentiation and repair [1,60]. Stem cells in their respective niches receive a myriad of information including oxygen and nutrient levels, circadian input, adhesion molecules, cell–cell contacts, growth factors, etc., to decide to maintain quiescence or to enter the cell cycle and undergo either symmetric or asymmetric division [1,61]. The extreme N-terminal 111 amino acids of CBP and p300, decidedly the most divergent regions of the two Kat3 coactivators [2], contain binding domains for β-catenin, nuclear receptors [9] and Stat1, an interferon-dependent transcription factor [62], as well as approximately 20 serine/threonine residues [1,2,63,64]. Post-translational modifications of these serine/threonine residues (by phosphorylation or dephosphorylation) [21–24] and combinatorial interactions, both antagonistic and synergistic [9], of multiple transcription factor families (i.e., β-catenin/TCF/LEF, β-catenin/FOXO, nuclear receptors, e.g., RAR, VDR, PPAR, etc., Stat1, 2 as well as others), provide a unique mechanism to integrate a diverse array of signal inputs. We previously demonstrated that a highly evolutionarily conserved 27bp/9aa insertion in the N-terminus of p300, which is not present in CBP, between the conserved β-catenin-binding region (DELI-sequence) and the nuclear receptor binding sequence (LXXLL), determines if the interaction will be potentially synergistic or purely antagonistic between the Wnt/β-catenin and nuclear receptor signaling cascades [2,9].

To further investigate mechanisms of signal integration effected by this domain of the Kat3 family, we generated p300 S89A knock-in mice. Based upon our earlier pharmacologic studies, p300 S89 is critical for controlling differential coactivator usage by β-catenin via post-translational phosphorylation in stem/progenitor populations [1,20,26] and Serine 89 appears to be a target for a number of kinase cascades [21–24]. Although, the p300 S89A polymorphism has not been reported in humans, to the best of our knowledge, homozygous p300 S89A mice, albeit born at sub-Mendelian ratios and exhibiting slightly decreased body weights, were relatively normal and fertile. However, after insult/stress and with aging (to be published separately later), we have found a range of interesting phenotypes associated with this single point mutation. Herein we report our initial findings regarding the intestinal phenotype of the p300 S89A mice. We first investigated the interaction of β-catenin with p300 in intestinal crypts, a region associated with activated Wnt signaling and found as anticipated that it was significantly reduced in S89A mice (Figure 2, right panel). Decreased β-catenin/p300 interaction in the p300 S89A mice did not manifest itself in obvious defects in either ileal or colonic architecture under normal homeostatic conditions (Figure 3C). However, treatment with a mild insult (2% DSS), while having minimal effects on wild type C57BL/6 mice, had a striking effect on the p300 S89A mice as evidenced by the development in the p300 S89A mice of severe colitis, a significant risk factor predisposing to colorectal cancer [27,28] (Figure 3A,B).

Further investigation demonstrated cell intrinsic differences in the intestinal epithelium, based upon RNA-seq of intestinal organoids, as well as microbiome compositional differences and differential immune responses in the intestine. Interestingly, S89A mice separately housed were dramatically more sensitive (Figure 4A) than when co-housed with WT mice (Figure 4A, left panel and Figure 4B). However, when separated again for four weeks after being co-housed for four weeks, S89A mice demonstrated intermediate sensitivity to DSS treatment (Figure 4C). These results point to a complex interplay between host intrinsic differences in the epithelium and extrinsic interaction with the intestinal microbiome associated with differential microbiome colonization and metabolite production [65,66] the host immune response, both innate and adaptive [67], related to a single amino acid variance within the highly conserved and critical region of signal integration in p300 [1,68].

Global genomic and proteomic analysis showed a number of prominent pathway differences including lipid metabolism, oxidative stress response, mitochondrial function and oxidative phosphorylation. We have found in further analyses of other organ systems (liver, brain and adipose tissue) that these are fundamental differences generally associated with differential Kat3/β-catenin coactivator usage. Notably, sulfate transporter *SLC13A1*, an FXR transcriptional target was significantly down-regulated in both organoids and ileum of S89A mice, consistent with the importance of p300 Ser89 phosphorylation on p300/nuclear receptor interactions [44,45]. Sulfate insufficiency impedes detoxification, heightens the risk of xenobiotic toxicity, and modifies the activity and metabolism of numerous physiologic compounds, including proteoglycans, hormones, and neurotransmitters [69] and very recently integrated microbiota and metabolite profiles linked Crohn's disease with sulfur metabolism [65]. Interestingly, the levels of both p-cresol sulfate and phenol sulfate, potentially toxic intestinal bacterial fermentation products [70], were significantly upregulated in the liver metabolome of S89A mice (to be published separately). Given the importance of cellular metabolism and mitochondrial function in the regulation of the immune response [71,72], further investigations with regard to intestinal immunity in the p300 S89A mice and the effects in other organ systems are ongoing and will be reported in due course. Additionally, mitochondrial activity has been linked to maintaining a state of physiological hypoxia at the colonic surface. Limiting the amount of oxygen at the mucosal surface controls the aerobic growth of facultative anaerobic bacteria [73], whereas reduced mitochondrial bioenergetics decreases epithelial oxygen consumption, thereby increasing epithelial oxygenation and the diffusion of oxygen into the intestinal lumen [74–76]. Recent experimental evidence [77] has provided support for the hypothesis that an expansion of facultative anaerobic bacteria in IBD patients are secondary to changes in epithelial energy metabolism [78]. Furthermore, it was demonstrated that treating mitochondrial dysfunction in the colon using the PPAR agonist 5-ASA [79], consistent with the dysfunctional PPAR signaling associated with S89A mutation, ameliorated signs of disease in mice with pre-IBD and normalized the microbiota composition by restoring epithelial hypoxia [77].

The diverse array of effects on fundamental processes including epithelial differentiation, metabolism, immune response and microbiome colonization, all brought about by a single amino acid modification S89A, highlights the role of this region in the Kat3 coactivator p300 as a critical signaling nexus and the rationale for conservation of this residue and surrounding region for hundreds of million years of vertebrate evolution. Additional studies related to the fundamental regulation of metabolism via differential Kat3/β-catenin usage and its roles in development and disease will be reported in due course.

5. Conclusions

We describe the generation of novel p300 S89A knock-in mice carrying a single site directed amino acid mutation in p300, changing the highly evolutionarily conserved serine 89 to alanine, thus enhancing Wnt/CBP/catenin signaling (at the expense of Wnt/p300/catenin signaling). We show that S89A mice are extremely sensitive to intestinal insult resulting in colitis, which is known to significantly predispose to colorectal cancer. We demonstrate cell intrinsic differences, and microbiome compositional differences and differential immune responses, in the intestines of S89A versus wild type mice. Genomic and proteomic analyses reveal pathway differences, including lipid metabolism, oxidative stress response, mitochondrial function and oxidative phosphorylation. The diverse effects on fundamental processes including epithelial differentiation, metabolism, immune response and microbiome colonization, all brought about by a single amino acid modification S89A, highlights the critical role of this region in p300 as a signaling nexus in development and disease (e.g., inflammation and cancer) and the rationale for conservation of this residue and surrounding region for hundreds of million years of vertebrate evolution.

Supplementary Materials: The following are available online at https://www.mdpi.com/2072-6694/13/6/1288/s1, Figure S1: Schematic of flip-excision switch construct used to create p300 S89A germ line mice, Figure S2: Body weight and blood count did not show any major abnormalities between p300 S89A mice and wild type mice, Figure S3: p300 S89A mice show differential usage of Kat3 coactivators CBP and p300 by β-catenin, Figure S4: Immunoblot analysis of Duox2 protein levels in intestinal tissue of S89A and WT mice, Figure S5: Bray–Curtis (beta) diversity between wild type and p300 S89A mutant mouse groups, Figure S6: Jaccard (beta) diversity between wild type and p300 S89A mutant mouse groups, Figure S7: Association of 14-3-3ε with p300 is decreased in intestinal tissue from p300 S89A mice, Table S1: Comparison of Blood Chemistry between p300 S89A and Wild Type Mice, Table S2: Organoids RNA-seq, Table S3: Intestine RNA-seq, Table S4: Intestine co-IP of CBP vs. p300 proteomics, Table S5: Intestine global proteomics, Table S6: Proteomic Identification of Differentially Expressed Proteins in p300 S89A vs. Wild Type Mice.

Author Contributions: K.K.Y.L.: formal analysis, funding acquisition, writing. X.H.: formal analysis, investigation, visualization, review and editing. K.C.: formal analysis, investigation, visualization, review and editing. C.N.: formal analysis, investigation, visualization, review and editing. D.P.L.: visualization, review and editing. K.K.L.: formal analysis, writing. N.K.: formal analysis, review and editing. Y.H.: formal analysis, review and editing. S.K.H.: formal analysis, review and editing. E.M.: investigation, review and editing. Y.E.: formal analysis, investigation, visualization, review and editing. P.T.F.: formal analysis, review and editing. A.J.O.: formal analysis, review and editing. N.-O.C.: formal analysis, visualization, writing. M.O.: formal analysis, investigation, writing. M.K.: conceptualization, formal analysis, funding acquisition, project administration, resources, supervision, writing. All authors have read and agreed to the published version of the manuscript.

Funding: K.K.Y.L. has been supported by NIH K08AA025112. M.K. has been supported by City of Hope Comprehensive Cancer Center Support Grant NIH P30CA033572, NIH R01CA166161, R21NS074392, R21AI105057, and R01HL112638, and the Rotary Coins for Alzheimer's Research Trust (CART).

Institutional Review Board Statement: Animal studies were approved by the University of Southern California Institutional Animal Care and Use Committee (IACUC) as per protocol #11023.

Data Availability Statement: Proteomics data have been deposited in the ProteomeXchange Consortium via the jPOST [35] partner repository with the data set identifier PXD021750. Additional genomics and proteomics data have been included in Supplementary Materials. All other data supporting the findings of this study are available from the corresponding author on reasonable request.

Acknowledgments: The authors thank Tomoyo Sasaki for her technical contributions to the project.

Conflicts of Interest: M.K. has an equity position in 3 + 2 Pharma. The other authors declare no conflict of interest. The funders had no role in the design of the study; in the collection, analyses, or interpretation of data; in the writing of the manuscript, or in the decision to publish the results.

References

1. Thomas, P.D.; Kahn, M. Kat3 coactivators in somatic stem cells and cancer stem cells: Biological roles, evolution, and pharmacologic manipulation. *Cell Biol. Toxicol.* **2016**, *32*, 61–81. [CrossRef] [PubMed]
2. Kahn, M. Wnt Signaling in Stem Cells and Cancer Stem Cells: A Tale of Two Coactivators. *Prog. Mol. Biol. Transl. Sci.* **2018**, *153*, 209–244. [CrossRef]
3. Trosko, J.E.; Kang, K.-S. Evolution of Energy Metabolism, Stem Cells and Cancer Stem Cells: How the Warburg and Barker Hypotheses Might Be Linked. *Int. J. Stem Cells* **2012**, *5*, 39–56. [CrossRef] [PubMed]
4. Arany, Z.; Sellers, W.R.; Livingston, D.M.; Eckner, R. E1A-associated p300 and CREB-associated CBP belong to a conserved family of coactivators. *Cell* **1994**, *77*, 799–800. [CrossRef]
5. Eckner, R.; Ewen, M.E.; Newsome, D.; Gerdes, M.; DeCaprio, J.A.; Lawrence, J.B.; Livingston, D.M. Molecular cloning and functional analysis of the adenovirus E1A-associated 300-kD protein (p300) reveals a protein with properties of a transcriptional adaptor. *Genes Dev.* **1994**, *8*, 869–884. [CrossRef]
6. Kung, A.L.; Rebel, V.I.; Bronson, R.T.; Ch'Ng, L.-E.; Sieff, C.A.; Livingston, D.M.; Yao, T.-P. Gene dose-dependent control of hematopoiesis and hematologic tumor suppression by CBP. *Genome Res.* **2000**, *14*, 272–277.
7. Yamauchi, T.; Oike, Y.; Kamon, J.; Waki, H.; Komeda, K.; Tsuchida, A.; Date, Y.; Li, M.-X.; Miki, H.; Akanuma, Y.; et al. Increased insulin sensitivity despite lipodystrophy in Crebbp heterozygous mice. *Nat. Genet.* **2002**, *30*, 221–226. [CrossRef]
8. Roth, J.-F.; Shikama, N.; Henzen, C.; Desbaillets, I.; Lutz, W.; Marino, S.; Wittwer, J.; Schorle, H.; Gassmann, M.; Eckner, R. Differential role of p300 and CBP acetyltransferase during myogenesis: p300 acts upstream of MyoD and Myf5. *EMBO J.* **2003**, *22*, 5186–5196. [CrossRef] [PubMed]
9. Ono, M.; Lai, K.K.Y.; Wu, K.; Nguyen, C.; Lin, D.P.; Murali, R.; Kahn, M. Nuclear receptor/Wnt beta-catenin interactions are regulated via differential CBP/p300 coactivator usage. *PLoS ONE* **2018**, *13*, e0200714. [CrossRef]
10. Ma, H.; Nguyen, C.; Lee, K.-S.; Kahn, M. Differential roles for the coactivators CBP and p300 on TCF/β-catenin-mediated survivin gene expression. *Oncogene* **2005**, *24*, 3619–3631. [CrossRef]
11. Moon, R.T. Wnt/-Catenin Pathway. *Sci. Signal.* **2005**, *2005*, cm1. [CrossRef]
12. Teo, J.-L.; Kahn, M. The Wnt signaling pathway in cellular proliferation and differentiation: A tale of two coactivators. *Adv. Drug Deliv. Rev.* **2010**, *62*, 1149–1155. [CrossRef]
13. McMillan, M.; Kahn, M. Investigating Wnt signaling: A chemogenomic safari. *Drug Discov. Today* **2005**, *10*, 1467–1474. [CrossRef]
14. Emami, K.H.; Nguyen, C.; Ma, H.; Kim, D.H.; Jeong, K.W.; Eguchi, M.; Moon, R.T.; Teo, J.-L.; Oh, S.W.; Kim, H.Y.; et al. A small molecule inhibitor of -catenin/CREB-binding protein transcription. *Proc. Natl. Acad. Sci. USA* **2004**, *101*, 12682–12687. [CrossRef] [PubMed]
15. Higuchi, Y.; Nguyen, C.; Yasuda, S.-Y.; McMillan, M.; Hasegawa, K.; Kahn, M. Specific Direct Small Molecule p300/?-Catenin Antagonists Maintain Stem Cell Potency. *Curr. Mol. Pharmacol.* **2016**, *9*, 272–279. [CrossRef]
16. Torchia, J.; Rose, D.W.; Inostroza, J.; Kamei, Y.; Westin, S.; Glass, C.K.; Rosenfeld, M.G. The transcriptional co-activator p/CIP binds CBP and mediates nuclear-receptor function. *Nat. Cell Biol.* **1997**, *387*, 677–684. [CrossRef]
17. Dillard, A.C.; Lane, M.A. Retinol decreases β-catenin protein levels in retinoic acid-resistant colon cancer cell lines. *Mol. Carcinog.* **2007**, *46*, 315–329. [CrossRef] [PubMed]
18. Easwaran, V.; Pishvaian, M.; Salimuddin; Byers, S. Cross-regulation of beta-catenin-LEF/TCF and retinoid signaling pathways. *Curr. Biol.* **1999**, *9*, 1415–1418. [CrossRef]
19. Larriba, M.J.; Martín-Villar, E.; Garcia, J.M.; Pereira, F.; Peña, C.; De Herreros, A.G.; Bonilla, F.; Munoz, A. Snail2 cooperates with Snail1 in the repression of vitamin D receptor in colon cancer. *Carcinogen* **2009**, *30*, 1459–1468. [CrossRef] [PubMed]
20. Miyabayashi, T.; Teo, J.-L.; Yamamoto, M.; McMillan, M.; Nguyen, C.; Kahn, M. Wnt/beta-catenin/CBP signaling maintains long-term murine embryonic stem cell pluripotency. *Proc. Natl. Acad. Sci. USA* **2007**, *104*, 5668–5673. [CrossRef]
21. Yuan, L.W.; Gambee, J.E. Phosphorylation of p300 at Serine 89 by Protein Kinase C. *J. Biol. Chem.* **2000**, *275*, 40946–40951. [CrossRef]

22. Yuan, L.W.; Soh, J.W.; Weinstein, I.B. Inhibition of histone acetyltransferase function of p300 by PKCdelta. *Biochim. Biophys. Acta* **2002**, *1592*, 205–211. [CrossRef]
23. Yang, W.; Hong, Y.H.; Shen, X.-Q.; Frankowski, C.; Camp, H.S.; Leff, T. Regulation of Transcription by AMP-activated Protein Kinase. *J. Biol. Chem.* **2001**, *276*, 38341–38344. [CrossRef]
24. Liu, Y.; Dentin, R.; Chen, D.; Hedrick, S.; Ravnskjaer, K.; Schenk, S.; Milne, J.; Meyers, D.J.; Cole, P.; Iii, J.Y.; et al. A fasting inducible switch modulates gluconeogenesis via activator/coactivator exchange. *Nat. Cell Biol.* **2008**, *456*, 269–273. [CrossRef]
25. Gusterson, R.J.; Yuan, L.; Latchman, D.S. Distinct serine residues in CBP and p300 are necessary for their activation by phenylephrine. *Int. J. Biochem. Cell Biol.* **2004**, *36*, 893–899. [CrossRef] [PubMed]
26. Rieger, M.E.; Zhou, B.; Solomon, N.; Sunohara, M.; Li, C.; Nguyen, C.; Liu, Y.; Pan, J.-H.; Minoo, P.; Crandall, E.D.; et al. p300/β-Catenin Interactions Regulate Adult Progenitor Cell Differentiation Downstream of WNT5a/Protein Kinase C (PKC). *J. Biol. Chem.* **2016**, *291*, 6569–6582. [CrossRef]
27. Lai, K.K.; Horvath, B.; Xie, H.; Wu, X.; Lewis, B.L.; Pai, R.K.; Plesec, T.; Patil, D.T.; Gordon, I.O.; Wang, Y.; et al. Risk for Colorectal Neoplasia in Patients with Inflammatory Bowel Disease and Mucosa Indefinite for Dysplasia. *Inflamm. Bowel Dis.* **2015**, *21*, 378–384. [CrossRef]
28. Chen, R.; Rabinovitch, P.S.; Crispin, D.A.; Emond, M.J.; Bronner, M.P.; Brentnall, T.A. The initiation of colon cancer in a chronic inflammatory setting. *Carcinogen* **2005**, *26*, 1513–1519. [CrossRef] [PubMed]
29. Yao, T.-P.; Oh, S.P.; Fuchs, M.; Zhou, N.-D.; Ch'Ng, L.-E.; Newsome, D.; Bronson, R.T.; Li, E.; Livingston, D.M.; Eckner, R. Gene Dosage–Dependent Embryonic Development and Proliferation Defects in Mice Lacking the Transcriptional Integrator p300. *Cell* **1998**, *93*, 361–372. [CrossRef]
30. O'Rourke, K.; Ackerman, S.; Dow, L.; Lowe, S. Isolation, Culture, and Maintenance of Mouse Intestinal Stem Cells. *Bio Protocol* **2016**, *6*, 6. [CrossRef] [PubMed]
31. Haas, B.J.; Gevers, D.; Earl, A.M.; Feldgarden, M.; Ward, D.V.; Giannoukos, G.; Ciulla, D.; Tabbaa, D.; Highlander, S.K.; Sodergren, E.; et al. Chimeric 16S rRNA sequence formation and detection in Sanger and 454-pyrosequenced PCR amplicons. *Genome Res.* **2011**, *21*, 494–504. [CrossRef] [PubMed]
32. Edgar, R.C. UPARSE: Highly accurate OTU sequences from microbial amplicon reads. *Nat. Methods* **2013**, *10*, 996–998. [CrossRef] [PubMed]
33. Sato, T.; Clevers, H. Primary Mouse Small Intestinal Epithelial Cell Cultures. *Adv. Struct. Saf. Stud.* **2012**, *945*, 319–328. [CrossRef]
34. Ring, A.; Nguyen, C.; Smbatyan, G.; Tripathy, D.; Yu, M.; Press, M.; Kahn, M.; Lang, J.E. CBP/β-Catenin/FOXM1 Is a Novel Therapeutic Target in Triple Negative Breast Cancer. *Cancers* **2018**, *10*, 525. [CrossRef]
35. Okuda, S.; Watanabe, Y.; Moriya, Y.; Kawano, S.; Yamamoto, T.; Matsumoto, M.; Takami, T.; Kobayashi, D.; Araki, N.; Yoshizawa, A.C.; et al. jPOSTrepo: An international standard data repository for proteomes. *Nucleic Acids Res.* **2017**, *45*, D1107–D1111. [CrossRef]
36. Whittem, C.G.; Williams, A.D.; Williams, C.S. Murine Colitis Modeling using Dextran Sulfate Sodium (DSS). *J. Vis. Exp.* **2010**, e1652. [CrossRef] [PubMed]
37. Kaser, A.; Zeissig, S.; Blumberg, R.S. Inflammatory Bowel Disease. *Annu. Rev. Immunol.* **2010**, *28*, 573–621. [CrossRef]
38. Sartor, R.B.; Wu, G.D. Roles for Intestinal Bacteria, Viruses, and Fungi in Pathogenesis of Inflammatory Bowel Diseases and Therapeutic Approaches. *Gastroenterology* **2017**, *152*, 327–339.e4. [CrossRef]
39. Lee, K.-A.; Cho, K.-C.; Kim, B.; Jang, I.-H.; Nam, K.; Kwon, Y.E.; Kim, M.; Hyeon, D.Y.; Hwang, D.; Seol, J.-H.; et al. Inflammation-Modulated Metabolic Reprogramming Is Required for DUOX-Dependent Gut Immunity in Drosophila. *Cell Host Microbe* **2018**, *23*, 338–352.e5. [CrossRef]
40. Rigoni, A.; Poulsom, R.; Jeffery, R.; Mehta, S.; Lewis, A.; Yau, C.; Giannoulatou, E.; Feakins, R.; Lindsay, J.O.; Colombo, M.P.; et al. Separation of Dual Oxidase 2 and Lactoperoxidase Expression in Intestinal Crypts and Species Differences May Limit Hydrogen Peroxide Scavenging During Mucosal Healing in Mice and Humans. *Inflamm. Bowel Dis.* **2017**, *24*, 136–148. [CrossRef]
41. Thompson, C.A.; Wojta, K.; Pulakanti, K.; Rao, S.; Dawson, P.; Battle, M.A. GATA4 Is Sufficient to Establish Jejunal Versus Ileal Identity in the Small Intestine. *Cell. Mol. Gastroenterol. Hepatol.* **2017**, *3*, 422–446. [CrossRef] [PubMed]
42. Cash, H.L.; Whitham, C.V.; Behrendt, C.L.; Hooper, L.V. Symbiotic Bacteria Direct Expression of an Intestinal Bactericidal Lectin. *Science* **2006**, *313*, 1126–1130. [CrossRef]
43. Wu, F.; Dassopoulos, T.; Cope, L.; Maitra, A.; Brant, S.R.; Harris, M.L.; Bayless, T.M.; Parmigiani, G.; Chakravarti, S. Genome-wide gene expression differences in Crohn's disease and ulcerative colitis from endoscopic pinch biopsies: Insights into distinctive pathogenesis. *Inflamm. Bowel Dis.* **2007**, *13*, 807–821. [CrossRef] [PubMed]
44. Ghosh, A.K.; Varga, J. The transcriptional coactivator and acetyltransferase p300 in fibroblast biology and fibrosis. *J. Cell. Physiol.* **2007**, *213*, 663–671. [CrossRef] [PubMed]
45. Kemper, J.K.; Xiao, Z.; Ponugoti, B.; Miao, J.; Fang, S.; Kanamaluru, D.; Tsang, S.; Wu, S.-Y.; Chiang, C.-M.; Veenstra, T.D. FXR Acetylation Is Normally Dynamically Regulated by p300 and SIRT1 but Constitutively Elevated in Metabolic Disease States. *Cell Metab.* **2009**, *10*, 392–404. [CrossRef] [PubMed]
46. Kawazoe, Y.; Sekimoto, T.; Araki, M.; Takagi, K.; Araki, K.; Yamamura, K.-I. Region-specific gastrointestinal Hox code during murine embryonal gut development. *Dev. Growth Differ.* **2002**, *44*, 77–84. [CrossRef]

47. Giles, E.M.; Sanders, T.J.; McCarthy, N.E.; Lung, J.; Pathak, M.; Macdonald, T.T.; Lindsay, J.O.; Stagg, A.J. Regulation of human intestinal T-cell responses by type 1 interferon-STAT1 signaling is disrupted in inflammatory bowel disease. *Mucosal Immunol.* **2016**, *10*, 184–193. [CrossRef]
48. Eckhardt, E.R.M.; Witta, J.; Zhong, J.; Arsenescu, R.; Arsenescu, V.; Wang, Y.; Ghoshal, S.; De Beer, M.C.; De Beer, F.C.; De Villiers, W.J.S. Intestinal Epithelial Serum Amyloid A Modulates Bacterial Growth In Vitro and Pro-Inflammatory Responses in Mouse Experimental Colitis. *BMC Gastroenterol.* **2010**, *10*, 133–139. [CrossRef]
49. Sasaki, M.; Yoshitane, H.; Du, N.-H.; Okano, T.; Fukada, Y. Preferential Inhibition of BMAL2-CLOCK Activity by PER2 Reemphasizes Its Negative Role and a Positive Role of BMAL2 in the Circadian Transcription. *J. Biol. Chem.* **2009**, *284*, 25149–25159. [CrossRef]
50. Shi, S.; Hida, A.; McGuinness, O.P.; Wasserman, D.H.; Yamazaki, S.; Johnson, C.H. Circadian Clock Gene Bmal1 Is Not Essential; Functional Replacement with its Paralog, Bmal2. *Curr. Biol.* **2010**, *20*, 316–321. [CrossRef]
51. Etchegaray, J.-P.; Lee, C.; Wade, P.A.; Reppert, S.M. Rhythmic histone acetylation underlies transcription in the mammalian circadian clock. *Nat. Cell Biol.* **2002**, *421*, 177–182. [CrossRef]
52. Zhong, X.; Yu, J.; Frazier, K.; Weng, X.; Li, Y.; Cham, C.M.; Dolan, K.; Zhu, X.; Hubert, N.; Tao, Y.; et al. Circadian Clock Regulation of Hepatic Lipid Metabolism by Modulation of m6A mRNA Methylation. *Cell Rep.* **2018**, *25*, 1816–1828.e4. [CrossRef]
53. Yang, X.; Downes, M.; Yu, R.T.; Bookout, A.L.; He, W.; Straume, M.; Mangelsdorf, D.J.; Evans, R.M. Nuclear Receptor Expression Links the Circadian Clock to Metabolism. *Cell* **2006**, *126*, 801–810. [CrossRef]
54. Venkatachalam, A.B.; Sawler, D.L.; Wright, J.M. Tissue-specific transcriptional modulation of fatty acid-binding protein genes, fabp2, fabp3 and fabp6, by fatty acids and the peroxisome proliferator, clofibrate, in zebrafish (Danio rerio). *Gene* **2013**, *520*, 14–21. [CrossRef] [PubMed]
55. Ding, L.; Yang, L.; Wang, Z.; Huang, W. Bile acid nuclear receptor FXR and digestive system diseases. *Acta Pharm. Sin. B* **2015**, *5*, 135–144. [CrossRef] [PubMed]
56. Ohkuro, M.; Kim, J.-D.; Kuboi, Y.; Hayashi, Y.; Mizukami, H.; Kobayashi-Kuramochi, H.; Muramoto, K.; Shirato, M.; Michikawa-Tanaka, F.; Moriya, J.; et al. Calreticulin and integrin alpha dissociation induces anti-inflammatory programming in animal models of inflammatory bowel disease. *Nat. Commun.* **2018**, *9*, 1–10. [CrossRef]
57. Krysko, D.V.; Ravichandran, K.S.; Vandenabeele, P. Macrophages regulate the clearance of living cells by calreticulin. *Nat. Commun.* **2018**, *9*, 4644. [CrossRef]
58. Pennington, K.L.; Chan, T.Y.; Torres, M.P.; Andersen, J.L. The dynamic and stress-adaptive signaling hub of 14-3-3: Emerging mechanisms of regulation and context-dependent protein–protein interactions. *Oncogene* **2018**, *37*, 5587–5604. [CrossRef]
59. Johnson, C.; Crowther, S.; Stafford, M.J.; Campbell, D.G.; Toth, R.; Mackintosh, C. Bioinformatic and experimental survey of 14-3-3-binding sites. *Biochem. J.* **2010**, *427*, 69–78. [CrossRef]
60. Teo, J.-L.; Ma, H.; Nguyen, C.; Lam, C.; Kahn, M. Specific inhibition of CBP/ -catenin interaction rescues defects in neuronal differentiation caused by a presenilin-1 mutation. *Proc. Natl. Acad. Sci. USA* **2005**, *102*, 12171–12176. [CrossRef]
61. Kahn, M. Symmetric division versus asymmetric division: A tale of two coactivators. *Futur. Med. Chem.* **2011**, *3*, 1745–1763. [CrossRef]
62. Zhang, J.J.; Vinkemeier, U.; Gu, W.; Chakravarti, D.; Horvath, C.M.; Darnell, J.E. Two contact regions between Stat1 and CBP/p300 in interferon signaling. *Proc. Natl. Acad. Sci. USA* **1996**, *93*, 15092–15096. [CrossRef]
63. Horvai, A.E.; Xu, L.; Korzus, E.; Brard, G.; Kalafus, D.; Mullen, T.-M.; Rose, D.W.; Rosenfeld, M.G.; Glass, C.K. Nuclear integration of JAK/STAT and Ras/AP-1 signaling by CBP and p300. *Proc. Natl. Acad. Sci. USA* **1997**, *94*, 1074–1079. [CrossRef]
64. Kurokawa, R.; Kalafus, D.; Ogliastro, M.-H.; Kioussi, C.; Xu, L.; Torchia, J.; Rosenfeld, M.G.; Glass, C.K. Differential Use of CREB Binding Protein-Coactivator Complexes. *Science* **1998**, *279*, 700–703. [CrossRef]
65. Metwaly, A.; Dunkel, A.; Waldschmitt, N.; Raj, A.C.D.; Lagkouvardos, I.; Corraliza, A.M.; Mayorgas, A.; Martinez-Medina, M.; Reiter, S.; Schloter, M.; et al. Integrated microbiota and metabolite profiles link Crohn's disease to sulfur metabolism. *Nat. Commun.* **2020**, *11*, 1–15. [CrossRef] [PubMed]
66. Alexander, M.; Turnbaugh, P.J. Deconstructing Mechanisms of Diet-Microbiome-Immune Interactions. *Immunology* **2020**, *53*, 264–276. [CrossRef]
67. Hernandez, J.B.; Chang, C.; Leblanc, M.; Grimm, D.; Le Lay, J.; Kaestner, K.H.; Zheng, Y.; Montminy, M. The CREB/CRTC2 pathway modulates autoimmune disease by promoting Th17 differentiation. *Nat. Commun.* **2015**, *6*, 7216. [CrossRef]
68. Mazmanian, S.K.; Liu, C.H.; Tzianabos, A.O.; Kasper, D.L. An Immunomodulatory Molecule of Symbiotic Bacteria Directs Maturation of the Host Immune System. *Cell* **2005**, *122*, 107–118. [CrossRef] [PubMed]
69. Markovich, D. Physiological Roles and Regulation of Mammalian Sulfate Transporters. *Physiol. Rev.* **2001**, *81*, 1499–1533. [CrossRef] [PubMed]
70. Williams, H.R.T.; Cox, I.J.; Walker, D.G.; North, B.V.; Patel, V.M.; Marshall, S.E.; Jewell, D.P.; Ghosh, S.; Thomas, H.J.W.; Teare, J.P.; et al. Characterization of Inflammatory Bowel Disease With Urinary Metabolic Profiling. *Am. J. Gastroenterol.* **2009**, *104*, 1435–1444. [CrossRef] [PubMed]
71. Weinberg, S.E.; Sena, L.A.; Chandel, N.S. Mitochondria in the Regulation of Innate and Adaptive Immunity. *Immunology* **2015**, *42*, 406–417. [CrossRef]
72. Rambold, A.S.; Pearce, E.L. Mitochondrial Dynamics at the Interface of Immune Cell Metabolism and Function. *Trends Immunol.* **2018**, *39*, 6–18. [CrossRef] [PubMed]

73. Litvak, Y.; Byndloss, M.X.; Bäumler, A.J. Colonocyte metabolism shapes the gut microbiota. *Science* **2018**, *362*, eaat9076. [CrossRef]
74. Byndloss, M.X.; Olsan, E.E.; Rivera-Chávez, F.; Tiffany, C.R.; Cevallos, S.A.; Lokken, K.L.; Torres, T.P.; Byndloss, A.J.; Faber, F.; Gao, Y.; et al. Microbiota-activated PPAR-γ signaling inhibits dysbiotic Enterobacteriaceae expansion. *Science* **2017**, *357*, 570–575. [CrossRef] [PubMed]
75. Furuta, G.T.; Turner, J.R.; Taylor, C.T.; Hershberg, R.M.; Comerford, K.; Narravula, S.; Podolsky, D.K.; Colgan, S.P. Hypoxia-Inducible Factor 1–Dependent Induction of Intestinal Trefoil Factor Protects Barrier Function during Hypoxia. *J. Exp. Med.* **2001**, *193*, 1027–1034. [CrossRef] [PubMed]
76. Kelly, C.J.; Zheng, L.; Campbell, E.L.; Saeedi, B.; Scholz, C.C.; Bayless, A.J.; Wilson, K.E.; Glover, L.E.; Kominsky, D.J.; Magnuson, A.; et al. Crosstalk between Microbiota-Derived Short-Chain Fatty Acids and Intestinal Epithelial HIF Augments Tissue Barrier Function. *Cell Host Microbe* **2015**, *17*, 662–671. [CrossRef]
77. Lee, J.-Y.; Cevallos, S.A.; Byndloss, M.X.; Tiffany, C.R.; Olsan, E.E.; Butler, B.P.; Young, B.M.; Rogers, A.W.; Nguyen, H.; Kim, K.; et al. High-Fat Diet and Antibiotics Cooperatively Impair Mitochondrial Bioenergetics to Trigger Dysbiosis that Exacerbates Pre-inflammatory Bowel Disease. *Cell Host Microbe* **2020**, *28*, 273–284.e6. [CrossRef] [PubMed]
78. Rigottier-Gois, L. Dysbiosis in inflammatory bowel diseases: The oxygen hypothesis. *ISME J.* **2013**, *7*, 1256–1261. [CrossRef]
79. Rousseaux, C.; El-Jamal, N.; Fumery, M.; Dubuquoy, C.; Romano, O.; Chatelain, D.; Langlois, A.; Bertin, B.; Buob, D.; Colombel, J.F.; et al. The 5-aminosalicylic acid antineoplastic effect in the intestine is mediated by PPARγ. *Carcinogen* **2013**, *34*, 2580–2586. [CrossRef] [PubMed]

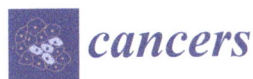

Article

The Hepatitis B Virus Pre-Core Protein p22 Activates Wnt Signaling

Bang Manh Tran [1], Dustin James Flanagan [1,2], Gregor Ebert [3,4], Nadia Warner [5], Hoanh Tran [3,4], Theodora Fifis [6], Georgios Kastrappis [6], Christopher Christophi [6], Marc Pellegrini [3,4], Joseph Torresi [7], Toby James Phesse [1,8,*] and Elizabeth Vincan [1,5,9,*]

1. The Peter Doherty Institute for Infection and Immunity, The University of Melbourne, Melbourne 3000, Australia; manht@unimelb.edu.au (B.M.T.); D.Flanagan@beatson.gla.ac.uk (D.J.F.)
2. Cancer Research UK Beatson Institute, Glasgow G61 1BD, UK
3. The Walter and Eliza Hall Institute of Medical Research, Parkville 3052, Australia; ebert@wehi.edu.au (G.E.); tran.h@wehi.edu.au (H.T.); pellegrini@wehi.edu.au (M.P.)
4. Department of Medical Biology, The University of Melbourne, Melbourne 3010, Australia
5. Victorian Infectious Diseases Reference Laboratory, The Peter Doherty Institute for Infection and Immunity, Melbourne 3000, Australia; Nadia.Warner@vidrl.org.au
6. Department of Surgery, Austin Health, The University of Melbourne, Melbourne 3010, Australia; tfifis@unimelb.edu.au (T.F.); g.kastrappis@student.unimelb.edu.au (G.K.); c.christophi@unimelb.edu.au (C.C.)
7. Department of Microbiology and Immunology, The Peter Doherty Institute for Infection and Immunity, The University of Melbourne, Melbourne 3000, Australia; josepht@unimelb.edu.au
8. European Cancer Stem Cell Research Institute, Cardiff University, Cardiff CF24 4HQ, UK
9. School of Pharmacy and Biomedical Sciences, Curtin University, Perth, WA 6102, Australia
* Correspondence: phesset@cardiff.ac.uk (T.J.P.); evincan@unimelb.edu.au (E.V.); Tel.: +44-0-29-2068-849 (T.J.P.); +613 9342 9348 (E.V.)

Received: 21 April 2020; Accepted: 27 May 2020; Published: 31 May 2020

Abstract: An emerging theme for Wnt-addicted cancers is that the pathway is regulated at multiple steps via various mechanisms. Infection with hepatitis B virus (HBV) is a major risk factor for liver cancer, as is deregulated Wnt signaling, however, the interaction between these two causes is poorly understood. To investigate this interaction, we screened the effect of the various HBV proteins for their effect on Wnt/β-catenin signaling and identified the pre-core protein p22 as a novel and potent activator of TCF/β-catenin transcription. The effect of p22 on TCF/β-catenin transcription was dose dependent and inhibited by dominant-negative TCF4. HBV p22 activated synthetic and native Wnt target gene promoter reporters, and TCF/β-catenin target gene expression in vivo. Importantly, HBV p22 activated Wnt signaling on its own and in addition to Wnt or β-catenin induced Wnt signaling. Furthermore, HBV p22 elevated TCF/β-catenin transcription above constitutive activation in colon cancer cells due to mutations in downstream genes of the Wnt pathway, namely *APC* and *CTNNB1*. Collectively, our data identifies a previously unappreciated role for the HBV pre-core protein p22 in elevating Wnt signaling. Understanding the molecular mechanisms of p22 activity will provide insight into how Wnt signaling is fine-tuned in cancer.

Keywords: Wnt signaling; hepatitis B virus; HBV; cancer; liver cancer; β-catenin; TCF/LEF

1. Introduction

Liver cancer is the second most common cause of cancer deaths worldwide and is projected to increase by ~40% by 2030 [1]. The most common type of liver cancer is hepatocellular carcinoma (HCC), which has very limited treatment options and a poor prognosis because it is usually diagnosed at a late stage [2]. The Wnt signal transduction pathway is aberrantly activated in most cases of HCC and mutations to the catenin beta 1 (*CTNNB1*) gene, the gene that codes for β-catenin, occurs in up to 40% of cases making it the most frequent mutation in HCC [3,4]. β-Catenin is the main effector of the canonical Wnt signaling pathway [5] and these mutations to *CTNNB1* lead to constitutive activation of Wnt signaling [6,7]. Liver cancer is also linked to chronic infection with the hepatitis B virus (HBV) that leads to cirrhosis and accounts for 50% of HCC cases [8]. Here, we investigated the oncogenic interplay between these two drivers of liver cancer, namely HBV and Wnt signaling.

Wnt/β-catenin signaling is activated by the coupling of Wnt to its cognate receptor, Frizzled (FZD), which initiates a series of events in the cytoplasm that leads to the activation of (TCF)/lymphoid enhancer factor (LEF)/β-catenin (referred to as TCF/β-catenin for simplicity from here on) mediated gene transcription. In the absence of Wnt, β-catenin is primarily engaged at cell-cell adherens junctions and any free β-catenin is cleared by a cytoplasmic destruction complex that contains several proteins, including Axin, adenomatous polyposis coli (APC), glycogen synthase kinase 3 (GSK3) and casein kinase 1 (CK1) [5]. Free, cytoplasmic β-catenin associates with the destruction complex and is sequentially phosphorylated by CK1 and GSK3 at its N-terminus, a post-translational modification that targets it for ubiquitylation and proteasomal degradation. However, upon activation of Wnt-FZD signaling, GSK3 enzyme activity is inhibited and β-catenin escapes phosphorylation and subsequent degradation, accumulates in the cytoplasm and translocates into the nucleus where it complexes with the enhanceosome to initiate the TCF/β-catenin target gene transcription [9]. In liver cancer, the phosphorylation sites of β-catenin are absent due to mutations to the *CTNNB1* gene, leading to the constitutive activation of Wnt/β-catenin signaling [3,4,10].

Another common etiologic factor in liver cancer is HBV infection [10,11]. HBV is an enveloped DNA virus whose genome codes for four overlapping genes, namely the envelope or surface (*S*) gene, the core (*C*) gene, the *X* gene and the polymerase (*P*) gene. The protein products include the surface antigens coded by the *S* gene, the capsid core proteins coded by the *C* gene and the HBx protein coded by the *X* gene. Post-translational processing of the HBV pre-core protein (p25) yields the HBV e antigen (HBeAg, p17) via a p22 intermediate [12]. The HBx protein has been extensively studied for its effects on Wnt/β-catenin signaling [13], however, much less is known about the potential oncogenic interplay with the other HBV proteins. Here, we performed a screen to determine the effects of HBV proteins on Wnt/β-catenin signaling and identified p22, the HBe precursor protein, as a potent activator on its own and in conjunction with active Wnt signaling. Importantly, p22 activated Wnt/β-catenin signaling in colon cancer cells that harbor mutations in intracellular components of the Wnt signaling cascade that result in constitutive activation of signaling. Concomitant regulation of Wnt signaling at multiple levels of the signaling cascade via various mechanisms (genetic, epigenetic, post-translational etc.) to achieve the "just right" level of Wnt signaling for a particular process is a common theme emerging for Wnt-addicted cancers [14–16] and here, we demonstrate that HBV p22 might contribute to our understanding of this fine tuning in cancer.

2. Results

2.1. Effect of HBV Proteins on TCF-β-Catenin Transcription

To investigate novel mechanisms of oncogenic interaction between HBV and Wnt signaling we screened the ability of various HBV proteins (Figure S1) for their effect of TCF/β-catenin transcription in the presence of Wnt stimulation (Wnt3a conditioned medium). TCF/β-catenin transcription was detected using the TCF reporter, super TOPflash (sTOPflash), which contains eight TCF response elements upstream of a minimal TK (Thymidine Kinase) promoter and sFOPflash, which has the TCF sites mutated [17,18]. The HBx protein activated TCF/β-catenin transcription above Wnt stimulation, however, the pre-core protein p22 was able to increase Wnt activity to a level markedly greater than the HBx protein (Figure 1a). The HBV envelope proteins did not activate reporter activity, nor did the pre-core precursor p25 or core p21, despite significant overlap in the amino acid sequence between the core/precore proteins (Figure S1). The precore contains the genetic sequence of two different proteins, the core protein HBc (p21) (183 amino acids) and precore polypeptide p25 (212 amino acids). They differ only by 29 amino acids at the N-terminus as p25 retains the signal sequence. The cleavage of 19 amino acids from this signal sequence releases cytosolic p22. P22 is further truncated, losing the arginine-rich C-terminal domain, to yield HBe (p17), which is secreted [19]. Expression of p22 was confirmed by immunoblot on whole cell lysates prepared from transfected Huh7 cells using an anti-HBc antibody and, as shown by others [19], neither p17 nor p25 were detected by immunoblot (Figures 1b and S2). HBV p17 and p25 were detected by confocal immunofluorescence in transfected Huh7 cells (Figure S3). Confocal microscopy of Huh7 cells transfected with pCI-p22 and the same anti-core antibody showed diffuse cytoplasmic, diffuse nuclear and, cytoplasmic puncta (Figures 1c and S3) placing p22 in the cellular compartments where Wnt signaling components are found [20].

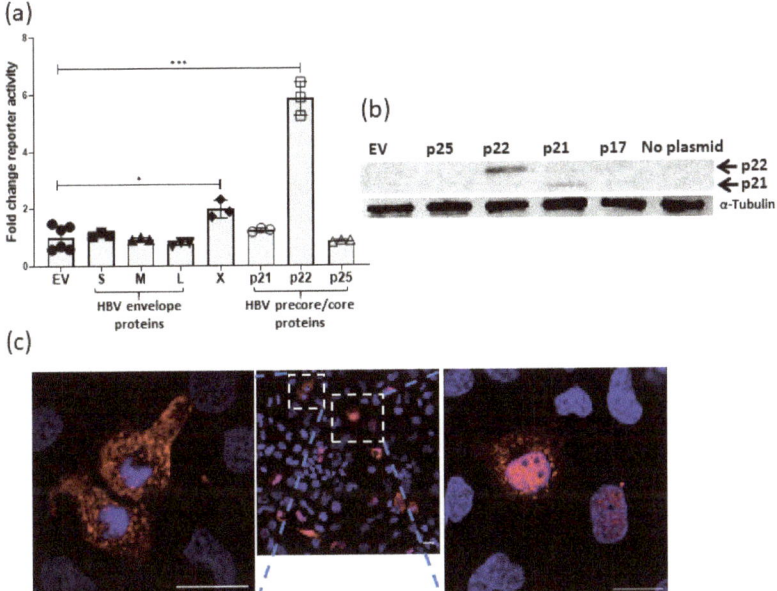

Figure 1. Wnt signaling activation is induced by hepatitis B virus (HBV) precore protein p22. (**a**) Effect of various HBV proteins on TCF/β-catenin transcription activity in Huh7 cells, was determined by reporter activity (sTOPflash reporter) and is shown as fold change relative to empty vector (EV) (mean ± SEM, * $p < 0.05$, *** $p < 0.0001$ Student *t*-test, $n \geq 3$ independent experiments for each data point) (**b**) Expression of protein from the indicated plasmids transfected in Huh7 cells was confirmed by immunoblot. Lysates prepared from Huh7 cells transfected with EV and the parental, un-transfected cells served as negative controls. Lysate from HBV core p21 transfected Huh7 cells was used as a positive control. The membrane was stained with anti-HBc antibody first, then re-probed with anti α-tubulin antibody. (**c**) Huh7 cells were transfected with p22 plasmid and p22 protein expression (red) and localization detected with anti-HBV core antibody and confocal microscopy (nuclei are blue). Scale bars = 20 µM.

2.2. HBV p22 Activates TCF-β-Catenin Transcription

Next, we demonstrated that p22 activates Wnt signaling on its own and can increase Wnt signaling activity in cells, which are stimulated with either Wnt3a or ectopic over-expression of full length, wild type β-catenin (β-cat-WT) (Figure 2a). The stimulatory effect of p22 on reporter activity was dose-dependent (Figure 2b) and decreased at the higher levels of p22 in the presence of β-cat-WT (Figure 2c). Notably, the levels of transcriptionally active non-phosphorylated β-catenin (β-cat-ACT) [21,22] were increased above that seen with β-cat-WT when p22 was co-expressed

(Figures 2d and S4). In the presence of active Wnt signaling, β-catenin escapes phosphorylation and subsequent degradation, and the elevated levels of β-cat-ACT confirm this mechanism for p22 activation of TCF/β-catenin transcription. Data to illustrate the comparative reporter activity between the different conditions is shown in Figure S5.

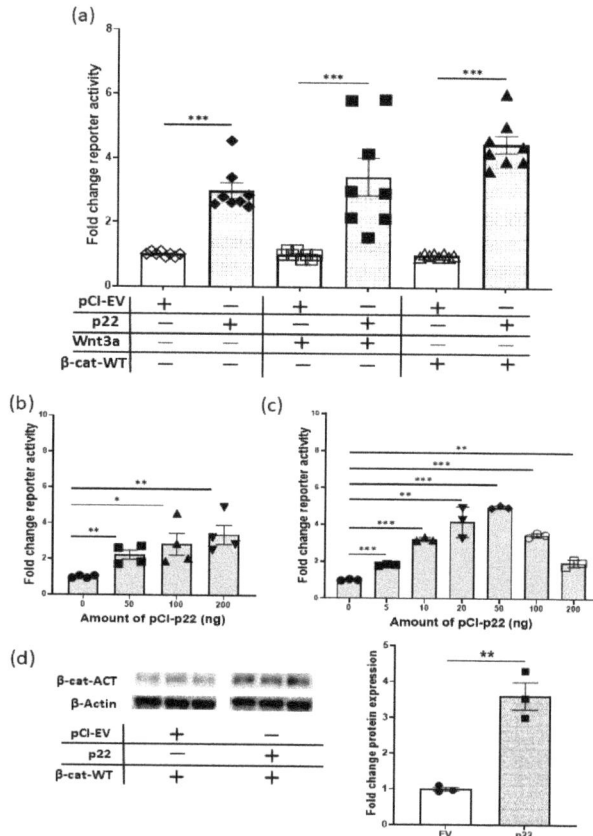

Figure 2. HBV p22 stimulates Wnt signaling in Huh7 cells. (**a**) The effect of HBV p22 alone or in addition to stimulation by Wnt 3a or wildtype β-catenin (β-cat-WT) on TCF/β-catenin transcription in Huh7 cells, was determined by reporter activity (sTOPflash reporter) and is shown as fold change relative to empty vector (EV) (mean ± SEM, *** $p < 0.0001$ Student t-test, $n = 8$ independent experiments). (**b**) Huh7 cells were transfected with the indicated amounts of p22 expression plasmid. The figure shows the dose-dependent effect of HBV p22 on TCF/β-catenin transcription activity (sTOPflash reporter) (mean ± SEM, * $p < 0.05$, ** $p < 0.001$ Student t-test, $n = 4$ independent experiments). (**c**) Huh7 cells were transfected with the indicated amounts of p22 and 100 ng of wild-type β-catenin expression plasmids. Co-expression of 5–50 ng p22 increased TCF/β-catenin transcription activity (sTOPflash reporter) mediated by wild-type β-catenin; reporter activity decreased when 100 or 200 ng p22 was co-transfected with wild-type β-catenin (mean ± SEM, ** $p < 0.001$, *** $p < 0.0001$ Student t-test, $n = 3$ independent experiments). (**d**) Immunoblot analysis for the transcriptionally active form of β-catenin (β-cat-ACT) on lysates prepared from Huh7 cells co-transfected with 100 ng wild-type β-catenin, 100 ng of p22 or equivalent EV expression plasmids. The membrane was stripped and re-probed with anti-actin antibody. The bar graph shows quantitative analysis for the levels of detected active β-catenin using Image Lab software and normalized for β-actin levels (mean ± SEM, ** $p < 0.001$ Student t-test, $n = 3$ samples).

During natural HBV infection, p22 is processed to p17 or HBV e antigen (HBeAg) and secreted into the extracellular space [19]. We confirmed that the transfected p22 is processed to p17 by detecting and quantifying HBeAg in the supernatant of transfected Huh7 cells (Figure S6). Notably, ectopically expressed p17 or p25 did not activate sTOPflash reporter activity above activation by β-catenin (Figure S7).

2.3. HBV p22 Activates Native TCF/β-Catenin Promoters

Next, we tested the ability of p22 to activate native TCF/β-catenin target gene promoters. First, we used our previously characterized Frizzled-7 (FZD7) promoter reporter, pFz7-prom [23]. FZD7 is a TCF/β-catenin target gene [23,24] and forms a positive feedback loop in various cancers, including HCC [25–27]. As shown above with the sTOPflash reporter (Figure 2a), HBV p22 activated the pFz7-prom on its own, and in the context of Wnt3a stimulation or β-cat-WT over-expression (Figure 3a).

Secondly, given that Wnt signaling is dependent on a three-dimentional tissue context [28], we tested the ability of p22 to activate native TCF/β-catenin target gene promoters in the liver in vivo. HBV is an exquisitely human hepatotropic virus and does not infect mouse hepatocytes. However, using hydrodynamic tail vein injection (HDI) plasmids can be introduced into mouse hepatocytes in live animals [29]. A large volume of plasmid containing saline was intravenously injected into mice. This volume overwhelms the heart and is shunted into the hepatic vein and the hepatocytes take up the injected solution (Figure 3b). The mice were culled 6 days and 20 days post HDI and their livers processed for mRNA gene expression analyses using quantitative RT-PCR (qRT-PCR). Expression of Wnt target genes (e.g., Fzd7, Glul) and those that are not target genes (e.g., SOCS3) was determined. At 6 days post-HDI, cyclin D2 and SOCS3 were upregulated by p22 (Figure S8a). Cyclin D2 is upregulated upon activation of Wnt signaling via truncating the *APC* gene and regulates proliferation in this setting [30], suggesting it is a Wnt target gene, however this may be indirect. Fzd7, a Wnt target gene [23,24] shows a trend in upregulation in response to p22 at 6 days post HDI, which was significantly different by 20 days post-HDI (Figures 3c and S8), whilst the expression of another TCF/β-catenin target gene glutamine synthetase (Glul, Figures 3c and S8b) was only upregulated by p22 at day 20, suggesting early and late regulation or signaling thresholds. There were trends towards increased expression of other TCF/β-catenin target genes but these changes did not reach significance (full qRT-PCR gene analyses are shown in Figure S8 and primer sequences in Table S1). Collectively, these data show p22 activates natural promoters of TCF/β-catenin target genes in the context of a human liver cancer cell line Huh7 (Figure 3a) and normal liver hepatocytes in vivo (Figures 3c and S8).

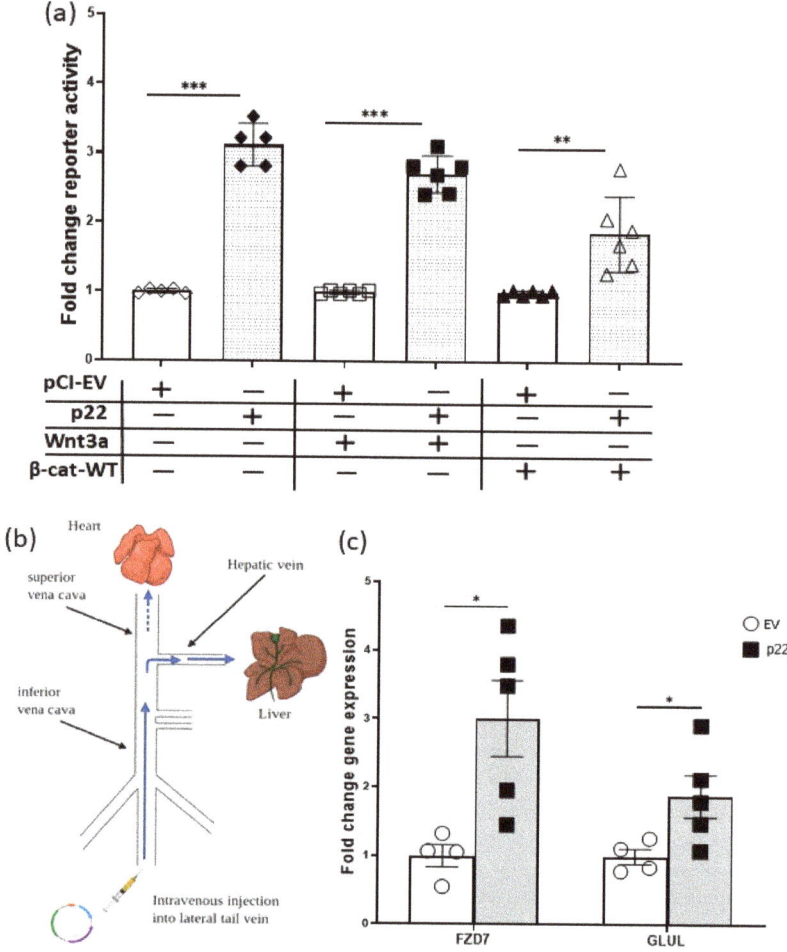

Figure 3. HBV p22 activates TCF/β-target gene native promoters. (**a**) Effect of HBV p22 on FZD7-native promoter reporter activity, with and without stimulation with Wnt3a or 100 ng wild-type β-catenin (β-cat-WT), in Huh7 cells was determined by luciferase activity (pFz7-prom reporter) and is shown as fold change relative to empty vector (EV) (mean ± SEM, ** $p < 0.001$, *** $p < 0.0001$ Student t-test, $n = 6$ independent experiments). (**b**) Schematic diagram of hydrodynamic tail-vein injection in mice (adapted from [31]). (**c**) Expression of TCF/β-target genes Fzd7 and glutamine synthase (Glul) was increased in mouse livers 20 days post HDI injection of p22. Gene expression was determined by qRT-PCR and is shown relative to empty vector (EV) (mean ± SEM, * $p < 0.05$ Student t-test, $n ≥ 4$ mice).

2.4. HBV p22 Activates TCF/β-Catenin Transcription in Addition to a Mutation to Downstream Wnt Pathway Components

Thus far, we have demonstrated that p22 activates TCF/β-catenin transcription on its own and in the context of Wnt stimulation and β-cat-WT over-expression. This mimics one scenario of additional Wnt signaling in cancer i.e., signaling from the ligand-receptor complex. Next, we investigated p22 activity in other cancer contexts, namely in the context of mutant intracellular components that constitutively activate the Wnt pathway i.e., truncated APC and stabilized, mutant β-catenin.

The role of Wnt signaling in cancer has been most extensively studied in colon cancer as Wnt signaling is frequently deregulated in these cancers [32]. Thus, to investigate the effect of p22 in cancer cells with endogenous mutations to intracellular Wnt pathway components, we used colon cancer cell lines SW480 and HCT116 that harbor truncated APC and mutated β-catenin, respectively [18,33]. We also tested the effect of p22 in HEK293T cells that have no known mutations in the Wnt pathway and are known to respond to Wnt [34]. In each cell line (HEK293T, SW480 and HCT116) p22 activated TCF/β-catenin transcription (sTOPflash) above the basal level (Figure 4a).

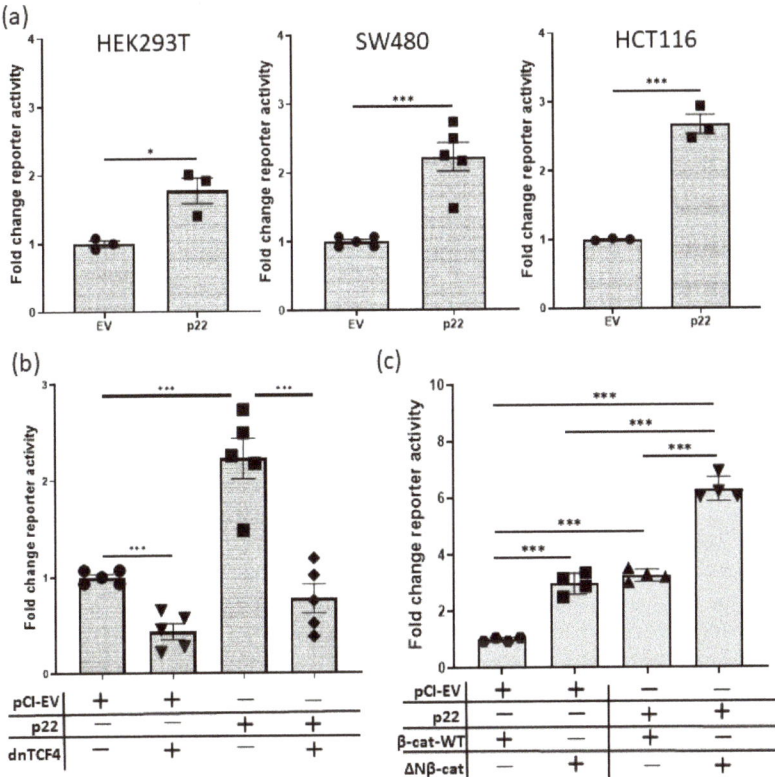

Figure 4. HBV p22 increases TCF/β-catenin signaling in the context of oncogenic activation of the Wnt pathway. (**a**) Effect of 100 ng p22 expression plasmid on TCF/β-catenin transcription activity (sTOPflash reporter) in HEK293T cells with no known mutation or aberrant modulation of Wnt signaling; SW480 cells with truncated, mutant APC, rendering Wnt signaling constitutively active and HCT116 cells with mutation at the N-terminus of β-catenin, making Wnt signaling constitutively active (mean ± SEM, * $p < 0.05$, *** $p < 0.0001$ Student t-test, $n = 3$, 5 and 3 experiments, respectively). Reporter activity is expressed relative to empty vector (EV). (**b**) HBV p22 upregulates TCF/β-catenin transcription (sTOPflash reporter) in the context of truncated APC and this upregulation is blocked by dnTCF4. SW480 cells were co-transfected with 100 ng of p22 and dnTCF4 expression plasmids and the reporter activity is expressed relative to EV (mean ± SEM, *** $p < 0.0001$ Student t-test, $n = 5$ experiments). (**c**) HBV p22 upregulates TCF/β-catenin transcription (sTOPflash reporter) in the context of mutant, oncogenic β-catenin in Huh7 cells. The effect of co-transfection of 100 ng p22 expression plasmid with 100 ng of wild-type or mutant β-catenin on TCF/β-catenin is shown relative to EV (mean ± SEM, *** $p < 0.0001$ t-test, $n = 4$ experiments).

There are four mammalian TCF genes and TCF4 is known to be expressed by SW480 cells [18]. Thus, we tested the ability of a dominant negative form of TCF4 (dnTCF4) [18] to inhibit TCF/β-catenin transcription (sTOPflash) in this cell line. As expected, dnTcf4 decreased constitutive Wnt signaling in SW480 cells. HBV p22 increased Wnt signaling in SW480 cells and this increase was reduced by dnTcf4 (Figure 4b). Collectively, these data show p22 regulates Wnt/β-catenin signaling in the context of genetic mutations that initiate Wnt-addicted cancers.

Next, to further test p22 activity in the context of mutant β-catenin compared to β-cat-WT, we used the N-terminally truncated, oncogenic form of β-catenin (ΔN-β-cat) that lacks the regulatory domains [33]. ΔN-β-Cat increased TCF/β-catenin transcription (sTOPflash) above β-cat-WT to a similar level as p22, while ΔN-β-cat and p22 together elevated reporter activity above either alone (Figure 4c). Data to illustrate comparative reporter activity between some of these different conditions is shown in Figure S5.

3. Discussion

The emerging theme for Wnt-addicted cancers is that the pathway is regulated via multiple mechanisms [16]. This has been extensively investigated in colon cancer. Colon cancers frequently harbor truncating mutations to *APC* that yield proteins with impeded function in degrading β-catenin; or oncogenic mutations to the *CTNNB1* gene that remove the destruction complex phosphorylation sites in the N-terminus of β-catenin [35]. The end result of either mutation is the constitutive activation of Wnt signaling and adenoma formation [6,18,33,36,37]. However, Wnt signaling is also deregulated at the level of the ligand/receptor in colon cancer. Naturally occurring inhibitors of Wnt-FZD interaction are silenced by promoter hypermethylation, while Wnts and FZDs are over-expressed (reviewed in [15,25]). Thus, transcription of TCF/β-catenin target genes can be increased or decreased despite a mutation to downstream components of the pathway. Indeed, all Wnt-addicted cancers show concomitant deregulation to Wnt signaling via intracellular and cell surface mechanisms [16]. Consistent with this, a potent anti-tumor effect was demonstrated by blocking FZD7 function in gastric cancer cells with and without mutant *APC* [38].

Notably, liver cancer displays similar Wnt-addicted mechanisms to colon and gastric cancer [16]. Constitutive activation of Wnt signaling in HCC is primarily via mutations to the *CTNNB1* gene that remove the regulatory phosphorylation sites from the N-terminus of β-catenin [3]. However, as in colon and gastric cancer, there is additional regulation of the pathway via over-expression of Wnts and FZDs and epigenetic silencing of naturally occurring inhibitors of Wnt-FZD interaction, for example secreted frizzled related proteins (sFRP) [16,39]. Furthermore, most cases of HCC have a viral etiology and are the culmination of chronic infection with HBV leading to liver disease where HBV proteins, such as HBx, are hypothesized to exert their oncogenic activity, at least in part, through activation of Wnt/β-catenin signaling [8]. Here, we screened the various HBV proteins for their impact on Wnt signaling and demonstrated that another HBV protein, p22, was more potent than HBx. HBV surface proteins (small, middle or large) did not activate TCF/β-catenin transcription. Interestingly, the other pre-core/core proteins (p25, p21 or p17) also did not activate TCF/β-catenin transcription despite significant overlap in their amino acid sequence with p22. Clinical studies show HBe-positivity is a significant independent risk factor of HCC and fatality in chronic HBV-infected patients [40,41]. Furthermore, HBe is produced within the first week after HBV infection in experimental models [42], and thus p22 has the potential to contribute to early events in the transition to cancer. Here, we showed ectopically expressed p22 was localized diffusely in the cytoplasm and nucleus, and in cytoplasmic puncta, indicating potential co-localization with various levels of the Wnt signaling machinery [20]. We also demonstrated Fzd7 and GLUL are induced by p22 in vivo; this shows that genes associate with liver cancer (*Fzd7* [39]) and β-catenin-mediated liver zonation and regeneration (*GLUL*, [43]) are induced by p22 in normal hepatocytes. Furthermore, we demonstrated that p22 can increase TCF/β-catenin transcription on its own and in conjunction with ectopically expressed wild-type or mutant β-catenin; and in colon cancer cells with endogenous mutant *APC* (SW480 cells) or *CTNNB1* (HCT116 cells). Activation of TCF/β-catenin transcription in the SW480 cells by p22 was blocked by dnTCF4, confirming impact specifically on Wnt signaling.

Collectively, our data identifies HBV p22 as a novel regulator of Wnt signaling in the context of cancer and provides insight into the mechanisms of 'just right' Wnt signaling in cancer. Identifying the molecular interactors of p22 will not only be relevant to HCC but to all Wnt-addicted cancers as it is a new tool to investigate context-dependent Wnt signaling. Immunohistochemical studies in colon cancer carcinomas show variable β-catenin staining where β-catenin is primarily membrane-bound in central areas of the tumor, and intense cytoplasmic and nuclear staining in localized regions that are referred to as the invasive front associated with metastasis [44,45]. This implies that Wnt signaling is constrained in cancer cells allowing for bursts of intense signaling for various processes such as metastasis. It remains to be determined if this localized hyperactive Wnt signaling is due to loss of transcriptional repression or activation of transcription. Further investigation of the p22 mechanism of action in ex vivo models systems for example that do not have the limitations of continuous, transformed cell lines and mouse models with respect to human disease [27], might reveal novel avenues of research to help identify new components to selectively harness different aspects of Wnt signaling; for example, blocking oncogenic Wnt signaling while preserving the critical role Wnt signaling provides to ensure the correct regulation of stem cells and homeostasis of many epithelial tissues. Selective regulation of Wnt signaling is at the core of identifying druggable Wnt pathway targets, as the desired outcome for a cancer specific drug that inhibits Wnt is for the drug to allow normal physiological processes to proceed thus reducing the toxicity of a blanket approach of inhibiting Wnt signaling.

4. Materials and Methods

4.1. Hydrodynamic Injection of Mice

C57BL/6 mice used in experiments were between 6 and 10 weeks old, and age- and sex-matched (both sexes were used). Hydrodynamic injection (HDI) was performed as we previously described [29]. Briefly, unanesthetized mice were injected intravenously (iv) through the tail vein with 10 μg pCI-p22 or pCI-EV (pCI, Promega, Madison, WI, USA) in a volume of saline equivalent to 8% of the mouse body weight. The injection was performed within 5 s. Mice were killed 6- and 20-days post HDI, their liver resected and processed for analysis. The Walter and Eliza Hall Institute of Medical Research Animal Ethics Committee (AEC) reviewed and approved all animal experiments (AEC number 2017.016).

4.2. RNA Extraction and Quantitative RT-PCR (qRT-PCR)

Mouse liver tissues were homogenized in TRizol (Invitrogen, Carlsbad, CA, USA) and total RNA purified, DNAse treated and quantified as previously described [46]. cDNA was synthesized and subjected to qPCR using SYBR green (ABI). Gene expression was calculated relative to the housekeeping gene β2M ($2^{-\Delta\Delta Ct}$) as described previously [46] and was expressed as fold change over empty vector (EV).

4.3. Cell Lines and Wnt3a Conditioned Medium

The human cell lines (SW480, HCT116, HEK293T and Huh7) were purchased from ATCC. SW480, HCT116 and HEK293T were maintained in RPMI-1640 supplemented with 20 mM HEPES, 10% (v/v) heat-inactivated fetal bovine serum (FBS), L-glutamine and antibiotics (penicillin and streptomycin). Wnt3a producing L-cells (L-3a) and the parental L-cells (L) were a generous gift from Prof Karl Willert [34]. L-3a, L and the Huh7 cells were maintained in DMEM, 10% (v/v) heat-inactivated FBS, supplemented with L-glutamine and antibiotics. Conditioned medium was prepared from L-3a and L cells in parallel as previously described [34].

4.4. Transfection and Reporter Assays

Cells were seeded into 24-well plates to reach 60–70% confluence overnight. Cells were transfected with 400 ng total plasmid (empty vector added to keep total plasmid constant) that included 100 ng sTOPflash or sFOPflash (generous gift from Prof Randall T Moon [17]); or 100 ng pGL or pGL-FZD7 promoter [23] and 2 ng *Renilla* luciferase plasmid (phRG-TK, Promega). The pDNA3.1 plasmids expressing β-catenin, ΔNβ-catenin and dnTCF4 were generous gifts from Professor Hans Clevers [18,22] and added at 100 ng/well. The pCI HBV protein expression plasmids were a generous gift from Professor Stephen Locarnini and added at 100 ng, unless indicated otherwise in the text. Cells were transfected using plasmids in OptiMEM (Life Technologies, Grand Island, NY, USA) and Lipofectamine LTX with Plus reagent (Invitrogen) according to the manufacturer's instructions. Cells were harvested 48 h later and analyzed using the dual luciferase reporter assay system (Promega). For Wnt3a stimulation, cells were treated with 200 µl L-3a or L conditioned medium for 6 h before harvesting in passive lysis buffer. Luciferase activity with control reporters sFOPflash and pGL, and L conditioned medium were negligible. Reporter activity was expressed relative to *Renilla* to the control for transfection efficiency and plotted as fold change over empty vector (EV) as previously described [38].

4.5. Immunoblot Analysis

Pre-cast 4–20% polyacrylamide gels (Mini-Protein TGX, Biorad, Hercules, CA, USA were used to separate proteins (Mini-Protein Tetra Cell, Biorad) and transferred onto nitrocellulose membranes using the Transblot-Turbo instrument (Biorad). The membranes were air-dried and blocked overnight in 1% skim milk at 4 °C. The following day, the membranes were incubated in primary antibody for 1 h and bound antibody detected with secondary antibody and ECL (Western Lightening Plus ECL, Perkin Elmer, Waltham, MA, USA). Primary antibody used were mouse anti-HBcAg [C1] (1:1000, Abcam ab8637, Cambridge, UK), mouse anti-αTubulin (1:1000, Abcam ab7291), mouse anti-active β-catenin (1:1000, Merck Millipore 05-665) and mouse anti-β-actin (1:5000, ThermoFisher AM4302, Waltham, MA, USA). Secondary antibody was rabbit anti-mouse polyclonal antibody HRP (1:10,000 Dako P0260, Glostrup, Denmark).

4.6. Immunofluorescenc Confocal Microscopy

Cells were seeded into two-well Nunc Lab-Tek (Thermofisher) chamber slides to reach 60–70% confluence overnight. Cells were transfected with 200 ng plasmid as described above. After 48 h, cells were fixed with 4% paraformaldehyde, permeabilized with 1% Triton-X100 and blocked with 1% FBS and stained with control antibody or anti-HBcAg [C1] (1:400, Abcam ab8637) primary antibody and detected with goat anti-mouse alexa fluor 488 (1:1000 Invitrogen A11029). DAPI (1:2000) was used for nuclear staining and the cells analyzed using Zeiss LSM700 as previously described [38].

4.7. Statistical Analysis

The data represent mean ± SEM, where n is at least three independent experiments with cell lines or tissue from at least three mice per cohort, unless stated otherwise. The Student t-test was used for comparisons and significance was defined as $p < 0.5$.

5. Conclusions

Mutations to *APC* and *CTNNB1* are the most frequent mutations in colon and liver cancer, respectively, and are thought to initiate cancer. Here we demonstrate that the HBV precore protein p22 can activate Wnt signaling in these cancer contexts. The ability of p22 to additionally activate Wnt signaling in the context of these mutations indicates oncogenic interplay between HBV infection and Wnt signaling in liver cancer. Furthermore, it is now clear that Wnt-addicted cancers harbor aberrations to Wnt signaling via both intracellular and cell-surface mechanisms [16], thus our findings identify HBV p22 as a novel tool to understand "additional" regulation and "fine-tuning" of Wnt signaling in the context of cancer [14,25]. Understanding the mechanisms that underly normal, wanted Wnt signaling and pathological, unwanted Wnt signaling is an important step for exploiting the Wnt pathway for anti-cancer treatment.

Supplementary Materials: The following are available online at http://www.mdpi.com/2072-6694/12/6/1435/s1, Figure S1: Schematic of the HBV genome and the genes encoding various HBV proteins. The HBV genome, depicted as a long purple continuous strand, encodes 7 proteins from 4 open reading frames (ORFs) (surface [S], core [C], polymerase [P], and the X gene [X]), which are shown as large arrows in different colors, and 3 upstream regions [precore (preC), preS1, and preS2]. The transcripts, ORFs, gene regions and protein products are also shown on the right, Figure S2: Expression of protein from the indicated plasmids. Huh7 cells were transfected with the indicated plasmids and protein expression confirmed by immunoblot. Lysates prepared from Huh7 cells transfected with EV and the parental, un-transfected cells served as negative controls. Lysate from HBV core p21 transfected Huh7 cells was used as a positive control. (**a**) The membrane was stained with anti-HBc antibody first, then (**b**) re-probed with anti-tubulin antibody. The boxed areas were used for the cropped blots in Figure 1, Figure S3: Sub-cellular localization of HBV p22. The indicated expression plasmids were transfected into Huh7 and the cells subjected to confocal microscopy following staining with control anti-body and anti-HBV core antibody (red, while DAPI stained nuclei are blue). A higher magnification of the boxed area of the p22 transfected cells is also shown. Scale bars = 20 μM, Figure S4: HBV p22 stimulates Wnt signaling in Huh7 cells. Huh7 cells were co-transfected with 100 ng wild-type β-catenin and the indicated amounts of p22 plasmid and the cell lysates subjected to immunoblot for (**a**) active β-catenin. The membrane was stripped and re-probed with (**b**) anti-actin antibody. The boxed regions in (a) and (b) were used the cropped immunoblots in Figure 2d, Figure S5: Comparative reporter activity in Huh7 cells across the various conditions. The TOPflash and FOPflash reporter activities in Huh7 cells transfected with the indicated plasmids and treated with the indicated conditioned media [L-cell conditioned medium (CM) or L-cell-Wnt3a conditioned medium (Wnt3a CM)] are plotted on the same Y-axis to demonstrate the relative reporter activity between controls [(FOPflash, CM, empty vector (EV)] and test samples (TOPflash, expression plasmids, Wnt3a CM) and are shown as fold change reporter activity relative to FOPflash/EV (Mean ± SEM, Student t test, $n = 3$ experiments). Reporter activity in control samples was negligible, Figure S6: Quantitation of HBeAg levels in the supernatant of transfected Huh7 cells. HBeAg levels in the supernatant fluid of transfected cells were determined (**a**) two days and (**b**) three days after transfection using a commercial Roche anti-HBe kit and Cobas e411 instrument. Cells were transfected with increasing amounts of HBV p22-containing plasmid, from 0 - 200 ng per well, with or without co-transfected 100 ng wild type β-catenin (Mean ± SD, $n = 3$ replicate wells). Transfected p22 was processed to HBeAg and detected in the supernatant, confirming normal processing, Figure S7: Effect HBV p25 and p17 on Wnt signalling. Effect of increasing amounts of transfected HBV precore p17 (**a**) and p25 (**b**) expression plasmids on TCF/β-catenin transcription (sTOPflash reporter) in Huh7 cells co-transfected with 100 ng wild type β-catenin was determined and is shown relative to no p17 and p25, respectively (Mean ± SEM, * $p < 0.05$, Student *t*-test, $n = 3$ experiments), Figure S8: HBV p22 upregulates gene expression in vivo. (**a**) Quantitative RT-PCR analysis of gene expression in livers of mice tail-vein-injected with EV or HBV p22 containing plasmids at 6 days post injection (mean ± SEM, * $p < 0.05$, $n = 7$ and 8 for EV and p22 injected mice, respectively). (**b**) Quantitative RT-PCR analysis of gene expression in livers of mice tail-vein-injected with EV or p22 containing plasmids at 20 days post injection (mean ± SEM, * $p < 0.05$, $n = 4$ and 5 for EV and p22 injected mice, respectively), Table S1: qRT-PCR Primer sequences.

Author Contributions: Conceptualization, B.M.T.; T.J.P.; and E.V.; formal analysis, B.M.T.; D.J.F.; T.J.P.; and E.V.; funding acquisition, D.J.F.; G.E.; N.W.; H.T.; T.F.; C.C.; J.T.; and E.V.; investigation, B.M.T.; D.J.F.; and G.E.; methodology, B.M.T.; D.J.F.; G.E.; T.J.P.; and E.V.; resources, N.W.; H.T.; T.F.; C.C.; M.P.; and J.T.; supervision, E.V.; visualization, B.M.T.; D.J.F.; and E.V.; writing—original draft, B.M.T.; and E.V.; writing—review and editing, D.J.F.; N.W.; H.T.; T.F.; C.C.; M.P.; and T.J.P. All authors have read and agreed to the published version of the manuscript.

Funding: This research was funded by Melbourne Health through a project grant number PG-002-2016 awarded to E.V.; T.J.P.; G.E.; N.W.; T.F.; and C.C.; and a post-graduate scholarship to B.M.T.; E.V.; and T.J.P. were funded, in part, by grants from the National Health and Medical Research Council (NHMRC), project grant number APP1099302 and investigator grant number APP1181580. T.J.P. was funded by BLS/CMU Fellowship and MRC (MR/R026424/1). D.J.F.; was funded, in part, by a Cancer Council of Victoria fellowship and a Melbourne Health early career grant GIA-033-2016.

Acknowledgments: We thank Damian Neate, Danni Colledge and Jean Moselen for technical assistance. We also thank Randall T. Moon, Hans Clevers, Thomas Brabletz, Peter Revill, Stephen Locarnini and Karl Willert for gifting cell lines and plasmids; and the staff at the Walter and Eliza Hall Institute Biological Resource Facility (mice) and the Biological Optical Microscopy Platform (BOMP), University of Melbourne for their assistance.

Conflicts of Interest: The authors declare no conflicts of interest.

References

1. Cancer Research UK. Liver Cancer Statisitcs. Available online: https://www.cancerresearchuk.org/health-professional/cancer-statistics/statistics-by-cancer-type/liver-cancer (accessed on 10 September 2019).
2. Llovet, J.M.; Ricci, S.; Mazzaferro, V.; Hilgard, P.; Gane, E.; Blanc, J.F.; De Oliveira, A.C.; Santoro, A.; Raoul, J.L.; Forner, A.; et al. Sorafenib in advanced hepatocellular carcinoma. *N. Engl. J. Med.* **2008**, *359*, 378–390. [CrossRef] [PubMed]

3. Schulze, K.; Imbeaud, S.; Letouzé, E.; Alexandrov, L.B.; Calderaro, J.; Rebouissou, S.; Couchy, G.; Meiller, C.; Shinde, J.; Soysouvanh, F.; et al. Exome sequencing of hepatocellular carcinomas identifies new mutational signatures and potential therapeutic targets. *Nat. Genet* **2015**, *47*, 505–511. [CrossRef] [PubMed]
4. De La Coste, A.; Romagnolo, B.; Billuart, P.; Renard, C.A.; Buendia, M.A.; Soubrane, O.; Fabre, M.; Chelly, J.; Beldjord, C.; Kahn, A.; et al. Somatic mutations of the beta-catenin gene are frequent in mouse and human hepatocellular carcinomas. *Proc. Natl. Acad. Sci. USA* **1998**, *95*, 8847–8851. [CrossRef]
5. Nusse, R.; Clevers, H. Wnt/beta-Catenin Signaling, Disease, and Emerging Therapeutic Modalities. *Cell* **2017**, *169*, 985–999. [CrossRef] [PubMed]
6. Van Noort, M.; van de Wetering, M.; Clevers, H. Identification of Two Novel Regulated Serines in the N Terminus of beta-Catenin. *Exp. Cell Res.* **2002**, *276*, 264–272. [CrossRef] [PubMed]
7. Ding, Y.; Dale, T. Wnt signal transduction: Kinase cogs in a nano-machine? *Trends Biochem. Sci.* **2002**, *27*, 327–329. [CrossRef]
8. Levrero, M.; Zucman-Rossi, J. Mechanisms of HBV-induced hepatocellular carcinoma. *J. Hepatol.* **2016**, *64* (Suppl. 1), S84–S101. [CrossRef]
9. Lyou, Y.; Habowski, A.N.; Chen, G.T.; Waterman, M.L. Inhibition of nuclear Wnt signalling: Challenges of an elusive target for cancer therapy. *Br. J. Pharmacol.* **2017**, *174*, 4589–4599. [CrossRef]
10. Kim, S.S.; Cho, H.J.; Lee, H.Y.; Park, J.H.; Noh, C.K.; Shin, S.J.; Lee, K.M.; Yoo, B.M.; Lee, K.J.; Cho, S.W.; et al. Genetic polymorphisms in the Wnt/beta-catenin pathway genes as predictors of tumor development and survival in patients with hepatitis B virus-associated hepatocellular carcinoma. *Clin. Biochem.* **2016**, *49*, 792–801. [CrossRef]
11. MacLachlan, J.H.; Locarnini, S.; Cowie, B.C. Estimating the global prevalence of hepatitis B. *Lancet* **2015**, *386*, 1515–1517. [CrossRef]
12. Garcia, P.D.; Ou, J.H.; Rutter, W.J.; Walter, P. Targeting of the hepatitis B virus precore protein to the endoplasmic reticulum membrane: After signal peptide cleavage translocation can be aborted and the product released into the cytoplasm. *J. Cell Biol.* **1988**, *106*, 1093–1104. [CrossRef] [PubMed]
13. Geng, M.; Xin, X.; Bi, L.Q.; Zhou, L.T.; Liu, X.H. Molecular mechanism of hepatitis B virus X protein function in hepatocarcinogenesis. *World J. Gastroenterol.* **2015**, *21*, 10732–10738. [CrossRef] [PubMed]
14. Flanagan, D.J.; Vincan, E.; Phesse, T.J. Winding back Wnt signalling: Potential therapeutic targets for treating gastric cancers. *Br. J. Pharmacol.* **2017**, *174*, 4666–4683. [CrossRef] [PubMed]
15. Vincan, E.; Barker, N. The upstream components of the Wnt signalling pathway in the dynamic EMT and MET associated with colorectal cancer progression. *Clin. Exp. Metastasis* **2008**, *25*, 657–663. [CrossRef]
16. Flanagan, D.J.; Vincan, E.; Phesse, T.J. Wnt Signaling in Cancer: Not a Binary ON: OFF Switch. *Cancer Res.* **2019**, *79*, 5901–5906. [CrossRef]
17. Biechele, T.L.; Moon, R.T. Assaying beta-catenin/TCF transcription with beta-catenin/TCF transcription-based reporter constructs. *Methods Mol. Biol.* **2008**, *468*, 99–110.
18. Korinek, V.; Barker, N.; Morin, P.J.; Van Wichen, D.; De Weger, R.; Kinzler, K.W.; Vogelstein, B.; Clevers, H. Constitutive transcriptional activation by a beta-catenin-Tcf complex in APC-/- colon carcinoma. *Science* **1997**, *275*, 1784–1787. [CrossRef]
19. Mitra, B.; Wang, J.; Kim, E.S.; Mao, R.; Dong, M.; Liu, Y.; Zhang, J.; Guo, H. Hepatitis B Virus Precore Protein p22 Inhibits Alpha Interferon Signaling by Blocking STAT Nuclear Translocation. *J. Virol.* **2019**, *93*, e00196-19. [CrossRef]
20. Gammons, M.; Bienz, M. Multiprotein complexes governing Wnt signal transduction. *Curr. Opin. Cell Biol.* **2018**, *51*, 42–49. [CrossRef]
21. Van Noort, M.; Meeldijk, J.; van der Zee, R.; Destree, O.; Clevers, H. Wnt signaling controls the phosphorylation status of beta-catenin. *J. Biol. Chem.* **2002**, *277*, 17901–17905. [CrossRef]
22. Van Noort, M.; Weerkamp, F.; Clevers, H.C.; Staal, F.J. Wnt signaling and phosphorylation status of beta-catenin: Importance of the correct antibody tools. *Blood* **2007**, *110*, 2778–2779. [CrossRef] [PubMed]
23. Vincan, E.; Flanagan, D.J.; Pouliot, N.; Brabletz, T.; Spaderna, S. Variable FZD7 expression in colorectal cancers indicates regulation by the tumour microenvironment. *Dev. Dyn.* **2010**, *239*, 311–317. [CrossRef] [PubMed]
24. Willert, J.; Epping, M.; Pollack, J.R.; Brown, P.O.; Nusse, R. A transcriptional response to Wnt protein in human embryonic carcinoma cells. *BMC Dev. Biol.* **2002**, *2*, 8–15. [CrossRef] [PubMed]

25. Phesse, T.; Flanagan, D.; Vincan, E. Frizzled7: A Promising Achilles' Heel for Targeting the Wnt Receptor Complex to Treat Cancer. *Cancers* **2016**, *8*, 50. [CrossRef]
26. Merle, P.; Kim, M.; Herrmann, M.; Gupte, A.; Lefrançois, L.; Califano, S.; Tre, C.; Tanaka, S.; Vitvitski, L.; de la Monte, S.; et al. Oncogenic role of the frizzled-7/beta-catenin pathway in hepatocellular carcinoma. *J. Hepatol.* **2005**, *43*, 854–862. [CrossRef]
27. Torresi, J.; Tran, B.M.; Christiansen, D.; Earnest-Silveira, L.; Schwab, R.H.M.; Vincan, E. HBV-related hepatocarcinogenesis: The role of signalling pathways and innovative ex vivo research models. *BMC Cancer* **2019**, *19*, 707. [CrossRef]
28. Van Amerongen, R.; Nusse, R. Towards an integrated view of Wnt signaling in development. *Development* **2009**, *136*, 3205–3214. [CrossRef]
29. Ebert, G.; Preston, S.; Allison, C.; Cooney, J.; Toe, J.G.; Stutz, M.D.; Ojaimi, S.; Scott, H.W.; Baschuk, N.; Nachbur, U.; et al. Cellular inhibitor of apoptosis proteins prevent clearance of hepatitis B virus. *Proc. Natl. Acad. Sci. USA* **2015**, *112*, 5797–5802. [CrossRef]
30. Cole, A.M.; Myant, K.; Reed, K.R.; Ridgway, R.A.; Athineos, D.; Van den Brink, G.R.; Muncan, V.; Clevers, H.; Clarke, A.R.; Sicinski, P.; et al. Cyclin D2-cyclin-dependent kinase 4/6 is required for efficient proliferation and tumorigenesis following Apc loss. *Cancer Res.* **2010**, *70*, 8149–8158. [CrossRef]
31. Casari, C.; Lenting, P.J.; Christophe, O.D.; Denis, C.V. Von Willebrand Factor Abnormalities Studied in the Mouse Model: What We Learned about VWF Functions. *Mediterr. J. Hematol. Infect. Dis.* **2013**, *5*, e2013047. [CrossRef]
32. Zhan, T.; Rindtorff, N.; Boutros, M. Wnt signaling in cancer. *Oncogene* **2017**, *36*, 1461–1473. [CrossRef] [PubMed]
33. Morin, P.J.; Sparks, A.B.; Korinek, V.; Barker, N.; Clevers, H.; Vogelstein, B.; Kinzler, K.W. Activation of beta-catenin-Tcf signaling in colon cancer by mutations in beta-catenin or APC. *Science* **1997**, *275*, 1787–1790. [CrossRef] [PubMed]
34. Willert, K.; Brown, J.D.; Danenberg, E.; Duncan, A.W.; Weissman, I.L.; Reya, T.; Yates, J.R.; Nusse, R. Wnt proteins are lipid-modified and can act as stem cell growth factors. *Nature* **2003**, *423*, 448–452. [CrossRef] [PubMed]
35. Cancer Genome Atlas Network. Comprehensivemolecular characterization of human colon and rectal cancer. *Nature* **2012**, *487*, 330–337. [CrossRef]
36. Harada, N.; Tamai, Y.; Ishikawa, T.O.; Sauer, B.; Takaku, K.; Oshima, M.; Taketo, M.M. Intestinal polyposis in mice with a dominant stable mutation of the beta-catenin gene. *EMBO J.* **1999**, *18*, 5931–5942. [CrossRef]
37. Su, L.K.; Kinzler, K.W.; Vogelstein, B.; Preisinger, A.C.; Moser, A.R.; Luongo, C.; Gould, K.A.; Dove, W.F. Multiple intestinal neoplasia caused by a mutation in the murine homolog of the APC gene. *Science* **1992**, *256*, 668–670. [CrossRef]
38. Flanagan, D.J.; Barker, N.; Di Costanzo, N.S.; Mason, E.A.; Gurney, A.; Meniel, V.S.; Koushyar, S.; Austin, C.R.; Ernst, M.; Pearson, H.B.; et al. Frizzled-7 Is Required for Wnt Signaling in Gastric Tumors with and Without Apc Mutations. *Cancer Res.* **2019**, *79*, 970–981. [CrossRef]
39. Bengochea, A.; De Souza, M.M.; Lefrancois, L.; Le Roux, E.; Galy, O.; Chemin, I.; Kim, M.; Wands, J.R.; Trepo, C.; Hainaut, P.; et al. Common dysregulation of Wnt/Frizzled receptor elements in human hepatocellular carcinoma. *Br. J. Cancer* **2008**, *99*, 143–150. [CrossRef]
40. Yang, H.I.; Lu, S.N.; Liaw, Y.F.; You, S.L.; Sun, C.A.; Wang, L.Y.; Hsiao, C.K.; Chen, P.J.; Chen, D.S.; Chen, C.J. Hepatitis B e antigen and the risk of hepatocellular carcinoma. *N. Engl. J. Med.* **2002**, *347*, 168–174. [CrossRef]
41. You, S.L.; Yang, H.I.; Chen, C.J. Seropositivity of hepatitis B e antigen and hepatocellular carcinoma. *Ann. Med.* **2004**, *36*, 215–224. [CrossRef]
42. Yan, H.; Zhong, G.; Xu, G.; He, W.; Jing, Z.; Gao, Z.; Huang, Y.; Qi, Y.; Peng, B.; Wang, H.; et al. Sodium taurocholate cotransporting polypeptide is a functional receptor for human hepatitis B and D virus. *eLife* **2012**, *1*, e00049. [CrossRef] [PubMed]
43. Burke, Z.D.; Reed, K.R.; Phesse, T.J.; Sansom, O.J.; Clarke, A.R.; Tosh, D. Liver zonation occurs through a beta-catenin-dependent, c-Myc-independent mechanism. *Gastroenterology* **2009**, *136*, e1–e3. [CrossRef] [PubMed]
44. Brabletz, T.; Jung, A.; Hermann, K.; Günther, K.; Hohenberger, W.; Kirchner, T. Nuclear overexpression of the oncoprotein beta-catenin in colorectal cancer is localized predominantly at the invasion front. *Pathol. Res. Pract.* **1998**, *194*, 701–704. [CrossRef]

45. Brabletz, T.; Jung, A.; Reu, S.; Porzner, M.; Hlubek, F.; Kunz-Schughart, L.A.; Knuechel, R.; Kirchner, T. Variable beta-catenin expression in colorectal cancers indicates tumor progression driven by the tumor environment. *Proc. Natl. Acad. Sci. USA* **2001**, *98*, 10356–10361. [CrossRef]
46. Vincan, E.; Darcy, P.K.; Farrelly, C.A.; Faux, M.C.; Brabletz, T.; Ramsay, R.G. Frizzled-7 dictates three-dimensional organization of colorectal cancer cell carcinoids. *Oncogene* **2007**, *26*, 2340–2352. [CrossRef]

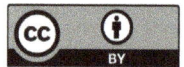

© 2020 by the authors. Licensee MDPI, Basel, Switzerland. This article is an open access article distributed under the terms and conditions of the Creative Commons Attribution (CC BY) license (http://creativecommons.org/licenses/by/4.0/).

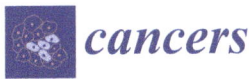

Review

β-Catenin Activation in Hepatocellular Cancer: Implications in Biology and Therapy

Yekaterina Krutsenko, Aatur D. Singhi and Satdarshan P. Monga *

Department of Pathology and Pittsburgh Liver Research Center, University of Pittsburgh and University of Pittsburgh Medical Center, Pittsburgh, PA 15261, USA; yek14@pitt.edu (Y.K.); singhiad@upmc.edu (A.D.S.)
* Correspondence: smonga@pitt.edu; Tel.: +1-(412)-648-9966; Fax: +1-(412)-648-1916

Simple Summary: Liver cancer is a dreadful tumor which has gradually increased in incidence all around the world. One major driver of liver cancer is the Wnt–β-catenin pathway which is active in a subset of these tumors. While this pathway is normally important in liver development, regeneration and homeostasis, it's excessive activation due to mutations, is detrimental and leads to tumor cell growth, making it an important therapeutic target. There are also some unique characteristics of this pathway activation in liver cancer. It makes the tumor addicted to specific amino acids and in turn to mTOR signaling, which can be treated by certain existing therapies. In addition, activation of the Wnt–β-catenin in liver cancer appears to alter the immune cell landscape making it less likely to respond to the new immuno-oncology treatments. Thus, Wnt–β-catenin active tumors may need to be treated differently than non-Wnt–β-catenin active tumors.

Abstract: Hepatocellular cancer (HCC), the most common primary liver tumor, has been gradually growing in incidence globally. The whole-genome and whole-exome sequencing of HCC has led to an improved understanding of the molecular drivers of this tumor type. Activation of the Wnt signaling pathway, mostly due to stabilizing missense mutations in its downstream effector β-catenin (encoded by *CTNNB1*) or loss-of-function mutations in *AXIN1* (the gene which encodes for Axin-1, an essential protein for β-catenin degradation), are seen in a major subset of HCC. Because of the important role of β-catenin in liver pathobiology, its role in HCC has been extensively investigated. In fact, *CTNNB1* mutations have been shown to have a trunk role. β-Catenin has been shown to play an important role in regulating tumor cell proliferation and survival and in tumor angiogenesis, due to a host of target genes regulated by the β-catenin transactivation of its transcriptional factor TCF. Proof-of-concept preclinical studies have shown β-catenin to be a highly relevant therapeutic target in *CTNNB1*-mutated HCCs. More recently, studies have revealed a unique role of β-catenin activation in regulating both tumor metabolism as well as the tumor immune microenvironment. Both these roles have notable implications for the development of novel therapies for HCC. Thus, β-catenin has a pertinent role in driving HCC development and maintenance of this tumor-type, and could be a highly relevant therapeutic target in a subset of HCC cases.

Keywords: β-catenin mutations; tumor metabolism; tumor immunology; molecular therapeutics; precision medicine

1. The Wnt–β-Catenin Signaling Pathway

The protein later termed Wnt1 was first identified almost 40 years ago in the context of its proto-oncogenic nature [1,2]. Subsequent studies have characterized Wnt1 itself, as well as other highly conserved components of Wnt signaling, as a key mediator involved not only in tumorigenesis, but also in the fundamental cellular processes governing embryonic development and adult tissue homeostasis [3,4]. Yet, the vital role of aberrant Wnt signaling in cancer initiation and progression remains one of the most intriguing and vital themes in the field. The Wnt pathway involves a multitude of components,

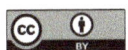

including ligands, receptors, and co-receptors acting in autocrine, paracrine, and endocrine fashion to regulate the processes of cell fate determination, proliferation, and polarity, among others [2,4,5]. Structural and functional classification has indicated the existence of several distinct Wnt signaling pathways, which can be broadly subdivided based on the involvement of β-catenin. β-Catenin-dependent canonical Wnt signaling remains arguably the most investigated branch.

In the canonical pathway, the control of the Wnt-dependent cellular processes is achieved by a tight regulation of the amount of β-catenin—a transcriptional co-activator and a regulator of cell–cell adhesion. Normally, in the absence of Wnt signals, cytosolic levels of β-catenin remain low due to continuous proteasomal degradation of the protein, initiated by its destruction complex. The complex, composed of the scaffold Axin, tumor-suppressor adenomatous polyposis coli (APC) gene product, and diversin, also includes two kinases, casein kinase 1 (CK1), and glycogen synthase kinase 3 (GSK3), which sequentially phosphorylate β-catenin, priming it for recognition by the ubiquitin ligase β-TrCP [1]. In the absence of negative regulation, the glycosylation and palmitoylation of Wnt glycoproteins allows their biological activity to in turn activate the Wnt–β-catenin signaling. The cascade is induced by the binding of secreted Wnts to the seven transmembrane G-protein-coupled Frizzled (Fz) receptors located at the plasma membrane [5]. The binding initiates the formation of a multicomponent complex consisting of Wnt ligand, Frizzled, and its co-receptor LRP (low-density lipoprotein receptor-related protein) 6 or 5 [6]. This, in turn, signals for the recruitment of Dishevelled (Dvl), and results in the phosphorylation of LRP5/6, thereby providing a docking site for the Axin and tethering it to the cell membrane, which eventually renders the β-catenin destruction complex inactive. Thus, the presence of Wnt ligands interferes with the sequestration of β-catenin and its subsequent ubiquitination, thereby stabilizing the protein in cytoplasm. This allows for the nuclear translocation of β-catenin, where it triggers the expression of Wnt-induced genes (i.e., Cyclin D1, c-Myc, vascular endothelial growth factor (VEGF), interleukin-8 (IL-8), etc.) by acting as transcriptional co-activator in conjunction with T-cell factor (TCF) and lymphoid enhancer factor (LEF) DNA-binding proteins [7].

2. Wnt–β-Catenin Signaling in Liver Pathophysiology

The central role of the canonical Wnt–β-catenin signaling pathway in multiple aspects of normal cell functioning and in pathobiological processes is especially eminent in liver [8–11]. There, β-catenin orchestrates embryonic development, patterning, adult tissue metabolism, proliferation, and regeneration. While discussing the many facets of β-catenin signaling as a component of the Wnt pathway is outside the scope of the current review, we would like to remind the readers of a few pertinent concepts that are also relevant in hepatocellular cancer (HCC).

2.1. Wnt–β-Catenin Signaling in Hepatic Development

β-Catenin was first reported to be active in normal mouse and chick embryonic liver development almost two decades ago [12–14]. β-Catenin was seen to be active in stages of hepatic development which showed proliferating hepatoblasts and immature hepatocytes. When mouse embryonic liver cultures were propagated in the presence of antisense oligonucleotides against the β-catenin gene, there was a notable deficit in the resident cell proliferation. This was later verified by conditional deletion of the β-catenin gene or via activation of β-catenin through APC gene loss from mouse hepatoblasts in vivo [15,16]. In addition to these observations, both in vitro and in vivo studies showed a dramatic compromise in hepatocyte maturation. This was seen as the maintenance of hepatoblast markers in the hepatocytes in the β-catenin absent or knocked-down livers, as well as by deficient markers of mature fetal hepatocytes, including glycogen [16]. Thus, β-catenin plays a role in both the proliferation of immature hepatocytes and hepatoblasts during earlier stages of hepatic development, but plays an equally important role in the maturation of immature hepatocytes during later stages. These temporal targets of β-catenin include c-myc and cyclin-D1 for proliferation, as well as CEBPα and as-yet unknown targets, which are likely distinct from its well-known zone-3 targets in adult liver [16]. It is also worth mentioning that, after birth, there is a postnatal growth spurt in livers from postnatal day 5 to about 25 days, after which the liver is mostly quiescent, showing minimal hepatocyte turnover [17]. β-Catenin signaling is also a major contributor of the postnatal wave of hepatocyte proliferation, and in its absence there is a decreased growth spurt which leaves liver-specific β-catenin knockout mice with around 15% lower liver-weight to body-weight ratio (LW/BW).

2.2. Wnt–β-Catenin Signaling in Liver Regeneration

Livers possess a unique feature of regeneration following surgical resection or toxicant-induced injury to regain its lost mass within days to weeks. The liver does so without any progenitor cell activation but via the replication of resident hepatocytes (and other cells) in the liver [18]. Wnt–β-Catenin signaling has been shown to be a key component of the normal molecular machinery of the liver following surgical resection [19]. Within hours of two-thirds hepatectomy, there is a nuclear translocation of β-catenin in hepatocytes and the appearance of β-catenin–TCF complex [20,21]. This is sustained for almost the first 48 h of regeneration. Using several genetic knockout mouse models, it appears that Wnt2 and Wnt9b are massively upregulated in hepatic sinusoidal endothelial cells and less so in monocytes/macrophages at 12 h after hepatectomy (earliest time point examined through individual cell-type isolation after surgery), followed by the engagement of Fzd-LRP5/6, resulting in the activation of β-catenin–TCF4 to regulate cyclin-D1 gene transcription [19]. The increased cyclin-D1 observed during this time allows for hepatocyte G1–S phase transition and eventually contributes to timely hepatocyte proliferation and the recovery of hepatic mass [22]. The absence of Wntless from endothelial cells (and less so macrophages) or the absence of LRP5 and 6 from hepatocytes or the absence of β-catenin from hepatocytes, all lead to a notable deficit in cyclin-D1 expression and a dramatically lower hepatocyte proliferation at 40–48 h after two-thirds hepatectomy [23–27]. Livers eventually recover in all models, despite a notable delay in restitution, and the mechanisms allowing for recovery in the absence of Wnt–β-catenin signaling remain unknown at this time. A similar role of the pathway during hepatocyte proliferation has also been reported after injury from acetaminophen, carbon-tetrachloride, diethoxycarbonyl dihydrocollidine, choline-deficient ethionine supplemented diet, and in Mdr2 knockout mice, making Wnt–β-catenin signaling a global hepatic repair pathway [28–33].

Intriguingly, a recent study also showed an important role of the Wnt–β-catenin pathway in serving a dual role of not only inducing hepatocyte proliferation but also maintaining hepatocyte function during liver regeneration after surgical resection, as well as after acetaminophen-induced injury and repair. Using single-cell RNA-sequencing, Walesky et al. showed a clever "division of labor" by the hepatocytes in the remnant liver following surgery or toxicant injury [34]. This strategy allows liver to maintain function even while it is proliferating, as distinct subsets of hepatocytes acquire proliferative versus hepatocyte-function phenotype, as shown by gene expression studies. Intriguingly, both these functions are regulated by the Wnt–β-catenin pathway; the cell source of the Wnt for regulating the hepatocyte function by β-catenin appears to be macrophages and not sinusoidal endothelial cells, which are likely the source of Wnts for β-catenin activation in hepatocytes for proliferative function.

2.3. Wnt–β-Catenin Signaling in Liver Zonation

Another unique characteristic of the liver is the expression of unique genes by the hepatocytes based on their location within a microscopic hepatic lobule. This disparate gene expression allows for the hepatocytes to perform distinct functions that are necessary for the delivery of optimal hepatic output in terms of metabolism, synthesis, and detoxification, which are the broad categories of around 500 functions that hepatocytes perform to maintain health and homeostasis. Toward this end, Wnt–β-catenin signaling is known to be the major regulator of the expression of genes in the zone-3 or pericentral region of the metabolic lobule [26,35,36]. These genes belong to the category of glutamine synthesis, glycolysis, lipogenesis, ketogenesis, bile acid synthesis, heme metabolism, and xenobiotic metabolism. Some of these target genes include Glul, which encodes glutamine synthetase (GS), and is specifically localized to 1–2 layers of hepatocytes around the central vein [37]. To prevent ammonia from leaving the liver, the zone-3 hepatocytes are efficient in its uptake and the high levels of GS in these cells are responsible for condensing ammonia to glutamate, leading to the formation of glutamine. Thus, intracellular levels of glutamine are highest in zone-3 hepatocytes. Some of the other key targets of β-catenin in zone-3 hepatocytes include Axin-2, Lect2, Cyp2e1, Cyp1a2, and others. Recently, choline transporter organic cation transporter 3 was also shown to be a target of the Wnt–β-catenin signaling, which led to the increased uptake of choline by HCC to promote phospholipid formation and DNA hypermethylation, and contributing to hepatocyte proliferation [38]. In fact, several of these β-catenin targets are upregulated in liver tumors where β-catenin signaling is highly activated in both preclinical models and in patients. Conversely, genetic knockout models that lack Wnt secretion from endothelial cells, lack LRP5 and 6 on hepatocytes, or lack β-catenin in hepatocytes, all lack zone-3 targets of the Wnt–β-catenin pathway [23,24,26,27,36]. Wnt2 and Wnt9b appear to be the major drivers of zonated β-catenin activation, and appear to be within the endothelial cells lining the central vein [39].

Thus, broadly, β-catenin seems to be playing a role in hepatocyte proliferation in physiological states including hepatic development (prenatal and postnatal) and liver regeneration (surgical and injury-driven), as well as in regulating hepatocyte functions including basally in the hepatocytes contained in zone-3 of the metabolic lobule. It is pertinent to mention the existence of regulators of the Wnt–β-catenin signaling that have been shown to play a role in the aforementioned hepatic processes. Factors like R-spondins and their receptors LGR4/5 have been shown to potentiate the effects of the Wnt–β-catenin pathways and have been specifically shown to positively impact the processes of both liver regeneration and metabolic zonation [40,41].

3. β-Catenin as a Component of the Adherens Junctions in Liver Pathophysiology

In addition to β-catenin being the major effector of Wnt signaling, it plays another evolutionarily conserved role at the adherens junctions (AJs), where it links the cytoplasmic tail of E-cadherin to α-catenin and F-actin [42]. Since the extracellular domain of E-cadherin of one cell binds to its counterpart on the next epithelial cell, the AJs are important mediators of intercellular adhesion. AJs are also present on hepatocytes, which are the predominant functioning epithelial cells of the liver. In fact, β-catenin and E-cadherin are mostly seen at the cell surface of hepatocytes. Immunohistochemistry is rarely sufficiently sensitive to detect β-catenin in cytoplasm or nuclei—even in zone-3 hepatocytes, where it is basally active. β-Catenin clearly associates with E-cadherin in the normal liver, and this association is likely part of maintaining junctional integrity, cell polarity, and epithelial identity, and plays a role in both cell adhesion in addition to providing some barrier function within this highly secretory and vascular organ.

3.1. β-Catenin–E-Cadherin Complex in the Liver and Its Regulation

The regulation of β-catenin at the AJs in the hepatocytes is not completely understood. There is an incomplete understanding of whether the same pool of β-catenin is allocated to Wnt signaling and AJs, of when and how this allocation occurs, and of how dynamic this process is [42]. The β-catenin–E-cadherin complex does not seem to be influenced by the Wnt signaling pathway. While liver-specific β-catenin knockout mice showed an absence of β-catenin–E-cadherin interactions, disruption of the Wnt–β-catenin signaling pathway did not impact this complex. This was evident when Wnt co-receptors LRP5/6 were conditionally deleted from hepatocytes, or when Wnt secretion was prevented from hepatic sinusoidal endothelial cells by loss of Wntless [24,27]. In both these models, β-catenin was intact at the AJs and was observed to be interacting with E-cadherin, thus maintaining cell–cell junctions and intact blood–bile barriers. This suggests that the absence of Wnt signaling does not impact the association. Interestingly, tyrosine phosphorylation of β-catenin, especially at tyrosine residue 654, has been shown to play an important role in negatively impacting β-catenin's association with E-cadherin [43]. Several receptor tyrosine kinases (RTKs), such as Src, EGFR, and Met, have been shown to phosphorylate β-catenin at these residues to negatively impact the AJ assembly, for which β-catenin tyrosine residues 654 and 670 have been shown to be important [44]. The fate of β-catenin following release from this complex is not completely clear, but may function as a co-activator for the TCF family, similar to its role in the Wnt signaling [45]. Indeed, RTKs like HGF and EGF can induce the nuclear translocation and activation of β-catenin signaling to cause liver growth, and can also be seen in a subset of tumors like hepatoblastomas and fibrolamellar HCCs [46–48]. Additionally, the cytoplasmic domain of E-cadherin in and around residues 685–699 contains several serine phosphorylation sites, and when these sites are phosphorylated, they interact extensively with armadillo repeats 3–4 of the β-catenin protein [49]. These phosphorylation events may be important in regulating β-catenin–E-cadherin interactions.

3.2. γ-Catenin Compensates for β-Catenin at AJs in the Absence of β-Catenin

Another important observation made in the livers of mice lacking β-catenin in hepatocytes was the maintenance of intact AJs. This coincided with an increase in γ-catenin or plakoglobin, a normal inhabitant of the desmosomes. Indeed, in the β-catenin knockouts, γ-catenin was shown to co-precipitate and thus bind to E-cadherin in lieu of β-catenin [50,51]. This was also previously observed in skin and heart [52,53]. To demonstrate the true functionality of the γ-catenin interaction with E-cadherin in the absence of β-catenin, we conditionally knocked out both β- and γ-catenin from liver epithelia using albumin-cre. This led to a severe cholestatic disease, progressive fibrosis, and mortality, which was associated with perturbations in cell–cell junctions, paracellular leaks, and a decrease in E-cadherin [54]. Indeed, β-catenin binds to the region of E-cadherin which contains the PEST sequence motifs, which allow for the recognition of E-cadherin by ubiquitin ligases as well as proteasomal degradation [49]. The binding of β-catenin to E-cadherin masks these motifs and allows for uneventful trafficking of the complex to the AJs. It is likely that γ-catenin binds to the same region of E-cadherin when β-catenin is absent, preventing E-cadherin degradation and successful delivery of the E-cadherin–γ-catenin complex to the cell surface. This also explains the notable decrease in E-cadherin in the β-γ-catenin double-knockout livers [54].

4. Hepatocellular Cancer
4.1. Alarming Trends in HCC Incidence

The incidence of hepatocellular carcinoma (HCC) has risen steadily in the US and worldwide over last decades [55,56]. Analysis of the NCI's (National Cancer Institute's) Surveillance, Epidemiology and End Results (SEER) database reveals alarming trends in HCC incidence. The rates for new liver and intrahepatic bile duct cancer cases have been rising on average 2.7% each year over the last 10 years. Death rates have risen on average 2.6% each year from 2005 to 2014. In 2014, there were an estimated 66,771 people living with liver tumors in USA. In 2020, liver tumors represented 2.4% of all new cancer cases in the US, with around 42,810 new diagnosed cases [55]. Globally, HCC is the 5th most common malignancy in men, 9th most common cause of cancer in women, and the overall 6th most common cancer worldwide [56].

4.2. Cellular and Molecular Pathogenesis of HCC

Most HCCs are a consequence of years of hepatic damage and wound healing. The events leading up to HCC are complex and involve bouts of cell injury and death, immune cell infiltration, oxidative stress, and stellate cell activation [57]. The liver tries to replace the dying hepatocytes through chronic regeneration via hepatocyte proliferation. Proliferating hepatocytes are susceptible to DNA damage and mutations, and the associated activation of signaling pathways. Any such alterations that provide proliferative and survival advantage to a cell lead to the initiation of the neoplastic transformation. Transcriptomic and whole-genome sequencing has validated that subsets of HCC are "driven" by key oncogenic signaling pathways [58–60]. The whole-exome sequencing of a large number of HCC cohorts has revealed common mutations that are the basis of the molecular classification of HCC [59]. Such analysis has revealed that irrespective of etiology, chronic injury, and downstream cellular events, HCC is driven by a few common genetic aberrations and molecular pathway activation, with only some preferential signaling evident in a few etiologies [60]. One common pathway activated in HCC independent of etiology is Wnt–β-catenin signaling.

5. β-Catenin and Hepatocellular Cancer

5.1. Mechanism of β-Catenin Activation in HCC

It is important to emphasize the key phosphorylation sites located in exon-3 of β-catenin, which are important in its eventual degradation. When the Wnt signals are absent, β-catenin is sequentially phosphorylated at serine-45 (S45), S33, S37, and threonine-41 (T41) by casein kinase I (CKI) and glycogen synthase kinase 3β (GSK3β) [61]. Phosphorylated β-catenin is recognized by β-transducin repeat-containing protein for ubiquitination and proteasomal degradation, and requires intact D32 and G34 sites [62]. When Wnt signaling is on, it inactivates the β-catenin degradation complex consisting of Axin-1 and adenomatous polyposis coli gene product (APC) in addition to CKI and GSK3β. Around 26–37% of all HCCs display *CTNNB1* mutations [8,63]. These missense mutations are localized to exon-3 of CTNNB1, the gene encoding for β-catenin, and affect phosphorylation and ubiquitination sites in the β-catenin promoter, making it resistant to degradation. This leads to β-catenin stabilization, nuclear translocation, and activation of the downstream target genes, playing important and unique roles in tumor biology in several subsets of HCC cases. There are several targets of β-catenin reported in HCC [8]. Some highly relevant ones include glutamine synthetase (GS), cyclin-D1, VEGF-A, lect2, Axin-2, and others.

Loss-of-function mutations in *AXIN1* are another major contributor to HCC development. AXIN1 is also among the top five mutated genes in HCC, seen in around 8% of human HCCs. This gene normally encodes for a protein essential for β-catenin degradation. In the absence of a functional Axin-1, β-catenin levels are increased and Wnt signaling is activated. Indeed, in preclinical models which used sleeping beauty transposon/transposase to express shRNA-*Axin1* along with Met proto-oncogene in either a hepatic β-catenin-sufficient or deficient liver, the requirement of β-catenin was unequivocally shown in this model [64]. Intriguingly, only a subset of targets of the β-catenin signaling are positive in these tumors, including cyclin-D1 and c-myc, and interestingly, these tumors are GS-negative.

Analysis of early HCC, multinodular HCC, and comparison of primary and metastatic HCC has also indicated that β-catenin has a trunk role in HCC similar to other major drivers such as mutations in *TERT* promoter or *TP53* [65].

5.2. Animal Models to Study β-Catenin Activation in HCC

The hepatic overexpression of β-catenin or the expression of mutated, constitutively-active β-catenin alone is insufficient for HCC development, as reported in many mouse models, suggesting cooperation with other pathways [37,66]. Indeed, *CTNNB1* mutations significantly correlate with the presence of other mutations such as in *TERT* promoter, *NFE2L2*, *MLL2*, *ARID2*, and *APOB* [59,67]. *CTNNB1* mutations also are seen to co-occur with the overexpression/activation of Met, Myc, or Nrf2 [63,68,69]. Using a reductionist approach, such concomitant alterations have been modeled in mice by the co-expression of various combinations in vivo using the sleeping beauty transposon/transposase or CRISPR/Cas9 approach and hydrodynamic tail vein injection [70]. For example, 11% of human HCCs show concomitant *CTNNB1* mutations and Met overexpression/activation, and their co-expression in murine liver in the Met–β-catenin model leads to clinically relevant HCC [63,71]. Likewise, Myc–β-catenin represents 6% of human HCCs [68]; and Nrf2–β-catenin represents 9–12% of HCC [69]. The continued generation and characterization of these models for their clinical relevance, biology, and for testing therapies, is of high value.

6. State of Therapies for HCC

The five-year survival of liver tumors is 19.6%, attributable partially to lack of effective therapies [55]. For localized disease, partial hepatectomy or liver transplantation are most beneficial. Loco-regional therapies like radio frequency ablation and transarterial chemoembolization are palliative or useful as neoadjuvants. Until recently, sorafenib was the only FDA-approved agent for unresectable HCC, and this non-specific tyrosine kinase inhibitor (TKI) improved survival by 3 months [72]. Several agents have been approved for HCC treatment in the last 5 years. Regorafenib was approved as second-line treatment, showing improvement in survival to 10.6 months vs. 7.8 months for placebo [73]. In 2017, the immune checkpoint inhibitor (ICI) nivolumab was approved by the FDA as second-line treatment, almost doubling overall survival to 15 months in the Checkmate trial [74]. More recently, another TKI, lenvatinib, was approved as first-line therapy, showing non-inferiority to sorafenib [75]. Cabozantinib, a Met inhibitor, also got approval for second-line use in HCC [76]. Another ICI, pembrolizumab, was awarded an accelerated approval as second-line therapy for HCC based on the KEYNOTE-224 trial [77]. More recently, the results of a phase III clinical trial (IMbrave150) showing higher efficacy to sorafenib and a response rate of around 35% to atezolizumab (anti PD-L1) plus bevacizumab (anti-VEGFA) led to their FDA approval as first-line therapy [78]. Some major existing challenges include a lack of biomarker-based therapy to select a proper subset of patients for a specific treatment and to improve response rates to ICIs, which have revolutionized oncology in general.

7. Targeting β-Catenin for HCC Treatment

7.1. Proof-of-Concept Studies

Because β-catenin is active in a notable subset of HCCs, and is also considered a trunk mutation, its inhibition could have a major impact on the treatment of a subset of these tumors. Several proof-of-concept studies in HCC, both in vitro and in vivo, have demonstrated the relevance of inhibiting β-catenin as a treatment strategy for HCC. siRNA-mediated *CTNNB1* knockdown resulted in a marked decrease in the viability and proliferation of human hepatoma cells in vitro [79]. Similarly, suppressing β-catenin via gamma-guanidine-based peptide nucleic acid antisense also reduced the viability, proliferation, metabolism, and survival of cells of an HCC line [80]. Interestingly, inhibition of β-catenin signaling also resulted in the diminished secretion of angiogenic factors, implying the dual positive effect of such suppression [80]. The DsiRNAs-mediated knockdown of β-catenin mRNA led to a significant decrease of tumor burden in mice bearing ectopic tumors originating from either Hep3B or HepG2 cells [81]. Using a chemical carcinogen (diethylnitrosamine) and tumor promotion (phenobarbital) model which selectively leads to *Ctnnb1*-mutation-driven HCC, β-catenin inhibition using locked nucleic acid antisense (LNA) had a profound impact on tumor development [82]. More recently, using Kras–β-catenin-driven HCC (which highly resembles the Met–β-catenin model), β-catenin was inhibited using EnCore lipid nanoparticles loaded with a Dicer substrate small interfering RNA targeting *CTNNB1*. This led to a notable decrease in tumor burden, also demonstrating β-catenin to be a highly relevant target in HCC for cases driven by *CTNNB1* mutations.

7.2. Where to Target Wnt–β-Catenin Signaling in HCC

The most important mechanism of β-catenin activation in HCC are the mutations in *CTNNB1* and the mutations in *AXIN1*. While there have been several other mechanisms identified to modulate β-catenin signaling, including the upregulation of certain Wnt genes, Frizzled genes, and epigenetic loss of negative regulators like DKK and FRPs and others, their true relevance remains unclear since Wnt–β-catenin signaling, like other signaling pathways, is able to regulate its overall activity via robust post-translational mechanisms. However, mutations in *CTNNB1* or *AXIN1* deem the β-catenin protein non-degradable and hence cannot be regulated by the normal mechanisms, which converge on β-catenin degradation to control the signaling pathway activity. This also suggests that several classes of Wnt inhibitors will not work in HCCs because they inhibit or impair Wnt activity upstream of the observed mutations in *CTNNB1* or *AXIN1*. Hence, the suppression of β-catenin itself using the RNA-based therapies discussed in the preceding section, or those impairing β-catenin nuclear translocation, impairing its interaction with TCF4 or preventing the β-catenin–TCF complex from transactivating target genes, would be most effective in treatment of some subsets of HCC. Finally, identifying unique opportunities related to β-catenin signaling in HCC is important, as it may help in selecting or excluding the right group of patients, and may help to identify innovative opportunities to target other mechanisms that are intimately related to β-catenin activation unique to HCC.

7.3. How to Target β-Catenin in HCC

Targeting β-catenin itself using RNA-based therapies is highly desirable. Several classes of siRNA- and antisense-based therapies have been described for use against β-catenin. The use of EnCore lipid nanoparticles along with Dicer substrate small interfering RNAs is especially innovative because it can be modified to specifically deliver the payload to liver tumors, and the safety of their use has been shown in patients [83]. Others such as peptide nucleic acid antisense, locked nucleic acid antisense, and other modalities have been reported, and may have eventual clinical use [80–82].

There may be an opportunity to identify the mechanisms of the nuclear transport or nuclear export of β-catenin. Targeting molecules that cargo β-catenin to the nucleus or activate its export out of the nucleus could have efficacy in the treatment of β-catenin-mutated HCCs. Pegylated interferon-α2a (peg-IFN), previously a first-line therapy for hepatitis C virus (HCV) patients, was shown to induce the levels of Ran-binding protein 3 (RanBP3), which is known to export β-catenin out of the nucleus [84]. Peg-IFN treatment was also shown to induce association between RanBP3 and β-catenin, and led to decreased TopFlash reporter activity that was abrogated by siRNA-mediated RanBP3 knockdown. In vivo, peg-IFN treatment led to increased nuclear RanBP3, decreased nuclear β-catenin and cyclin D1, and decreased GS, and eventually led to decreased tumor cell proliferation.

The use of small-molecule inhibitors that interfere with its interactions with TCF or other relevant co-factors or components of the transcriptional complex would be highly desirable. However, a high specificity of the small-molecule inhibitors will be required because of the overlap of the β-catenin–TCF4 binding site, and with the binding sites for APC and E-cadherin [85]. Even though a number of the identified compounds showed selectivity of inhibition in vitro (e.g., PKF115-584, CGP049090, and PKF118-310), none of them has entered clinical trials [85]. PR1-724, the next-generation compound of the original small-molecule ICG-001, interferes with β-catenin–TCF4 interactions with CBP, a histone acetyltransferase essential for transcriptional function of the complex [86,87]. PRI-724 has been shown to be safe in patients with HCV-related cirrhosis, and may be of high relevance in the treatment of subsets of HCC with known mutations in *CTNNB1* [88].

7.4. Unique and Exploitable Aspects of Targeting β-Catenin in Subsets of HCC

In addition to a general role of β-catenin in regulating tumor cell proliferation, survival, and angiogenesis, there are specific and unique aspects of β-catenin activation due to mutations in HCC which can have notable biological and therapeutic implications—especially related to a step towards precision medicine.

7.4.1. Role of β-Catenin in Tumor Immune Evasion

ICIs have revolutionized the treatment of many tumors, including HCC as can be seen by the FDA approval of nivolumab and pembrolizumab as second-line therapy and of atezolizumab (anti PD-L1) plus bevacizumab (anti-VEGFA), as first line treatment for unresectable HCC [78]. However, there are no available biomarkers which predict either the efficacy or lack thereof to ICIs. Clinical response to ICIs, most of which are T-cell-based therapies, depend on the presence of a CD8$^+$ T cell inflamed environment and chemokines and interferon signature within the tumor [89]. Intriguingly, activation of β-catenin signaling has been linked to immune evasion in tumors such as melanoma through T-cell exclusion from tumors [90]. This is shown in our own analysis as well (Figure 1). Several mechanisms underlie this observation, including the effect of β-catenin activation on CD8$^+$ T cell priming and infiltration by acting on Batf3-lineage CD103$^+$ dendritic cells (DCs) and decreasing CCL4 production by inducing the expression of transcription repressor ATF3 [91]; disruption of Foxp3 transcriptional activity, key for development and function of regulatory T cells [92]; and increased Treg survival, which can reduce CD8$^+$ T cell proliferation [93]. HCCs with β-catenin activation have been linked to immune cell exclusion [94,95]. We have shown that *CTNNB1*-mutated HCCs are resistant to anti-PD-1 [68], and hence may benefit from the inhibition of β-catenin or its downstream effectors to sensitize these tumors to ICIs.

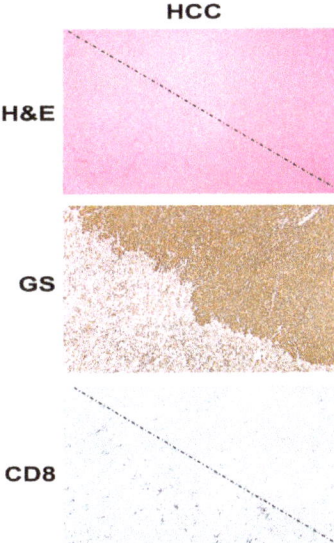

Figure 1. β-Catenin activation in HCC reduces CD8 T cell infiltration in the tumor. The top panel shows histology of explanted liver for hepatocellular cancer (HCC) showing the presence of two distinct tumors (separated by a dotted line) which are otherwise difficult to distinguish and demarcate by hematoxylin and eosin (H&E) staining (100×). The middle panel shows the immunohistochemistry of the adjacent tissue section to the top panel, for glutamine synthetase (GS), a surrogate marker of β-catenin activation due to mutations in *CTNNB1*. The staining for GS shows the presence of uniform positive staining in the upper-right part which decorates a β-catenin-active HCC, whereas the lower-left tumor is negative for this stain. Immunohistochemistry for CD8 for a subset of T cells, in the section adjacent to those shown in the top and middle panels, shows a general dearth of positive cells in the top-right (β-catenin-active) tumor, while there are notably more CD8-positive cells in the lower left or in the non-β-catenin-active HCC. The two tumors are separated by a dotted line.

One additional relevant mechanism in the liver might be through a known interaction of β-catenin with NF-κB in the hepatocytes and liver tumor cells [96]. This inhibitory association between the p65 subunit of NF-κB and β-catenin prevents NF-κB activation even when appropriate upstream effectors of NF-κB are present. In this study, we also showed that this association led to reduced p65-luciferase reporter activity when constitutively active β-catenin was transfected in hepatoma cells. Furthermore, β-catenin mutated HCCs showed decreased p65 nuclear translocation. Knowing that NF-κB signaling plays a major role in inducing inflammatory milieu [97], its suppression brought about by stable β-catenin due to mutations in *CTNNB1* may be one additional contributor of an immune-deficient tumor microenvironment which may in turn lead to resistance to ICIs.

7.4.2. Role of β-Catenin in Regulating Tumor Metabolism Through mTORC1 in HCC

The suppression of β-catenin in *CTNNB1*-mutant liver tumors decreases tumor burden in many models [71,82]. We made a unique discovery of how this response was mediated by the regulation of mTORC1 by β-catenin [98]. The Wnt–β-catenin pathway transcriptionally regulates the expression of *Glul*, which encodes GS in hepatocytes in zone-3 of the hepatic lobule [37], and leads to the highest glutamine in zone-3 hepatocytes [99] (Figure 2A,B). Glutamine directly phosphorylates mTOR at serine-2448 in lysosomes [100]. We identified p-mTOR-S2448 (active mTORC1) [101] in zone-3 hepatocytes basally, which was absent in hepatocyte-specific knockout (KO) of β-catenin, Wnt co-receptors LRP5-6, and GS (Figure 2B). We also found by immunohistochemistry (IHC) that HCCs with *CTNNB1* mutations are simultaneously positive for GS and p-mTOR-S2448 in preclinical models and patients (Figure 2B). We also showed a dependence of the CTNNB1-mutated HCCs to mTORC1 by their susceptibility to mTOR inhibition by rapamycin in a preclinical model. This may be a novel way to target β-catenin mutated liver tumors in patients until anti-β-catenin therapies become a reality.

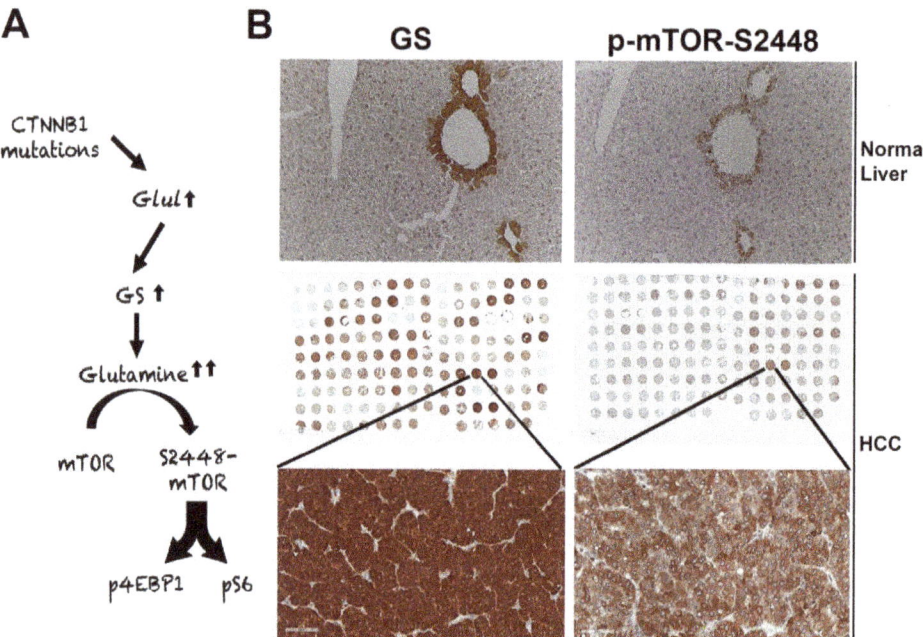

Figure 2. Unique mTORC1 addiction of *CTNNB1*-mutated HCCs due to glutamine. (**A**) The unique axis of mTORC1 activation in β-catenin gene mutated HCCs due to overexpression of *GLUL*, the gene encoding for glutamine synthetase (GS), which generates glutamine from ammonia and glutamate, and in turn glutamine activates mTORC1 in lysosomes. (**B**) The top panel shows immunohistochemistry for GS and p-mTOR-S2448 in adjacent sections from a normal mouse liver. Both proteins are localizing exclusively to zone-3 hepatocytes in the immediate proximity to the central vein (200×). The whole slide scans (middle row) of two adjacent tissue microarrays of human HCC samples stained for the same antibodies against GS and p-mTOR-S2448 also shows several HCCs to be simultaneously positive for GS and p-mTOR-S2448. A representative tissue array sample is magnified (400×) to show GS and p-mTOR-S2448-positive HCC (bottom panels).

Funding: This work was supported in part by NIH grants 1R01DK62277, 1R01DK116993, 1R01CA204586, 1R01CA251155, R01CA250227, and Endowed Chair for Experimental Pathology to S.P.M. The tissue samples for analysis were provided by the Clinical Biospecimen Repository and Processing Core of the Pittsburgh Liver Research Center and supported by 1P30DK120531.

Institutional Review Board Statement: The study was conducted according to the guidelines of the Declaration of Helsinki, and approved by the Institutional Review Board of the University of Pittsburgh (STUDY19070068, STUDY20010114, and STUDY20040276 on 3/23/2021).

Informed Consent Statement: Informed consent was obtained from all subjects involved in the study.

Data Availability Statement: Not applicable.

Conflicts of Interest: S.P.M. has research funding from Vicero Inc., Revolution Medicines, and ALIGOS Therapeutics. The funders had no role in the design of the study; in the collection, analyses, or interpretation of data; in the writing of the manuscript, or in the decision to publish the results.

References

1. MacDonald, B.T.; Tamai, K.; He, X. Wnt/beta-catenin signaling: Components, mechanisms, and diseases. *Dev. Cell* **2009**, *17*, 9–26. [CrossRef] [PubMed]
2. Polakis, P. Wnt signaling in cancer. *Cold Spring Harb. Perspect. Biol.* **2012**, *4*. [CrossRef] [PubMed]
3. Klaus, A.; Birchmeier, W. Wnt signalling and its impact on development and cancer. *Nat. Rev. Cancer* **2008**, *8*, 387–398. [CrossRef]
4. Taciak, B.; Pruszynska, I.; Kiraga, L.; Bialasek, M.; Krol, M. Wnt signaling pathway in development and cancer. *J. Physiol. Pharmacol.* **2018**, *69*. [CrossRef]
5. Clevers, H.; Nusse, R. Wnt/beta-catenin signaling and disease. *Cell* **2012**, *149*, 1192–1205. [CrossRef]
6. Tamai, K.; Zeng, X.; Liu, C.; Zhang, X.; Harada, Y.; Chang, Z.; He, X. A mechanism for Wnt coreceptor activation. *Mol. Cell* **2004**, *13*, 149–156. [CrossRef]
7. Cadigan, K.M.; Waterman, M.L. TCF/LEFs and Wnt signaling in the nucleus. *Cold Spring Harb. Perspect. Biol.* **2012**, *4*. [CrossRef]
8. Monga, S.P. β-catenin signaling and roles in liver homeostasis, injury, and tumorigenesis. *Gastroenterology* **2015**, *148*, 1294–1310. [CrossRef]
9. Perugorria, M.J.; Olaizola, P.; Labiano, I.; Esparza-Baquer, A.; Marzioni, M.; Marin, J.J.G.; Bujanda, L.; Banales, J.M. Wnt-beta-catenin signalling in liver development, health and disease. *Nat. Rev. Gastroenterol. Hepatol.* **2019**, *16*, 121–136. [CrossRef] [PubMed]
10. Russell, J.O.; Monga, S.P. Wnt/β-catenin signaling in liver development, homeostasis, and pathobiology. *Annu. Rev. Pathol.* **2018**, *13*, 351–378. [CrossRef] [PubMed]
11. Thompson, M.D.; Monga, S.P.S. WNT/β-catenin signaling in liver health and disease. *Hepatology* **2007**, *45*, 1298–1305. [CrossRef]
12. Micsenyi, A.; Tan, X.; Sneddon, T.; Luo, J.H.; Michalopoulos, G.K.; Monga, S.P. Beta-catenin is temporally regulated during normal liver development. *Gastroenterology* **2004**, *126*, 1134–1146. [CrossRef]
13. Monga, S.P.; Monga, H.K.; Tan, X.; Mule, K.; Pediaditakis, P.; Michalopoulos, G.K. Beta-catenin antisense studies in embryonic liver cultures: Role in proliferation, apoptosis, and lineage specification. *Gastroenterology* **2003**, *124*, 202–216. [CrossRef]
14. Suksaweang, S.; Lin, C.M.; Jiang, T.X.; Hughes, M.W.; Widelitz, R.B.; Chuong, C.M. Morphogenesis of chicken liver: Identification of localized growth zones and the role of beta-catenin/Wnt in size regulation. *Dev. Biol.* **2004**, *266*, 109–122. [CrossRef] [PubMed]
15. Decaens, T.; Godard, C.; de Reynies, A.; Rickman, D.S.; Tronche, F.; Couty, J.P.; Perret, C.; Colnot, S. Stabilization of beta-catenin affects mouse embryonic liver growth and hepatoblast fate. *Hepatology* **2008**, *47*, 247–258. [CrossRef]
16. Tan, X.; Yuan, Y.; Zeng, G.; Apte, U.; Thompson, M.D.; Cieply, B.; Stolz, D.B.; Michalopoulos, G.K.; Kaestner, K.H.; Monga, S.P. Beta-catenin deletion in hepatoblasts disrupts hepatic morphogenesis and survival during mouse development. *Hepatology* **2008**, *47*, 1667–1679. [CrossRef]
17. Apte, U.; Zeng, G.; Thompson, M.D.; Muller, P.; Micsenyi, A.; Cieply, B.; Kaestner, K.H.; Monga, S.P. beta-Catenin is critical for early postnatal liver growth. *Am. J. Physiol. Gastrointest. Liver Physiol.* **2007**, *292*, G1578–G1585. [CrossRef] [PubMed]
18. Michalopoulos, G.K.; Bhushan, B. Liver regeneration: Biological and pathological mechanisms and implications. *Nat. Rev. Gastroenterol. Hepatol.* **2021**, *18*, 40–55. [CrossRef] [PubMed]
19. Hu, S.; Monga, S.P. Wnt/beta-catenin signaling and liver regeneration: Circuit, biology and opportunities. *Gene Expr.* **2021**. [CrossRef]
20. Monga, S.P.; Pediaditakis, P.; Mule, K.; Stolz, D.B.; Michalopoulos, G.K. Changes in WNT/beta-catenin pathway during regulated growth in rat liver regeneration. *Hepatology* **2001**, *33*, 1098–1109. [CrossRef]
21. Nejak-Bowen, K.; Moghe, A.; Cornuet, P.; Preziosi, M.; Nagarajan, S.; Monga, S.P. Role and regulation of p65/beta-catenin association during liver injury and regeneration: A "complex" relationship. *Gene Expr.* **2017**, *17*, 219–235. [CrossRef] [PubMed]
22. Torre, C.; Benhamouche, S.; Mitchell, C.; Godard, C.; Veber, P.; Letourneur, F.; Cagnard, N.; Jacques, S.; Finzi, L.; Perret, C.; et al. The transforming growth factor-alpha and cyclin D1 genes are direct targets of beta-catenin signaling in hepatocyte proliferation. *J. Hepatol.* **2011**, *55*, 86–95. [CrossRef] [PubMed]

23. Leibing, T.; Geraud, C.; Augustin, I.; Boutros, M.; Augustin, H.G.; Okun, J.G.; Langhans, C.D.; Zierow, J.; Wohlfeil, S.A.; Olsavszky, V.; et al. Angiocrine Wnt signaling controls liver growth and metabolic maturation in mice. *Hepatology* **2018**, *68*, 707–722. [CrossRef] [PubMed]
24. Preziosi, M.; Okabe, H.; Poddar, M.; Singh, S.; Monga, S.P. Endothelial Wnts regulate beta-catenin signaling in murine liver zonation and regeneration: A sequel to the Wnt-Wnt situation. *Hepatol. Commun.* **2018**, *2*, 845–860. [CrossRef] [PubMed]
25. Sekine, S.; Gutierrez, P.J.; Lan, B.Y.; Feng, S.; Hebrok, M. Liver-specific loss of beta-catenin results in delayed hepatocyte proliferation after partial hepatectomy. *Hepatology* **2007**, *45*, 361–368. [CrossRef]
26. Tan, X.; Behari, J.; Cieply, B.; Michalopoulos, G.K.; Monga, S.P. Conditional deletion of beta-catenin reveals its role in liver growth and regeneration. *Gastroenterology* **2006**, *131*, 1561–1572. [CrossRef]
27. Yang, J.; Mowry, L.E.; Nejak-Bowen, K.N.; Okabe, H.; Diegel, C.R.; Lang, R.A.; Williams, B.O.; Monga, S.P. Beta-catenin signaling in murine liver zonation and regeneration: A Wnt-Wnt situation! *Hepatology* **2014**, *60*, 964–976. [CrossRef]
28. Apte, U.; Singh, S.; Zeng, G.; Cieply, B.; Virji, M.A.; Wu, T.; Monga, S.P. Beta-catenin activation promotes liver regeneration after acetaminophen-induced injury. *Am. J. Pathol.* **2009**, *175*, 1056–1065. [CrossRef]
29. Bhushan, B.; Walesky, C.; Manley, M.; Gallagher, T.; Borude, P.; Edwards, G.; Monga, S.P.; Apte, U. Pro-regenerative signaling after acetaminophen-induced acute liver injury in mice identified using a novel incremental dose model. *Am. J. Pathol.* **2014**, *184*, 3013–3025. [CrossRef]
30. Pradhan-Sundd, T.; Kosar, K.; Saggi, H.; Zhang, R.; Vats, R.; Cornuet, P.; Green, S.; Singh, S.; Zeng, G.; Sundd, P.; et al. Wnt/beta-catenin signaling plays a protective role in the Mdr2 knockout murine model of cholestatic liver disease. *Hepatology* **2020**, *71*, 1732–1749. [CrossRef]
31. Russell, J.O.; Lu, W.Y.; Okabe, H.; Abrams, M.; Oertel, M.; Poddar, M.; Singh, S.; Forbes, S.J.; Monga, S.P. Hepatocyte-specific beta-catenin deletion during severe liver injury provokes cholangiocytes to differentiate into hepatocytes. *Hepatology* **2019**, *69*, 742–759. [CrossRef]
32. Thompson, M.D.; Wickline, E.D.; Bowen, W.B.; Lu, A.; Singh, S.; Misse, A.; Monga, S.P. Spontaneous repopulation of beta-catenin null livers with beta-catenin-positive hepatocytes after chronic murine liver injury. *Hepatology* **2011**, *54*, 1333–1343. [CrossRef]
33. Zhao, L.; Jin, Y.; Donahue, K.; Tsui, M.; Fish, M.; Logan, C.Y.; Wang, B.; Nusse, R. Tissue repair in the mouse liver following acute carbon tetrachloride depends on injury-induced Wnt/beta-catenin signaling. *Hepatology* **2019**, *69*, 2623–2635. [CrossRef]
34. Walesky, C.M.; Kolb, K.E.; Winston, C.L.; Henderson, J.; Kruft, B.; Fleming, I.; Ko, S.; Monga, S.P.; Mueller, F.; Apte, U.; et al. Functional compensation precedes recovery of tissue mass following acute liver injury. *Nat. Commun.* **2020**, *11*, 5785. [CrossRef] [PubMed]
35. Benhamouche, S.; Decaens, T.; Godard, C.; Chambrey, R.; Rickman, D.S.; Moinard, C.; Vasseur-Cognet, M.; Kuo, C.J.; Kahn, A.; Perret, C.; et al. Apc tumor suppressor gene is the "zonation-keeper" of mouse liver. *Dev. Cell* **2006**, *10*, 759–770. [CrossRef] [PubMed]
36. Sekine, S.; Lan, B.Y.; Bedolli, M.; Feng, S.; Hebrok, M. Liver-specific loss of beta-catenin blocks glutamine synthesis pathway activity and cytochrome p450 expression in mice. *Hepatology* **2006**, *43*, 817–825. [CrossRef] [PubMed]
37. Cadoret, A.; Ovejero, C.; Terris, B.; Souil, E.; Levy, L.; Lamers, W.H.; Kitajewski, J.; Kahn, A.; Perret, C. New targets of beta-catenin signaling in the liver are involved in the glutamine metabolism. *Oncogene* **2002**, *21*, 8293–8301. [CrossRef]
38. Gougelet, A.; Sartor, C.; Senni, N.; Calderaro, J.; Fartoux, L.; Lequoy, M.; Wendum, D.; Talbot, J.N.; Prignon, A.; Chalaye, J.; et al. Hepatocellular carcinomas with mutational activation of beta-catenin require choline and can be detected by positron emission tomography. *Gastroenterology* **2019**, *157*, 807–822. [CrossRef]
39. Wang, B.; Zhao, L.; Fish, M.; Logan, C.Y.; Nusse, R. Self-renewing diploid Axin2(+) cells fuel homeostatic renewal of the liver. *Nature* **2015**, *524*, 180–185. [CrossRef]
40. Planas-Paz, L.; Orsini, V.; Boulter, L.; Calabrese, D.; Pikiolek, M.; Nigsch, F.; Xie, Y.; Roma, G.; Donovan, A.; Marti, P.; et al. The RSPO-LGR4/5-ZNRF3/RNF43 module controls liver zonation and size. *Nat. Cell. Biol.* **2016**, *18*, 467–479. [CrossRef]
41. Rocha, A.S.; Vidal, V.; Mertz, M.; Kendall, T.J.; Charlet, A.; Okamoto, H.; Schedl, A. The angiocrine factor Rspondin3 is a key determinant of liver zonation. *Cell Rep.* **2015**, *13*, 1757–1764. [CrossRef]
42. Van der Wal, T.; van Amerongen, R. Walking the tight wire between cell adhesion and WNT signalling: A balancing act for beta-catenin. *Open Biol.* **2020**, *10*, 200267. [CrossRef] [PubMed]
43. Roura, S.; Miravet, S.; Piedra, J.; Garcia de Herreros, A.; Dunach, M. Regulation of E-cadherin/catenin association by tyrosine phosphorylation. *J. Biol. Chem.* **1999**, *274*, 36734–36740. [CrossRef]
44. Zeng, G.; Apte, U.; Micsenyi, A.; Bell, A.; Monga, S.P. Tyrosine residues 654 and 670 in beta-catenin are crucial in regulation of Met-beta-catenin interactions. *Exp. Cell Res.* **2006**, *312*, 3620–3630. [CrossRef] [PubMed]
45. Monga, S.P.; Mars, W.M.; Pediaditakis, P.; Bell, A.; Mule, K.; Bowen, W.C.; Wang, X.; Zarnegar, R.; Michalopoulos, G.K. Hepatocyte growth factor induces Wnt-independent nuclear translocation of beta-catenin after Met-beta-catenin dissociation in hepatocytes. *Cancer Res.* **2002**, *62*, 2064–2071.
46. Apte, U.; Zeng, G.; Muller, P.; Tan, X.; Micsenyi, A.; Cieply, B.; Dai, C.; Liu, Y.; Kaestner, K.H.; Monga, S.P. Activation of Wnt/beta-catenin pathway during hepatocyte growth factor-induced hepatomegaly in mice. *Hepatology* **2006**, *44*, 992–1002. [CrossRef]
47. Cieply, B.; Zeng, G.; Proverbs-Singh, T.; Geller, D.A.; Monga, S.P. Unique phenotype of hepatocellular cancers with exon-3 mutations in beta-catenin gene. *Hepatology* **2009**, *49*, 821–831. [CrossRef] [PubMed]

48. Purcell, R.; Childs, M.; Maibach, R.; Miles, C.; Turner, C.; Zimmermann, A.; Sullivan, M. HGF/c-Met related activation of beta-catenin in hepatoblastoma. *J. Exp. Clin. Cancer Res.* **2011**, *30*, 96. [CrossRef] [PubMed]
49. Huber, A.H.; Weis, W.I. The structure of the beta-catenin/E-cadherin complex and the molecular basis of diverse ligand recognition by beta-catenin. *Cell* **2001**, *105*, 391–402. [CrossRef]
50. Wickline, E.D.; Du, Y.; Stolz, D.B.; Kahn, M.; Monga, S.P. Gamma-Catenin at adherens junctions: Mechanism and biologic implications in hepatocellular cancer after beta-catenin knockdown. *Neoplasia* **2013**, *15*, 421–434. [CrossRef]
51. Wickline, E.D.; Awuah, P.K.; Behari, J.; Ross, M.; Stolz, D.B.; Monga, S.P. Hepatocyte gamma-catenin compensates for conditionally deleted beta-catenin at adherens junctions. *J. Hepatol.* **2011**, *55*, 1256–1262. [CrossRef] [PubMed]
52. Posthaus, H.; Williamson, L.; Baumann, D.; Kemler, R.; Caldelari, R.; Suter, M.M.; Schwarz, H.; Muller, E. Beta-catenin is not required for proliferation and differentiation of epidermal mouse keratinocytes. *J. Cell Sci.* **2002**, *115*, 4587–4595. [CrossRef] [PubMed]
53. Zhou, J.; Qu, J.; Yi, X.P.; Graber, K.; Huber, L.; Wang, X.; Gerdes, A.M.; Li, F. Upregulation of gamma-catenin compensates for the loss of beta-catenin in adult cardiomyocytes. *Am. J. Physiol. Heart Circ. Physiol.* **2007**, *292*, H270–H276. [CrossRef] [PubMed]
54. Pradhan-Sundd, T.; Zhou, L.; Vats, R.; Jiang, A.; Molina, L.; Singh, S.; Poddar, M.; Russell, J.; Stolz, D.B.; Oertel, M.; et al. Dual catenin loss in murine liver causes tight junctional deregulation and progressive intrahepatic cholestasis. *Hepatology* **2018**, *67*, 2320–2337. [CrossRef] [PubMed]
55. National Cancer Institute. Cancer Stat Facts: Liver and Intrahepatic Bile Duct Cancer. Available online: https://seer.cancer.gov/statfacts/html/livibd.html (accessed on 28 February 2021).
56. American Institute for Cancer Research. Liver Cancer Statistics. Available online: https://www.wcrf.org/dietandcancer/cancer-trends/liver-cancer-statistics (accessed on 28 February 2021).
57. Farazi, P.A.; DePinho, R.A. Hepatocellular carcinoma pathogenesis: From genes to environment. *Nat. Rev. Cancer* **2006**, *6*, 674–687. [CrossRef]
58. Hoshida, Y.; Nijman, S.M.; Kobayashi, M.; Chan, J.A.; Brunet, J.P.; Chiang, D.Y.; Villanueva, A.; Newell, P.; Ikeda, K.; Hashimoto, M.; et al. Integrative transcriptome analysis reveals common molecular subclasses of human hepatocellular carcinoma. *Cancer Res.* **2009**, *69*, 7385–7392. [CrossRef]
59. Schulze, K.; Imbeaud, S.; Letouze, E.; Alexandrov, L.B.; Calderaro, J.; Rebouissou, S.; Couchy, G.; Meiller, C.; Shinde, J.; Soysouvanh, F.; et al. Exome sequencing of hepatocellular carcinomas identifies new mutational signatures and potential therapeutic targets. *Nat. Genet.* **2015**, *47*, 505–511. [CrossRef]
60. Zucman-Rossi, J.; Villanueva, A.; Nault, J.C.; Llovet, J.M. Genetic landscape and biomarkers of hepatocellular carcinoma. *Gastroenterology* **2015**, *149*, 1226–1239. [CrossRef]
61. Amit, S.; Hatzubai, A.; Birman, Y.; Andersen, J.S.; Ben-Shushan, E.; Mann, M.; Ben-Neriah, Y.; Alkalay, I. Axin-mediated CKI phosphorylation of beta-catenin at Ser 45: A molecular switch for the Wnt pathway. *Genes Dev.* **2002**, *16*, 1066–1076. [CrossRef] [PubMed]
62. Winston, J.T.; Strack, P.; Beer-Romero, P.; Chu, C.Y.; Elledge, S.J.; Harper, J.W. The SCFbeta-TRCP-ubiquitin ligase complex associates specifically with phosphorylated destruction motifs in IkappaBalpha and beta-catenin and stimulates IkappaBalpha ubiquitination in vitro. *Genes Dev.* **1999**, *13*, 270–283. [CrossRef]
63. Tao, J.; Xu, E.; Zhao, Y.; Singh, S.; Li, X.; Couchy, G.; Chen, X.; Zucman-Rossi, J.; Chikina, M.; Monga, S.P. Modeling a human HCC subset in mice through co-expression of met and point-mutant beta-catenin. *Hepatology* 2016. [CrossRef]
64. Qiao, Y.; Wang, J.; Karagoz, E.; Liang, B.; Song, X.; Shang, R.; Evert, K.; Xu, M.; Che, L.; Evert, M.; et al. Axis inhibition protein 1 (Axin1) deletion-induced hepatocarcinogenesis requires intact beta-catenin but not notch cascade in mice. *Hepatology* **2019**, *70*, 2003–2017. [CrossRef]
65. Torrecilla, S.; Sia, D.; Harrington, A.N.; Zhang, Z.; Cabellos, L.; Cornella, H.; Moeini, A.; Camprecios, G.; Leow, W.Q.; Fiel, M.I.; et al. Trunk mutational events present minimal intra- and inter-tumoral heterogeneity in hepatocellular carcinoma. *J. Hepatol.* **2017**, *67*, 1222–1231. [CrossRef]
66. Nejak-Bowen, K.N.; Thompson, M.D.; Singh, S.; Bowen, W.C., Jr.; Dar, M.J.; Khillan, J.; Dai, C.; Monga, S.P. Accelerated liver regeneration and hepatocarcinogenesis in mice overexpressing serine-45 mutant beta-catenin. *Hepatology* **2010**, *51*, 1603–1613. [CrossRef] [PubMed]
67. National Cancer Institute. The Cancer Genome Atlas. Available online: http://cancergenome.nih.gov/ (accessed on 28 February 2021).
68. de Galarreta, M.R.; Bresnahan, E.; Molina-Sanchez, P.; Lindblad, K.E.; Maier, B.; Sia, D.; Puigvehi, M.; Miguela, V.; Casanova-Acebes, M.; Dhainaut, M.; et al. Beta-catenin activation promotes immune escape and resistance to anti-PD-1 therapy in hepatocellular carcinoma. *Cancer Discov.* **2019**, *9*, 1124–1141. [CrossRef] [PubMed]
69. Tao, J.; Krutsenko, Y.; Moghe, A.; Singh, S.; Poddar, M.; Bell, A.; Oertel, M.; Singhi, A.D.; Geller, D.; Chen, X.; et al. Nrf2 and beta-catenin coactivation in hepatocellular cancer: Biological and therapeutic implications. *Hepatology* 2021. [CrossRef]
70. Chen, X.; Calvisi, D.F. Hydrodynamic transfection for generation of novel mouse models for liver cancer research. *Am. J. Pathol.* **2014**, *184*, 912–923. [CrossRef]
71. Tao, J.; Zhang, R.; Singh, S.; Poddar, M.; Xu, E.; Oertel, M.; Chen, X.; Ganesh, S.; Abrams, M.; Monga, S.P. Targeting beta-catenin in hepatocellular cancers induced by coexpression of mutant beta-catenin and K-Ras in mice. *Hepatology* **2017**, *65*, 1581–1599. [CrossRef] [PubMed]

72. Bruix, J.; Raoul, J.L.; Sherman, M.; Mazzaferro, V.; Bolondi, L.; Craxi, A.; Galle, P.R.; Santoro, A.; Beaugrand, M.; Sangiovanni, A.; et al. Efficacy and safety of sorafenib in patients with advanced hepatocellular carcinoma: Subanalyses of a phase III trial. *J. Hepatol.* **2012**, *57*, 821–829. [CrossRef] [PubMed]
73. Bruix, J.; Qin, S.; Merle, P.; Granito, A.; Huang, Y.H.; Bodoky, G.; Pracht, M.; Yokosuka, O.; Rosmorduc, O.; Breder, V.; et al. Regorafenib for patients with hepatocellular carcinoma who progressed on sorafenib treatment (RESORCE): A randomised, double-blind, placebo-controlled, phase 3 trial. *Lancet* **2017**, *389*, 56–66. [CrossRef]
74. El-Khoueiry, A.B.; Sangro, B.; Yau, T.; Crocenzi, T.S.; Kudo, M.; Hsu, C.; Kim, T.Y.; Choo, S.P.; Trojan, J.; Welling, T.H.R.; et al. Nivolumab in patients with advanced hepatocellular carcinoma (CheckMate 040): An open-label, non-comparative, phase 1/2 dose escalation and expansion trial. *Lancet* **2017**, *389*, 2492–2502. [CrossRef]
75. Kudo, M.; Finn, R.S.; Qin, S.; Han, K.H.; Ikeda, K.; Piscaglia, F.; Baron, A.; Park, J.W.; Han, G.; Jassem, J.; et al. Lenvatinib versus sorafenib in first-line treatment of patients with unresectable hepatocellular carcinoma: A randomised phase 3 non-inferiority trial. *Lancet* **2018**, *391*, 1163–1173. [CrossRef]
76. Abou-Alfa, G.K.; Meyer, T.; Cheng, A.L.; El-Khoueiry, A.B.; Rimassa, L.; Ryoo, B.Y.; Cicin, I.; Merle, P.; Chen, Y.; Park, J.W.; et al. Cabozantinib in patients with advanced and progressing hepatocellular carcinoma. *N. Engl. J. Med.* **2018**, *379*, 54–63. [CrossRef] [PubMed]
77. Zhu, A.X.; Finn, R.S.; Edeline, J.; Cattan, S.; Ogasawara, S.; Palmer, D.; Verslype, C.; Zagonel, V.; Fartoux, L.; Vogel, A.; et al. Pembrolizumab in patients with advanced hepatocellular carcinoma previously treated with sorafenib (KEYNOTE-224): A non-randomised, open-label phase 2 trial. *Lancet Oncol.* **2018**, *19*, 940–952. [CrossRef]
78. Finn, R.S.; Qin, S.; Ikeda, M.; Galle, P.R.; Ducreux, M.; Kim, T.Y.; Kudo, M.; Breder, V.; Merle, P.; Kaseb, A.O.; et al. Atezolizumab plus Bevacizumab in unresectable hepatocellular carcinoma. *N. Engl. J. Med.* **2020**, *382*, 1894–1905. [CrossRef] [PubMed]
79. Zeng, G.; Apte, U.; Cieply, B.; Singh, S.; Monga, S.P. siRNA-mediated beta-catenin knockdown in human hepatoma cells results in decreased growth and survival. *Neoplasia* **2007**, *9*, 951–959. [CrossRef]
80. Delgado, E.; Bahal, R.; Yang, J.; Lee, J.M.; Ly, D.H.; Monga, S.P. β-Catenin knockdown in liver tumor cells by a cell permeable gamma guanidine-based peptide nucleic acid. *Curr. Cancer Drug Targets* **2013**, *13*, 867–878. [CrossRef]
81. Dudek, H.; Wong, D.H.; Arvan, R.; Shah, A.; Wortham, K.; Ying, B.; Diwanji, R.; Zhou, W.; Holmes, B.; Yang, H.; et al. Knockdown of β-catenin with dicer-substrate siRNAs reduces liver tumor burden in vivo. *Mol. Ther.* **2014**, *22*, 92–101. [CrossRef] [PubMed]
82. Delgado, E.; Okabe, H.; Preziosi, M.; Russell, J.O.; Alvarado, T.F.; Oertel, M.; Nejak-Bowen, K.N.; Zhang, Y.; Monga, S.P. Complete response of Ctnnb1-mutated tumours to beta-catenin suppression by locked nucleic acid antisense in a mouse hepatocarcinogenesis model. *J. Hepatol.* **2015**, *62*, 380–387. [CrossRef]
83. Ganesh, S.; Koser, M.L.; Cyr, W.A.; Chopda, G.R.; Tao, J.; Shui, X.; Ying, B.; Chen, D.; Pandya, P.; Chipumuro, E.; et al. Direct pharmacological inhibition of beta-catenin by RNA interference in tumors of diverse origin. *Mol Cancer Ther.* **2016**, *15*, 2143–2154. [CrossRef]
84. Thompson, M.D.; Dar, M.J.; Monga, S.P. Pegylated interferon alpha targets Wnt signaling by inducing nuclear export of beta-catenin. *J. Hepatol.* **2011**, *54*, 506–512. [CrossRef] [PubMed]
85. Yan, M.; Li, G.; An, J. Discovery of small molecule inhibitors of the Wnt/β-catenin signaling pathway by targeting β-catenin/Tcf4 interactions. *Exp. Biol. Med.* **2017**, *242*, 1185–1197. [CrossRef] [PubMed]
86. Emami, K.H.; Nguyen, C.; Ma, H.; Kim, D.H.; Jeong, K.W.; Eguchi, M.; Moon, R.T.; Teo, J.L.; Kim, H.Y.; Moon, S.H.; et al. A small molecule inhibitor of beta-catenin/CREB-binding protein transcription. *Proc. Natl. Acad. Sci. USA* **2004**, *101*, 12682–12687. [CrossRef] [PubMed]
87. Lenz, H.J.; Kahn, M. Safely targeting cancer stem cells via selective catenin coactivator antagonism. *Cancer Sci.* **2014**, *105*, 1087–1092. [CrossRef] [PubMed]
88. Kimura, K.; Ikoma, A.; Shibakawa, M.; Shimoda, S.; Harada, K.; Saio, M.; Imamura, J.; Osawa, Y.; Kimura, M.; Nishikawa, K.; et al. Safety, tolerability, and preliminary efficacy of the anti-fibrotic small molecule PRI-724, a CBP/beta-catenin inhibitor, in patients with hepatitis C virus-related cirrhosis: A single-center, open-label, dose escalation phase 1 trial. *EBioMedicine* **2017**, *23*, 79–87. [CrossRef] [PubMed]
89. Gajewski, T.F. The next hurdle in cancer immunotherapy: Overcoming the non-T-cell-inflamed tumor microenvironment. *Semin. Oncol.* **2015**, *42*, 663–671. [CrossRef] [PubMed]
90. Pai, S.G.; Carneiro, B.A.; Mota, J.M.; Costa, R.; Leite, C.A.; Barroso-Sousa, R.; Kaplan, J.B.; Chae, Y.K.; Giles, F.J. Wnt/beta-catenin pathway: Modulating anticancer immune response. *J. Hematol. Oncol.* **2017**, *10*, 101. [CrossRef]
91. Spranger, S.; Gajewski, T.F. A new paradigm for tumor immune escape: Beta-catenin-driven immune exclusion. *J. Immunother. Cancer* **2015**, *3*, 43. [CrossRef]
92. Van Loosdregt, J.; Fleskens, V.; Tiemessen, M.M.; Mokry, M.; van Boxtel, R.; Meerding, J.; Pals, C.E.; Kurek, D.; Baert, M.R.; Delemarre, E.M.; et al. Canonical Wnt signaling negatively modulates regulatory T cell function. *Immunity* **2013**, *39*, 298–310. [CrossRef]
93. Hong, Y.; Manoharan, I.; Suryawanshi, A.; Majumdar, T.; Angus-Hill, M.L.; Koni, P.A.; Manicassamy, B.; Mellor, A.L.; Munn, D.H.; Manicassamy, S. Beta-catenin promotes regulatory T-cell responses in tumors by inducing vitamin A metabolism in dendritic cells. *Cancer Res.* **2015**, *75*, 656–665. [CrossRef]
94. Pinyol, R.; Sia, D.; Llovet, J.M. Immune exclusion-Wnt/CTNNB1 class predicts resistance to immunotherapies in HCC. *Clin. Cancer Res.* 2019. [CrossRef]

95. Sia, D.; Jiao, Y.; Martinez-Quetglas, I.; Kuchuk, O.; Villacorta-Martin, C.; de Moura, M.C.; Putra, J.; Camprecios, G.; Bassaganyas, L.; Akers, N.; et al. Identification of an immune-specific class of hepatocellular carcinoma, based on molecular features. *Gastroenterology* **2017**, *153*, 812–826. [CrossRef]
96. Nejak-Bowen, K.; Kikuchi, A.; Monga, S.P. Beta-catenin-NF-kappaB interactions in murine hepatocytes: A complex to die for. *Hepatology* **2013**, *57*, 763–774. [CrossRef] [PubMed]
97. Oeckinghaus, A.; Ghosh, S. The NF-kappaB family of transcription factors and its regulation. *Cold Spring Harb. Perspect. Biol.* **2009**, *1*, a000034. [CrossRef] [PubMed]
98. Michael, A.; Ko, S.; Tao, J.; Moghe, A.; Yang, H.; Xu, M.; Russell, J.O.; Pradhan-Sundd, T.; Liu, S.; Singh, S.; et al. Inhibiting glutamine-dependent mTORC1 activation ameliorates liver cancers driven by beta-catenin mutations. *Cell Metab.* **2019**, *29*, 1135–1150. [CrossRef] [PubMed]
99. Gebhardt, R.; Coffer, P.J. Hepatic autophagy is differentially regulated in periportal and pericentral zones–A general mechanism relevant for other tissues? *Cell Commun. Signal* **2013**, *11*, 21. [CrossRef]
100. Jewell, J.L.; Kim, Y.C.; Russell, R.C.; Yu, F.X.; Park, H.W.; Plouffe, S.W.; Tagliabracci, V.S.; Guan, K.L. Metabolism Differential regulation of mTORC1 by leucine and glutamine. *Science* **2015**, *347*, 194–198. [CrossRef]
101. Laplante, M.; Sabatini, D.M. mTOR signaling in growth control and disease. *Cell* **2012**, *149*, 274–293. [CrossRef]

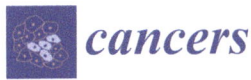

Communication

Targeting the CBP/β-Catenin Interaction to Suppress Activation of Cancer-Promoting Pancreatic Stellate Cells

Mingtian Che [1], Soo-Mi Kweon [1], Jia-Ling Teo [1], Yate-Ching Yuan [2], Laleh G. Melstrom [3], Richard T. Waldron [4,5], Aurelia Lugea [4,5], Raul A. Urrutia [6], Stephen J. Pandol [4,5] and Keane K. Y. Lai [7,8,*]

[1] Department of Molecular Medicine, Beckman Research Institute of City of Hope, Duarte, CA 91010, USA; Mingtian.Che@cshs.org (M.C.); skweon@coh.org (S.-M.K.); jteo@coh.org (J.-L.T.)
[2] Department of Computational and Quantitative Medicine, Beckman Research Institute of City of Hope, Duarte, CA 91010, USA; YYuan@coh.org
[3] Department of Surgery, City of Hope National Medical Center, Duarte, CA 91010, USA; lmelstrom@coh.org
[4] Pancreatic Research Program, Cedars-Sinai Medical Center, Los Angeles, CA 90048, USA; Richard.Waldron@cshs.org (R.T.W.); Aurelia.Lugea@cshs.org (A.L.); Stephen.Pandol@cshs.org (S.J.P.)
[5] Department of Medicine, University of California, Los Angeles (UCLA), Los Angeles, CA 90095, USA
[6] Department of Surgery and the Genomic Sciences and Precision Medicine Center (GSPMC), Medical College of Wisconsin, Milwaukee, WI 53226, USA; rurrutia@mcw.edu
[7] Department of Pathology, City of Hope National Medical Center, and Department of Molecular Medicine, Beckman Research Institute of City of Hope, Duarte, CA 91010, USA
[8] City of Hope Comprehensive Cancer Center, Duarte, CA 91010, USA
* Correspondence: klai@coh.org

Received: 2 May 2020; Accepted: 2 June 2020; Published: 5 June 2020

Abstract: Background: Although cyclic AMP-response element binding protein-binding protein (CBP)/β-catenin signaling is known to promote proliferation and fibrosis in various organ systems, its role in the activation of pancreatic stellate cells (PSCs), the key effector cells of desmoplasia in pancreatic cancer and fibrosis in chronic pancreatitis, is largely unknown. Methods: To investigate the role of the CBP/β-catenin signaling pathway in the activation of PSCs, we have treated mouse and human PSCs with the small molecule specific CBP/β-catenin antagonist ICG-001 and examined the effects of treatment on parameters of activation. Results: We report for the first time that CBP/β-catenin antagonism suppresses activation of PSCs as evidenced by their decreased proliferation, down-regulation of "activation" markers, e.g., α-smooth muscle actin (α-SMA/Acta2), collagen type I alpha 1 (Col1a1), Prolyl 4-hydroxylase, and Survivin, up-regulation of peroxisome proliferator activated receptor gamma (Ppar-γ) which is associated with quiescence, and reduced migration; additionally, CBP/β-catenin antagonism also suppresses PSC-induced migration of cancer cells. Conclusion: CBP/β-catenin antagonism represents a novel therapeutic strategy for suppressing PSC activation and may be effective at countering PSC promotion of pancreatic cancer.

Keywords: pancreatic cancer; pancreatic stellate cells; Wnt signaling; CBP; p300; pancreatitis; fibrosis

1. Introduction

Pancreatic cancer, predominantly comprised of pancreatic ductal adenocarcinoma (PDAC), ranks as the 4th leading cause of cancer deaths in both men and women in the United States, with ~52% of pancreatic cancer patients being diagnosed at an advanced stage of disease for which 5-year survival is a dismal 3% [1]. As such, there is an urgent need for treatments that offer durable benefits to PDAC patients. Treatments for PDAC, which traditionally have focused on targeting pancreatic tumor cells (i.e., parenchymal cells), have been insufficient or have failed for the most part [2,3]. More recently, it has been recognized that activated pancreatic stellate cells (PSCs) (i.e., stromal cells), which are characterized by increased proliferation, up-regulation of "activation" markers, and enhanced migration, promote PDAC progression [2–4]. Moreover, the "desmoplasia" of PDAC, i.e., the extensive pro-tumorigenic fibrosis effected by activated PSCs [2–5], has been found to correlate negatively with patient survival and to be present at similar levels in both primary tumors and metastatic lesions [6]. Thus, activated PSCs represent an attractive therapeutic target to aid in combating PDAC.

The Wnt signaling pathway is an incredibly complex and critical controller of a myriad of processes in mammals, intricately regulating cellular proliferation and cellular differentiation [7,8]. "Canonical" Wnt signaling (or Wnt/β-catenin signaling) is the arm of the pathway associated with β-catenin accumulation in the nucleus and β-catenin forming a complex with members of the TCF/LEF family of transcription factors to regulate target gene transcription. A previous study has shown that retinoic acid-mediated suppression of Wnt/β-catenin signaling suppresses PSC activation in mice with chronic pancreatitis, leading to amelioration of chronic pancreatitis (which itself is a predominant risk factor for PDAC [9,10]) and associated fibrosis [11]. It has been previously demonstrated that, in Wnt/β-catenin signaling, β-catenin recruits either of the Kat3 transcriptional coactivators, cyclic AMP-response element binding protein-binding protein (CBP) or its closely related homolog, p300, to effect transcription and expression of respective target genes [12–15]. CBP/β-catenin signaling is associated with symmetric non-differentiative proliferation in cancer and fibrosis, whereas p300/β-catenin signaling initiates differentiation and a decrease in cellular potency [12–15]. Recently, it has been reported that the small molecule specific CBP/β-catenin antagonist ICG-001 [16] suppresses the activation of hepatic stellate cells, which are developmentally and functionally analogous to PSCs [17,18], as well as suppressing associated fibrogenesis in an acute CCl$_4$-induced liver injury mouse model [19]. However, the significance of the CBP/β-catenin signaling pathway in PSCs is largely unknown. Thus, the CBP/β-catenin signaling pathway represents a potentially viable, but not yet characterized therapeutic opportunity to target in activated PSCs.

Based on the aforementioned observations, we set out to investigate whether antagonizing the CBP/β-catenin signaling pathway would suppress activation of PSCs and may be useful for combating PDAC and chronic pancreatitis. Herein, we report for the first time that the small molecule specific CBP/β-catenin antagonist ICG-001 suppresses activation of PSCs as evidenced by their decreased proliferation, down-regulation of activation markers, e.g., α-smooth muscle actin (α-SMA/Acta2), collagen type I alpha 1 (Col1a1), Prolyl 4-hydroxylase, and Survivin, up-regulation of peroxisome proliferator activated receptor gamma (Ppar-γ), which is associated with quiescence, and reduced migration; and that migration of PDAC cells is reduced when co-cultured with PSCs which have been pre-treated with ICG-001. Hence, CBP/β-catenin antagonist ICG-001 represents a novel therapeutic option for suppressing PSC activation and promotion of PDAC.

2. Results

2.1. CBP/β-Catenin Antagonism Suppresses Proliferation of Pancreatic Stellate Cells

Activated pancreatic stellate cells (PSCs) are known to promote pancreatic ductal adenocarcinoma (PDAC) progression and are characterized by increased proliferation [2–4]. To investigate whether inhibition of CBP/β-catenin signaling would suppress proliferation of PSCs, the small molecule specific CBP/β-catenin antagonist ICG-001 [16] versus control (DMSO) was used to treat immortalized mouse PSC line (imPSC) and immortalized human PSC line (ihPSC), which were established as previously described [20,21]. We found that ICG-001 inhibited proliferation of imPSC and ihPSC, as assessed by CellTiter-Glo proliferation assay (Figure 1A,B), microscopy (Figure 1C,D), and cell counting (Figure 1E,F). In addition, ICG-001 IC$_{50}$ of ~25 μM and ranging from ~5 to ~25 uM, for imPSC and ihPSC, respectively, were estimated based on CellTiter-Glo proliferation assay (Figure 1A,B). Furthermore, ICG-001 treatment induces imPSC and ihPSC to change from a more spread out morphology to a thinner or more round, quiescent morphology (Figure 1C,D). Collectively, our results demonstrate that ICG-001 suppresses activation of PSC by inhibiting proliferation and inducing quiescent morphology.

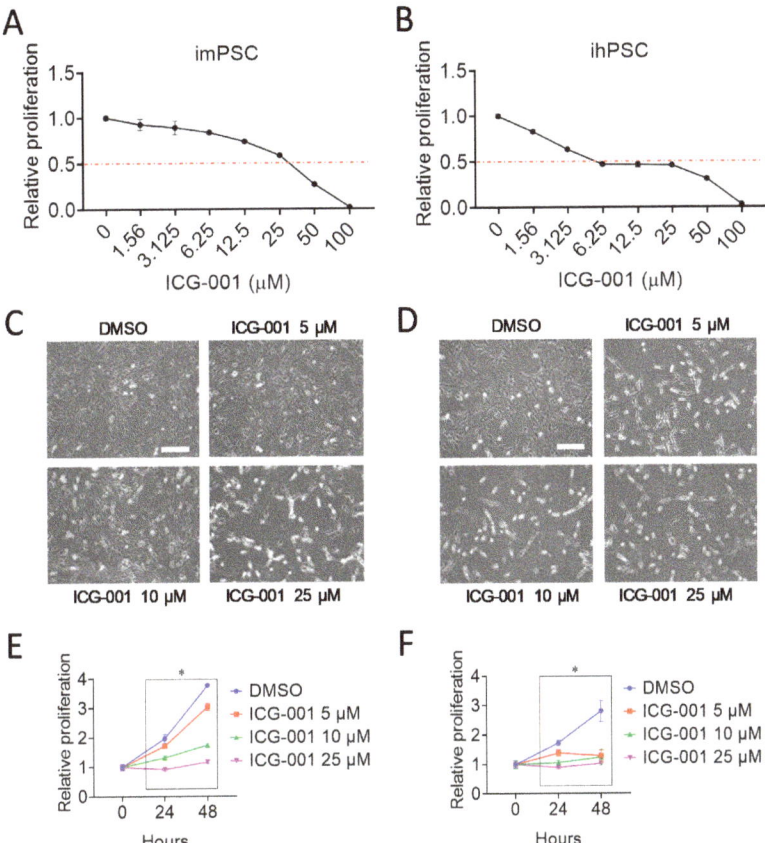

Figure 1. Cyclic AMP-response element binding protein-binding protein (CBP)/β-catenin antagonism suppresses proliferation of pancreatic stellate cells. Effect of CBP/β-catenin antagonist ICG-001 versus control (DMSO) treatment for 48 h on proliferation of immortalized mouse pancreatic stellate cells (imPSC) (**A**) and immortalized human pancreatic stellate cells (ihPSC) (**B**) as assessed by CellTiter-Glo assay. imPSC, immortalized mouse pancreatic stellate cells; ihPSC, immortalized human pancreatic stellate cells. Effect of ICG-001 treatment for 48 h on proliferation of imPSC (**C**) and ihPSC (**D**) as assessed by microscopy. Scale bar: 150 μm. Effect of ICG-001 treatment for 24 h and 48 h on proliferation of imPSC (**E**) and ihPSC (**F**) as assessed by cell counting. $n = 3$, * $p < 0.05$ when each ICG-001 group compared to control (DMSO) at respective time point.

2.2. CBP/β-Catenin Antagonism Suppresses Activation Markers of PSCs

We next tested whether inhibition of CBP/β-catenin signaling would suppress established activation markers of PSCs, such as *Acta2*, *Col1a1*, and *Survivin (Birc5)* [2–4,22–24] at the level of mRNA expression. We found that CBP/β-catenin antagonist ICG-001 versus control (DMSO) suppressed in a dose dependent manner, Acta2, Col1a1, and Survivin (Birc5) mRNA expression by up to ~60%, 70%, and 50%, respectively, in imPSC (Figure 2A–C), as assessed by qPCR. Consistent with these findings, we found that ICG-001 also induced mRNA expression of Ppar-γ, which is associated with PSC quiescence [4,22,25,26], up to ~2.1-fold in imPSC. ICG-001 also suppressed *COL1A1* and *SURVIVIN*

(BIRC5) mRNA expression by up to ~75% and 90%, respectively, in ihPSC, but interestingly ACTA2 mRNA expression was induced up to ~1.9-fold, whereas PPAR-γ mRNA expression was not detected (Ct value > 35) (Figure 2E–G).

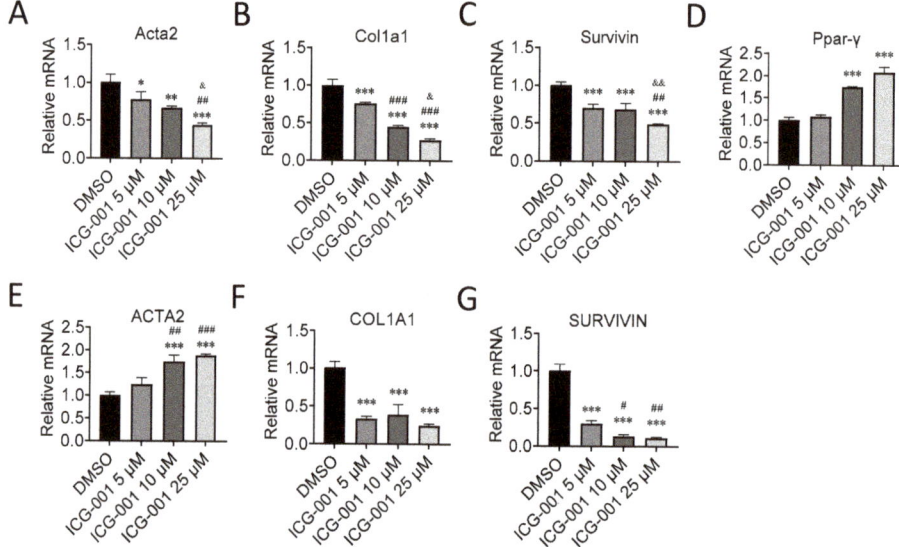

Figure 2. CBP/β-catenin antagonism suppresses gene expression of activation markers of pancreatic stellate cells. Effect of CBP/β-catenin antagonist ICG-001 versus control (DMSO) treatment for 48 h of immortalized mouse pancreatic stellate cells (imPSC) on mRNA expression of activation markers, Acta2 (**A**); Col1a1 (**B**); Survivin (**C**); and Ppar-γ which is associated with quiescence (**D**). Effect of ICG-001 treatment for 48 h of immortalized human pancreatic stellate cells (ihPSC) on mRNA expression of activation markers, ACTA2 (**E**); COL1A1 (**F**); and SURVIVIN (**G**). $n = 3$, * $p < 0.05$, ** $p < 0.01$, *** $p < 0.001$ compared to control (DMSO), # $p < 0.05$, ## $p < 0.01$, ### $p < 0.001$ compared to ICG-001 5 μM, & $p < 0.05$, && $p < 0.01$ compared to ICG-001 10 μM.

We next assessed the effect of ICG-001 on PSC activation and quiescence markers at the level of protein expression, by immunofluorescence or immunoblot. We found that ICG-001 reduced the expression of Acta2 (α-SMA) and Survivin and induced the expression of Ppar-γ in imPSC (Figure 3A,B,D), and similar results were obtained for SURVIVIN and PPAR-γ in ihPSC (Figure 3C,E), as assayed by immunofluorescence. Interestingly, α-SMA was not detected by immunofluorescence in ihPSC, consistent with previous findings, which failed to detect α-SMA at the protein level in this cell line (data not shown) and another immortalized human PSC cell line [27]. Consistent with the immunofluorescence results, ICG-001 reduced the expression of α-SMA by up to ~40% in imPSC (Figure 4A). Given that Prolyl 4-hydroxylase is a central enzyme in the hydroxylation of proline residues in procollagen, serving as a functional indicator of collagen synthesis and thus as another PSC activation marker [26,28], we next tested the effect of ICG-001 on the expression of this marker at the protein level. Immunoblot shows that ICG-001 suppresses Prolyl 4-hydroxylase (P4HA2) by up to ~50% in imPSC (Figure 4B). Thus, based on these protein expression data, along with the aforementioned mRNA expression data, we conclude that CBP/β-catenin antagonism suppresses activation and induces quiescence markers of PSCs.

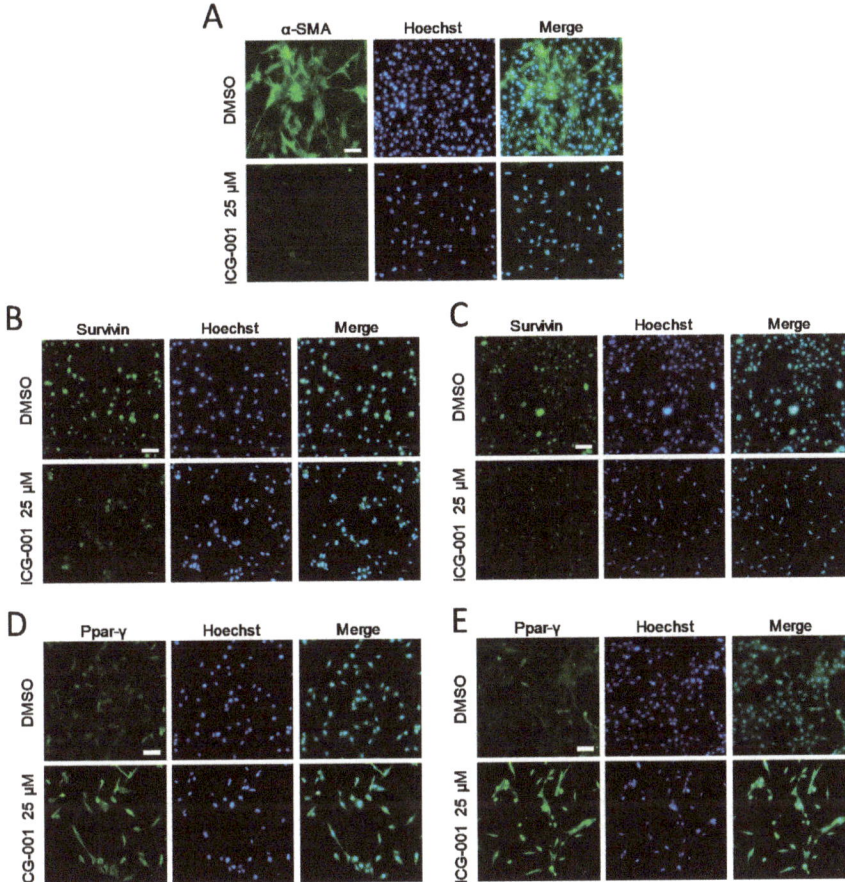

Figure 3. CBP/β-catenin antagonism suppresses protein expression of activation markers of pancreatic stellate cells as assessed by immunofluorescence. Effect of CBP/β-catenin antagonist ICG-001 versus control (DMSO) treatment for 72 h of immortalized mouse pancreatic stellate cells (imPSC) on protein expression of activation markers, Acta2 (α-SMA) (**A**); and Survivin (**B**); and Ppar-γ which is associated with quiescence (**D**); Effect of ICG-001 treatment for 72 h of immortalized human pancreatic stellate cells (ihPSC) on protein expression of activation markers, SURVIVIN (**C**); and PPAR-γ (**E**); Scale bar: 100 μm. Hoechst: Hoechst 33342.

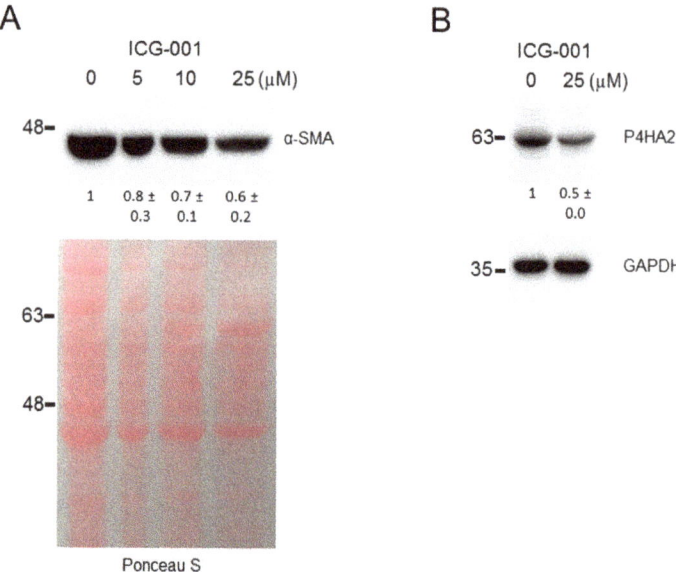

Figure 4. CBP/β-catenin antagonism suppresses protein expression of activation markers of pancreatic stellate cells as assessed by immunoblot. Effect of CBP/β-catenin antagonist ICG-001 versus control (DMSO) treatment for 72 h of immortalized mouse pancreatic stellate cells (imPSC) on protein expression of activation markers, Acta2 (α-SMA) (**A**) and Prolyl 4-hydroxylase (P4HA2) (**B**). Numerical values below protein bands indicate densitometric quantitation normalized to Ponceau S or GAPDH as indicated and then to control (DMSO). Numerical values and associated horizontal marks to the left of protein bands indicate relative position of molecular weight (kDa) markers. (Whole immunoblots are presented in Figure S1.).

2.3. CBP/β-Catenin Antagonism Suppresses Migration of PSCs and PSC-Induced Migration of Cancer Cells

Next, we tested whether inhibition of CBP/β-catenin signaling would suppress PSC migration which is another established characteristic of activated PSCs [2–4]. To do so, we treated imPSC with CBP/β-catenin antagonist ICG-001 versus control (DMSO) and found that ICG-001 treatment suppressed migration by up to ~90%, as assessed by Transwell migration assay (Figure 5A,B). ICG-001 also suppressed migration of ihPSC by up to ~50% (Figure 5C,D). Activated PSCs are known to induce pancreatic cancer cell migration [2–4,29–31], possibly via PSC-mediated induction of epithelial-mesenchymal transition in cancer cells [31]. Accordingly, we reasoned that pancreatic cancer cells, co-cultured with PSCs, which have been pre-treated with and thus presumably "de-activated" by ICG-001, would exhibit decreased migration compared with pancreatic cancer cells co-cultured with PSCs pre-treated with vehicle control. To test this notion, we co-cultured mouse pancreatic cancer cell line Panc02 with imPSC, which had been pre-treated for 72 h with ICG-001 or control, and assessed Transwell migration of the pancreatic cancer cells. We found that ICG-001 pre-treatment of imPSC, which were subsequently co-cultured with Panc02 cancer cells, suppressed PSC-induced migration of Panc02 cancer cells by up to ~60% (Figure 5E,F). Similarly, we found that ICG-001 pre-treatment of ihPSC, which were subsequently co-cultured with human pancreatic cancer cell line PANC-1, suppressed PSC-induced migration of PANC-1 cancer cells by up to ~70% (Figure 5G,H).

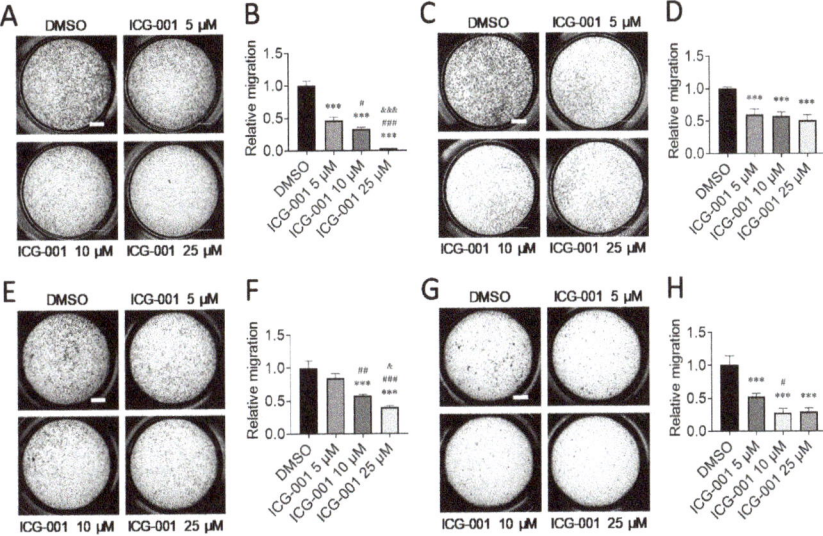

Figure 5. CBP/β-catenin antagonism suppresses migration of pancreatic stellate cells and pancreatic stellate cell-induced migration of pancreatic cancer cells. Effect of CBP/β-catenin antagonist ICG-001 versus control (DMSO) on migration of immortalized mouse pancreatic stellate cells (imPSC) ((**A**), Crystal Violet staining of cells which migrated; and (**B**), relative migration) and on migration of immortalized human pancreatic stellate cells (ihPSC) ((**C**), Crystal Violet staining of cells which migrated; and (**D**), relative migration), as assessed by Transwell migration assay. Note: imPSC and ihPSC were treated with ICG-001 for 48 h, after which time cells were seeded in serum-free medium onto 8-μm Transwell insert, and the lower chamber was filled with 10% FBS medium. Cells were then allowed to migrate for 6 h (imPSC) or 24 h (ihPSC) and kept in corresponding concentrations of ICG-001 versus control (DMSO) during migration. Effect of ICG-001 on imPSC-induced migration of mouse pancreatic cancer cells Panc02 ((**E**), Crystal Violet staining of cells which migrated; and (**F**), relative migration) and on ihPSC-induced migration of human pancreatic cancer cells PANC-1 ((**G**), Crystal Violet staining of cells which migrated; and (**H**), relative migration), as assessed by Transwell migration assay. Note: For PSC-induced Panc02 and PANC-1 cell migration, imPSC and ihPSC were pre-treated with ICG-001 for 72 h, after which time respective PSCs were seeded in 10% FBS medium into the lower chamber and respective cancer cells were seeded in 10% FBS medium onto Transwell insert. Cells were then allowed to migrate for 24 h. Relative migration was determined by counting the number of cells which had migrated across the Transwell insert as assessed by Crystal Violet staining and then normalizing to control (DMSO). $n = 3$, *** $p < 0.001$ compared to control (DMSO), # $p < 0.05$, ## $p < 0.01$, ### $p < 0.001$ compared to ICG-001 5 μM, & $p < 0.05$, &&& $p < 0.001$ compared to ICG-001 10 μM. Scale bar: 1 mm.

3. Discussion

Given that pancreatic cancer, predominantly comprised of pancreatic ductal adenocarcinoma (PDAC), ranks as the 4th leading cause of cancer deaths in the United States with a 5-year survival for advanced stage disease of only 3% [1], there is an urgent need for treatments that offer durable benefits to PDAC patients. With increasing recognition that PDAC treatments traditionally focused on targeting pancreatic tumor cells have been insufficient or failed [2,3] and that activated pancreatic stellate cells (PSCs) promote PDAC progression [2–4] and are the key effector cells of desmoplasia [2–5], which correlates negatively with patient survival [6], there has been an increasing focus on developing novel therapeutic strategies which target activated PSCs to aid in combatting PDAC [2–5].

We now report for the first time that the small molecule specific CBP/β-catenin antagonist ICG-001 suppresses activation of PSCs as evidenced by their decreased proliferation, down-regulation of activation markers, e.g., Acta2 (in imPSC but apparently not in ihPSC), Col1a1, Prolyl 4-hydroxylase, and Survivin, up-regulation of Ppar-γ which is associated with quiescence, and reduced migration of PSC, as well as by reduced PSC-induced migration of pancreatic cancer cells. Our results are consistent with those of a previous study showing that retinoic acid-mediated suppression of Wnt/β-catenin signaling suppresses PSC activation as evidenced by inhibition of PSC proliferation and Col1a1 expression in vitro and by amelioration of PSC-mediated chronic pancreatitis and associated fibrosis in mice [11]. Our results are also consistent with those of a recent report revealing that ICG-001 suppresses the activation of hepatic stellate cells (which are developmentally and functionally analogous to PSCs) as evidenced by inhibition of α-SMA and collagen-I expression and migration by hepatic stellate cells in vitro, as well as by suppression of associated fibrogenesis in an acute CCl_4-induced liver injury mouse model [19]. Expression of Acta2, Col1a1, Prolyl 4-hydroxylase, and Survivin is associated with activated PSCs [2–4,22–24,26,28] which actively proliferate and migrate [4], whereas expression of Ppar-γ is associated with quiescent PSCs [4,22,25,26]. Activated PSCs are the key effector cells for producing the collagen stroma of PDAC, with the resulting fibrous stroma capable of impeding chemotherapeutics/drugs from reaching targets [3]. The interplay between activated PSCs and PDAC cells enhances cancer progression [3], e.g., activated PSCs induce PDAC cell migration which has previously been correlated with epithelial-mesenchymal transition (EMT) [3,31]. Hence, based on our results, we would expect that suppressing activation and inducing quiescence of PSCs by treatment with ICG-001 would have a therapeutically beneficial effect on PSCs and PSC-associated PDAC progression in vivo.

Interestingly, we found in our current study that Acta2 mRNA expression differed between imPSC and ihPSC in response to ICG-001 treatment, with imPSC showing down-regulation and ihPSC showing apparent up-regulation in expression. The exact cause of the observed apparent discrepancy is unknown. A possible explanation for the discrepancy is that imPSC originates from relatively normal tissue whereas ihPSC originates from cancer tissue. Additionally, the Ct value of Acta2 for imPSC treated with control (DMSO) was ~21, whereas the Ct value for ihPSC treated with control (DMSO) was ~27, suggesting that perhaps Acta2 is not substantially expressed at the mRNA level in ihPSC versus imPSC, so that the observed up-regulation in mRNA expression with ICG-001 treatment in ihPSC may not be entirely comparable to the down-regulation in imPSC, given that the baseline Ct values between the two cell lines are so different. Moreover, the immortalization process, together with the difference in tissue of origin, in addition to the inherent biological variability between the different cells, may explain the differential regulation of Acta2 mRNA expression. An analogous explanation could be offered for the observed difference in Ppar-γ mRNA expression between imPSC and ihPSC. Thus and as recently underscored by Lenggenhager et al., cognizance of differences in PSC origin, condition of the pancreas from which PSCs were derived, and whether PSC cultures were primary or immortalized, is important given that such differences may explain apparently contradictory results between experiments using different types of PSCs [27].

In a broader, more fundamental context, Acta2 [32,33], Col1a1 [34], and Survivin [35] have all been previously identified as direct or indirect targets of the CBP/β-catenin signaling pathway and associated with a proliferative and pro-fibrotic phenotype which characterizes activated PSCs [2–4,22–24]. Furthermore, Ppar-γ, a nuclear receptor which is associated with PSC quiescence [4,22,25,26], is known to have anti-inflammatory/anti-fibrotic activity [36] and should compete with β-catenin for binding to CBP's N-terminal region, thereby phenocopying ICG-001 antagonism of CBP/β-catenin binding and associated signaling [37]. As such, it is not surprising that various studies have shown that treatment with CBP/β-catenin antagonist ICG-001 (or the structurally related derivative PRI-724) is effective pre-clinically at ameliorating fibrosis in the peritoneum [38], endometrium [39], lung [13], kidney [32], skin [40], heart [41], and liver [19,42]. Importantly, a recent phase 1 trial utilizing PRI-724 demonstrated that treatment of patients safely improved liver histology and Child–Pugh scores for cirrhosis [43], suggesting that CBP/β-catenin antagonism is a viable therapeutic for combating fibrotic diseases in general. Moreover, it is known that chronic pancreatitis is a pathological syndrome characterized by persistent fibrosis effected by activated PSCs and is itself a predominant risk factor for PDAC [9,10], conferring a ~8 to 12-fold increased risk of developing PDAC to chronic pancreatitis patients [44]. These observations, in conjunction with the results of our current study, have overarching therapeutic implications, namely: CBP/β-catenin antagonism would be expected not only to be effective at suppressing activation of PSCs and thereby ameliorating already existing PDAC, but also to be effective as a "PDAC prophylactic" by inhibiting activation of PSCs during the early pre-cancerous stage of pancreatic fibrosis/chronic pancreatitis.

Given the pressing need to develop and implement better treatment strategies for combatting PDAC, we now present in this Communication our novel results on the effectiveness of CBP/β-catenin antagonism in suppressing PSC activation, with broad therapeutic implications for treating PDAC and chronic pancreatitis, both of which are known to be promoted by activated PSCs. Because of the limitation in scope of our current study, future studies (e.g., using primary PSCs and in vivo models) would be required to further validate the effect of CBP/β-catenin antagonism on PSC biology/pathobiology, including the interaction between PSCs and PDAC cells.

4. Materials and Methods

4.1. Cell Lines and Culture Conditions

Immortalized mouse pancreatic stellate cell line (imPSC) and immortalized human pancreatic stellate cell line (ihPSC) were kindly provided by Richard T. Waldron, Aurelia Lugea, and Raul A. Urrutia and were established as previously described [20,21]. imPSC were grown and cultivated in Dulbecco's Modified Eagle Medium (DMEM) with low glucose (1000 mg/L) while ihPSC were grown and cultivated in DMEM with high glucose (4500 mg/L). All culture medium was supplemented with 10% fetal bovine serum (FBS) and 1% penicillin-streptomycin unless otherwise indicated. Cells were maintained in an incubator at 37 °C with 5% CO_2.

4.2. Pharmacologic Agents

Small molecule specific CBP/β-catenin antagonist ICG-001 as previously described [16] was donated by Professor Michael Kahn and used at concentrations as indicated.

4.3. Cell Proliferation Assays

CellTiter-Glo assay (Promega) was performed according to the manufacturer's protocol. Cells were plated in triplicate in 96-well plates at 1×10^4 cells/well in 100 µL of medium. Plates were incubated at 37 °C in 5% CO_2. The next day, cells were treated with ICG-001 at 100 µM, 50 µM, 25 µM, 12.5 µM, 6.25 µM, 3.13 µM 1.56 µM or control (DMSO) and were incubated for an additional 48 h. Then, 50 µL CellTiter-Glo reagent and 50 µL of DMEM were added to the wells and incubated for 10 min protected from the light. Luminescence signal was assayed using EnVision Multilabel Plate Reader (Perkin-Elmer).

Cell proliferation was also assessed by cell counting using a hemocytometer. Briefly, imPSC or ihPSC were seeded in 6-well plates at 5×10^4 cells/well and incubated at 37 °C in 5% CO_2. The next day, cells were treated with ICG-001 at 5 µM, 10 µM, 25 µM or control (DMSO) for 24 h or 48 h. Cell numbers were counted at 0, 24, and 48 h after treatment.

4.4. Quantitative Polymerase Chain Reaction (qPCR)

Cells were treated with ICG-001 for 48 h. Total mRNA was extracted by TRIzol reagent (Invitrogen) according to the manufacturer's protocol. cDNA was synthesized using qScript cDNA Synthesis Kit (Quantabio) and used as template for qPCR with SYBR Green detection method. The PCR primer sequences used for mouse cells were as follows:

Acta2 (F: 5′-GTCCCAGACATCAGGGAGTAA-3′, R: 5′-TCGGATACTTCAGCGTCAGGA-3′); Col1a1 (F: 5′-GCTCCTCTTAGGGGCCACT-3′, R: 5′-CCACGTCTCACCATTGGGG-3′); Survivin (F: 5′-GAGGCTGGCTTCATCCACTG, R: 5′-ATGCTCCTCTATCGGGTTGTC-3′); Ppar-γ (F: 5′-TTTTCCGAAGAACCATCCGATT-3′, R: 5′-ATGGCATTGTGAGACATCCCC-3′). The PCR primer sequences used for human cells were as follows: ACTA2 (F: 5′-CTATGAGGGCTATGCCTTGCC-3′, R: 5′-GCTCAGCAGTAGTAACGAAGGA-3′); COL1A1 (F: 5′-GAGGGCCAAGACGAAGACATC-3′, R: 5′-CAGATCACGTCATCGCACAAC-3′); SURVIVIN (F: 5′-AGGACCACCGCATCTCTACAT-3′, R: 5′-AAGTCTGGCTCGTTCTCAGTG-3′); PPAR-γ (F: 5′-CTATGGAGTTCATGCTTGTG-3′, R: 5′-GTACTGACATTTATTT-3′). Housekeeping gene PCR primer sequences used were GAPDH for mouse cells (F: 5′-GGTGCTGAGTATGTCGTGGA-3′, R: 5′-ACAGTCTTCTGGGTGGCAGT-3′) and GAPDH for human cells (F: 5′-AGAAGGCTGGGGCTCATTTG-3′, R: 5′-AGGGGCCATCCACAGTCTTC-3′).

4.5. Immunofluorescence

Cells were plated, and the next day cells were treated with ICG-001 or control (DMSO) for 72 h, followed by 4% PFA fixation for 10 min. After 3 times of PBS washing, 1% BSA with 0.1% Triton X-100 was used for blocking nonspecific binding. Primary antibodies for α-SMA (Cell Signaling Technology, #19245s; 1:100), Survivin (Cell Signaling Technology, #2808s; 1:250), and Ppar-γ (Affinity BioReagents, #PA3-821; 1:50) were used for overnight incubation at 4 °C. Secondary antibody anti-rabbit IgG-Alexa Fluor 488 (Invitrogen, #A11034; 1:1000) was incubated for 40 min at room temperature. Hoechst 33342 was used for nuclear staining for 10 min. A fluorescence microscope (Eclipse Ti2, Nikon) was used to observe target protein expression.

4.6. Western Blot

2×10^5 of imPSC were plated in 10 cm plates. The next day, cells were treated with ICG-001 or control (DMSO) and were incubated for an additional 72 h. Then, cells were collected, and total cellular proteins were extracted using M-PER Mammalian Protein Extraction Reagent (ThermoFisher). After protein quantification by Bradford assay method, protein samples were separated by 10% SDS PAGE, followed by transfer to nitrocellulose membrane. Next, the membranes were blocked with 5% milk in Tris-Buffered Saline with 0.1% Tween. The membranes were incubated with primary antibody overnight at 4 °C and incubated with secondary antibody for 1 h the following day. Primary antibodies for α-SMA (Cell Signaling Technology, #19245s), Prolyl 4-hydroxylase (P4HA2) (ThermoFisher, #PA5-96280), and GAPDH (Santa Cruz Biotechnologies, #sc-32233), and secondary antibody anti-rabbit IgG-HRP (Santa Cruz Biotechnologies, #sc-2357) were used. Protein bands were detected using ECL prime Western blotting detection reagent (Amersham) and visualized by Chemidoc Imaging System (Bio-Rad). Each protein band of interest was digitized by densitometry program ImageJ (NIH) or ImageLab (Bio-Rad). Densitometric quantitation of protein bands was normalized to Ponceau S or GAPDH and then to control (DMSO).

4.7. Transwell Migration Assay

For PSC Transwell migration assay, imPSC and ihPSC were treated with ICG-001 for 48 h. Then, 1×10^4 cells were seeded in serum-free DMEM onto 8-μm Transwell insert (Corning). The lower chamber was filled with 10% FBS supplemented DMEM. Cells were then allowed to migrate while incubated at 37 °C with 5% CO_2 for 6 h (imPSC) or 24 h (ihPSC) and kept in corresponding concentrations of ICG-001 versus control (DMSO) during migration.

For PSC-induced Panc02 and PANC-1 cancer cell Transwell migration assay, imPSC and ihPSC were pre-treated with ICG-001 for 72 h, and then seeded in 10% FBS DMEM into the lower chamber of 24-well plate at a total number of 5×10^4 (imPSC) or 1×10^5 (ihPSC) cells per well. Panc02 or PANC-1 cells (1×10^4) were seeded in 10% FBS DMEM onto Transwell insert. Cells were then incubated and allowed to migrate for 24 h.

For both PSC Transwell migration assay and PSC-induced Panc02 and PANC-1 cancer cell Transwell migration assay, after incubation, cells were stained with 1% Crystal Violet solution (Sigma) for 30 min. The cells on the upper surface of the Transwell insert were gently removed by cotton swab, and the cells which had migrated to the bottom surface of the insert were counted under bright field microscopy. Relative migration was determined by normalizing the number of cells which had migrated with ICG-001 treatment to the number of cells which had migrated with control (DMSO) treatment.

4.8. Statistical Analysis

Numerical data were expressed as the means ± SD unless otherwise noted. Student's t-test was performed to assess the statistical significance between two sets of data as appropriate. One-way ANOVA followed by post-hoc Tukey test was performed for multiple comparisons when appropriate. p values less than 0.05 were considered significant.

5. Conclusions

We report for the first time that the small molecule specific CBP/β-°C antagonist ICG-001 suppresses activation of PSCs as evidenced by their decreased proliferation, down-regulation of activation markers, e.g., Acta2, Col1a1, Prolyl 4-hydroxylase, and Survivin, up-regulation of Ppar-γ which is associated with quiescence, and reduced migration; furthermore, migration of PDAC cells is reduced when co-cultured with PSCs which have been pre-treated with ICG-001. Hence, CBP/β-catenin antagonism represents a novel therapeutic strategy for suppressing PSC activation and may be effective at treating PDAC and "pre-cancerous" chronic pancreatitis, both of which are known to be promoted by activated PSCs.

Supplementary Materials: The following are available online at http://www.mdpi.com/2072-6694/12/6/1476/s1, Figure S1: CBP/β-catenin antagonism suppresses protein expression of activation markers of pancreatic stellate cells as assessed by immunoblot (Whole immunoblots).

Author Contributions: M.C., methodology, formal analysis, investigation, writing—original draft preparation, visualization; S.-M.K., methodology, formal analysis, investigation, writing—original draft preparation, visualization; J.-L.T., methodology, investigation, writing—review and editing; Y.-C.Y., investigation, writing—review and editing; L.G.M., investigation, writing—review and editing; R.T.W., methodology, investigation, resources, writing—review and editing; A.L., methodology, investigation, resources, writing—review and editing; R.A.U., methodology, resources, writing—review and editing, funding acquisition; S.J.P., methodology, investigation, resources, writing—original draft preparation, funding acquisition; K.K.Y.L., conceptualization, methodology, formal analysis, investigation, resources, writing—original draft preparation, writing—review and editing, visualization, supervision, project administration, funding acquisition. All authors have read and agreed to the published version of the manuscript.

Funding: K.K.Y. Lai has been supported by NIH K08AA025112. S.J. Pandol has been supported by NIH U01DK108314, P01CA233452, and P01CA236585. R.A. Urrutia has been supported by NIH R01DK052913.

Conflicts of Interest: The authors declare no conflict of interest. The funders had no role in the design of the study; in the collection, analyses, or interpretation of data; in the writing of the manuscript, or in the decision to publish the results.

References

1. American Cancer Society. *Cancer Facts & Figures 2019*; American Cancer Society: Atlanta, AT, USA, 2019; pp. 1–71.
2. Apte, M.V.; Wilson, J.S.; Lugea, A.; Pandol, S.J. A starring role for stellate cells in the pancreatic cancer microenvironment. *Gastroenterology* **2013**, *144*, 1210–1219. [CrossRef] [PubMed]
3. Pothula, S.P.; Pirola, R.C.; Wilson, J.S.; Apte, M.V. Pancreatic stellate cells: Aiding and abetting pancreatic cancer progression. *Pancreatology* **2020**, *20*, 409–418. [CrossRef]
4. Xue, R.; Jia, K.; Wang, J.; Yang, L.; Wang, Y.; Gao, L.; Hao, J. A rising star in pancreatic diseases: Pancreatic stellate cells. *Front Physiol.* **2018**, *9*, 754. [CrossRef]

5. Apte, M.V.; Park, S.; Phillips, P.A.; Santucci, N.; Goldstein, D.; Kumar, R.K.; Ramm, G.A.; Buchler, M.; Friess, H.; McCarroll, J.A.; et al. Desmoplastic reaction in pancreatic cancer: Role of pancreatic stellate cells. *Pancreas* **2004**, *29*, 179–187. [CrossRef] [PubMed]
6. Whatcott, C.J.; Diep, C.H.; Jiang, P.; Watanabe, A.; LoBello, J.; Sima, C.; Hostetter, G.; Shepard, H.M.; Von Hoff, D.D.; Han, H. Desmoplasia in primary tumors and metastatic lesions of pancreatic cancer. *Clin. Cancer Res.* **2015**, *21*, 3561–3568. [CrossRef]
7. Clevers, H.; Nusse, R. Wnt/β-catenin signaling and disease. *Cell* **2012**, *149*, 1192–1205. [CrossRef]
8. Monga, S.P. β-Catenin Signaling and Roles in Liver Homeostasis, Injury, and Tumorigenesis. *Gastroenterology* **2015**, *148*, 1294–1310. [CrossRef] [PubMed]
9. Lew, D.; Afghani, E.; Pandol, S. Chronic pancreatitis: Current status and challenges for prevention and treatment. *Dig. Dis. Sci.* **2017**, *62*, 1702–1712. [CrossRef] [PubMed]
10. Whitcomb, D.C.; Shelton, C.A.; Brand, R.E. Genetics and genetic testing in pancreatic cancer. *Gastroenterology* **2015**, *149*, 1252–1264. [CrossRef]
11. Xiao, W.; Jiang, W.; Shen, J.; Yin, G.; Fan, Y.; Wu, D.; Qiu, L.; Yu, G.; Xing, M.; Hu, G.; et al. Retinoic acid ameliorates pancreatic fibrosis and inhibits the activation of pancreatic stellate cells in mice with experimental chronic pancreatitis via suppressing the Wnt/β-catenin signaling pathway. *PLoS ONE* **2015**, *10*, e0141462. [CrossRef]
12. Teo, J.L.; Ma, H.; Nguyen, C.; Lam, C.; Kahn, M. Specific inhibition of CBP/beta-catenin interaction rescues defects in neuronal differentiation caused by a presenilin-1 mutation. *Proc. Natl. Acad. Sci. USA* **2005**, *102*, 12171–12176. [CrossRef] [PubMed]
13. Henderson, W.R.; Chi, E.Y.; Ye, X.; Nguyen, C.; Tien, Y.T.; Zhou, B.; Borok, Z.; Knight, D.A.; Kahn, M. Inhibition of Wnt/beta-catenin/CREB binding protein (CBP) signaling reverses pulmonary fibrosis. *Proc. Natl. Acad. Sci. USA* **2010**, *107*, 14309–14314. [CrossRef] [PubMed]
14. Lai, K.K.Y.; Nguyen, C.; Lee, K.S.; Lee, A.; Lin, D.P.; Teo, J.L.; Kahn, M. Convergence of canonical and Non-canonical Wnt signal: Differential Kat3 coactivator usage. *Curr. Mol. Pharmacol.* **2019**. [CrossRef] [PubMed]
15. Thomas, P.D.; Kahn, M. Kat3 coactivators in somatic stem cells and cancer stem cells: Biological roles, evolution, and pharmacologic manipulation. *Cell Biol. Toxicol.* **2016**, *32*, 61–81. [CrossRef] [PubMed]
16. Emami, K.H.; Nguyen, C.; Ma, H.; Kim, D.H.; Jeong, K.W.; Eguchi, M.; Moon, R.T.; Teo, J.L.; Oh, S.W.; Kim, H.Y.; et al. A small molecule inhibitor of beta-catenin/CREB-binding protein transcription [corrected]. *Proc. Natl. Acad. Sci. USA* **2004**, *101*, 12682–12687. [CrossRef]
17. Omary, M.B.; Lugea, A.; Lowe, A.W.; Pandol, S.J. The pancreatic stellate cell: A star on the rise in pancreatic diseases. *J. Clin. Investig.* **2007**, *117*, 50–59. [CrossRef]
18. Buchholz, M.; Kestler, H.A.; Holzmann, K.; Ellenrieder, V.; Schneiderhan, W.; Siech, M.; Adler, G.; Bachem, M.G.; Gress, T.M. Transcriptome analysis of human hepatic and pancreatic stellate cells: Organ-specific variations of a common transcriptional phenotype. *J. Mol. Med. (Berl)* **2005**, *83*, 795–805. [CrossRef]
19. Akcora, B.; Storm, G.; Bansal, R. Inhibition of canonical WNT signaling pathway by β-catenin/CBP inhibitor ICG-001 ameliorates liver fibrosis in vivo through suppression of stromal CXCL12. *Biochim. Biophys. Acta Mol. Basis Dis.* **2018**, *1864*, 804–818. [CrossRef]
20. Cao, Y.; Szabolcs, A.; Dutta, S.K.; Yaqoob, U.; Jagavelu, K.; Wang, L.; Leof, E.B.; Urrutia, R.A.; Shah, V.H.; Mukhopadhyay, D. Neuropilin-1 mediates divergent R-Smad signaling and the myofibroblast phenotype. *J. Biol. Chem.* **2010**, *285*, 31840–31848. [CrossRef]
21. Mathison, A.; Liebl, A.; Bharucha, J.; Mukhopadhyay, D.; Lomberk, G.; Shah, V.; Urrutia, R. Pancreatic stellate cell models for transcriptional studies of desmoplasia-associated genes. *Pancreatology* **2010**, *10*, 505–516. [CrossRef]
22. Apte, M.V.; Pirola, R.C.; Wilson, J.S. Pancreatic stellate cells: A starring role in normal and diseased pancreas. *Front Physiol.* **2012**, *3*, 344. [CrossRef] [PubMed]
23. De Minicis, S.; Seki, E.; Uchinami, H.; Kluwe, J.; Zhang, Y.; Brenner, D.A.; Schwabe, R.F. Gene expression profiles during hepatic stellate cell activation in culture and in vivo. *Gastroenterology* **2007**, *132*, 1937–1946. [CrossRef] [PubMed]

24. Mantoni, T.S.; Schendel, R.R.; Rödel, F.; Niedobitek, G.; Al-Assar, O.; Masamune, A.; Brunner, T.B. Stromal SPARC expression and patient survival after chemoradiation for non-resectable pancreatic adenocarcinoma. *Cancer Biol. Ther.* **2008**, *7*, 1806–1815. [CrossRef]
25. Jaster, R.; Lichte, P.; Fitzner, B.; Brock, P.; Glass, A.; Karopka, T.; Gierl, L.; Koczan, D.; Thiesen, H.J.; Sparmann, G.; et al. Peroxisome proliferator-activated receptor gamma overexpression inhibits pro-fibrogenic activities of immortalised rat pancreatic stellate cells. *J. Cell Mol. Med.* **2005**, *9*, 670–682. [CrossRef]
26. Masamune, A.; Kikuta, K.; Satoh, M.; Sakai, Y.; Satoh, A.; Shimosegawa, T. Ligands of peroxisome proliferator-activated receptor-gamma block activation of pancreatic stellate cells. *J. Biol. Chem.* **2002**, *277*, 141–147. [CrossRef]
27. Lenggenhager, D.; Amrutkar, M.; Sántha, P.; Aasrum, M.; Löhr, J.M.; Gladhaug, I.P.; Verbeke, C.S. Commonly used pancreatic stellate cell cultures differ phenotypically and in their interactions with pancreatic cancer cells. *Cells* **2019**, *8*, 23. [CrossRef] [PubMed]
28. Masamune, A.; Satoh, M.; Kikuta, K.; Suzuki, N.; Shimosegawa, T. Establishment and characterization of a rat pancreatic stellate cell line by spontaneous immortalization. *World J. Gastroenterol.* **2003**, *9*, 2751–2758. [CrossRef]
29. Hwang, R.F.; Moore, T.; Arumugam, T.; Ramachandran, V.; Amos, K.D.; Rivera, A.; Ji, B.; Evans, D.B.; Logsdon, C.D. Cancer-associated stromal fibroblasts promote pancreatic tumor progression. *Cancer Res.* **2008**, *68*, 918–926. [CrossRef]
30. Vonlaufen, A.; Joshi, S.; Qu, C.; Phillips, P.A.; Xu, Z.; Parker, N.R.; Toi, C.S.; Pirola, R.C.; Wilson, J.S.; Goldstein, D.; et al. Pancreatic stellate cells: Partners in crime with pancreatic cancer cells. *Cancer Res.* **2008**, *68*, 2085–2093. [CrossRef]
31. Kikuta, K.; Masamune, A.; Watanabe, T.; Ariga, H.; Itoh, H.; Hamada, S.; Satoh, K.; Egawa, S.; Unno, M.; Shimosegawa, T. Pancreatic stellate cells promote epithelial-mesenchymal transition in pancreatic cancer cells. *Biochem. Biophys. Res. Commun.* **2010**, *403*, 380–384. [CrossRef]
32. Hao, S.; He, W.; Li, Y.; Ding, H.; Hou, Y.; Nie, J.; Hou, F.F.; Kahn, M.; Liu, Y. Targeted inhibition of β-catenin/CBP signaling ameliorates renal interstitial fibrosis. *J. Am. Soc. Nephrol.* **2011**, *22*, 1642–1653. [CrossRef] [PubMed]
33. Zhou, B.; Liu, Y.; Kahn, M.; Ann, D.K.; Han, A.; Wang, H.; Nguyen, C.; Flodby, P.; Zhong, Q.; Krishnaveni, M.S.; et al. Interactions between β-catenin and transforming growth factor-β signaling pathways mediate epithelial-mesenchymal transition and are dependent on the transcriptional co-activator cAMP-response element-binding protein (CREB)-binding protein (CBP). *J. Biol. Chem.* **2012**, *287*, 7026–7038. [CrossRef] [PubMed]
34. Rong, M.; Chen, S.; Zambrano, R.; Duncan, M.R.; Grotendorst, G.; Wu, S. Inhibition of β-catenin signaling protects against CTGF-induced alveolar and vascular pathology in neonatal mouse lung. *Pediatr. Res.* **2016**, *80*, 136–144. [CrossRef]
35. Ma, H.; Nguyen, C.; Lee, K.S.; Kahn, M. Differential roles for the coactivators CBP and p300 on TCF/beta-catenin-mediated survivin gene expression. *Oncogene* **2005**, *24*, 3619–3631. [CrossRef]
36. Belvisi, M.G.; Hele, D.J.; Birrell, M.A. Peroxisome proliferator-activated receptor gamma agonists as therapy for chronic airway inflammation. *Eur. J. Pharmacol.* **2006**, *533*, 101–109. [CrossRef]
37. Ono, M.; Lai, K.K.Y.; Wu, K.; Nguyen, C.; Lin, D.P.; Murali, R.; Kahn, M. Nuclear receptor/Wnt beta-catenin interactions are regulated via differential CBP/p300 coactivator usage. *PLoS ONE* **2018**, *13*, e0200714. [CrossRef]
38. Ji, S.; Deng, H.; Jin, W.; Yan, P.; Wang, R.; Pang, L.; Zhou, J.; Zhang, J.; Chen, X.; Zhao, X.; et al. Beta-catenin participates in dialysate-induced peritoneal fibrosis. *FEBS Open Bio.* **2017**, *7*, 265–273. [CrossRef]
39. Hirakawa, T.; Nasu, K.; Miyabe, S.; Kouji, H.; Katoh, A.; Uemura, N.; Narahara, H. β-catenin signaling inhibitors ICG-001 and C-82 improve fibrosis in preclinical models of endometriosis. *Sci. Rep.* **2019**, *9*, 20056. [CrossRef]
40. Beyer, C.; Reichert, H.; Akan, H.; Mallano, T.; Schramm, A.; Dees, C.; Palumbo-Zerr, K.; Lin, N.Y.; Distler, A.; Gelse, K.; et al. Blockade of canonical Wnt signalling ameliorates experimental dermal fibrosis. *Ann. Rheum. Dis.* **2013**, *72*, 1255–1258. [CrossRef]

41. Blyszczuk, P.; Müller-Edenborn, B.; Valenta, T.; Osto, E.; Stellato, M.; Behnke, S.; Glatz, K.; Basler, K.; Lüscher, T.F.; Distler, O.; et al. Transforming growth factor-β-dependent Wnt secretion controls myofibroblast formation and myocardial fibrosis progression in experimental autoimmune myocarditis. *Eur. Heart J.* **2017**, *38*, 1413–1425. [CrossRef]
42. Tokunaga, Y.; Osawa, Y.; Ohtsuki, T.; Hayashi, Y.; Yamaji, K.; Yamane, D.; Hara, M.; Munekata, K.; Tsukiyama-Kohara, K.; Hishima, T.; et al. Selective inhibitor of Wnt/β-catenin/CBP signaling ameliorates hepatitis C virus-induced liver fibrosis in mouse model. *Sci. Rep.* **2017**, *7*, 325. [CrossRef]
43. Kimura, K.; Ikoma, A.; Shibakawa, M.; Shimoda, S.; Harada, K.; Saio, M.; Imamura, J.; Osawa, Y.; Kimura, M.; Nishikawa, K.; et al. Safety, Tolerability, and preliminary efficacy of the anti-fibrotic small molecule PRI-724, a CBP/β-catenin inhibitor, in patients with hepatitis C virus-related cirrhosis: A single-center, open-label, dose escalation phase 1 trial. *EBioMedicine* **2017**, *23*, 79–87. [CrossRef]
44. Kirkegård, J.; Mortensen, F.V.; Cronin-Fenton, D. Chronic pancreatitis and pancreatic cancer risk: A systematic review and meta-analysis. *Am. J. Gastroenterol.* **2017**, *112*, 1366–1372. [CrossRef]

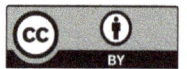

© 2020 by the authors. Licensee MDPI, Basel, Switzerland. This article is an open access article distributed under the terms and conditions of the Creative Commons Attribution (CC BY) license (http://creativecommons.org/licenses/by/4.0/).

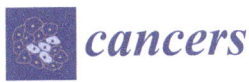

Article

Feasibility of Targeting Traf2-and-Nck-Interacting Kinase in Synovial Sarcoma

Tetsuya Sekita [1,2], Tesshi Yamada [3,*], Eisuke Kobayashi [4], Akihiko Yoshida [5], Toru Hirozane [2], Akira Kawai [4], Yuko Uno [6], Hideki Moriyama [6], Masaaki Sawa [6], Yuichi Nagakawa [3], Akihiko Tsuchida [3], Morio Matsumoto [2], Masaya Nakamura [2], Robert Nakayama [2] and Mari Masuda [1]

1. Laboratory of Collaborative Research, Division of Cellular Signaling, National Cancer Center Research Institute, Tokyo 104-0045, Japan; tsekita@ncc.go.jp (T.S.); mamasuda@ncc.go.jp (M.M.)
2. Department of Orthopedic Surgery, Keio University School of Medicine, Tokyo 160-8582, Japan; t.hirozane@gmail.com (T.H.); morio@a5.keio.jp (M.M.); masa@keio.jp (M.N.); robert.a2@keio.jp (R.N.)
3. Department of Gastrointestinal and Pediatric Surgery, Tokyo Medical University, Tokyo 160-0023, Japan; ynagakawa@gmail.com (Y.N.); akihikot@tokyo-med.ac.jp (A.T.)
4. Division of Musculoskeletal Oncology, National Cancer Center Hospital, Tokyo 104-0045, Japan; ekobayas@ncc.go.jp (E.K.); akawai@ncc.go.jp (A.K.)
5. Department of Diagnostic Pathology, National Cancer Center Hospital, Tokyo 104-0045, Japan; akyoshid@ncc.go.jp
6. Carna Biosciences, Inc., Kobe 650-0047, Japan; yuko.uno@carnabio.com (Y.U.); hideki.moriyama@carnabio.com (H.M.); masaaki.sawa@carnabio.com (M.S.)
* Correspondence: tesshi.yamada@gmail.com

Received: 22 April 2020; Accepted: 10 May 2020; Published: 16 May 2020

Abstract: Background: The treatment of patients with metastatic synovial sarcoma is still challenging, and the development of new molecular therapeutics is desirable. Dysregulation of Wnt signaling has been implicated in synovial sarcoma. Traf2-and-Nck-interacting kinase (TNIK) is an essential transcriptional co-regulator of Wnt target genes. We examined the efficacy of a small interfering RNA (siRNA) to *TNIK* and a small-molecule TNIK inhibitor, NCB-0846, for synovial sarcoma. Methods: The expression of TNIK was determined in 20 clinical samples of synovial sarcoma. The efficacy of NCB-0846 was evaluated in four synovial sarcoma cell lines and a mouse xenograft model. Results: We found that synovial sarcoma cell lines with Wnt activation were highly dependent upon the expression of *TNIK* for proliferation and survival. NCB-0846 induced apoptotic cell death in synovial sarcoma cells through blocking of Wnt target genes including *MYC*, and oral administration of NCB-846 induced regression of xenografts established by inoculation of synovial sarcoma cells. Discussion: It has become evident that activation of Wnt signaling is causatively involved in the pathogenesis of synovial sarcoma, but no molecular therapeutics targeting the pathway have been approved. This study revealed for the first time the therapeutic potential of TNIK inhibition in synovial sarcoma.

Keywords: Wnt signaling; synovial sarcoma; TNIK; NCB-0846; MYC

1. Introduction

Synovial sarcoma is a rare aggressive neoplasm that accounts for 10–20% of soft tissue sarcomas. It affects mainly adolescents and young adults [1,2], and 40–50% of patients are under the age of 30 at diagnosis [3]. The mainstay of treatment is wide surgical excision and conventional chemotherapy [4,5]. However, the disease tends to show early or late recurrence and often becomes resistant to cytotoxic agents. The 10 year disease-free survival rate of patients with distant metastases remains around

50% [6]. It is desirable to develop new molecular therapeutics targeting pathways essential for the growth and survival of synovial sarcoma. The fusion *SS18-SSX* (*SSX1*, *SSX2*, or *SSX4*) gene produced by a chromosomal translocation, t (X;18) (p11.2; q11.2), is detectable in ~95% of synovial sarcomas [7–9]. Although dysregulation of the BAF chromatin-remodeling complex has been shown to be involved in the oncogenic activity of SS18-SSX [10,11], no therapeutics that can target the product of SS18-SSX or the BAF complex have yet been developed.

The canonical (β-catenin-dependent) Wnt signaling pathway plays crucial roles in the regulation of diverse biological processes including cell proliferation, survival, migration, and polarity, specification of cell fate, and self-renewal of embryonic stem cells, and its dysregulation has been implicated in the generation and progression of various malignancies [12]. Wnt signaling is also implicated in the pathogenesis of synovial sarcoma; synovial sarcoma cells frequently show accumulation of β-catenin protein in the nucleus [13], and express Wnt target gene products such as AXIN2 (axis inhibition protein 2), DKK1 (dickkopf1), survivin, c-MYC, and cyclinD1 [14]. SS18-SSX is responsible for the nuclear translocation of β-catenin [15,16], and Wnt signaling is aberrantly activated by SS18-SSX in a transgenic mouse model; inhibition of Wnt signaling through genetic loss of β-catenin blocks synovial sarcoma tumor formation [17]. *SS18-SSX2*-specific small interfering RNA (siRNA) reduces the expression of Wnt target gene products [14]. Together, these studies have highlighted the Wnt signaling pathway as a potential therapeutic target for synovial sarcoma.

Through comprehensive mass spectrometry analysis of the nuclear proteins of colorectal cancer cells, we previously identified Traf2-and-Nck-interacting kinase (TNIK) as a component of the T-cell factor-4 (TCF4) and β-catenin transcriptional complex, the most downstream effector of the Wnt signaling pathway [18]. More than 80% of colorectal cancers carry inactive mutations in the *APC* tumor-suppressor gene, and Wnt signaling is activated downstream of it. We found that TNIK was essential for transactivation of Wnt target genes and that colorectal cancer cells were highly sensitive to TNIK inhibition [19,20]. We screened a compound library and identified a novel small-molecule TNIK inhibitor named NCB-0846. NCB-0846 suppresses the transcriptional co-regulator function of TNIK by modifying its conformational structure [21,22]. NCB-0846 exhibited marked anti-tumor and anti-stem-cell activities in colorectal cancer cells and patient-derived xenografts through blocking of Wnt target gene expression [21].

Based on these findings, we speculated that TNIK inhibition would be effective for treatment of synovial sarcoma. Here, we report the therapeutic potential of TNIK inhibition in synovial sarcoma.

2. Results

2.1. Activation of Wnt Signaling and TNIK in Synovial Sarcoma

To evaluate the activation of Wnt signaling, four synovial sarcoma cell lines were transfected with a pair of reporters (super-TOP and super-FOP luciferase reporter plasmids), and their luciferase activity was measured. Active transcription of T-cell factor (TCF)/lymphoid enhancer factor (LEF) was detected in two synovial sarcoma cell lines, HS-SY-II and SYO-1 (Figure 1A). Expression of a Wnt target gene product (AXIN2 protein) (Figure 1B) and nuclear expression of β-catenin (red, Figure 1C) were detected in these two cell lines. Nuclear translocation of TNIK is indicative of its active status [19]. Nuclear expression of TNIK was detected in all four cell lines examined (green, Figure 1C), and TNIK was co-localized with β-catenin in the nuclei of synovial sarcoma cell lines with Wnt activation (merge, Figure 1C). Using immunohistochemistry, the expression of β-catenin and TNIK was then examined in tissue specimens resected from 20 patients with synovial sarcoma. We detected nuclear staining of β-catenin in 90% (18/20) of the examined cases, and these tumors also exhibited nuclear expression of TNIK (Figure 1D and Table S1).

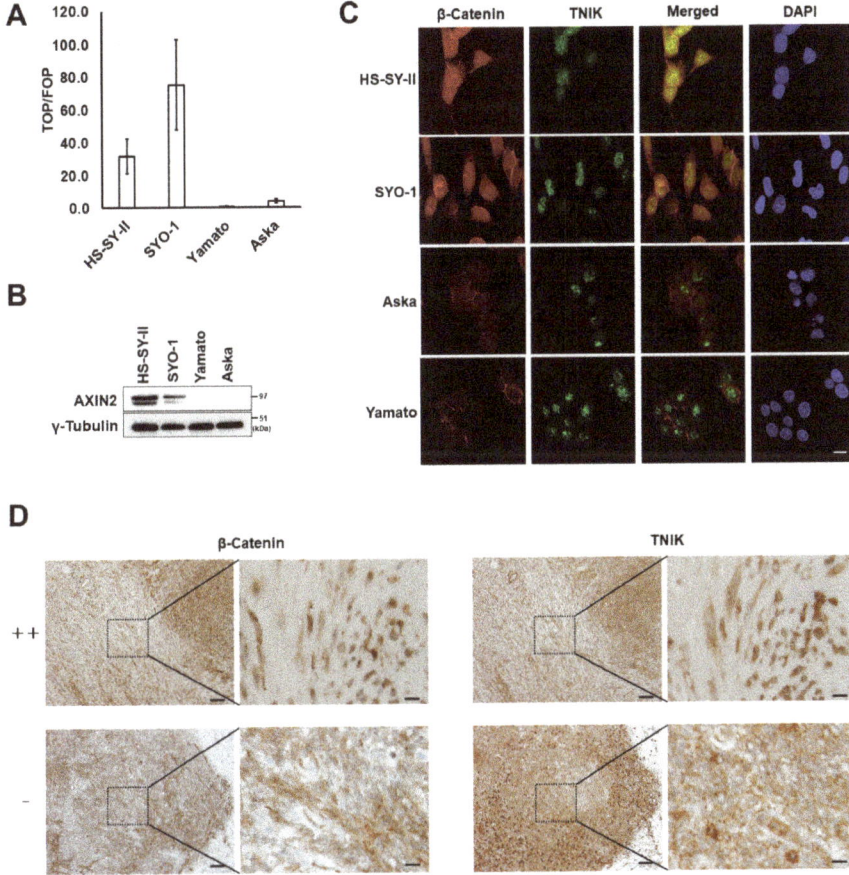

Figure 1. Wnt activation in synovial sarcoma. (**A**) T-cell factor (TCF)/lymphoid enhancer factor (LEF) transcriptional activity of synovial sarcoma cells. Four synovial sarcoma cell lines (HS-SY-II, SYO-1, Yamato, and Aska) were transfected with the super-TOP flash or super-FOP flash luciferase reporter, and their luciferase activity was measured 24 h later. Data represent the mean TOP/FOF ratio (± S.D.) of three replicates. (**B**) Expression of the axis inhibition protein 2 (AXIN2) and γ-tubulin (loading control) proteins determined by immunoblotting. (**C**) Dual immunofluorescence analysis of β-catenin and Traf2-and-Nck-interacting kinase (TNIK) protein expression in synovial sarcoma cells. Scale bar: 20 μm. (**D**) Immunohistochemical analysis of the β-catenin and TNIK proteins in clinical specimens of synovial sarcoma. Representative cases with strong positive (++) and negative (−) nuclear β-catenin expression are shown. Scale bars: 100 μm in low-power views (left) and 10 μm in high-power views (right).

2.2. Growth Suppression of Synovial Sarcoma Cells Through Silencing of TNIK

Transfection of three siRNA constructs targeting *TNIK* (siTNIK#1, #2, and #3) into HS-SY-II and SYO-1 synovial sarcoma cells was confirmed to reduce the levels of *TNIK* gene expression relative to cells transfected with control siRNA (Ctrl) (Figure 2A). Real-time monitoring revealed that knockdown of *TNIK* induced the almost complete growth arrest of HS-SY-II and SYO-1 cells (Figure 2B) and significantly reduced TCF/LEF transcription in HS-SY-II cells lentivirally engineered to stably carry a TOP-driven green fluorescent protein (GFP) reporter construct (Figure 2C), even after being normalized to cell viability (Figure 2D). The four synovial sarcoma cell lines were transfected with siRNA to *TNIK* (siTNIK#2) or control siRNA (siCtrl), and their viability was assessed 72 h later.

TNIK knockdown significantly suppressed the viability of HS-SY-II, SYO-1, and Yamato cells, but not that of Aska cells (Figure 2E). Aska cells lack Wnt activation or *MYC* gene amplification (discussed later). *TNIK* knockdown induced cleavage of poly (ADP-ribose) polymerase-1 (PARP-1) in HS-SY-II cells (Figure 2F), indicating induction of apoptosis.

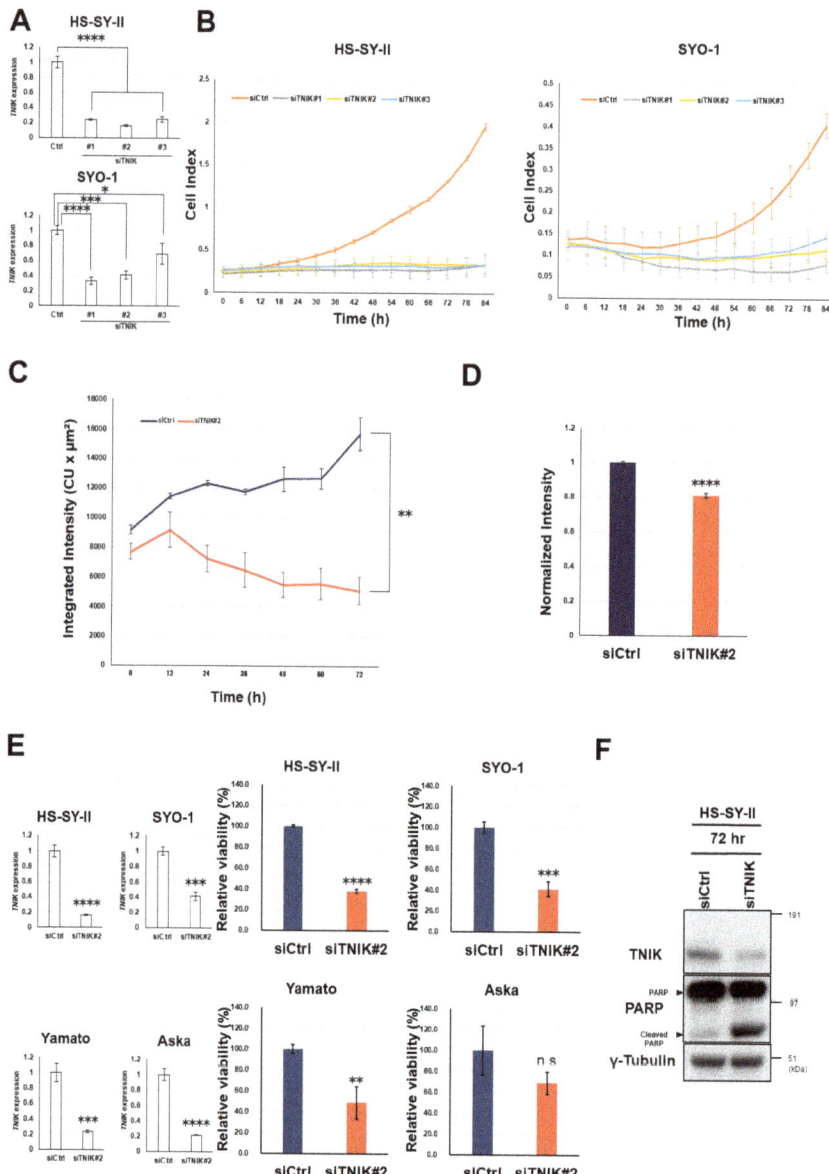

Figure 2. Growth suppression and apoptosis induction in synovial sarcoma cells by knockdown of *TNIK*. (**A**) HS-SY-II and SYO-1 cells were transfected with control small interfering RNA (siRNA) (siCtrl) and siRNA to *TNIK* (siTNIK#1, #2, and #3), and their relative expression of *TNIK* (normalized to *ACTB*) was quantified in triplicate by real-time RT-PCR 72 h after transfection. The expression level in cells

transfected with siCtrl was set at 1. * $p < 0.05$, *** $p < 0.0005$, **** $p < 0.0005$ (multiple t-test corrected using the Holm–Sidak method). (**B**) Real-time growth monitoring of HS-SY-II and SYO-1 cells transfected with siCtrl and siRNA to TNIK (siTNIK#1, #2, and #3). Data represent the mean cell index (https://www.aceabio.com/products/icelligence/) ± S.D. of three replicates. (**C,D**) Suppression of TCF/LEF transcription by *TNIK* knockdown. HS-SY-II cells engineered to stably carry a TOP-driven green fluorescent protein (GFP) reporter were transfected with siCtrl or siTNIK#2. Average integrated intensity (summed fluorescence intensity per cell) (https://www.essenbioscience.com/media/uploads/files/8000-0193-A00_ZOOM_Fluorescence_Processing_Tech_Note.pdf#search=%27Average+Integrated+Intensity%27) was monitored every 6 h for 72 h (**C**). Total integrated intensity (total sum of fluorescence intensity per well) was normalized to ATP production 24 h after transfection (D). Data represent the mean ± S.D. of three replicates. ** $p < 0.005$, **** $p < 0.0005$ (multiple t-test corrected using the Holm–Sidak method). (**E**) Synovial sarcoma cells were transfected with siCtrl or siTNIK#2, and their expression of *TNIK* (normalized to *ACTB*) was quantified by real-time RT-PCR 72 h after transfection (left). Their relative viability to siCtrl (set to one) was assessed in terms of ATP production (right). ** $p < 0.005$, *** $p < 0.0005$, **** $p < 0.0005$, n.s. not significant (multiple t-test corrected using the Holm–Sidak method). Data represent the mean ± S.D. of three replicates. (**F**) Expression of the poly (ADP-ribose) polymerase-1 (PARP-1) and γ-tubulin (loading control) proteins determined by immunoblotting for 72 h.

2.3. Sensitivity of Synovial Sarcoma to NCB-0846

Based on the remarkable growth suppression and apoptosis induction in synovial sarcoma cells by silencing of the *TNIK* gene, the sensitivity of synovial sarcoma cell lines to a small-molecule TNIK inhibitor, NCB-0846, was then evaluated. Consistent with the siRNA to *TNIK*, NCB-0846 reduced the viability of HS-SY-II, SYO-1, and Yamato cells with a half maximal inhibitory concentration (IC$_{50}$) of 339, 356, and 767 nM, respectively. Aska cells were insensitive to NCB-0846 and had an IC$_{50}$ value exceeding 2.0 µM (Figure 3A). The water-soluble hydrochloride salt of NCB-0846 (named NCB-1055) [21] was administered orally to immune-deficient mice subcutaneously inoculated with HS-SY-II cells. The xenografts regressed below the baseline (before administration) even after the first administration of NCB-1055 and did not re-grow (Figure 3B). Real-time monitoring of cell-surface phosphatidylserine (PS) revealed that NCB-0846, but not its diastereomer (named NCB-0970), induced apoptotic cell death of HS-SY-II cells within 6 h after the start of drug treatment (Figure 3C). NCB-0970 was used as a negative control, i.e., a compound having the same chemical structure as NCB-0846 except for an opposite configuration of one terminal hydroxyl group [21]. An increase of the sub-G1 cell population (Figure 3D) and cleavage of PARP-1 (Figure 3E) confirmed the induction of apoptotic cell death by NCB-0846.

2.4. Gene Expression Profiling

We then examined the changes in gene expression associated with the early induction of apoptosis by NCB-0846. HS-SY-II cells were exposed to NCB-0846 or NCB-0970 for 6 h, and their relative RNA expression (FPKM, fragments per kilobase of exon per million mapped reads) was determined using a next-generation sequencer. We found that the expression of a large number (6710/14,611) of genes was suppressed more than 2-fold by treatment with NCB-0846 in comparison to that with NCB-0970 (Figure 4A,B), indicating that this compound had a large impact on gene transcription beyond the suppression of Wnt target gene expression. Gene set enrichment analysis (GSEA) (Table S2) revealed significantly concordant alteration of a group of genes annotated to the Wnt signaling pathway (Figure 4C). The differentially expressed genes were mapped to the Wnt signaling pathway deposited in the Kyoto Encyclopedia of Genes and Genomes (KEGG) database (Figure 4D). We previously reported that TNIK was required for the tumor-initiating function of colorectal cancer stem cells [21,22]. Consistently, a significant proportion of downregulated genes were mapped to the signaling pathways regulating stem cell pluripotency (Figure S1). The entire RNA sequencing dataset has been deposited in the DNA Data Bank of Japan (DDBJ) Sequence Read Archive (SRA) database with the accession number DRA010051.

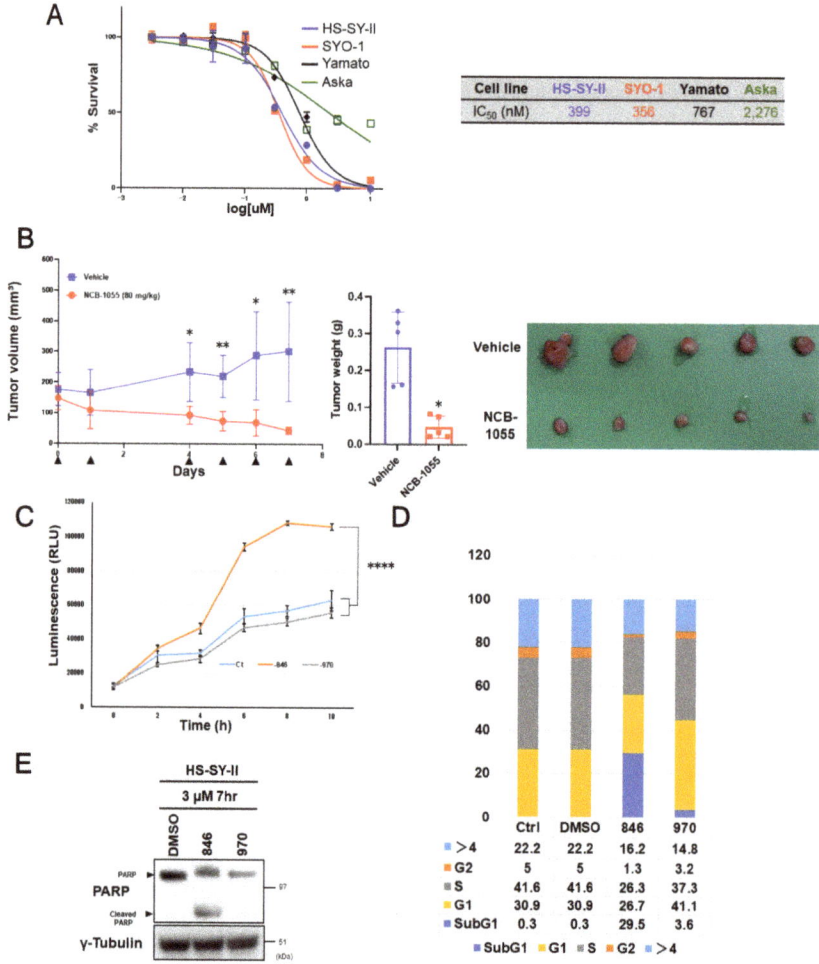

Figure 3. Sensitivity of synovial sarcoma to NCB-0846. (**A**) ATP production by four synovial sarcoma cell lines cultured with increasing doses of NCB-0846 for 72 h. Data represent the mean (relative to no treatment) of three replicates. (**B**) HS-SY-II cells were inoculated into the subcutaneous tissues of 6 week old female NOD.CB17-$Prkdc^{scid}$/J (NOD/SCID) mice. When the average volume of the xenografts reached ~200 mm^3, water (vehicle, $n = 5$) or 80 mg/kg ($n = 5$) NCB-0846 hydrochloride (NCB-1055) [21] was administered orally on the days indicated by ▼. Tumor volume was measured on the days of drug administration (left), and tumors were excised (lower right) and weighed (upper right) 7 days after the start of drug administration. * $p < 0.05$, ** $p < 0.005$ (multiple *t*-test corrected using the Holm–Sidak method). Error bars represent S.E.M. (**C**) HS-SY-II cells were cultured with dimethyl sulfoxide (DMSO) (vehicle), NCB-0846 (3 μM) or NCB-0970 (3 μM) in the presence of the Real-time-Glo™ Annexin V Apoptosis Assay Reagent (Promega), and relative luminescence unit (URL) data were collected at every 2 h over a 10 h time course. **** $p < 0.0005$ (multiple *t*-test corrected using the Holm–Sidak method). Data represent the mean of three readings for each replicate ± S.D. (**D**) HS-SY-II cells were untreated (Ctrl) or treated with DMSO, NCB-0846 (3 μM), or NCB-0970 (3 μM) for 6 h. The percentage of cells in each cell cycle fraction was determined by flow cytometry. (**E**) HS-SY-II cells were treated with DMSO (control), NCB-0846 (3 μM), or NCB-0970 (3 μM) for 7 h. The expression levels of PARP-1 and γ-tubulin (loading control) were determined by immunoblotting.

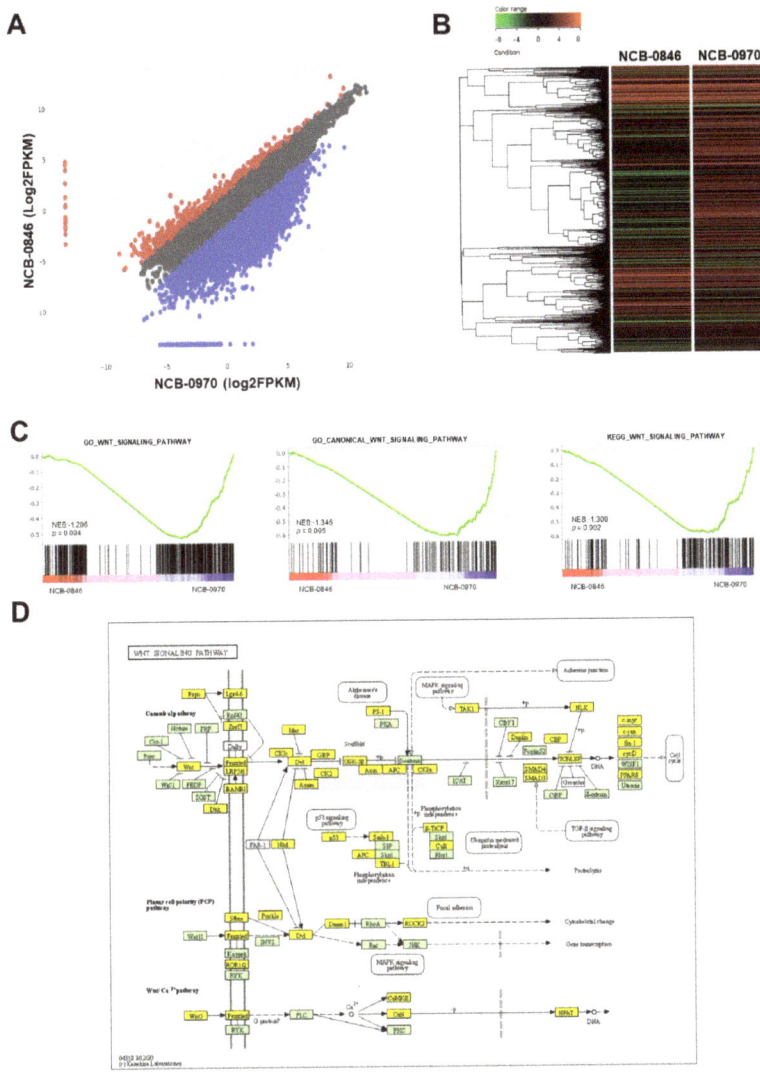

Figure 4. Gene expression profiling of synovial sarcoma cells treated with NCB-0846. (**A**) Scatter plot of genes differentially expressed between cells treated with NCB-0846 and NCB-0970 (negative control). Red dots represent genes upregulated more than 2-fold, and blue dots represent genes downregulated more than 2-fold in cells treated with NCB-0846. (**B**) Heat map plot of genes differentially expressed between NCB-0846 and NCB-0970. The upper color bar represents the degree of differential expression. (**C**) Gene set enrichment analysis (GSEA) showing the significant enrichment of genes annotated to the gene ontology (GO) terms "Wnt signaling pathway" ($p = 0.004$) and "canonical Wnt signaling pathway" ($p = 0.005$) and to "Wnt signaling pathway" deposited in the KEGG database ($p = 0.002$). NES: normalized enrichment score (http://software.broadinstitute.org/gsea/index.jsp). (**D**) Mapping of differentially expressed genes onto the Wnt signaling pathway. Yellow boxes indicate genes downregulated (>2-fold) by NCB-0846.

2.5. NCB-0846 Suppresses MYC Gene Expression

Using real-time RT-PCR, we then confirmed the differential expression of Wnt target genes. The expression of 88% (78/88) of known Wnt target genes (https://web.stanford.edu/group/nusselab/cgi-bin/wnt/target_genes) was found to be downregulated (Table S3). Among these genes, *MYC* showed the most significant degree of downregulation (Figure 5A). *MYC* encodes the c-MYC protein, a transcription factor that regulates as many as 10–15% of genes in the genome [23]. We confirmed the significant enrichment of c-MYC transcriptional targets among genes regulated by NCB-0846 (Figure 5B). This marked downregulation of *MYC* was also observed in other synovial sarcoma cell lines (Figure 5C).

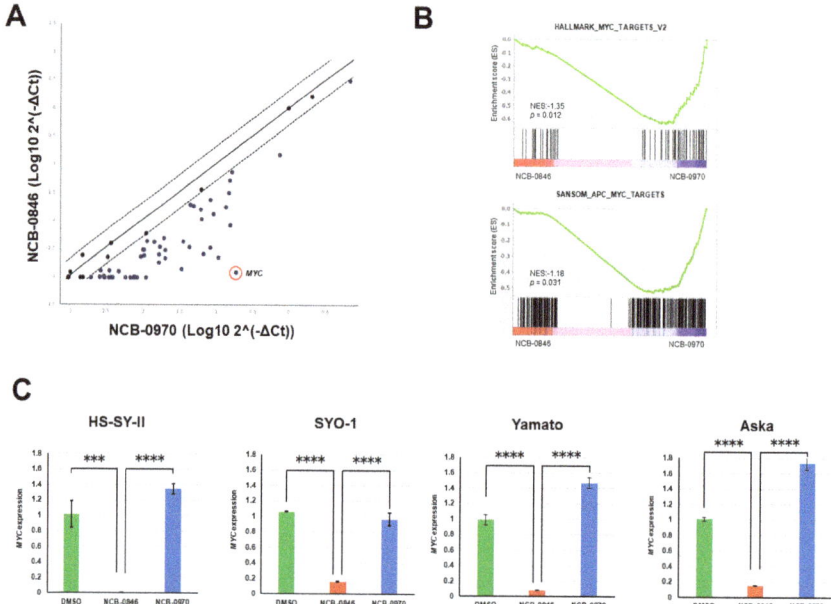

Figure 5. NCB-0846 suppresses *MYC* gene expression. (**A**) Comparison of Wnt target gene expression (normalized to *GAPDH* and log-transformed) of HS-SY-II cells treated with NC-0846 and NCB-0970 for 6 h. (**B**) Significant enrichment of c-MYC target genes revealed by RNA sequencing and Gene set enrichment analysis (GSEA). (**C**) Four synovial sarcoma cell lines were treated with dimethyl sulfoxide (DMSO) (control), NCB-0846 (3 µM), or NCB-0970 (3 µM) for 6 h, and expression of the *MYC* gene (relative to DMSO) was quantified by real-time RT-PCR and normalized to that of *ACTB*. *** $p < 0.0005$, **** $p < 0.0005$ (multiple *t*-test corrected using the Holm–Sidak method). Data represent the mean ± S.D. of three replicates.

2.6. Dependency of Synovial Sarcoma Cells on MYC

MYC is one of the targets of TCF/LEF transcription factors [24], and Wnt signaling is known to exert its oncogenic activity primarily through transactivation of the *MYC* gene [25]. We found that synovial sarcoma HS-SY-II cells with active Wnt target gene expression were highly dependent on *MYC* gene expression for proliferation (Figure 6A). However, Yamato cells also expressed the c-MYC protein (Figure 6B) in spite of inactive Wnt signaling (Figure 1A–C). We found that an increase (2.2-fold) in the copy number of the *MYC* gene (Figure 6C) appeared to be responsible for the upregulation. A high degree (>2.0-fold) of *MYC* oncogene amplification is known to be infrequent in synovial sarcoma [26]. However, nuclear expression of c-MYC was detected in 85% (17/20) of clinical specimens and was frequent (≥30% of tumor cells) in 15% of them (3/20) (Figure S2 and Table S1). The Aska cell line carried the normal copy number (1.0-fold) of *MYC* (Figure 6C), and its level of c-MYC expression was lower than in other cell lines (Figure 6B). Knockdown of *MYC* gene expression by siRNA reduced the viability of HS-SY-II, SYO-1, and Yamato cells, but Aska cells were insensitive to silencing of *MYC* (Figure 6D) and NCB-0846 (Figure 3A), suggesting that NCB-0846 induces apoptotic cell death of synovial sarcoma at least partially through transcriptional suppression of *MYC*.

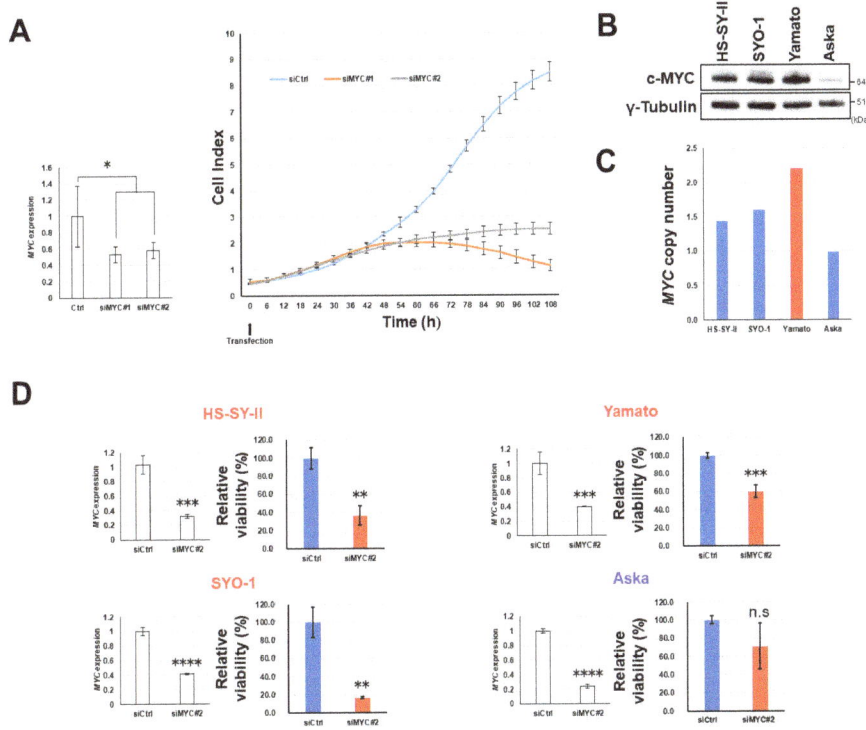

Figure 6. Dependence of synovial sarcoma cells on *MYC*. (**A**) Relative *MYC* expression (left) and real-time growth monitoring (right) of HS-SY-II cells transfected with control small interfering (siRNA) (siCtrl) and siRNA to *MYC* (siMYC#1 and #2). Data represent the mean *MYC* expression (normalized to *ACTB*) (left) and cell index (right) ± S.D. of three replicates. * $p < 0.05$ (multiple *t*-test corrected using the Holm–Sidak method). (**B**) The expression of c-MYC and γ-tubulin (loading control) in four synovial sarcoma cell lines was determined by immunoblotting. (**C**) Relative copy numbers of the *MYC* gene (normalized to the RNase P gene) in four synovial sarcoma cell lines determined by digital PCR. (**D**) Four synovial sarcoma cell lines were transfected with control siRNA (siCtrl) and siRNA to *MYC* (siMYC#2) in triplicate. Seventy-two hours later, their relative expression of *MYC* (normalized to *ACTB*) was quantified by real-time RT-PCR (left), and their relative viability was assessed in terms of ATP production (right). Data represent the mean ± S.D. of three replicates. ** $p < 0.005$, *** $p < 0.0005$, **** $p < 0.0005$, n.s. not significant (multiple *t*-test corrected using the Holm–Sidak method).

3. Discussion

Conventional cytotoxic chemotherapeutic agents including anthracycline, ifomide, and trabectedin have proven to be effective for the treatment of metastatic synovial sarcoma [27], but their usage and efficacy are often limited by the emergence of adverse events and drug resistance. Pazopanib is the first and only molecular therapeutic agent approved for the treatment of multiple histological subtypes of soft tissue sarcoma [28]. Pazopanib is a multi-tyrosine kinase inhibitor, and its main mode of action is believed to be inhibition of vascular endothelial growth factor receptor (VEGF)-mediated tumor angiogenesis [29]. The median survival of synovial sarcoma patients treated with pazopanib, however, was only 10.6 months, and the pazopanib treatment was associated with a high frequency of adverse events including hypertension, thrombocytopenia, and pneumothorax [28,30]. Early clinical trials of T lymphocytes genetically engineered to target the NY-ESO-1 cancer/testis antigen have yielded promising results [31,32], but this cancer immunotherapy is applicable only to patients with the human leukocyte antigen (HLA)-A*0201 or -A*0206 type as well as expression of NY-ESO-1 in tumors. Moreover, autologous lymphocyte cultivation is incurs significant costs and requires long-term discontinuation of ongoing treatment, potentially leading to fatal disease progression. Frizzled homolog 10 (FZD10) has attracted attention as a promising therapeutic target for synovial sarcoma [33], as its expression is limited to the cell membrane of synovial sarcoma and absent from vital organs [34]. A recent first-in-human clinical trial clarified the biodistribution, safety, and recommended dose of a radiolabeled humanized monoclonal antibody to FZD10 [35], but its efficacy has not been established.

Synovial sarcoma is uniquely characterized by the balanced chromosomal translocation t[X, 18; p11, q11], demonstrable in virtually all cases and not found in any other human neoplasms [2,8]. This translocation creates an in-frame fusion of SS18 to SSX1, SSX2, or SSX4, whereby all but the eight C-terminal amino acids of SS18 are replaced by the 78 C-terminal amino acids of the SSX partner. Kadoch and Crabtree observed that SS18-SSX was incorporated into the SWI/SNF (SWItch/Sucrose Non-Fermentable) complex [36]. Middeljans and colleagues reported that expression of the fusion oncogene induced depletion of the BAF47 (*SMARCB1*) subunit from the SWI/SNF complex [37]. Potential convergence may exist between the SWI/SNF complex and Wnt signaling, as loss of *SMARCB1* reportedly activates Wnt signaling [38]. Barham and colleagues [17] provided direct evidence for involvement of Wnt signaling in the SS18-SSX-mediated carcinogenesis of synovial sarcoma. The Wnt signaling pathway is aberrantly activated in an SS18-SSX2 transgenic mouse model, and genetic loss of β-catenin (*Ctnnb1*) blocks tumor formation in this model. Trautmann and colleagues [14] found that introduction of SS18-SSX into untransformed cells induced transactivation of Wnt target genes. Synovial sarcoma cell lines (SYO-1, CME-1, and HS-SY-II) showed sensitivity to three small-molecule inhibitors of the TCF/β-catenin complex (PKF115–584, CGP049090, and PKF118–310). β-Catenin stabilization in a transgenic animal model reportedly enhanced SS18-SSX-driven tumorigenesis and produced more dedifferentiated tumors [39]. Based on these findings, it is considered feasible to target a signaling molecule of the Wnt signaling pathway in synovial sarcoma.

TNIK is a component of the TCF4 and β-catenin transcriptional complex and functions as an essential co-regulator of Wnt target gene expression [19,40]. We screened a chemical library and identified a small-molecule TNIK-inhibitory compound named NCB-0846. This compound inhibited the expression of various Wnt target genes (such as *MYC*, *AXIN2*, and *CD44*) through conformational modification of TNIK and abrogated the stemness of colorectal cancer cells [21]. The *MYC* oncogene is a direct target of TCF/LEF family transcription factors [24] and centrally mediates the oncogenic activity of Wnt signaling [25]. In the present study, we revealed that Wnt signaling is activated in synovial sarcoma cells (Figure 1) and that siRNA-mediated or pharmacological TNIK inhibition reduced their viability and induced apoptosis (Figures 2 and 3). NCB-0846 suppressed the expression of *MYC* and other Wnt target genes (Figure 5). Synovial sarcoma cell lines with high c-MYC protein expression were sensitive to the compound (Figure 3) and to the gene silencing of *MYC* (Figure 6). These results suggest that transcriptional *MYC* gene suppression is the central mode of action (MOA) of NCB-0846.

c-MYC is a versatile transcription factor that regulates the expression of genes involved in various biological functions such as cell proliferation, apoptosis, differentiation, and metabolism [41], and its inhibition would be expected to have a huge impact on the cancer transcriptome [42]. Aberrant expression or gene amplification of *MYC* has been implicated in the aggressiveness of various malignancies [43,44]. Shen and colleagues examined 32 cases of limb synovial sarcoma immunohistochemically and revealed a significant association of c-MYC expression with poor patient prognosis [45]. Synovial sarcoma is histologically divided into monophasic, biphasic, and poorly differentiated subtypes. We previously revealed the significant association of poorly differentiated synovial sarcoma with the expression of *MYC* [46]. Patients with poorly differentiated synovial sarcoma showed a high risk of recurrence [47]. NCB-0846 may be effective for the treatment of aggressive poorly differentiated synovial sarcoma.

In conclusion, we demonstrated for the first time that TNIK is a feasible drug target in synovial sarcoma. No effective molecular therapeutics have yet been approved for this lethal disease. We observed marked regression of xenografts even after the first oral administration of NCB-846, confirming its high efficacy. The compound is now under preclinical development aimed at investigational new drug (IND) application.

4. Materials and Methods

4.1. Ethical Issues

All of the animal experimental protocols in this study were reviewed and approved by the ethics and recombination safety committees of the National Cancer Center Research Institute (Tokyo, Japan) (T-17-022-m01, approved on 21 July 2017). The minimum number of animals necessary to obtain reliable results was used, and maximum attention was paid to animal rights and welfare protection. The use of human materials was reviewed and approved by the Institutional Review Board (IRB) of the National Cancer Center (Tokyo, Japan) (2004-050, approved on 30 October 2014 and revised on 7 November 2019). All patients gave their informed consent at the time. The IRB waived the requirement for obtaining new informed consent for this retrospective study. The investigations were carried out in accordance with the Declaration of Helsinki (https://www.wma.net/what-we-do/medical-ethics/declaration-of-helsinki/).

4.2. Cell Lines

Human synovial sarcoma HS-SY-II, Aska [48], and Yamato [48] cell lines were obtained from the Riken BioResource Center (Tsukuba, Japan). The SYO-1 cell line was established by one of the authors (A.K.) [49]. All cell lines were maintained in Dulbecco's modified Eagle medium (Thermo Fisher Scientific, Waltham, MA, USA) supplemented with 10–20% fetal calf serum (Thermo Fisher Scientific). Absence of mycoplasma contamination was routinely confirmed using the e-Myco VALiD Mycoplasma PCR Detection Kit (iNtRon Biotechnology, Seoul, Korea).

4.3. Luciferase Reporter Assay

A pair of luciferase reporter constructs, super TOP-FLASH and super FOP-FLASH (Addgene, Watertown, MA, USA), was used to evaluate TCF/LEF transcriptional activity. Cells were transiently transfected in triplicate with one of the luciferase reporters and phRL-TK (Promega, Madison, WI, USA) (internal control) [18]. Luciferase activity was measured using the Dual-Luciferase Reporter Assay System (Promega) and normalized to that of *Renilla reniformis*. Data are presented as the ratio of TOP-FLASH to FOP-FLASH (TOP/FOP ratio).

4.4. Antibodies

Antibodies used in this study are listed in Table S4.

4.5. Immunoblot Analysis

Protein samples were fractionated by SDS–PAGE and blotted onto Immobilon-P membranes (Millipore, Burlington, MA, USA) as described previously [50]. After incubation with the primary antibodies at 4 °C overnight, the blots were detected with the relevant horseradish-peroxidase-conjugated anti-mouse or anti-rabbit IgG antibody (Cell Signaling Technology, Danvers, MA, USA) and Western lighting ECL Pro (PerkinElmer, Waltham, MA, USA). Signals were visualized with the LAS-4010 system (GE Healthcare, Chicago, IL, USA) and quantified using the ImageJ software package [51]. The uncropped images and relative quantification of blots in Figures 1B, 2F, 3E and 6B are shown in Figures S3–S6, respectively.

4.6. Immunofluorescence Microscopy

Cells were fixed with 4% paraformaldehyde (PFA) for 10 min and permeabilized in 0.5% Triton X-100 for 3 min. The fixed cells were incubated with a primary antibody overnight at 4 °C and subsequently with a relevant secondary antibody (AlexaFluor 488-conjugated anti-rabbit IgG or AlexaFluor 568-conjugated anti-mouse IgG, Invitrogen, Waltham, MA, USA) for 1 h at 37 °C. The nuclei were stained with DAPI (Vectashield HardSet Mounting Medium with DAPI, Vector Laboratories, Burlingame, CA, USA). Images were captured using a TCS SP8 confocal microscope (Leica Microsystems, Wetzlar, Germany).

4.7. Patients and Tumor Samples

The study included tumor tissues surgically resected from 20 patients with synovial sarcoma (10 women and 10 men; median age at diagnosis 50 years, range 5–71 years). Clinicopathological characteristics are summarized in Table S1. The diagnosis of synovial sarcoma was made by a pathologist specialized in soft tissue sarcomas (A.Y.) and confirmed by the detection of *SS18* rearrangement by fluorescence in situ hybridization (FISH) or RT-PCR and/or the reduced expression of SMARCB1 [52,53].

4.8. Immunohistochemistry

Immunoperoxidase staining was performed using the Ventana DABMap detection kit and an automated slide stainer (Discovery XT, Ventana Medical Systems, Oro Valley, AZ, USA) [54]. The stained tissues were scored as strong positive (++, ≥30%), positive (+, <30%), or negative (−) according to the percentage of tumor cells with nuclear expression (Figure S7).

4.9. Gene Silencing by RNA Interference

Cells seeded at 50–70% confluency were transfected with siTNIK (s22905, s22906, and s22907; Thermo Fisher Scientific) and siMYC (s9129 and s9130; Thermo Fisher Scientific) at a final concentration of 50 nM in accordance with the manufacturer's instructions.

4.10. Real-Time RT-PCR

Total RNA was prepared with a RNeasy Plus Mini Kit and treated with RNase-free DNase (Qiagen, Hilden, Germany). The cDNA was synthesized using a High-Capacity cDNA reverse transcription kit (Thermo Fisher Scientific) and subjected to TaqMan gene expression assay using pre-designed primer and probe sets (listed in Table S5). Amplification data measured as an increase in reporter fluorescence were collected using the StepOne™ Real-Time PCR System (Thermo Fisher Scientific). The relative mRNA expression level normalized to the internal control (human β-actin (*ACTB*) gene) was calculated using the comparative threshold cycle (CT) method [18]. Experiments were performed in triplicate and repeated at least two times. Wnt Signaling Targets RT^2 Profiler PCR Arrays (Qiagen) were used for pathway-focused gene expression analyses.

4.11. Digital PCR

Total DNA was extracted from 5×10^6 cells using the DNA Easy Blood and Tissue kit (Qiagen), in accordance with the manufacturer's instructions. Copy number variation (CNV) data were obtained by the QuantStudio 3D digital PCR system (Life Technologies, Carlsbad, CA, USA) using pre-designed primer and probe sets (listed in Table S6) and analyzed with the QuantStudio 3D Analysis Suite Cloud software (Thermo Fisher Scientific). RNase P (*RPPH1*) was selected as an internal standard gene (Table S6).

4.12. Real-Time Cell Analysis (RTCA)

Cells were seeded at 5000 cells per well in 96 well clusters one day before transfection with control RNA (siCtrl) or siRNA to *TNIK* (siTNIK) or *MYC* (siMYC) using Lipofectamine RNAiMAX

(Invitrogen). Cell growth was monitored periodically by a real-time cell electronic sensing analyzer (xCELLigence, ACEA Biosciences, Santa Clara, CA, USA) for 108 h via calculation of cell index (https://www.aceabio.com/products/icelligence/). Experiments were performed in triplicate and repeated two times.

4.13. Real-Time Monitoring of Transcriptional Activity

Lentiviral reporter gene transfer was used to evaluate the TCF/LEF transcriptional activity of HS-SY-II after transfection with siCtrl or siTNIK. Cells were infected with TCF/LEF reporter lentiviral particles encoding the GFP gene under control of the TCF/LEF-responsive promoter (Signal Lenti TCF/LEF Reporter (GFP) (Qiagen)) at a multiplicity of infection of 10 in the presence of 4 µg/mL SureEntry Transduction Reagent (Qiagen) for 24 h. GFP-positive cells were cloned by limiting dilution in the presence of 2 µg/mL puromycin (Sigma-Aldrich, St. Louis, MO, USA) and sorted with an S3e cell sorter (BIO-RAD, Hercules, CA, USA). The cells were seeded at a density of 20,000 per well in 96 well plates (Corning, Corning, NY, USA) and transfected with siCtrl or siTNIK. The amount of fluorescence was measured using Incucyte ZOOM (Essen BioScience, Tokyo, Japan).

4.14. Drug Sensitivity

Cells were seeded at a density of 3000 per well in 96 well plates. Twenty-four hours after seeding, the cells were exposed to serially diluted compounds (0.003, 0.01, 0.03, 0.1, 0.3, 1, 3, and 10 µM) and incubated for 72 h. ATP production was measured using a Cell Titer-Glo Luminescent Cell Viability Assay kit (Promega).

4.15. Xenografts

Five million HS-SY-II cells suspended in PBS containing 25% Matrigel (BD Biosciences, Franklin Lakes, NJ, USA) were inoculated into the subcutaneous tissues of 6 week old female NOD/SCID (NOD.CB17-Prkdcscid/J) mice. When the average tumor volume reached ~200 mm^3, the mice were randomized according to tumor volume (five mice/group) and administered water (vehicle alone) or 80 mg/kg (body weight) NCB-0846 HCl (NCB-1055) dissolved in water by oral gavage twice a day in a 7 day schedule of 5 days on and 2 days off.

4.16. Real-Time Monitoring of Apoptosis Induction

The Real-Time-Glo™ Annexin V Apoptosis and Necrosis Assay reagent (Promega) was prepared as instructed in its technical manual and added to culture media at the beginning of drug treatment. Luciferase activity was measured every 2 h using the GloMax Discover System (Promega).

4.17. Cell Cycle Analysis

Cells were dissociated with Accutase, fixed with 70% EtOH at 4 °C, stained with Guava Cell Cycle reagent (Merck-Millipore, Burlington, MA, USA) in accordance with the manufacturer's instructions, and analyzed using a Guava easy Cyte HT flow cytometer (Merck-Millipore). Cell doublets were eliminated by doublet discrimination gating. Data were analyzed using the FLOWJO version 10 software package (Treestar, Ashland, OR, USA).

4.18. RNA Sequencing

Total RNAs were extracted from HS-SY-II cells treated with 3 µM NCB-0846 or 3 µM NCB-0970 for 6 h. After confirming the absence of contamination with genomic DNA using a 2200 TapeStation (Agilent, Santa Clara, CA, USA), the TruSeq Stranded mRNA SamplePrep Kit was used to construct the sequencing library (Illumina, San Diego, CA, USA), and the libraries were sequenced using Illumina NovaSeq 6000 using a NovaSeq 6000 S4 Reagent Kit. Base calling was performed using the Illumina Basecall Software (bcl2fastq2 v2.20) with default parameters. Gene lists extracted from the transcriptome analyses were uploaded to the Database for Annotation, Visualization, and Integrated Discovery (DAVID) Bioinformatics database (https://david.ncifcrf.gov/), and the statistical significance of functional annotation was evaluated. The pathway analysis was performed by displaying the DAVID data on a pathway map of KEGG (Kyoto Encyclopedia of Genes and Genomes (http://www.genome.jp/kegg/). Clustering analysis was performed with MeV (http://mev.tm4.org). GSEA software was used to evaluate the statistical significance of pathway enrichment and to calculate the NES.

4.19. Statistical Analysis

All statistical analyses were performed using GraphPad Prism 8 (GraphPad, San Diego, CA, USA). Unless otherwise indicated, two-tailed Student's *t*-tests of two groups assuming equal variances were used to calculate *p* values. Differences at $p < 0.05$ were considered significant.

5. Conclusions

Synovial sarcoma is highly dependent upon the expression of TNIK for cell proliferation and survival, and a small-molecule TNIK inhibitor NCB-0846 induced rapid apoptotic death of synovial sarcoma cells. This study demonstrated for the first time the therapeutic potential of TNIK inhibition in synovial sarcoma.

Supplementary Materials: The following are available online at http://www.mdpi.com/2072-6694/12/5/1258/s1, Figure S1: Mapping of differentially expressed genes onto the signaling pathways regulating pluripotency of stem cells. Yellow boxes indicate genes downregulated (>2-fold) by NCB-0846, Figure S2: Immunohistochemical analysis of the c-MYC proteins in clinical specimens of synovial sarcoma. Representative cases with strong positive (++) and negative (−) nuclear c-MYC expression are shown. Scale bars: 100 µm in low-power views (left) and 20 µm in high-power views (right), Figure S3. Uncropped immunoblots of Figure 1B. The expression levels of axis inhibition protein 2 (AXIN2) were normalized to those of γ-tubulin, and quantification relative to HS-SY-II is shown below the blots, Figure S4. Uncropped immunoblots of Figure 2F. The expression levels of Traf2-and-Nck-interacting kinase (TNIK) and cleaved poly (ADP-ribose) polymerase-1 (PARP-1) were normalized to those of γ-tubulin, and quantification relative to siCtrl is shown below the blots, Figure S5. Uncropped immunoblots of Figure 3E. The expression levels of cleaved PARP-1 were normalized to those of γ-tubulin, and quantification relative to the dimethyl sulfoxide (DMSO) control is shown below the blots, Figure S6. Uncropped immunoblots of Figure 6B. The expression levels of c-MYC were normalized to those of γ-tubulin, and quantification relative to HS-SY-II is shown below the blots, Figure S7. Scoring of immunohistochemistry. The 20 tissue samples of synovial sarcoma were scored as strong positive (++, ≥30%), positive (+, <30%), or negative (−) according to the percentage of tumor cells with nuclear β-catenin (top), TNIK (middle), and c-MYC (bottom) expression. Scale bars: 20 µm, Table S1: Expression of the β-catenin, TNIK, and c-MYC proteins in clinical specimens, Table S2: Pathway analysis of genes regulated by NCB-0846, Table S3: Regulation of Wnt target genes by NCB-0846, Table S4: List of antibodies used in this study, Table S5: Pre-designed primer and probe sets used for real-time RT-PCR, Table S6: Pre-designed primer and probe sets used for digital PCR.

Author Contributions: Conceptualization, T.S., T.Y., E.K. and M.M. (Mari Masuda); Material and clinical data provision, E.K., A.Y., A.K., Y.U., H.M., and M.S.; Methodology development, T.S. and M.M. (Mari Masuda); Experiments, T.S., T.H., and M.M. (Mari Masuda); Writing, T.S., T.Y., and E.K.; Supervision, Y.N., A.T., M.M. (Morio Matsumoto), M.N. and R.N.; Project Administration, M.M. (Mari Masuda); Funding Acquisition, T.S., T.Y. and M.M. (Mari Masuda). All authors have read and agreed to the published version of the manuscript.

Funding: This study was supported by the National Cancer Center Research and Development Fund (30-A-2 to M.M. (Mari Masuda)), the Acceleration Transformative Research for Medical Innovation (ACT-MS) program of the Japan Agency for Medical Research and Development (AMED) (16im0210804h0001 to T.Y.), the Kobayashi Foundation for Cancer Research (to T.Y.), a KAKENHI Grant-in-Aid for Challenging Research (16K14627 to M.M. (Mari Masuda) and 19H05566 to T.Y.), a Grant-in Aid for Scientific Research (B) (17H03603 to M.M. (Mari Masuda)) from the Japan Society for the Promotion of Science (JSPS), a Cancer Research Grant from the Foundation for Promotion of Cancer Research in Japan (to M.M. (Mari Masuda)), a Research Grant from the Princess Takamatsu Cancer Research Fund (to M.M. (Mari Masuda)), and a Grant-in-Aid for Early-Career Scientists (19J21415 to T.S.) of the Japan Society for the Promotion of Science (JSPS).

Conflicts of Interest: U.Y., H.M., and M.S. are employees of Carna Biosciences, Inc. T.Y. and M.M. (Mari Masuda) have received a research grant from Carna Biosciences, Inc. The remaining authors have no conflicts of interest to declare.

References

1. Herzog, C.E. Overview of sarcomas in the adolescent and young adult population. *J. Pediatr. Hematol. Oncol.* **2005**, *27*, 215–218. [CrossRef]
2. Ferrari, A.; Dirksen, U.; Bielack, S. Sarcomas of Soft Tissue and Bone. *Prog. Tumor Res.* **2016**, *43*, 128–141.
3. Ladanyi, M.; Antonescu, C.R.; Leung, D.H.; Woodruff, J.M.; Kawai, A.; Healey, J.H.; Brennan, M.F.; Bridge, J.A.; Neff, J.R.; Barr, F.G.; et al. Impact of SYT-SSX fusion type on the clinical behavior of synovial sarcoma: A multi-institutional retrospective study of 243 patients. *Cancer Res.* **2002**, *62*, 135–140.
4. Al-Hussaini, H.; Hogg, D.; Blackstein, M.E.; O'Sullivan, B.; Catton, C.N.; Chung, P.W.; Griffin, A.M.; Hodgson, D.; Hopyan, S.; Kandel, R.; et al. Clinical features, treatment, and outcome in 102 adult and pediatric patients with localized high-grade synovial sarcoma. *Sarcoma* **2011**, *2011*, 231789. [CrossRef] [PubMed]
5. Outani, H.; Kakunaga, S.; Hamada, K.; Takenaka, S.; Imura, Y.; Nagata, S.; Tanaka, T.; Tamiya, H.; Oshima, K.; Naka, N.; et al. Favorable outcomes of localized synovial sarcoma patients with a high utilization rate of neoadjuvant and/or adjuvant chemotherapy. *Mol. Clin. Oncol.* **2019**, *11*, 151–156. [CrossRef] [PubMed]
6. Sultan, I.; Rodriguez-Galindo, C.; Saab, R.; Yasir, S.; Casanova, M.; Ferrari, A. Comparing children and adults with synovial sarcoma in the Surveillance, Epidemiology, and End Results program, 1983 to 2005: An analysis of 1268 patients. *Cancer* **2009**, *115*, 3537–3547. [CrossRef] [PubMed]
7. Clark, J.; Rocques, P.J.; Crew, A.J.; Gill, S.; Shipley, J.; Chan, A.M.; Gusterson, B.A.; Cooper, C.S. Identification of novel genes, SYT and SSX, involved in the t(X;18)(p11.2;q11.2) translocation found in human synovial sarcoma. *Nat. Genet.* **1994**, *7*, 502–508. [CrossRef] [PubMed]
8. Panagopoulos, I.; Mertens, F.; Isaksson, M.; Limon, J.; Gustafson, P.; Skytting, B.; Akerman, M.; Sciot, R.; Dal Cin, P.; Samson, I.; et al. Clinical impact of molecular and cytogenetic findings in synovial sarcoma. *Genes Chromosomes Cancer* **2001**, *31*, 362–372. [CrossRef]
9. Carmody Soni, E.E.; Schlottman, S.; Erkizan, H.V.; Uren, A.; Toretsky, J.A. Loss of SS18-SSX1 inhibits viability and induces apoptosis in synovial sarcoma. *Clin. Orthop. Relat. Res.* **2014**, *472*, 874–882. [CrossRef]
10. McBride, M.J.; Pulice, J.L.; Beird, H.C.; Ingram, D.R.; D'Avino, A.R.; Shern, J.F.; Charville, G.W.; Hornick, J.L.; Nakayama, R.T.; Garcia-Rivera, E.M.; et al. The SS18-SSX Fusion Oncoprotein Hijacks BAF Complex Targeting and Function to Drive Synovial Sarcoma. *Cancer Cell* **2018**, *33*, 1128–1141. [CrossRef]
11. Banito, A.; Li, X.; Laporte, A.N.; Roe, J.S.; Sanchez-Vega, F.; Huang, C.H.; Dancsok, A.R.; Hatzi, K.; Chen, C.C.; Tschaharganeh, D.F.; et al. The SS18-SSX Oncoprotein Hijacks KDM2B-PRC1.1 to Drive Synovial Sarcoma. *Cancer Cell* **2018**, *34*, 346–348. [CrossRef] [PubMed]
12. Anastas, J.N.; Moon, R.T. WNT signalling pathways as therapeutic targets in cancer. *Nat. Rev. Cancer* **2013**, *13*, 11–26. [CrossRef] [PubMed]
13. Sato, H.; Hasegawa, T.; Kanai, Y.; Tsutsumi, Y.; Osamura, Y.; Abe, Y.; Sakai, H.; Hirohashi, S. Expression of cadherins and their undercoat proteins (α-, β-, and γ-catenins and p120) and accumulation of β-catenin with no gene mutations in synovial sarcoma. *Virchows Arch.* **2001**, *438*, 23–30. [PubMed]
14. Trautmann, M.; Sievers, E.; Aretz, S.; Kindler, D.; Michels, S.; Friedrichs, N.; Renner, M.; Kirfel, J.; Steiner, S.; Huss, S.; et al. SS18-SSX fusion protein-induced Wnt/β-catenin signaling is a therapeutic target in synovial sarcoma. *Oncogene* **2014**, *33*, 5006–5016. [CrossRef] [PubMed]
15. Pretto, D.; Barco, R.; Rivera, J.; Neel, N.; Gustavson, M.D.; Eid, J.E. The synovial sarcoma translocation protein SYT-SSX2 recruits β-catenin to the nucleus and associates with it in an active complex. *Oncogene* **2006**, *25*, 3661–3669. [CrossRef] [PubMed]
16. Cironi, L.; Petricevic, T.; Fernandes Vieira, V.; Provero, P.; Fusco, C.; Cornaz, S.; Fregni, G.; Letovanec, I.; Aguet, M.; Stamenkovic, I. The fusion protein SS18-SSX1 employs core Wnt pathway transcription factors to induce a partial Wnt signature in synovial sarcoma. *Sci. Rep.* **2016**, *6*, 22113. [CrossRef]
17. Barham, W.; Frump, A.L.; Sherrill, T.P.; Garcia, C.B.; Saito-Diaz, K.; VanSaun, M.N.; Fingleton, B.; Gleaves, L.; Orton, D.; Capecchi, M.R.; et al. Targeting the Wnt pathway in synovial sarcoma models. *Cancer Discov.* **2013**, *3*, 1286–1301. [CrossRef]
18. Shitashige, M.; Naishiro, Y.; Idogawa, M.; Honda, K.; Ono, M.; Hirohashi, S.; Yamada, T. Involvement of splicing factor-1 in β-catenin/T-cell factor-4-mediated gene transactivation and pre-mRNA splicing. *Gastroenterology* **2007**, *132*, 1039–1054. [CrossRef]

19. Shitashige, M.; Satow, R.; Jigami, T.; Aoki, K.; Honda, K.; Shibata, T.; Ono, M.; Hirohashi, S.; Yamada, T. Traf2- and Nck-interacting kinase is essential for Wnt signaling and colorectal cancer growth. *Cancer Res.* **2010**, *70*, 5024–5033. [CrossRef]

20. Masuda, M.; Sawa, M.; Yamada, T. Therapeutic targets in the Wnt signaling pathway: Feasibility of targeting TNIK in colorectal cancer. *Pharmacol. Ther.* **2015**, *156*, 1–9. [CrossRef]

21. Masuda, M.; Uno, Y.; Ohbayashi, N.; Ohata, H.; Mimata, A.; Kukimoto-Niino, M.; Moriyama, H.; Kashimoto, S.; Inoue, T.; Goto, N.; et al. TNIK inhibition abrogates colorectal cancer stemness. *Nat. Commun.* **2016**, *7*, 12586. [CrossRef] [PubMed]

22. Yamada, T.; Masuda, M. Emergence of TNIK inhibitors in cancer therapeutics. *Cancer Sci.* **2017**, *108*, 818–823. [CrossRef] [PubMed]

23. Knoepfler, P.S. Myc goes global: New tricks for an old oncogene. *Cancer Res.* **2007**, *67*, 5061–5063. [CrossRef] [PubMed]

24. He, T.C.; Sparks, A.B.; Rago, C.; Hermeking, H.; Zawel, L.; da Costa, L.T.; Morin, P.J.; Vogelstein, B.; Kinzler, K.W. Identification of c-MYC as a target of the APC pathway. *Science* **1998**, *281*, 1509–1512. [CrossRef]

25. Sansom, O.J.; Meniel, V.S.; Muncan, V.; Phesse, T.J.; Wilkins, J.A.; Reed, K.R.; Vass, J.K.; Athineos, D.; Clevers, H.; Clarke, A.R. Myc deletion rescues Apc deficiency in the small intestine. *Nature* **2007**, *446*, 676–679. [CrossRef]

26. Barrios, C.; Castresana, J.S.; Ruiz, J.; Kreicbergs, A. Amplification of the c-myc proto-oncogene in soft tissue sarcomas. *Oncology* **1994**, *51*, 13–17. [CrossRef]

27. Vlenterie, M.; Litière, S.; Rizzo, E.; Marréaud, S.; Judson, I.; Gelderblom, H.; Le Cesne, A.; Wardelmann, E.; Messiou, C.; Gronchi, A.; et al. Outcome of chemotherapy in advanced synovial sarcoma patients: Review of 15 clinical trials from the European Organisation for Research and Treatment of Cancer Soft Tissue and Bone Sarcoma Group; setting a new landmark for studies in this entity. *Eur. J. Cancer* **2016**, *58*, 62–72. [CrossRef]

28. van der Graaf, W.T.; Blay, J.Y.; Chawla, S.P.; Kim, D.W.; Bui-Nguyen, B.; Casali, P.G.; Schöffski, P.; Aglietta, M.; Staddon, A.P.; Beppu, Y.; et al. Pazopanib for metastatic soft-tissue sarcoma (PALETTE): A randomised, double-blind, placebo-controlled phase 3 trial. *Lancet* **2012**, *379*, 1879–1886. [CrossRef]

29. Lee, A.T.J.; Jones, R.L.; Huang, P.H. Pazopanib in advanced soft tissue sarcomas. *Signal Transduct. Target. Ther.* **2019**, *4*, 16. [CrossRef]

30. Nakamura, T.; Matsumine, A.; Kawai, A.; Araki, N.; Goto, T.; Yonemoto, T.; Sugiura, H.; Nishida, Y.; Hiraga, H.; Honoki, K.; et al. The clinical outcome of pazopanib treatment in Japanese patients with relapsed soft tissue sarcoma: A Japanese Musculoskeletal Oncology Group (JMOG) study. *Cancer* **2016**, *122*, 1408–1416. [CrossRef]

31. Robbins, P.F.; Morgan, R.A.; Feldman, S.A.; Yang, J.C.; Sherry, R.M.; Dudley, M.E.; Wunderlich, J.R.; Nahvi, A.V.; Helman, L.J.; Mackall, C.L.; et al. Tumor regression in patients with metastatic synovial cell sarcoma and melanoma using genetically engineered lymphocytes reactive with NY-ESO-1. *J. Clin. Oncol.* **2011**, *29*, 917–924. [CrossRef] [PubMed]

32. D'Angelo, S.P.; Melchiori, L.; Merchant, M.S.; Bernstein, D.; Glod, J.; Kaplan, R.; Grupp, S.; Tap, W.D.; Chagin, K.; Binder, G.K.; et al. Antitumor Activity Associated with Prolonged Persistence of Adoptively Transferred NY-ESO-1 (c259)T Cells in Synovial Sarcoma. *Cancer Discov.* **2018**, *8*, 944–957. [CrossRef] [PubMed]

33. Nagayama, S.; Fukukawa, C.; Katagiri, T.; Okamoto, T.; Aoyama, T.; Oyaizu, N.; Imamura, M.; Toguchida, J.; Nakamura, Y. Therapeutic potential of antibodies against FZD 10, a cell-surface protein, for synovial sarcomas. *Oncogene* **2005**, *24*, 6201–6212. [CrossRef] [PubMed]

34. Li, H.K.; Sugyo, A.; Tsuji, A.B.; Morokoshi, Y.; Minegishi, K.; Nagatsu, K.; Kanda, H.; Harada, Y.; Nagayama, S.; Katagiri, T.; et al. α-particle therapy for synovial sarcoma in the mouse using an astatine-211-labeled antibody against frizzled homolog 10. *Cancer Sci.* **2018**, *109*, 2302–2309. [CrossRef]

35. Giraudet, A.L.; Cassier, P.A.; Iwao-Fukukawa, C.; Garin, G.; Badel, J.N.; Kryza, D.; Chabaud, S.; Gilles-Afchain, L.; Clapisson, G.; Desuzinges, C.; et al. A first-in-human study investigating biodistribution, safety and recommended dose of a new radiolabeled MAb targeting FZD10 in metastatic synovial sarcoma patients. *BMC Cancer* **2018**, *18*, 646. [CrossRef]

36. Kadoch, C.; Crabtree, G.R. Reversible disruption of mSWI/SNF (BAF) complexes by the SS18-SSX oncogenic fusion in synovial sarcoma. *Cell* **2013**, *153*, 71–85. [CrossRef]

37. Middeljans, E.; Wan, X.; Jansen, P.W.; Sharma, V.; Stunnenberg, H.G.; Logie, C. SS18 together with animal-specific factors defines human BAF-type SWI/SNF complexes. *PLoS ONE* **2012**, *7*, e33834. [CrossRef]

38. Mora-Blanco, E.L.; Mishina, Y.; Tillman, E.J.; Cho, Y.J.; Thom, C.S.; Pomeroy, S.L.; Shao, W.; Roberts, C.W. Activation of β-catenin/TCF targets following loss of the tumor suppressor SNF5. *Oncogene* **2014**, *33*, 933–938. [CrossRef]
39. Barrott, J.J.; Illum, B.E.; Jin, H.; Zhu, J.F.; Mosbruger, T.; Monument, M.J.; Smith-Fry, K.; Cable, M.G.; Wang, Y.; Grossmann, A.H.; et al. β-Catenin stabilization enhances SS18-SSX2-driven synovial sarcomagenesis and blocks the mesenchymal to epithelial transition. *Oncotarget* **2015**, *6*, 22758–22766. [CrossRef]
40. Mahmoudi, T.; Li, V.S.; Ng, S.S.; Taouatas, N.; Vries, R.G.; Mohammed, S.; Heck, A.J.; Clevers, H. The kinase TNIK is an essential activator of Wnt target genes. *EMBO J.* **2009**, *28*, 3329–3340. [CrossRef]
41. Meichle, A.; Philipp, A.; Eilers, M. The functions of Myc proteins. *Biochim. Biophys. Acta* **1992**, *1114*, 129–146. [CrossRef]
42. Levens, D. Cellular MYCro economics: Balancing MYC function with MYC expression. *Cold Spring Harb. Perspect. Med.* **2013**, *3*, a014233. [CrossRef]
43. Riou, G.; Barrois, M.; Le, M.G.; George, M.; Le Doussal, V.; Haie, C. C-myc proto-oncogene expression and prognosis in early carcinoma of the uterine cervix. *Lancet* **1987**, *1*, 761–763. [CrossRef]
44. Garte, S.J. The c-myc oncogene in tumor progression. *Crit. Rev. Oncog.* **1993**, *4*, 435–449.
45. Shen, J.; Scotlandi, K.; Baldini, N.; Manara, M.C.; Benini, S.; Cerisano, V.; Picci, P.; Serra, M. Prognostic significance of nuclear accumulation of c-myc and mdm2 proteins in synovial sarcoma of the extremities. *Oncology* **2000**, *58*, 253–260. [CrossRef] [PubMed]
46. Nakayama, R.; Mitani, S.; Nakagawa, T.; Hasegawa, T.; Kawai, A.; Morioka, H.; Yabe, H.; Toyama, Y.; Ogose, A.; Toguchida, J.; et al. Gene expression profiling of synovial sarcoma: Distinct signature of poorly differentiated type. *Am. J. Surg. Pathol.* **2010**, *34*, 1599–1607. [CrossRef] [PubMed]
47. Machen, S.K.; Easley, K.A.; Goldblum, J.R. Synovial sarcoma of the extremities: A clinicopathologic study of 34 cases, including semi-quantitative analysis of spindled, epithelial, and poorly differentiated areas. *Am. J. Surg. Pathol.* **1999**, *23*, 268–275. [CrossRef]
48. Naka, N.; Takenaka, S.; Araki, N.; Miwa, T.; Hashimoto, N.; Yoshioka, K.; Joyama, S.; Hamada, K.; Tsukamoto, Y.; Tomita, Y.; et al. Synovial sarcoma is a stem cell malignancy. *Stem Cells* **2010**, *28*, 1119–1131. [CrossRef]
49. Kawai, A.; Naito, N.; Yoshida, A.; Morimoto, Y.; Ouchida, M.; Shimizu, K.; Beppu, Y. Establishment and characterization of a biphasic synovial sarcoma cell line, SYO-1. *Cancer Lett.* **2004**, *204*, 105–113. [CrossRef]
50. Masuda, M.; Chen, W.Y.; Miyanaga, A.; Nakamura, Y.; Kawasaki, K.; Sakuma, T.; Ono, M.; Chen, C.L.; Honda, K.; Yamada, T. Alternative mammalian target of rapamycin (mTOR) signal activation in sorafenib-resistant hepatocellular carcinoma cells revealed by array-based pathway profiling. *Mol. Cell. Proteom.* **2014**, *13*, 1429–1438. [CrossRef]
51. Schneider, C.A.; Rasband, W.S.; Eliceiri, K.W. NIH Image to ImageJ: 25 years of image analysis. *Nat. Methods* **2012**, *9*, 671–675. [CrossRef] [PubMed]
52. Ito, J.; Asano, N.; Kawai, A.; Yoshida, A. The diagnostic utility of reduced immunohistochemical expression of SMARCB1 in synovial sarcomas: A validation study. *Hum. Pathol.* **2016**, *47*, 32–37. [CrossRef] [PubMed]
53. Amary, M.F.; Berisha, F.; Bernardi Fdel, C.; Herbert, A.; James, M.; Reis-Filho, J.S.; Fisher, C.; Nicholson, A.G.; Tirabosco, R.; Diss, T.C.; et al. Detection of SS18-SSX fusion transcripts in formalin-fixed paraffin-embedded neoplasms: Analysis of conventional RT-PCR, qRT-PCR and dual color FISH as diagnostic tools for synovial sarcoma. *Mod. Pathol.* **2007**, *20*, 482–496. [CrossRef] [PubMed]
54. Miyanaga, A.; Honda, K.; Tsuta, K.; Masuda, M.; Yamaguchi, U.; Fujii, G.; Miyamoto, A.; Shinagawa, S.; Miura, N.; Tsuda, H.; et al. Diagnostic and prognostic significance of the alternatively spliced ACTN4 variant in high-grade neuroendocrine pulmonary tumours. *Ann. Oncol.* **2013**, *24*, 84–90. [CrossRef]

© 2020 by the authors. Licensee MDPI, Basel, Switzerland. This article is an open access article distributed under the terms and conditions of the Creative Commons Attribution (CC BY) license (http://creativecommons.org/licenses/by/4.0/).

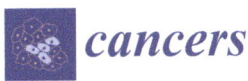

Review

Wnt/β-Catenin Signaling and Immunotherapy Resistance: Lessons for the Treatment of Urothelial Carcinoma

Alexander Chehrazi-Raffle, Tanya B. Dorff, Sumanta K. Pal and Yung Lyou *

Department of Medical Oncology & Experimental Therapeutics, City of Hope Comprehensive Cancer Center, Duarte, CA 91010, USA; achehraziraffle@coh.org (A.C.-R.); tdorff@coh.org (T.B.D.); spal@coh.org (S.K.P.)
* Correspondence: ylyou@coh.org; Tel.: +1-626-256-4673; Fax: +1-626-301-8233

Simple Summary: Metastatic urothelial cell carcinoma (UCC) is a significant public health burden with a median survival estimated at about 15 months. The use of immunotherapy with immune checkpoint inhibitors has greatly improved outcomes but only benefits a minority (~20%) of patients. In this review we discuss the evidence showing how a key molecular pathway known as Wnt/β-catenin signaling can be a driver of immunotherapy resistance and how these insights can serve as lessons for improving future treatment of urothelial carcinoma.

Abstract: Urothelial cell carcinoma (UCC) is a significant public health burden. It accounts for approximately 90 percent of all bladder cancers with an estimated 200,000 annual deaths globally. Platinum based cytotoxic chemotherapy combinations are the current standard of care in the frontline setting for metastatic UCC. Even with these treatments the median overall survival is estimated to be about 15 months. Recently, immune checkpoint inhibitors (ICIs) have demonstrated superior clinical benefits compared to second line chemotherapy in UCC treatment. However only a minority of patients (~20%) respond to ICIs, which highlights the need to better understand the mechanisms behind resistance. In this review, we (i) examine the pathophysiology of Wnt/β-catenin signaling, (ii) discuss pre-clinical evidence that supports the combination of Wnt/β-catenin inhibitors and ICI, and (iii) propose future combination treatments that could be investigated through clinical trials.

Keywords: Wnt; β-catenin; urothelial cancer; immune checkpoint inhibitor; immunotherapy resistance

1. Introduction

Urothelial cell carcinoma (UCC) is the most common malignancy of the urinary system. It accounts for approximately 90 percent of all bladder cancers with an estimated 200,000 annual deaths globally [1,2]. UCC is also an aggressive histology as 25% of patients who receive potentially curative treatment for localized disease will unfortunately succumb to tumor metastasis.

Cytotoxic chemotherapy is the current standard of care in the frontline setting for metastatic UCC. The median overall survival is estimated to be about 15 months with modern chemotherapy regimens containing platinum-based agents [3,4]. Once patients progress on first line chemotherapy treatments the second line chemotherapies have limited efficacy with median progression-free survival periods of 3–4 months (Figure 1) [5,6].

More recently, immune checkpoint inhibitors (ICIs) have demonstrated superior clinical benefits compared to second line chemotherapy in UCC treatment [7,8]. However, only a minority of patients (~20%) respond to ICIs in the treatment of UCCs and other malignancies [7–9]. It has also been noted that those patients who respond to ICIs can often maintain an impressive durable response lasting more than 14–15 months [7,8]. This phenomenon has been observed across numerous cancer subtypes [10], highlighting the need to better understand the mechanisms behind ICI resistance.

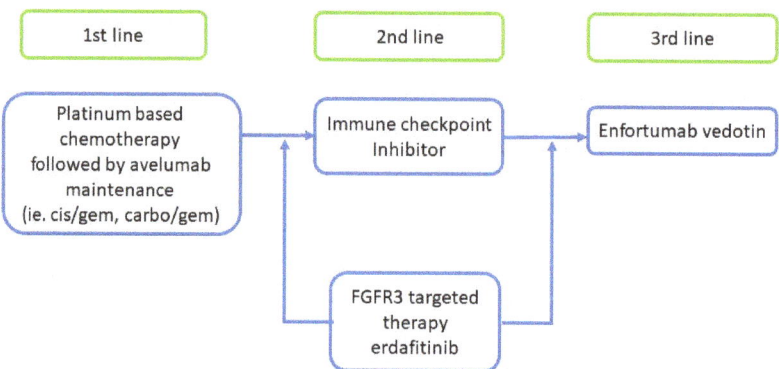

Figure 1. Current systemic treatments in metastatic urothelial cell carcinoma.

Several mechanisms of ICI resistance in cancers have been reviewed extensively elsewhere [11,12]. Previously proposed resistance pathways include PTEN, FGF, MYC, TGFB, TP53, WNT, VEGF, and ANG2 [11,12]. The majority of studies investigating immunotherapy resistance mechanisms have been done in non-UCC studies; as a result, the proposals in this review extrapolate data derived from both urothelial and non-urothelial studies. In this review, we will (i) examine the pathophysiology of Wnt/β-catenin signaling, (ii) discuss pre-clinical evidence that supports the combination of Wnt/β-catenin inhibitors and ICI, and (iii) propose future combination treatments that could be investigated through clinical trials.

2. Canonical Wnt Signaling

Wnt signaling is a highly coordinated and conserved signaling cascade that occurs at the cell surface and within the cytoplasm. This pathway mediates an array of biological functions, including cell fate decisions during embryonic development, stem cell equipoise, and immune system homeostasis [13–16]. Recent reviews published elsewhere provide a more exhaustive discussion on the β-catenin dependent and independent pathways [17–22]. For the purposes of this review (which is most relevant to ICI resistance) we will focus primarily on β-catenin-dependent Wnt signaling.

Canonical, or β-catenin-dependent, Wnt signaling is one of the primary sources of dysregulated transcription in cancer. In the "on-state", the signal cascade begins at the cell surface with Wnt ligands binding to the Frizzled:LRP5/LRP6 receptor complexes, and culminates in the nucleus with the formation of a transcription-activating complex [23]. The primary mediator of this cell surface-to-nucleus signal is β-catenin, a membrane/cytoplasmic armadillo repeat protein which lacks the ability to independently promote DNA transcription [17,20,24]. Instead, β-catenin is trafficked into the nucleus to DNA-binding T-cell factor (TCF)/lymphoid enhancer binding factor (LEF) transcription factors [24,25].

Once bound to DNA by TCF/LEFs, β-catenin recruits other co-activators and regulatory components that collectively activate transcription of the downstream genes known as the Wnt target genes. These sets of Wnt target genes drive cells to proliferate, self-renew, differentiate and survive in a variety of tissues and contexts. In normal cells, feedback inhibition results in this activity occurring only transiently, which in turn prevents overactivation of Wnt target gene transcription. Signal transduction is thus "turned off" in cells with low or absent Wnt because β-catenin becomes unstable by being tagged in the cytoplasm for ubiquitination by the destruction complex, which then leads to proteasome degradation.

However, in various cancers (i.e., colon cancer) mutations in the destruction complex components (e.g., *APC*, *AXIN2* and *FAM123B/WTX*) or regulators of the receptors/ligand (e.g., *RNF43/ZNRF3*, *RSPO2*, or *RSPO3*) components can lead to unchecked Wnt signaling.

These mutations negate the cytoplasmic feedback controls and create cells with constitutive, high levels of β-catenin and aberrantly high levels of Wnt target gene transcription that can initiate carcinogenesis and immune suppression [20,26–29].

3. Upregulation of Wnt/β-Catenin in Bladder Carcinogenesis

Several correlative studies have shown conflicting evidence between upregulation of Wnt/β-catenin signaling and UCC carcinogenesis [30–34]. For instance, The Cancer Genome Atlas (TCGA) Research Network detected Wnt signaling alterations in 73% of UCC tumors [35]. However, Ahmad et al. noted Wnt signaling in only 33% of their clinical UCC samples [36–38]. The discrepancy could most likely be due to comparisons using different methods and patient populations. For example, one Ahmad et al. study used a tissue microarray array with core biopsy samples, whereas a TCGA study detected aberrations in Wnt signaling through genomics using RNA-seq and whole exome sequencing [35–38]. Also there was a difference in sample size with TCGA and Ahmad et al. studies using 131 and 60 patient samples respectively [35–38]. Additionally it was noted that β-catenin expression's correlation to tumor grade and muscle invasion has been inconsistent [39]. Despite these discrepancies between studies, it is evident that a substantial proportion of UCC develops in the context of Wnt signaling aberrations.

From a pathophysiologic perspective, numerous pre-clinical studies have implicated the silencing of endogenous Wnt inhibitors as potential oncogenic events. CpG hypermethylation of the WIF1 (Wnt inhibitory factor-1) promoter was found to lead to decreased transcription and increased Wnt signaling activity in human bladder cancer cell lines [40]. Knockdown of WIF1 by siRNA in bladder cancer cell lines led to increased activity in c-myc and cyclin D1 mRNA transcription and increased cell growth [40]. These results suggested that Wnt signaling via WIF1 could potentially promote development of UCC [40]. Another proposed mechanism involves aberrations in the oncogene activation-induced cytidine deaminase, which upregulates the Wnt/β-catenin pathway and thereby promotes UCC growth [41]. More studies are needed to better understand how Wnt signaling can drive urothelial carcinogenesis.

4. Wnt/β-Catenin Induces Immune Cell Exclusion in Urothelial Cancer

Due to the limited efficacy of ICI treatments, much effort is being dedicated to developing predictive biomarkers of response and understanding the biological mechanisms for resistance. One widely established predictive biomarker for ICI response is intratumoral enrichment of CD8+ T-cells prior to treatment [42,43]. Therefore, many studies have used the presence and quantity of CD8+ T-cell infiltration as a surrogate marker when performing correlative studies to determine if other molecular pathways may be involved in predicting the ICI response.

A recent study by Sweis et al. used a bioinformatics approach to correlate CD8+ T-cell infiltration with various signaling pathways [44]. The investigators analyzed the whole exome sequencing (WES) and RNA-seq transcriptional profile data from the 267 samples of urothelial bladder cancer collected for the TCGA study. The investigators stratified these tumors based on a 160-gene T-cell inflamed expression signature indicative of a T-cell inflamed and non-inflamed microenvironment. This T-cell inflamed gene signature was then validated by performing immunohistochemistry (IHC) staining for CD8+ T-cell infiltration on a sample of 19 tumors (7.1%).

Once stratified into inflamed vs. non-inflamed phenotypes, the investigators uncovered that 730 genes were preferentially expressed in the non-T-cell-inflamed tumors. Ingenuity pathway analysis then showed that one of the top upstream regulators for these groups of differentially expressed genes were those that were regulated by β-catenin/Wnt signaling. The authors then went back to the 19 samples which they had initially performed CD8+ T-cell IHC staining and co-stained for nuclear β-catenin as a marker for active β-catenin dependent Wnt signaling. The investigators found a statistically significant inverse relationship between nuclear β-catenin and the density of CD8+ T cells infiltrating the tumor.

To further validate the Wnt signaling pathway as a mediator of non-T-cell-inflamed tumor microenvironments, a follow up study done by Luke et al. employed a similar approach (WES genomics and RNA-seq transcriptional profiling) and analyzed 9244 samples across 31 different types of cancers [45]. The investigators used their previously developed 160-gene T-cell inflamed expression signature to segregate the samples into T-cell inflamed, intermediate, or non-T-cell inflamed. The investigators defined Wnt/β-catenin signaling activation at three different levels: assessment of somatic mutations or copy number alterations in *CTNNB1* (gene for β-catenin) and other regulatory genes predicted to result in pathway activation, expression of downstream Wnt target genes, and β-catenin protein levels which were assessed through reverse phase protein array (RPPA). With respect to the 363 UCC samples included in this cohort, all three levels correlated with a non-T-cell inflamed tumor signature, the most pronounced of which was CTNNB1 protein level. Taken together, these findings suggest that there is a significant correlation between upregulation of Wnt signaling and a non-T-cell-inflamed microenvironment in UCC.

5. ICI Attenuation via CCL4

As previously discussed, translational studies have suggested that Wnt/β-catenin signaling may induce a non-T-cell-inflamed tumor phenotype thereby excluding immune cells from the tumor microenvironment and dampening the therapeutic effect of ICIs. To elucidate molecular mediators, the Gajewski group used a genetically engineered melanoma mouse model with active β-catenin signaling (BRAF/PTEN/CAT-STA) in the tumors [46].

In their mouse model, the authors found that β-catenin signaling activation was associated with low levels of tumor infiltrating CD8+ T-cells. Conversely, mice in which β-catenin signaling was absent contained a high density of CD8+ T-cell infiltration. In order to discern if this was due to differences in neo-antigens, the authors introduced a neo-antigen (SIY) expressing construct genetically into the tumors and adoptively transferred T-cells with SIY T cell receptor. They found that the transferred T-cells accumulated in the BRAF/PTEN-STA tumors but not the β-catenin expressing BRAF/PTEN/Bcat-STA tumors despite both tumors now expressing the neo-antigen. Furthermore, anti-PD-1 and anti-CTLA-4 agents were rendered ineffective in the Wnt-activated (BRAF/PTEN/Bcat-STA) mice but remained effective in Wnt-inactivated (BRAF/PTEN-STA) mice. These results suggested that upregulation of Wnt/β-catenin may indeed induce resistance to immune checkpoint inhibition.

The investigators then queried whether this blunted response to ICIs could be dependent on antigen presentation from CD103+ dendritic cells (DC). Within Wnt/β-catenin-activated T-cell-depleted tumors, they found that CD103+ DCs were nearly absent and IFN-β cytokine expression was reduced. The investigators then found that intratumoral injection of CD103+ DCs led to restoration of T-cells infiltration within the tumor. This supported the role of CD103+ dendritic cells as key mediators of an antitumor immune response. To characterize the mechanism of failed recruitment of the CD103+ DCs, the investigators analyzed the gene expression of these two tumor types and found that four chemokines (CCL3, CXCL1, CXCL2, and CCL4) were lower in the non-T-cell inflamed BRAF/PTEN/Bcat-STA tumors. Of these four chemokines, only CCL4 was found on an in vitro DC migration assay to possess the ability to effectively modulate cell migration.

Furthermore, the investigators found that the Wnt signaling target gene ATF3–which also binds at the promoter region of the CCL4 gene—was expressed at higher levels in the β-catenin activated melanoma tumors. This negative feedback was substantiated by then demonstrating that gene knockdown of ATF3 and CTNNB1 in melanoma cell lines led to upregulation of CCL4 expression (Figure 2).

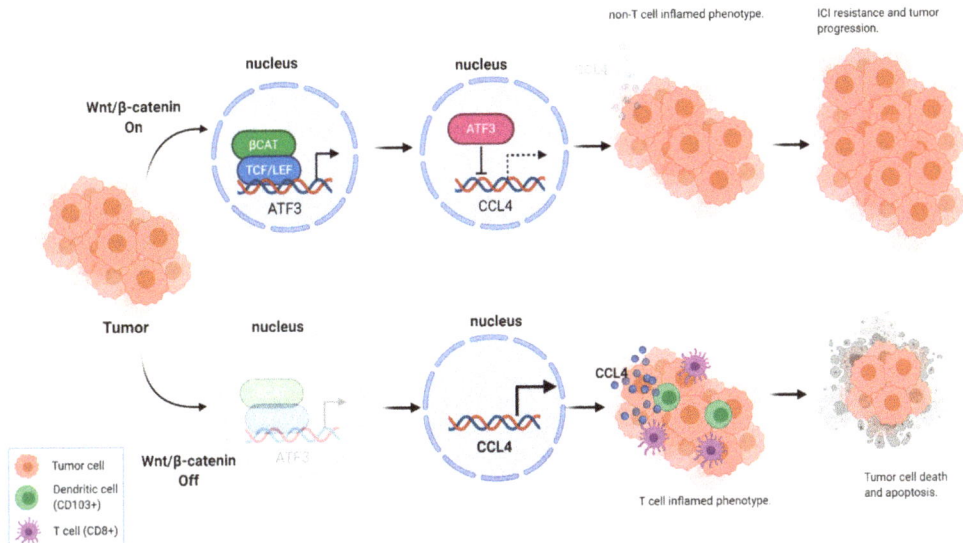

Figure 2. Wnt/β-catenin signaling can alter T-cell infiltration status and ICI response via CCL4. (Created with BioRender®).

6. Wnt/β-Catenin Signaling Induces Immune Cell Exclusion by Affecting the Tumor Microenvironment (TME)

Tumor-associated macrophages (TAMs) are amongst the most common tumor immune infiltrating cells in the tumor microenvironment (TME) [47]. TAMs are classically thought to exist in two polarized states with the activated M1 and M2 subtypes [47]. The M1 subtypes are thought to play a significant role in the anti-tumor immune response by producing reactive oxygen species (ROS) and pro-inflammatory cytokines [47]. The M2 subtype has been found to have an opposite immunosuppressive function by producing anti-inflammatory cytokines (i.e., IL1, IL-13, and TGF-β) which can promote tumor growth and ICI resistance [47]. These anti-inflammatory cytokines and chemokines can also induce the production of regulatory T-cells which directly inhibit cytotoxic T cells further driving immunosuppression [47–49].

It has been shown that Wnt/β-catenin signaling can modulate the TAMs population in the TME leading to a protumoral phenotype which may be ICI resistant [50,51]. In a study done by Kaler et al. using isogenic colon cancer cell lines (HCT116 and Hke-3 cells) with mutated active β-catenin, the investigators found that TAMs could further enhance the pre-existing Wnt/β-catenin signaling present and protect the cancer cells from TRAIL-induced apoptosis [50]. In contrast, when HCT116 cancer cells with an inactive β-catenin allele were cultured with TAMs, the investigators noted that these cells were susceptible to TRAIL induced apoptosis and were unable to increase their Wnt/β-catenin signaling levels [50]. The investigators also found that the isogenic colon cancer cell lines (HCT116 and Hke-3 cells) with mutated active β-catenin when cultured with TAMs would produce more snail protein, which is a known Wnt/β-catenin signaling target gene and driver of tumor mesenchymal transition [50]. These results suggested that the increased Wnt/β-catenin signaling from the TAMs could induce snail gene expression and drive a tumor mesenchymal transition phenotype [50]. Of note this nail driven tumor mesenchymal transition has recently been reported to be a possible mechanism for ICI resistance [50–52].

Another potential mechanism for ICI resistance is through the tumor's ability to create a hostile TME that is acidic from increased lactic acid production which can lead to impaired cytotoxic T-cell function [53–55]. A detailed discussion on how tumors create a hostile hypoxic and acidic TME which leads to suppression of the T-cells' cytotoxic function is beyond the scope of this manuscript. For a more comprehensive review on this topic there are many excellent reviews which can be found in the reference section of this manuscript [53,56,57]. Briefly, the oncogenic mutations that drive carcinogenesis (i.e., Akt/PI3k/mTOR and Wnt/β-catenin signaling) have also been shown to drive a metabolic reprogramming of cells from oxidative phosphorylation towards aerobic glycolysis [56,58]. This phenomenon wherein cancer cells prefer to undergo the more inefficient aerobic glycolysis even in the presence of oxygen has been known for almost 100 years since it was first described by Dr. Otto Heinrich Warburg [57,59]. It is thought that cancer cells have evolved this shift towards aerobic glycolysis as a way to produce metabolic byproducts which can then be converted to provide the needed biomass to use as building blocks for its rapid cell proliferation [56,57]. As the tumor grows larger in size its metabolic demands also increase in an unregulated manner which often outstrips the local oxygen and nutrient supply [53,56]. This imbalance in metabolic demand and available supply of local resources creates a hostile TME that is hypoxic, acidic (due to lactic acid build up), and nutrient deficient [53,56]. In addition, to the existing overactive oncogenic signaling pathways present in the cancer cells (i.e., Akt/PI3k/mTOR and Wnt/β-catenin signaling) these hostile TME conditions will further drive the tumors to adapt by increasing angiogenesis and glycolysis via the VEGF and HIF signaling pathways [53,56]. These same acidic and hypoxic TME conditions will then inhibit the oxidative phosphorylation that is needed by T-cells in order to perform their cytotoxic functions potentially leading to immunosuppression and ICI resistance [53]. In fact it has been shown that high lactate concentrations in the TME can impede the CD8+ T-cells ability to export lactate and suppress their natural cytotoxic function [60].

As discussed above, the Wnt/β-catenin signaling pathway was found to initially play a central role in carcinogenesis by driving cell proliferation [20]. More recently, it has also been found to play an additional role in cancer metabolism by metabolically reprogramming cancer cells to promote aerobic glycolysis and lactic acid production [58,61–63]. In a study done by Pate et al. the investigators found that by using genetically engineered human colon cancer cell lines that overactive Wnt/β-catenin signaling drives aerobic glycolysis and lactic acid production by upregulating the genes pyruvate dehydrogenase kinase 1 (PDK1) and monocarboxylate transporter 1 (MCT1/SLC16A1) [58,61]. They also found that when this metabolic shift towards glycolysis occurred that there was also a corresponding inhibition in the gene expression of pyruvate dehydrogenase (PDH) and oxidative phosphorylation [58,61]. Other independent studies have also provided further supporting evidence that Wnt/β-catenin signaling can drive the metabolic reprogramming of cancer cells towards lactic acid production and aerobic glycolysis [62,63].

It has also been shown that the lactic acid in the TME can play a role in immunosuppression and drive further tumor growth [53,54,64]. In a study done by Brand et al. the investigators found that patients who had melanoma tumors with increased LDHA gene expression and lactic acid levels were more likely to have findings of impaired T and NK cell infiltration consistent with an immunosuppressed or immune deficient tumor phenotype [54]. The investigators then used shRNA to create LDH_{low} murine melanoma and pancreatic cancer cell lines [54]. Through the use of various clever control experiments the investigators showed that knockdown of the LDHA gene resulted in a stable tumor cell phenotype that produced low levels of lactate with no effects on the other metabolic pathways analyzed [54]. They then proceeded to inject these murine melanoma and pancreatic cells lines which were either LDH_{high} or LDH_{low} into syngeneic mice [54]. They found that the LDH_{low} had impaired tumor growth and higher T-cell and NK cell infiltration compared to the LDH_{high} tumors [54]. These findings suggested that the acidic TME created by uncontrolled lactate production led to impaired immunosurveillance and T-cell and NK cell infiltration leading to an immune deficient TME [54]. In another independent study done by Harel et al. the investigators found that increased oxidative phosphorylation and lipid metabolism in melanoma tumors by proteomic analysis were more likely to have potentiated antigen presentation and response to anti-PD1 immune checkpoint inhibitor or TIL-based immunotherapy [64]. The investigators of the Harel et al. study concluded that the tumors with increased oxidative phosphorylation were undergoing less glycolysis, secreting less lactate, and creating a more favorable TME for immune cells [64].

The above studies provide evidence supporting the hypothesis that the presence of lactic acid in the TME can be immunosuppressive by inhibiting the needed oxidative phosphorylation of cytotoxic T-cells. As a result, this has led to the proposal that targeting lactic acid production could be a potential way to overcome ICI resistance [55]. In summary, the above findings provide evidence that Wnt/β-catenin signaling can drive ICI resistance by modulating the TME through the interaction with TAMs or driving lactic acid production and creating a local immunosuppressive environment for cytotoxic T-cells (Figure 3) [50,53–58,61,64].

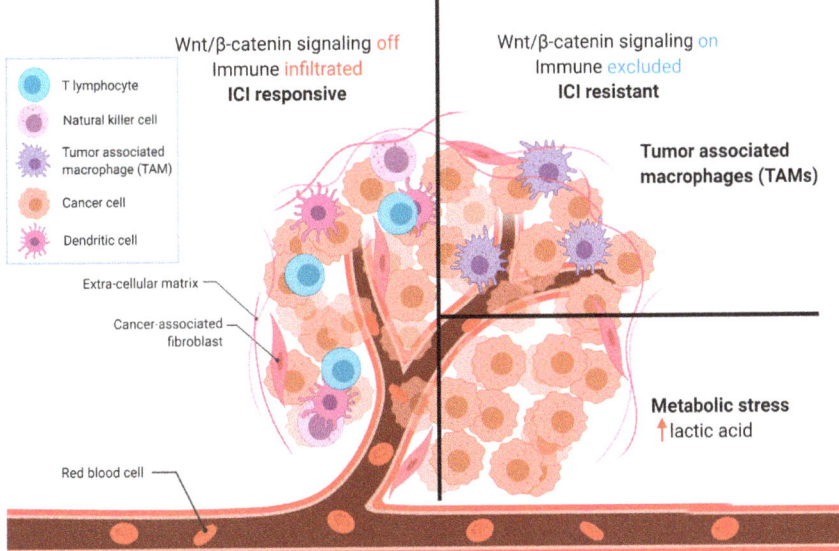

Figure 3. Wnt/β-catenin signaling can alter tumor microenvironment. (Adapted from "Tumor Microenvironment", by BioRender.com (2020). Retrieved from https://app.biorender.com/biorender-templates).

7. Overcoming ICI Resistance with β-Catenin Inhibition

The above mentioned studies provide strong evidence that the Wnt/β-catenin signaling pathway drives immune cell exclusion which can then lead to immune checkpoint inhibitor resistance in cancer treatment [44,45,65]. As a result, one could reason that combining a Wnt/β-catenin signaling inhibitor and ICI may lead to overcoming this resistance mechanism (Figure 4).

Early therapeutic efforts primarily centered on finding targets for Wnt inhibition [23,66–68]. However, one of the major hurdles that researchers encountered was developing a molecule small enough to penetrate the nuclear membranes yet robust enough to counteract the large β-catenin regulatory complex [23,68,69]. Another challenging adverse class effect was on-target bone toxicity, which ultimately led to the early termination of several Phase I studies [23,68,70–72].

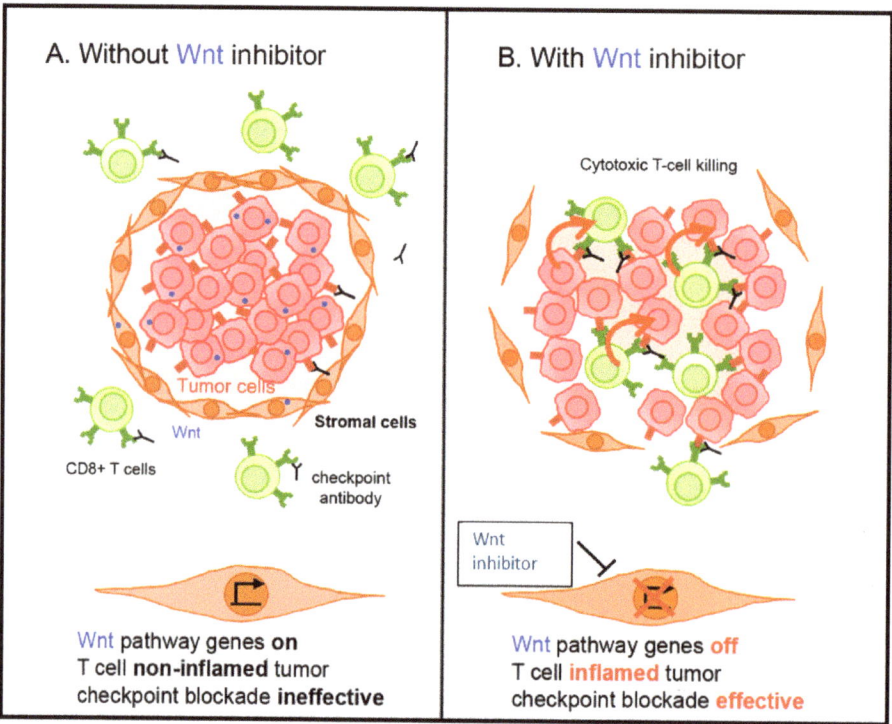

Figure 4. Proposed model for overcoming Wnt signaling driven immune checkpoint inhibitor resistance. (**A**) Immune cell exclusion driven by Wnt signaling. (**B**) Combination of Wnt signaling inhibitor and immune checkpoint inhibitor can overcome resistance.

More recently, several studies have shifted focus toward downstream inhibition of the intranuclear transcriptional β-catenin complex to enhance immune cell infiltration within the tumor microenvironment. For instance, Ganesh et al. designed a β-catenin inhibitor (DCR-BCAT) that selectively silenced CTNNB1 (the gene which transcribes/β-catenin) in tumors using an RNAi oligonucleotide [73]. Using allografted B16F10 mouse melanoma cells on immunocompetent C57BL/6 mice, which are known to be refractory to ICI treatments through T-cell exclusion [73], Ganesh et al. found that treatment with DCR-BCAT significantly increased the intratumoral density of CD8+ T-cells compared to the placebo control. Quantitative analysis of tumor RNA detected a decrease in β-catenin gene expression as well as a concomitant increase in CCL4 expression. Furthermore, single-cell flow cytometry of the DCR-BCAT mouse tumors showed a significant increase in CD8+, CD3+, CD103+, and PD-1 positive cells, suggesting that these tumors were transitioning to a T-cell-inflamed phenotype.

Encouraged by these results, the investigators subsequently examined if their β-catenin inhibitor could reconstitute an immune response within their T-cell-excluded tumor model. Although monotherapy with either the DCR-BCAT or an ICI was minimally effective, the combination of DCR-BCAT plus ICI elicited a synergistic effect with reductions in tumor size by as much as 87% [73]. Moreover, the authors confirmed that this combination was effective in another model, the Neuro2A (neuroblastoma) cell lines, which are also non-T-cell-inflamed at baseline [73]. These findings suggest that a β-catenin inhibitor can effectively downregulate Wnt/β-catenin signaling and induce a T-cell-inflamed phenotype that can potentiate a response to immune checkpoint inhibitors [73].

8. Ongoing Clinical Trials and Future Directions

In recent years, several novel agents with varied mechanisms of action have attempted to mitigate the immunosuppressive tumor microenvironment through WNT/β-catenin inhibition (Figure 5, Table 1). One such therapeutic effort in development is DKN-01, an antibody that antagonizes the WNT/β-catenin pathway through inhibition of DKK1 [74]. Preliminary results from a Phase 1b/2a study of DKN-01 plus pembrolizumab (NCT02013154) demonstrated a disease control rate of 80% in patients who had tumors with high DKK1 expression as compared to a disease control rate of 20% in patients with low DKK1 expression [74].

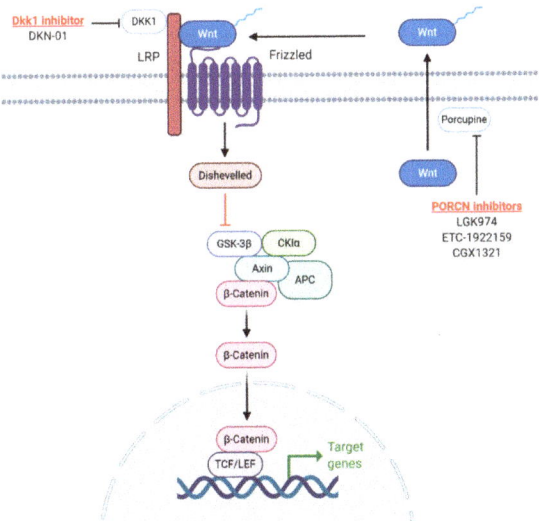

Figure 5. Current WNT/β-catenin inhibitors being used in combination with ICI for human clinical trial. (Adapted from "Wnt//β-catenin signaling", by BioRender.com (2020). Retrieved from https://app.biorender.com/biorender-templates).

Table 1. Current clinical trials combining Wnt inhibitor and immune checkpoint inhibitor.

Drug	ICI Agent	Mechanism of Action of Wnt Inhibitor	Disease	Clinical Trial	Trial Phase
LGK974	PDR001 (anti-PD-1)	PORCN inhibitor	Solid tumors	NCT01351103	Phase I
ETC-1922159	pembrolizumab (anti-PD-1)	PORCN inhibitor	Solid tumors	NCT02521844	Phase IA/B
CGX1321	pembrolizumab (anti-PD-1)	PORCN inhibitor	Advanced GI Tumors	NCT02675946	Phase I/Ib
DKN-01	nivolumab (anti-PD-1)	DKK1 inhibitor	Advanced Biliary Tract Cancer	NCT04057365	Phase II
DKN-01 ± chemotherapy	tislelizumab (anti-PD-1)	DKK1 inhibitor	Advanced Esophagogastric Cancer	NCT04363801	Phase IIa
DKN-01	pembrolizumab (anti-PD-1)	DKK1 inhibitor	Advanced Esophagogastric Cancer	NCT02013154	Phase I

Another class of WNT/β-catenin inhibitors disrupt PORCN, an enzyme that facilitates WNT secretion [75]. A recent Phase I study of the PORCN inhibitor WNT974 combined with the PD-1 monoclonal antibody spartalizumab (NCT01351103) reported impressive results across several solid tumors, including stable disease in 53% of patients who were previously refractory to ICIs [76]. Of note, neither one of these trials included urothelial carcinoma and focused on other malignancies such as GI cancers, melanoma, and NSCLC. However, seeing how the combination of ICIs with WNT/β-catenin inhibitors has produced some signal of efficacy even in the early phase clinical trials, this combination warrants further investigation for the treatment of UCC.

9. Conclusions

In summary, WNT/β-catenin signaling can drive immune cell exclusion and may be a resistance mechanism for immune checkpoint inhibitors. Several preclinical studies have shown that inhibition of the WNT/β-catenin pathway in conjunction with an ICI can effectively overcome this resistance mechanism. With respect to UCC, this combination is particularly promising given the high frequency of WNT/β-catenin aberrations in correlative studies as well as its potential role in upregulating urothelial oncogenesis. Thus, to complement ongoing clinical trials across other solid tumors, additional studies that validate the synergistic relationship of ICIs and WNT/β-catenin inhibitors in UCC are urgently needed.

Author Contributions: Y.L., A.C.-R., S.K.P. and T.B.D. wrote and revised the manuscript. All authors have read and agreed to the published version of the manuscript.

Funding: Y.L. is supported by the American Cancer Society.

Conflicts of Interest: Y.L., T.B.D. and A.C.-R. have no conflicts of interest that might be relevant to the contents of this manuscript. S.K.P.: Consulting or Advisory Role: Genentech, Bristol-Myers Squibb.

References

1. Siegel, R.L.; Miller, K.D.; Jemal, A. Cancer statistics, 2020. *CA Cancer J. Clin.* **2020**, *70*, 7–30. [CrossRef]
2. Bray, F.; Ferlay, J.; Soerjomataram, I.; Siegel, R.L.; Torre, L.A.; Jemal, A. Global cancer statistics 2018: GLOBOCAN estimates of incidence and mortality worldwide for 36 cancers in 185 countries. *CA Cancer J. Clin.* **2018**, *68*, 394–424. [CrossRef] [PubMed]
3. von der Maase, H.; Hansen, S.W.; Roberts, J.T.; Dogliotti, L.; Oliver, T.; Moore, M.J.; Bodrogi, I.; Albers, P.; Knuth, A.; Lippert, C.M.; et al. Gemcitabine and cisplatin versus methotrexate, vinblastine, doxorubicin, and cisplatin in advanced or metastatic bladder cancer: Results of a large, randomized, multinational, multicenter, phase III study. *J. Clin. Oncol.* **2000**, *18*, 3068–3077. [CrossRef]
4. von der Maase, H.; Sengelov, L.; Roberts, J.T.; Ricci, S.; Dogliotti, L.; Oliver, T.; Moore, M.J.; Zimmermann, A.; Arning, M. Long-term survival results of a randomized trial comparing gemcitabine plus cisplatin, with methotrexate, vinblastine, doxorubicin, plus cisplatin in patients with bladder cancer. *J. Clin. Oncol.* **2005**, *23*, 4602–4608. [CrossRef] [PubMed]
5. Albers, P.; Park, S.-I.; Niegisch, G.; Fechner, G.; Steiner, U.; Lehmann, J.; Heimbach, D.; Heidenreich, A.; Fimmers, R.; Siener, R. Randomized phase III trial of 2nd line gemcitabine and paclitaxel chemotherapy in patients with advanced bladder cancer: Short-term versus prolonged treatment [German Association of Urological Oncology (AUO) trial AB 20/99]. *Ann. Oncol.* **2011**, *22*, 288–294. [CrossRef] [PubMed]
6. Bellmunt, J.; Théodore, C.; Demkov, T.; Komyakov, B.; Sengelov, L.; Daugaard, G.; Caty, A.; Carles, J.; Jagiello-Gruszfeld, A.; Karyakin, O.; et al. Phase III trial of vinflunine plus best supportive care compared with best supportive care alone after a platinum-containing regimen in patients with advanced transitional cell carcinoma of the urothelial tract. *J. Clin. Oncol.* **2009**, *27*, 4454–4461. [CrossRef]
7. Bellmunt, J.; de Wit, R.; Vaughn, D.J.; Fradet, Y.; Lee, J.-L.; Fong, L.; Vogelzang, N.J.; Climent, M.A.; Petrylak, D.P.; Choueiri, T.K.; et al. Pembrolizumab as second-line therapy for advanced urothelial carcinoma. *N. Engl. J. Med.* **2017**, *376*, 1015–1026. [CrossRef]
8. Rosenberg, J.E.; Hoffman-Censits, J.; Powles, T.; van der Heijden, M.S.; Balar, A.V.; Necchi, A.; Dawson, N.; O'Donnell, P.H.; Balmanoukian, A.; Loriot, Y.; et al. Atezolizumab in patients with locally advanced and metastatic urothelial carcinoma who have progressed following treatment with platinum-based chemotherapy: A single-arm, multicentre, phase 2 trial. *Lancet* **2016**, *387*, 1909–1920. [CrossRef]
9. Ribas, A.; Wolchok, J.D. Cancer immunotherapy using checkpoint blockade. *Science* **2018**, *359*, 1350–1355. [CrossRef]
10. Fares, C.M.; Van Allen, E.M.; Drake, C.G.; Allison, J.P.; Hu-Lieskovan, S. Mechanisms of resistance to immune checkpoint blockade: Why does checkpoint inhibitor immunotherapy not work for all patients? *Am. Soc. Clin. Oncol. Educ. Book* **2019**, *39*, 147–164. [CrossRef]
11. Sharma, P.; Hu-Lieskovan, S.; Wargo, J.A.; Ribas, A. Primary, adaptive, and acquired resistance to cancer immunotherapy. *Cell* **2017**, *168*, 707–723. [CrossRef]
12. Spranger, S.; Gajewski, T.F. Impact of oncogenic pathways on evasion of antitumour immune responses. *Nat. Rev. Cancer* **2018**, *18*, 139–147. [CrossRef] [PubMed]
13. Nusse, R.; Varmus, H.E. Many tumors induced by the mouse mammary tumor virus contain a provirus integrated in the same region of the host genome. *Cell* **1982**, *31*, 99–109. [CrossRef]
14. Bodmer, W.F.; Bailey, C.J.; Bodmer, J.; Bussey, H.J.; Ellis, A.; Gorman, P.; Lucibello, F.C.; Murday, V.A.; Rider, S.H.; Scambler, P. Localization of the gene for familial adenomatous polyposis on chromosome 5. *Nature* **1987**, *328*, 614–616. [CrossRef] [PubMed]
15. McMahon, A.P.; Moon, R.T. Ectopic expression of the proto-oncogene int-1 in Xenopus embryos leads to duplication of the embryonic axis. *Cell* **1989**, *58*, 1075–1084. [CrossRef]

16. Rocheleau, C.E.; Downs, W.D.; Lin, R.; Wittmann, C.; Bei, Y.; Cha, Y.H.; Ali, M.; Priess, J.R.; Mello, C.C. Wnt signaling and an APC-related gene specify endoderm in early C. elegans embryos. *Cell* **1997**, *90*, 707–716. [CrossRef]
17. Niehrs, C.; Acebron, S.P. Mitotic and mitogenic Wnt signalling. *EMBO J.* **2012**, *31*, 2705–2713. [CrossRef] [PubMed]
18. DeBruine, Z.J.; Xu, H.E.; Melcher, K. Assembly and architecture of the Wnt/β-catenin signalosome at the membrane. *Br. J. Pharmacol.* **2017**, *174*, 4564–4574. [CrossRef]
19. Driehuis, E.; Clevers, H. Wnt signalling events near the cell membrane and their pharmacological targeting for the treatment of cancer. *Br. J. Pharmacol.* **2017**, *174*, 4547–4563. [CrossRef] [PubMed]
20. Nusse, R.; Clevers, H. Wnt/β-catenin signaling, disease, and emerging therapeutic modalities. *Cell* **2017**, *169*, 985–999. [CrossRef]
21. Zimmerli, D.; Hausmann, G.; Cantù, C.; Basler, K. Pharmacological interventions in the Wnt pathway: Inhibition of Wnt secretion versus disrupting the protein-protein interfaces of nuclear factors. *Br. J. Pharmacol.* **2017**, *174*, 4600–4610. [CrossRef]
22. van Kappel, E.C.; Maurice, M.M. Molecular regulation and pharmacological targeting of the β-catenin destruction complex. *Br. J. Pharmacol.* **2017**, *174*, 4575–4588. [CrossRef]
23. Lyou, Y.; Habowski, A.N.; Chen, G.T.; Waterman, M.L. Inhibition of nuclear Wnt signalling: Challenges of an elusive target for cancer therapy. *Br. J. Pharmacol.* **2017**, *174*, 4589–4599. [CrossRef]
24. Masuda, T.; Ishitani, T. JB special review—Wnt signaling: Biological functions and its implications in diseases: Context-dependent regulation of the β-catenin transcriptional complex supports diverse functions of Wnt/β-catenin signaling. *J. Biochem.* **2017**, *161*, 9–17. [CrossRef]
25. Cadigan, K.M.; Waterman, M.L. TCF/LEFs and Wnt signaling in the nucleus. *Cold Spring Harb. Perspect. Biol.* **2012**, *4*, a007906. [CrossRef]
26. Mazzoni, S.M.; Fearon, E.R. AXIN1 and AXIN2 variants in gastrointestinal cancers. *Cancer Lett.* **2014**, *355*, 1–8. [CrossRef]
27. Polakis, P. Wnt signaling in cancer. *Cold Spring Harb. Perspect. Biol.* **2012**, *4*, a008052. [CrossRef]
28. Atlas, T.C.G.N.; Muzny, D.; Bainbridge, M.; Chang, K.; Dinh, H.; Drummond, J.; Fowler, G.; Kovar, C.; Lewis, L.; Morgan, M.; et al. Comprehensive molecular characterization of human colon and rectal cancer. *Nature* **2012**, *487*, 330–337. [CrossRef]
29. Grasso, C.S.; Giannakis, M.; Wells, D.K.; Hamada, T.; Mu, X.J.; Quist, M.; Nowak, J.A.; Nishihara, R.; Qian, Z.R.; Inamura, K.; et al. Genetic mechanisms of immune evasion in colorectal cancer. *Cancer Discov.* **2018**, *8*, 730–749. [CrossRef]
30. Kashibuchi, K.; Tomita, K.; Schalken, J.A.; Kume, H.; Takeuchi, T.; Kitamura, T. The prognostic value of E-cadherin, α-, β- and γ-catenin in bladder cancer patients who underwent radical cystectomy. *Int. J. Urol.* **2007**, *14*, 789–794. [CrossRef]
31. Nakopoulou, L.; Zervas, A.; Gakiopoulou-Givalou, H.; Constantinides, C.; Doumanis, G.; Davaris, P.; Dimopoulos, C. Prognostic value of E-cadherin, beta-catenin, P120ctn in patients with transitional cell bladder cancer. *Anticancer Res.* **2000**, *20*, 4571–4578.
32. Zhu, X.; Kanai, Y.; Saito, A.; Kondo, Y.; Hirohashi, S. Aberrant expression of β-catenin and mutation of exon 3 of the β-catenin gene in renal and urothelial carcinomas. *Pathol. Int.* **2000**, *50*, 945–952. [CrossRef] [PubMed]
33. Garcia Del Muro, X.; Torregrosa, A.; Muñoz, J.; Castellsagué, X.; Condom, E.; Vigués, F.; Arance, A.; Fabra, A.; Germà, J.R. Prognostic value of the expression of E-cadherin and β-catenin in bladder cancer. *Eur. J. Cancer* **2000**, *268*, 1335–1341. [CrossRef]
34. Shimazui, T.; Schalken, J.A.; Giroldi, L.A.; Jansen, C.F.J.; Akaza, H.; Koiso, K.; Debruyne, F.M.J.; Bringuier, P.P. Prognostic value of cadherin-associated molecules (α-, β-, and γ- catenins and p120cas) in bladder tumors. *Cancer Res.* **1996**, *56*, 4154–4158.
35. Weinstein, J.N.; Akbani, R.; Broom, B.M.; Wang, W.; Verhaak, R.G.W.; McConkey, D.; Lerner, S.; Morgan, M.; Creighton, C.J.; Smith, C.; et al. Comprehensive molecular characterization of urothelial bladder carcinoma. *Nature* **2014**, *507*, 315–322. [CrossRef]
36. Ahmad, I. The role of WNT signalling in urothelial cell carcinoma. *Ann. R. Coll. Surg. Engl.* **2015**, *97*, 481–486. [CrossRef] [PubMed]
37. Ahmad, I.; Patel, R.; Liu, Y.; Singh, L.B.; Taketo, M.M.; Wu, X.R.; Leung, H.Y.; Sansom, O.J. Ras mutation cooperates with β-catenin activation to drive bladder tumourigenesis. *Cell Death Dis.* **2011**, *13*, 2039–2045. [CrossRef]
38. Ahmad, I.; Morton, J.P.; Singh, L.B.; Radulescu, S.M.; Ridgway, R.A.; Patel, S.; Woodgett, J.; Winton, D.J.; Taketo, M.M.; Wu, X.R.; et al. B-Catenin activation synergizes with PTEN loss to cause bladder cancer formation. *Oncogene* **2011**, *12*, 6309–6322. [CrossRef]
39. Ren, J.; Yang, Y.; Peng, T.; Xu, D. Predictive value of β-catenin in bladder cancer: A systematic review and meta-analysis. *Biosci. Rep.* **2020**, *40*, BSR20202127. [CrossRef]
40. Urakami, S.; Shiina, H.; Enokida, H.; Kawakami, T.; Tokizane, T.; Ogishima, T.; Tanaka, Y.; Li, L.-C.; Ribeiro-Filho, L.A.; Terashima, M.; et al. Epigenetic inactivation of Wnt inhibitory factor-1 plays an important role in bladder cancer through aberrant canonical Wnt/beta-catenin signaling pathway. *Clin. Cancer Res.* **2006**, *12*, 383–391. [CrossRef] [PubMed]
41. Li, H.; Li, Q.; Ma, Z.; Zhou, Z.; Fan, J.; Jin, Y.; Wu, Y.; Cheng, F.; Liang, P. AID modulates carcinogenesis network via DNA demethylation in bladder urothelial cell carcinoma. *Cell Death Dis.* **2019**, *10*, 251. [CrossRef]
42. Harlin, H.; Meng, Y.; Peterson, A.C.; Zha, Y.; Tretiakova, M.; Slingluff, C.; McKee, M.; Gajewski, T.F. Chemokine expression in melanoma metastases associated with CD8 + T-Cell recruitment. *Cancer Res.* **2009**, *69*, 3077–3085. [CrossRef]
43. Ji, R.R.; Chasalow, S.D.; Wang, L.; Hamid, O.; Schmidt, H.; Cogswell, J.; Alaparthy, S.; Berman, D.; Jure-Kunkel, M.; Siemers, N.O.; et al. An immune-active tumor microenvironment favors clinical response to ipilimumab. *Cancer Immunol. Immunother.* **2012**, *61*, 1019–1031. [CrossRef]
44. Sweis, R.F.; Spranger, S.; Bao, R.; Paner, G.P.; Stadler, W.M.; Steinberg, G.; Gajewski, T.F. Molecular drivers of the non-T-cell-inflamed tumor microenvironment in urothelial bladder cancer. *Cancer Immunol. Res.* **2016**, *4*, 563–568. [CrossRef]

45. Luke, J.J.; Bao, R.; Sweis, R.F.; Spranger, S.; Gajewski, T.F. WNT/β-catenin pathway activation correlates with immune exclusion across human cancers. *Clin. Cancer Res.* **2019**, *25*, 3074–3083. [CrossRef]
46. Spranger, S.; Bao, R.; Gajewski, T.F. Melanoma-intrinsic β-catenin signalling prevents anti-tumour immunity. *Nature* **2015**, *523*, 231–235. [CrossRef] [PubMed]
47. Chen, Y.; Song, Y.; Du, W.; Gong, L.; Chang, H.; Zou, Z. Tumor-associated macrophages: An accomplice in solid tumor progression. *J. Biomed. Sci.* **2019**, *26*, 78. [CrossRef]
48. Movahedi, K.; Van Ginderachter, J.A. The ontogeny and microenvironmental regulation of tumor-associated macrophages. *Antioxid Redox Signal.* **2016**, *25*, 775–791. [CrossRef]
49. Komohara, Y.; Fujiwara, Y.; Ohnishi, K.; Takeya, M. Tumor-associated macrophages: Potential therapeutic targets for anti-cancer therapy. *Adv. Drug Deliv. Rev.* **2016**, *99*, 180–185. [CrossRef]
50. Kaler, P.; Augenlicht, L.; Klampfer, L. Activating mutations in β-catenin in colon cancer cells alter their interaction with macrophages; the role of snail. *PLoS ONE* **2012**, *7*, e45462. [CrossRef]
51. Ding, Y.; Shen, S.; Lino, A.C.; Curotto de Lafaille, M.A.; Lafaille, J.J. Beta-catenin stabilization extends regulatory T cell survival and induces anergy in nonregulatory T cells. *Nat. Med.* **2008**, *14*, 162–169. [CrossRef]
52. Horn, L.A.; Riskin, J.; Hempel, H.A.; Fousek, K.; Lind, H.; Hamilton, D.H.; McCampbell, K.K.; Maeda, D.Y.; Zebala, J.A.; Su, Z.; et al. Simultaneous inhibition of CXCR1/2, TGF-β, and PD-L1 remodels the tumor and its microenvironment to drive antitumor immunity. *J. Immunother. Cancer* **2020**, *8*, e000326. [CrossRef] [PubMed]
53. Lim, A.R.; Rathmell, W.K.; Rathmell, J.C. The tumor microenvironment as a metabolic barrier to effector T cells and immunotherapy. *eLife* **2020**, *9*, e55185. [CrossRef]
54. Brand, A.; Singer, K.; Koehl, G.E.; Kolitzus, M.; Schoenhammer, G.; Thiel, A.; Matos, C.; Bruss, C.; Klobuch, S.; Peter, K.; et al. LDHA-associated lactic acid production blunts tumor immunosurveillance by T and NK cells. *Cell Metab.* **2016**, *24*, 657–671. [CrossRef]
55. Murciano-Goroff, Y.R.; Warner, A.B.; Wolchok, J.D. The future of cancer immunotherapy: Microenvironment-targeting combinations. *Cell Res.* **2020**, *30*, 507–519. [CrossRef]
56. Pavlova, N.N.; Thompson, C.B. The emerging hallmarks of cancer metabolism. *Cell Metab.* **2016**, *23*, 27–47. [CrossRef]
57. Ward, P.S.; Thompson, C.B. Metabolic reprogramming: A cancer hallmark even warburg did not anticipate. *Cancer Cell* **2012**, *21*, 297–308. [CrossRef]
58. Pate, K.T.; Stringari, C.; Sprowl-Tanio, S.; Wang, K.; TeSlaa, T.; Hoverter, N.P.; McQuade, M.M.; Garner, C.; Digman, M.A.; Teitell, M.A.; et al. Wnt signaling directs a metabolic program of glycolysis and angiogenesis in colon cancer. *EMBO J.* **2014**, *33*, 1454–1473. [CrossRef]
59. Warburg, O. On the origin of cancer cells. *Science* **1956**, *123*, 309–314. [CrossRef]
60. Fischer, K.; Hoffmann, P.; Voelkl, S.; Meidenbauer, N.; Ammer, J.; Edinger, M.; Gottfried, E.; Schwarz, S.; Rothe, G.; Hoves, S.; et al. Inhibitory effect of tumor cell-derived lactic acid on human T cells. *Blood* **2007**, *109*, 3812–3819. [CrossRef]
61. Sprowl-Tanio, S.; Habowski, A.N.; Pate, K.T.; McQuade, M.M.; Wang, K.; Edwards, R.A.; Grun, F.; Lyou, Y.; Waterman, M.L. Lactate/pyruvate transporter MCT-1 is a direct Wnt target that confers sensitivity to 3-bromopyruvate in colon cancer. *Cancer Metab.* **2016**, *4*, 20. [CrossRef]
62. Lee, S.Y.; Jeon, H.M.; Ju, M.K.; Kim, C.H.; Yoon, G.; Han, S.I.; Park, H.G.; Kang, H.S. Wnt/Snail signaling regulates cytochrome C oxidase and glucose metabolism. *Cancer Res.* **2012**, *72*, 3607–3617. [CrossRef] [PubMed]
63. Sherwood, V.; Chaurasiya, S.K.; Ekström, E.J.; Guilmain, W.; Liu, Q.; Koeck, T.; Brown, K.; Hansson, K.; Agnarsdóttir, M.; Bergqvist, M.; et al. WNT5A-mediated β-catenin-independent signalling is a novel regulator of cancer cell metabolism. *Carcinogenesis* **2014**, *35*, 784–794. [CrossRef] [PubMed]
64. Harel, M.; Ortenberg, R.; Varanasi, S.K.; Mangalhara, K.C.; Mardamshina, M.; Markovits, E.; Baruch, E.N.; Tripple, V.; Arama-Chayoth, M.; Greenberg, E.; et al. Proteomics of melanoma response to immunotherapy reveals mitochondrial dependence. *Cell* **2019**, *179*, 236–250.e18. [CrossRef]
65. Li, Y.; Yang, J.; Li, S.; Zhang, J.; Zheng, J.; Hou, W.; Zhao, H.; Guo, Y.; Liu, X.; Dou, K.; et al. N-myc downstream-regulated gene 2, a novel estrogen-targeted gene, is involved in the regulation of Na^+/K^+-ATPase. *J. Biol. Chem.* **2011**, *286*, 32289–32299. [CrossRef]
66. Le, P.; McDermott, J.D.; Jimeno, A. Targeting the Wnt pathway in human cancers: Therapeutic targeting with a focus on OMP-54F28. *Pharmacol. Ther.* **2015**, *146*, 1–11. [CrossRef]
67. Mita, M.M.; Becerra, C.; Richards, D.A.; Mita, A.C.; Shagisultanova, E.; Osborne, C.R.C.; O'Shaughnessy, J.; Zhang, C.; Henner, R.; Kapoun, A.M.; et al. Phase 1b study of WNT inhibitor vantictumab (VAN, human monoclonal antibody) with paclitaxel (P) in patients (pts) with 1st- to 3rd-line metastatic HER2-negative breast cancer (BC). *J. Clin. Oncol.* **2016**, *34*, 2516. [CrossRef]
68. Kahn, M. Can we safely target the WNT pathway? *Nat. Rev. Drug Discov.* **2014**, *13*, 513–532. [CrossRef] [PubMed]
69. El-Khoueiry, A.B.; Ning, Y.; Yang, D.; Cole, S.; Kahn, M.; Zoghbi, M.; Berg, J.; Fujimori, M.; Inada, T.; Kouji, H.; et al. A phase I first-in-human study of PRI-724 in patients (pts) with advanced solid tumors. *J. Clin. Oncol.* **2013**, *31*, 2501. [CrossRef]
70. Moore, K.N.; Gunderson, C.C.; Sabbatini, P.; McMeekin, D.S.; Mantia-Smaldone, G.; Burger, R.A.; Morgan, M.A.; Kapoun, A.M.; Brachmann, R.K.; Stagg, R.; et al. A phase 1b dose escalation study of ipafricept (OMP54F28) in combination with paclitaxel and carboplatin in patients with recurrent platinum-sensitive ovarian cancer. *Gynecol. Oncol.* **2019**, *154*, 294–301. [CrossRef]

71. Dotan, E.; Cardin, D.B.; Lenz, H.-J.; Messersmith, W.; O'Neil, B.; Cohen, S.J.; Denlinger, C.S.; Shahda, S.; Astsaturov, I.; Kapoun, A.M.; et al. Phase Ib study of Wnt inhibitor ipafricept with gemcitabine and nab-paclitaxel in patients with previously untreated stage IV pancreatic cancer. *Clin. Cancer Res.* **2020**, *26*, 5348–5352. [CrossRef]
72. Davis, S.L.; Cardin, D.B.; Shahda, S.; Lenz, H.-J.; Dotan, E.; O'Neil, B.H.; Kapoun, A.M.; Stagg, R.J.; Berlin, J.; Messersmith, W.A.; et al. A phase 1b dose escalation study of Wnt pathway inhibitor vantictumab in combination with nab-paclitaxel and gemcitabine in patients with previously untreated metastatic pancreatic cancer. *Invest. New Drugs* **2020**, *38*, 821–830. [CrossRef]
73. Ganesh, S.; Shui, X.; Craig, K.P.; Park, J.; Wang, W.; Brown, B.D.; Abrams, M.T. RNAi-mediated β-catenin inhibition promotes T cell infiltration and antitumor activity in combination with immune checkpoint blockade. *Mol. Ther.* **2018**, *26*, 2567–2579. [CrossRef]
74. Klempner, S.J.; Bendell, J.C.; Villaflor, V.M.; Tenner, L.L.; Stein, S.; Naik, G.S.; Sirard, C.A.; Kagey, M.; Chaney, M.F.; Strickler, J.H. DKN-01 in combination with pembrolizumab in patients with advanced gastroesophageal adenocarcinoma (GEA): Tumoral DKK1 expression as a predictor of response and survival. *J. Clin. Oncol.* **2020**, *38*, 357. [CrossRef]
75. Harb, J.; Lin, P.-J.; Hao, J. Recent development of Wnt signaling pathway inhibitors for cancer therapeutics. *Curr. Oncol. Rep.* **2019**, *21*, 12. [CrossRef] [PubMed]
76. Janku, F.; de Vos, F.; de Miguel, M.; Forde, P.; Ribas, A.; Nagasaka, M.; Argiles, G.; Arance, A.M.; Calvo, A.; Giannakis, M.; et al. Abstract CT034: Phase I study of WNT974 + spartalizumab in patients (pts) with advanced solid tumors. *Cancer Res.* **2020**, *80*, CT034. [CrossRef]

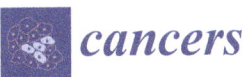

Article

Methylation Patterns of *DKK1*, *DKK3* and *GSK3β* Are Accompanied with Different Expression Levels in Human Astrocytoma

Anja Kafka [1,2,*], Anja Bukovac [1,2], Emilija Brglez [1], Ana-Marija Jarmek [1], Karolina Poljak [1], Petar Brlek [1], Kamelija Žarković [3,4], Niko Njirić [1,5] and Nives Pećina-Šlaus [1,2]

[1] Laboratory of Neuro-Oncology, Croatian Institute for Brain Research, School of Medicine, University of Zagreb, Šalata 12, 10 000 Zagreb, Croatia; anja.bukovac@mef.hr (A.B.); brglez.e@gmail.com (E.B.); anamarija.jarmek@gmail.com (A.-M.J.); k.poljak96@gmail.com (K.P.); pbrlek@gmail.com (P.B.); njiricn@gmail.com (N.N.); nina@mef.hr (N.P.-Š.)
[2] Department of Biology, School of Medicine, University of Zagreb, Šalata 3, 10 000 Zagreb, Croatia
[3] Department of Pathology, School of Medicine, University of Zagreb, Šalata 10, 10 000 Zagreb, Croatia; kamelijazarkovic@gmail.com
[4] Division of Pathology, University Hospital Center "Zagreb", Kišpatićeva 12, 10 000 Zagreb, Croatia
[5] Department of Neurosurgery, University Hospital Center "Zagreb", School of Medicine, University of Zagreb, Kišpatićeva 12, 10 000 Zagreb, Croatia
* Correspondence: anja.kafka@mef.hr

Citation: Kafka, A.; Bukovac, A.; Brglez, E.; Jarmek, A.-M.; Poljak, K.; Brlek, P.; Žarković, K.; Njirić, N.; Pećina-Šlaus, N. Methylation Patterns of *DKK1*, *DKK3* and *GSK3β* Are Accompanied with Different Expression Levels in Human Astrocytoma. *Cancers* **2021**, *13*, 2530. https://doi.org/10.3390/cancers13112530

Academic Editors: Michael Kahn and Keane Lai

Received: 2 May 2021
Accepted: 19 May 2021
Published: 21 May 2021

Publisher's Note: MDPI stays neutral with regard to jurisdictional claims in published maps and institutional affiliations.

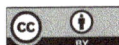

Copyright: © 2021 by the authors. Licensee MDPI, Basel, Switzerland. This article is an open access article distributed under the terms and conditions of the Creative Commons Attribution (CC BY) license (https://creativecommons.org/licenses/by/4.0/).

Simple Summary: Astrocytomas are the most common type of primary brain tumor in adults. In this study, 64 astrocytoma samples of grades II–IV were analyzed for genetic and epigenetic changes as well as protein expression patterns in order to explore the roles of the Wnt pathway components, such as DKK1, DKK3, GSK3β, β-catenin, and APC in astrocytoma initiation and progression. Our findings on *DKK1* and *DKK3* show the importance of methylation in the regulation of Wnt signaling activity and also indicate pro-oncogenic effects of GSK3β on astrocytoma development and progression. Close connections between large deletions and mutations in the APC gene and increased β-catenin expression in glioblastoma were also established. Our results suggest that Wnt pathway related genes and proteins play an active role in the etiology of astrocytic brain tumors.

Abstract: In the present study, we investigated genetic and epigenetic changes and protein expression levels of negative regulators of Wnt signaling, *DKK1*, *DKK3*, and *APC* as well as glycogen synthase kinase 3 (GSK3β) and β-catenin in 64 human astrocytomas of grades II–IV. Methylation-specific PCR revealed promoter methylation of *DKK1*, *DKK3*, and *GSK3β* in 38%, 43%, and 18% of samples, respectively. Grade IV comprised the lowest number of methylated *GSK3β* cases and highest of *DKK3*. Evaluation of the immunostaining using H-score was performed for β-catenin, both total and unphosphorylated (active) forms. Additionally, active (pY216) and inactive (pS9) forms of GSK3β protein were also analyzed. Spearman's correlation confirmed the prevalence of β-catenin's active form ($r_s = 0.634$, $p < 0.001$) in astrocytoma tumor cells. The Wilcoxon test revealed that astrocytoma with higher levels of the active pGSK3β-Y216 form had lower expression levels of its inactive form ($p < 0.0001$, $Z = -5.332$). Changes in *APC*'s exon 11 were observed in 44.44% of samples by PCR/RFLP. Astrocytomas with changes of *APC* had higher H-score values of total β-catenin compared to the group without genetic changes ($t = -2.264$, $p = 0.038$). Furthermore, a positive correlation between samples with methylated *DKK3* promoter and the expression of active pGSK3β-Y216 ($r_s = 0.356$, $p = 0.011$) was established. Our results emphasize the importance of methylation for the regulation of Wnt signaling. Large deletions of the *APC* gene associated with increased β-catenin levels, together with oncogenic effects of both β-catenin and GSK3β, are clearly involved in astrocytoma evolution. Our findings contribute to a better understanding of the etiology of gliomas. Further studies should elucidate the clinical and therapeutic relevance of the observed molecular alterations.

Keywords: astrocytic brain tumors; Wnt signaling; DKKs; GSK3β; APC; β-catenin

1. Introduction

Astrocytomas are glial cell tumors originating from astrocytes and account for nearly half of all primary brain tumors. According to the latest World Health Organization (WHO) classification, there are three different grades of astrocytoma, indicating their growth potential and aggressiveness [1,2]. Diffuse astrocytoma, defined as a grade II neoplasm, is a type of low-grade infiltrative glioma. Grade II astrocytomas have a tendency to progress toward high-grade malignancies called anaplastic astrocytomas (grade III) and eventually secondary glioblastomas (GBM, grade IV). The proliferative potential of diffuse astrocytomas and their growth rate are much lower than those of GBMs, which are a highly aggressive tumor with pronounced brain invasion and fast progression [1]. In addition to the biological behavior, an important criterion for the classification of diffuse glioma is the status of *IDH1* and *IDH2* gene mutations; astrocytomas are now defined as *IDH* mutant or *IDH* wild-type. Low-grade astrocytomas and secondary GBMs often carry *IDH* mutations, associated with younger age, as well as a much better prognosis [3,4]. *IDH* wild-type status refers to 90% of GBMs and indicates a primary tumor that arises de novo and carries a poorer prognosis than those classified as *IDH* mutant.

Despite new molecular findings that characterize tumors in the group of diffuse gliomas, the differences between individual pathohistological grades are still insufficiently investigated. For this reason, we decided to study the molecular characteristics of the WNT and AKT signaling pathway components in astrocytomas of different grades.

Signaling pathways form a complex network of molecular interaction in our cells, and a close connection between Wnt/β-catenin and PI3K/AKT/mTOR signaling has been described in many cancers [5]. One of the most prominent linking elements between these pathways is GSK3β (glycogen synthase kinase 3) [6]. The major mode of GSK3β activity regulation is through phosphorylation events. Activated Akt molecule phosphorylates GSK3β on the amino acid serine 9 (S9), leading to GSK3β inactivation. In contrast, GSK3β is activated by autophosphorylation or phosphorylation on tyrosine 216 (Y216) by other kinases [5,7]. In addition to S9 phosphorylation, promoter methylation may also be one of the mechanisms of GSK3β inactivation [8].

In the Wnt signaling pathway, GSK3β plays a key role in modulating β-catenin and TCF/LEF (T cell factor/lymphoid enhancer-binding factor) transcription factor activity [7]. Active GSK3β can act as a tumor suppressor as it participates, together with other members of the destruction complex including APC (Adenomatous Polyposis Coli), AXIN1 and CK1 (Casein Kinase 1), in phosphorylation and subsequent degradation of the oncogenic β-catenin protein. In the pathway's "off" state, TCF/LEF is inactive due to its interaction with the repressor Groucho. In contrast, inactive GSK3β stimulates cell proliferation in the pathway's "on" state. The pathway is activated upon binding of Wnt ligands to the Frizzled (Fz) receptor and the co-receptor lipoprotein receptor-related protein (LRP) 5/6, resulting in the disintegration of the destruction complex and β-catenin cytoplasmic accumulation. Afterward, unphosphorylated β-catenin enters the cell nucleus, where it interacts with transcription factors from the TCF/LEF family, leading to Wnt target gene transcription (*cyclin D1, c-myc, fra-1, c-jun*, etc.) thus stimulating tumor growth [9]. Except for phosphorylating β-catenin, GSK3β can phosphorylate LRP co-receptor, thus revealing a binding site for AXIN on LRP, which mimics pathway activation by a Wnt ligand [10] (Figure 1).

Wnt signaling activity is also regulated by evolutionarily conserved inhibitors and activators that antagonize Wnt signaling such as the Dickkopf (DKK) gene family. The family consists of four members (DKK 1–4) in humans that specifically inhibit the Wnt/β-catenin signaling cascade by preventing the Wnt ligand from binding to LRP 5/6 co-receptors. Some members of the DKK family interact with transmembrane proteins Kremen 1 and 2, also modulating the pathway's activity [11]. Not all DKK family members have consistent roles. Recent reports reveal that they can have dual agonistic and antagonistic functions, depending on the cellular context. Numerous studies report on changes in DKK protein expression within tumor tissues. DKK1 is differentially expressed in different types of human cancers, and its expression affects cell invasion, proliferation, and tumor growth. Some authors have reported on DKK1 overexpression [12–21], while others have noted its downregulation in tumors [22–24]. On the other hand, DKK3 is omnipresent in normal human tissues, including the brain; however, it is significantly depleted in various cancer cell types. DKK3 silencing due to epigenetic alterations has also been reported in multiple cancers [12]. However, there are few studies investigating the expression of DKK1 and DKK3 in gliomas [25–28].

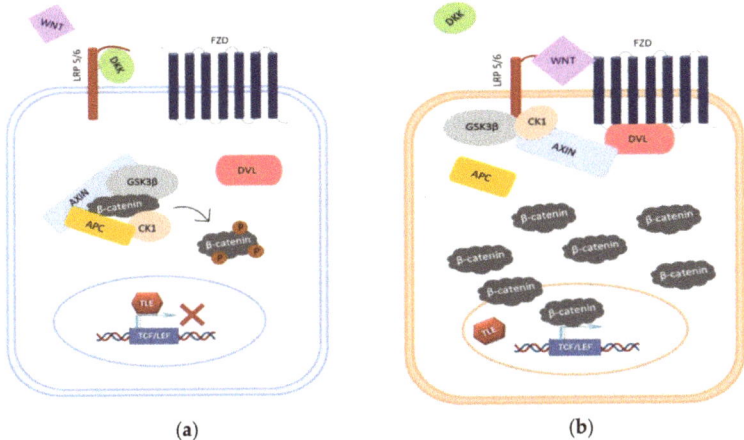

Figure 1. Overview of Wnt signaling pathway. (**a**) In the canonical Wnt pathway, DKK directly competes with Wnt for binding to LRP6. When DKK binds to the receptor, cytosolic pool of β-catenin is maintained at low levels through proteasomal degradation, due to its phosphorylation by the complex consisting of Axin/APC/CK1/GSK-3β. (**b**) Binding of Wnt to receptors Fz/LRP leads to the recruitment of components of the destruction complex to the membrane. This prevents phosphorylation and degradation of β-catenin, resulting in its accumulation in the cytoplasm. Stabilized β-catenin translocates into the nucleus and activates transcription of Wnt target genes.

These opposite reports indicate the need for further elucidation of the role of Wnt signaling molecules in cancer. Our study aims to contribute to the great efforts that are being made to clarify the genetic and epigenetic signatures in gliomas. Our goal was to clarify the behavior of *DKK1*, *DKK3*, and *GSK3β* and identify potential correlations to changes of *APC* and beta-catenin genes and proteins.

2. Materials and Methods

2.1. Tissue Samples

Sixty-four astrocytoma samples of different pathohistological types and grades, together with corresponding blood and formalin-fixed paraffin-embedded (FFPE) slides of brain tumor tissues, were collected with patients' consents from the Departments of Neurosurgery and Departments of Pathology University Hospital Centers "Zagreb" and "Sisters of Charity".

Chosen slides were reviewed by a certified pathologist (KŽ) to confirm the diagnosis (diffuse astrocytoma, anaplastic astrocytoma, glioblastoma). The diagnoses of astrocytic brain tumors were in concordance with the most recent WHO classification of the tumors of the central neural system [3]. In selected cases, additional immunohistochemical analyses (IDH1/2, ATRX, p53) were conducted in order to provide the correct diagnosis. The patients included in the study had no family history of brain tumors and did not undergo any cancer treatment prior to surgery, which could affect the results of molecular analyses. The sample consisted of 10 diffuse astrocytomas (grade II), 11 anaplastic astrocytomas (grade III), and 43 glioblastomas (grade IV). Twenty seven patients were female and 37 male.

The age of patients varied from 6 to 83 (mean age = 50.31, median = 54 years). The mean age at diagnosis for females was 54.85 (median 56) and for males, 47 years (median 49).

The study was approved by the Ethical Committees, School of Medicine University of Zagreb (Case number: 380-59-10106-14-55/147; Class: 641-01/14-02/01) and University Hospital Centers "Sisters of Mercy" (number EP-7426/14-9) and "Zagreb" (number 02/21/JG, class: 8.1.-14/54-2). Patients gave their informed consent.

2.2. DNA Extraction

The genomic DNA extraction from unfixed frozen tumor tissue was performed according to the protocol by Green and Sambrook [29]. Briefly, approximately 0.5 g of tumor tissue was homogenized with 1 mL extraction buffer (10 mM Tris–HCl, pH 8.0; 0.1 M EDTA, pH 8.0; 0.5% sodium dodecyl sulfate) and incubated with proteinase K (100 µg/mL; Sigma-Aldrich, St. Louis, MO, USA) overnight at 37 °C. Organic (phenol–chloroform) extraction and ethanol precipitation followed.

The salting-out method was used to extract DNA from peripheral blood leucocytes [30]. Five milliliters of blood was lysed with 15 mL RCLB (red blood cell lysis buffer) (0.16 M NH4Cl; 10 mM KHCO3; 10 mM EDTA; pH 7.6), centrifuged (15 min/5000× g), and incubated overnight with 2 mL SE buffer (sodium-EDTA; 75 mM NaCl; 25 mM Na2EDTA; pH 8), 200 µL 10% SDS (sodium dodecyl sulphate) and 15 µL proteinase K (Sigma, Darmstadt, Germany) (20 mg/mL) at 37 °C. The salting-out method and isopropanol precipitation followed. The method is based on the principle that proteins and other cellular components, except DNA, will precipitate in a saturated salt solution (5M NaCl) due to their relative hydrophobicity.

The extracted DNA was successfully used for genetic (PCR/RFLP) and epigenetic (MS-PCR) analysis.

2.3. Polymerase Chain Reaction (PCR), Restriction Fragment Length Polymorphism (RFLP), Loss of Heterozygosity (LOH)

2.3.1. Polymerase Chain Reaction

The PCR mixture (25 µL) for *APC*'s exon 11 amplification consisted of 10 pmol of each primer (5′-GGACTACAGGCCATTGCAGAA-3′ and 5′-GGCTACATCTCCAAAAGTCAA-3′), ~250 ng template DNA, 2.5 µL × 10x PicoMaxx reaction buffer, 2.5 mM of each dNTP, and 0.5 µL (1.25 U) of PicoMaxx high fidelity PCR system polymerase. PCR conditions were initial denaturation, 4 min/95 °C; denaturation, 1 min/94 °C; annealing, 2 min/58 °C; extension, 1.5 min/72 °C; for 35 cycles and final extension 7 min/72 °C. The PCR products were analyzed on 2% agarose gels.

2.3.2. Restriction Fragment Length Polymorphism/Loss of Heterozygosity

Loss of heterozygosity of the *APC* gene was detected on the basis of restriction fragment length polymorphism (RFLP) of the PCR products. RFLP was performed by using restriction enzyme Rsa I, which recognizes a polymorphic site in exon 11 of the *APC* gene. PCR amplification of exon 11 generated a fragment of 133 bp that Rsa I cleaves into 85 bp and 48 bp fragments if the polymorphic site is present, or leaves uncleaved if the site is absent. LOH/Rsa I was demonstrated only in informative (heterozygous) samples when the tumor DNA showed loss of either the single uncut band (133 bp) or of the two cut bands (85 + 48 bp) compared to autologous blood tissue. PCR aliquots (20 µL) were digested with 6 U Rsa I (New England BioLabs, SAD) overnight at 37 °C and were electrophoresed on Spreadex EL 400 Mini gels (Elchrom Scientific, AL-Diagnostic GmbH, Amstetten, Austria) in the ORIGINS electrophoresis system (AL-Diagnostic GmbH, Amstetten, Austria) at 120 V and 55 °C.

2.3.3. Methylation-Specific PCR (MSP)

After isolation from tumor tissue, DNA was treated with bisulfite using the MethylEdge Bisulfite Conversion System (Promega, Madison, WI, USA) following the manufacturer's instructions. Bisulfite-treated DNA was afterward used for methylation-specific PCR (MSP).

Primer sequences of *DKK1*, *DKK3*, and *GSK3β* promoter region for MSP were synthesized according to [31–33], respectively (Table 1).

Table 1. PCR primers used for MSP.

Gene	Primer	Sequence	Product Size
DKK1	MR-F	5′-CGTTCGTTGGTAGTTTTTATTTCGA-3′	175 bp
	MR-R	5′-GCGACTACCTTTATACCGCGAA-3′	
	UMR-F	5′-TGTTTGTTGGTAGTTTTTATTTTGA-3′	173 bp
	UMR-R	5′-ACCACAACTACCTTTATACCACAAA-3′	
DKK3	MR-F	5′-CGGTTTTTTTTCGTTTTCGGG-3′	154 bp
	MR-R	5′-CAAACCGCTACATCTCCGCT-3′	
	UMR-F	5′-TTTTGGTTTTTTTTTGTTTTTGGG-3′	155 bp
	UMR-R	5′-CCAA ACCACTACATCTCCACT-3′	
GSK3β	MR-F	5′ CGTCGTTATCGTTATCGTTC 3′	135 bp
	MR-R	5′ AATAACTCGAAAATACGACG 3′	
	UMR-F	5′ GAGGAGTTGTTGTTATTGTTATTGTTT 3′	136 bp
	UMR-R	5′ AAAAAAATAACTCAAAAATACAACA 3′	

MR-F and MR-R-primer set for methylated reaction; UMR-F and UMR-R-primer set for unmethylated reaction; bp-base pairs.

PCRs for bisulfite-treated DNA were performed using TaKaRa EpiTaq HS (TaKaRa Bio, USA): 1XEpiTaq PCR Buffer (Mg_2^+ free), 2.5 mM $MgCl_2$, 0.3 mM dNTPs, 20 pmol of each primer (Sigma-Aldrich, USA), 50 ng of DNA, and 1.5 units of TaKaRa EpiTaq HS DNA Polymerase in a 25 µL final reaction volume. PCR cycling conditions are shown in Table 2.

Table 2. MSP conditions for amplification of promoter region of *DKK1*, *DKK3*, and *GSK3β* genes.

Gene		Initial Denaturation	Cycle Conditions			Final Elongation
DKK1	MR	95 °C 5 min	95 °C 30 s	61 °C 30 s	72 °C 30 s	72 °C 7 min
	UMR	95 °C 5 min	95 °C 30 s	61 °C 30 s	72 °C 30 s	72 °C 7 min
DKK3	MR	95 °C 5 min	95 °C 30 s	61 °C 30 s	72 °C 30 s	72 °C 7 min
	UMR	95 °C 5 min	95 °C 30 s	61 °C 30 s	72 °C 30 s	72 °C 7 min
GSK3β	MR	95 °C 5 min	95 °C 30 s	55 °C 30 s	72 °C 30 s	72 °C 7 min
	UMR	95 °C 5 min	95 °C 30 s	56,5 °C 30 s	72 °C 30 s	72 °C 7 min

MR: methylated reaction; UMR: unmethylated reaction.

PCR products were separated on 2% agarose gel stained with Syber Safe nucleic acid stain (Invitrogen, Thermo Scientific, Waltham, MA, USA) and visualized on a UV transilluminator. Methylated Human Control (Promega, Madison, WI, USA) was used as a positive control for the methylated reaction, while unmethylated DNA EpiTect Control DNA (Qiagen, Hilden, Germany) served as a positive control for the unmethylated reaction.

2.4. Immunohistochemistry (IHC)

Immunohistochemical staining was performed on 4 µm thick paraffin embedded tissue sections placed on silanized glass slides (DakoCytomation, Glostrup, Denmark). Tissue sections were deparaffinized in xylene (3×, 5 min), rehydrated in a decreasing ethanol series, (100%, 96%, and 70% ethanol; 2×, 3 min), and placed in water (30 s). Antigen retrieval was performed by heating the sections in microwave oven 2 times for 10 min at 400 W and 3 times for 5 min at 350 W in 6 M citrate buffer. Afterward, the endogenous peroxidase activity was blocked using 3% hydrogen peroxide for 10 min in dark. Non-specific binding was blocked by incubating samples with protein block serum-free ready-to-use (Agilent Technologies, Santa Clara, CA, USA) for 30 min at 4 °C. Next, sections were incubated with primary antibody Anti-GSK3β (phospho Y216) (rabbit polyclonal; ab75745, Abcam, Cambridge, MA, USA; dilution 1:100), Anti-GSK3β (phospho S9) (rabbit polyclonal; ab131097, Abcam, Cambridge, MA, USA; dilution 1:100), Active β-Catenin (rabbit monoclonal, non-phospho (Ser33/37/Thr41), D131A1, Cell Signalling Technology, Danvers, MA, USA; dilution 1:800) and Anti-Human Beta-Catenin (mouse monoclonal; Clone b-Catenin-1, M3539, Dako, Santa Clara, CA, USA; dilution 1:200) overnight at 4 °C. Dako REAL Envision detection system Peroxidase/DAB, Rabbit/Mouse, HRP (Agilent Technologies, Santa Clara, CA, USA) was used for visualization according to the manufacturer's instructions, and the sections were counterstained with hematoxylin.

The level of expression of examined proteins in the healthy brain was determined by using the cerebral cortex of the human brain (Amsbio, Oxfordshire, UK). It was found that the level of immunoreactivity of all examined proteins in the healthy brain tissue was generally low, and the signal was detected only in the cytoplasm. Human placenta (decidual cells) and colon cancer served as positive controls. Negative controls underwent the same staining procedure but without incubating samples with primary antibodies.

2.5. Microscopic Analysis

In the tumor hot-spot area, 200 cells were counted and the intensity of protein expression was determined using the computer program ImageJ (National Institutes of Health, Bethesda, MD, USA). Astrocytic brain tumors stained for pGSK3β-Y216, pGSK3β-S9, β-catenin (non-phospho Ser33/37/Thr41), and total β-catenin protein were interpreted by 5 independent observers, of which 2 were pathologists using the following criteria: score 0 (no staining), score 1 (<10% tumor cells), score 2 (10–50% of tumor cells), and score 3 (>50% of tumor cells).

Next, a histological score (H-score) was calculated as the sum of the percentages of positively-stained tumor cells multiplied by the weighted intensity of staining:

$$\text{H-score} = [1 \times (\% \text{ of cells } 1+) + 2 \times (\% \text{ of cells } 2+) + 3 \times (\% \text{ of cells } 3+)].$$

The H-score, therefore, ranged from 0–300, where '% of cells' represents the percentage of stained cells for each intensity (1 = lack or weak expression, 2 = moderate expression, and 3 = strong expression).

Immunohistochemical results were interpreted blindly in regard to the genetic and epigenetic status.

2.6. Statistical Analysis

Statistical analysis was performed using SPSS v.19.0.1 (SPSS, Chicago, IL, USA) statistical program. The significance level was set at $p < 0.05$.

The distribution of the data was assessed by the Kolmogorov-Smirnov test and Shapiro-Wilk W-test. Depending on the results of the test of normality and the number of patients per group, differences in the values between the 3 grades were analyzed by one-way variance analysis (ANOVA) or Kruskal-Wallis test, while differences between the 2 groups were tested by Student's t-test or the Mann-Whitney test. Pearson χ^2 and Spearman's correlation were used to test the relationships between *DKK1*, *DKK3*, and *GSK3β* methylation, *APC* genetic change, GSK3β and β-catenin protein expression levels, localization, and other clinical and demographic features.

3. Results

3.1. Methylation Status of Promoter Regions of GSK3β, DKK1 and DKK3

Expression of *DKK1*, *DKK3*, and *GSK3β* genes is controlled, among other mechanisms, by DNA methylation (Figure 2).

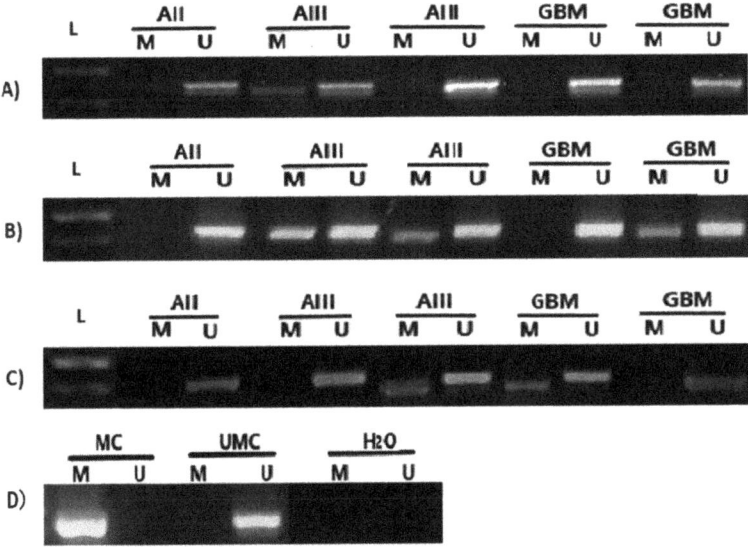

Figure 2. Methylation-specific PCR analysis for (**A**) *GSK3β*, (**B**) *DKK1*, and (**C**) *DKK3* promoter in astrocytic brain tumors grade II–IV. The presence of a visible PCR product in lanes marked M indicates the presence of methylated promoters, the presence of a product in lanes marked U indicates the presence of unmethylated promoters; (**D**) methylated human control (MC) was used as positive control for methylated reaction, unmethylated human control (UMC) was used as positive control for unmethylated reaction, and water served as negative control. L–standard DNA 50 bp ladder (Invitrogen).

Out of 50 analyzed astrocytoma samples of different grades, 41 (82%) had an unmethylated *GSK3β* gene promoter, while methylation of the promoter region was detected in nine samples (18%), including three AII (30%), three AIII (27%), and three GBM (10.34%) (Figure 3A). Furthermore, methylation of *DKK1* promoter was detected in 19 of 50 tumors (38%), including three AII (30%), five AIII (45.45%), and eleven GBM (37.93%), respectively. Similarly, *DKK3* promoter was methylated in 21 of 49 tumors (42.86%), including four AII (44.44%), four AIII (36.36%), and thirteen GBM (44.83%), respectively (Figure 3B,C). Although it was obvious that grade IV comprised the lowest number of methylated cases for *GSK3β* and highest for *DKK3*, the Kruskal-Wallis test showed no significant association of methylation patterns of *GSK3β* ($p = 0.235$), *DKK1* ($p = 0.771$), and *DKK3* ($p = 0.723$) promoter regions with the tumor malignancy grade.

Spearman test did not reveal a statistically significant association of promoter methylation between *DKK1* and *DKK3* ($p = 0.429$), *DKK1* and *GSK3β* ($p = 0.775$), or *DKK3* and *GSK3β* ($p = 0.121$) in our sample (Figures S1–S4).

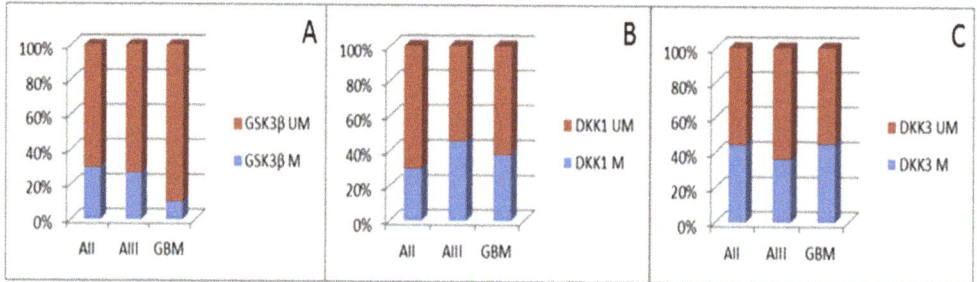

Figure 3. Graph showing the percentage of samples with methylated (M) and unmethylated (UM) promoter of (**A**) *GSK3β*, (**B**) *DKK1*, and (**C**) *DKK3* in astrocytic brain tumors grade II–IV.

3.2. pGSK3β-S9 and pGSK3β-Y216 Expression Levels

The effect of epigenetic changes on the protein expression levels was investigated in the same group of patients. When analyzing active pGSK3β-Y216 in the total sample, low expression was observed in 4% (2/50), moderate expression in 26% (13/50), and strong expression in 70% (35/50). Low expression of the inactive form, pGSK3β-S9, was present in 36% (18/50), moderate in 50% (25/50), and high in 14% (7/50) of total astrocytoma samples (Figure 4).

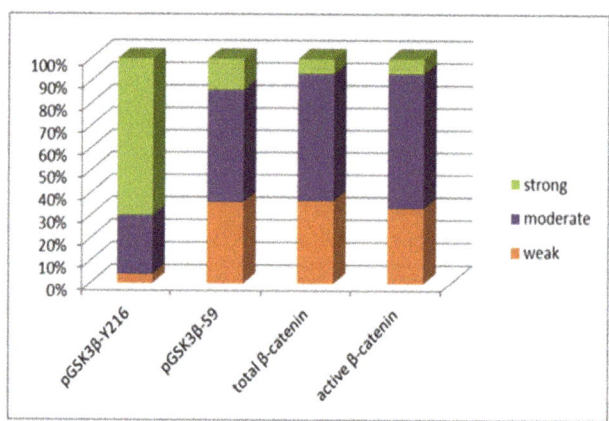

Figure 4. Graph illustrating the levels of expression of active (pGSK3β-Y216) and inactive (pGSK3β-S9) forms of GSK3β investigated in our total astrocytoma sample; and levels of expression of both forms of β-catenin (total and active) in glioblastoma group.

When analyzing both forms of GSK3β expression in specific astrocytoma types, diffuse astrocytoma revealed 50% (5/10) of the samples with a lack or low levels of pGSK3β-S9 expression, while 70% (7/10) of the samples showed high levels of pGSK3β-Y216. In anaplastic astrocytoma, moderate expression was observed in 60% (6/10) of analyzed cases for pGSK3β-S9, while 70% (7/10) of samples showed a high level of pGSK3β-Y216 expression. The majority of glioblastoma samples analyzed for active pGSK3β-Y216 showed high levels of expression (70%), while for the inactive pGSK3β-S9, moderate expression was observed in 50% of samples. The signal was co-localized in the cytoplasm and cell nucleus in all of the analyzed samples (Figure 5).

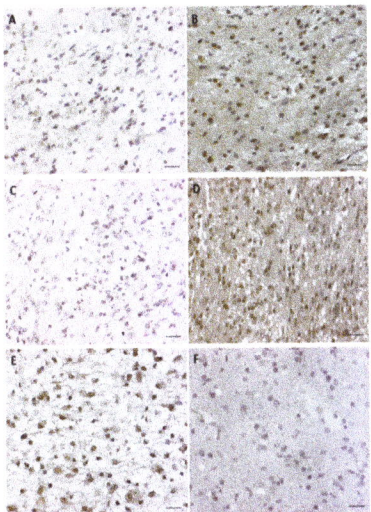

Figure 5. Characteristic immunohistochemical staining of active pGSK3β-Y216 and inactive pGSK3β-S9 protein in astrocytoma. (**A**) astrocytic brain tumor grade II with unmethylated GSK3β promoter showing weak cytoplasmic staining of pGSK3β-S9; (**B**) same astrocytic brain tumor grade II with unmethylated GSK3β promoter showing strong cytoplasmic and nuclear staining of pGSK3β-Y216; (**C**) glioblastoma (grade IV) with unmethylated GSK3β promoter showing lack of cytoplasmic staining of pGSK3β-S9; (**D**) same glioblastoma with unmethylated GSK3β promoter showing strong cytoplasmic and nuclear staining of pGSK3β-Y216; (**E**) glioblastoma (grade IV) with methylated GSK3β promoter showing moderate cytoplasmic and strong nuclear staining of pGSK3β-S9; (**F**) glioblastoma (grade IV) with methylated GSK3β promoter showing weak cytoplasmic staining of pGSK3β-Y216. Scale bar 50 µm.

Protein expressions of both active and inactive forms of GSK3β (pGSK3β-S9 ($p = 0.728$) and pGSK3β-Y216 ($p = 0.820$)) showed no significant association with any specific astrocytoma grade. Wilcoxon test revealed a statistically significant difference between the expression of pGSK3β-S9 and pGSK3β-Y216 protein in investigated astrocytoma ($p < 0.0001$, $Z = -5.332$). This result indicates that samples with a higher level of expression of active pGSK3β-Y216 have a lower expression level of inactive pGSK3β-S9 protein.

3.3. Total β-Catenin and Unphosphorylated β-Catenin Expression Levels in Glioblastoma

Expression and localization of total β-catenin (detects both phosphorylated and unphosphorylated form) and active (unphosphorylated) β-catenin were further examined in glioblastoma.

H-score analysis for total β-catenin revealed 36.66% (11/30) samples with weak, 56.67% with moderate (17/30) and 6.67% (2/30) with strong protein expression when compared to levels of β-catenin in a healthy brain (Figure 4). Grouped together, elevated expressions (2+ and 3+) were detected in 63.34% of samples. Most samples showed cytoplasmic expression (86.67%), while co-localization of the signal in cytoplasm and nucleus was present in only 4 cases (13.33%).

Unphosphorylated β-catenin showed a similar distribution of signal strengths. H-score analysis detected 33.33% (10/30) of samples with weak, 60% (18/30) with moderate, and 6.67% (2/30) with strong expression (Figure 4). When compared to cellular levels of β-catenin in a healthy brain, grouped elevated expressions (2+ and 3+) were observed in 66.67% of samples. Cytoplasmic and nuclear co-localization of unphosphorylated β-catenin was noticed in five samples (16.67%), and again in most samples, the expression was present exclusively in the cytoplasm (83.33%).

Spearman's correlation showed a statistically significant positive correlation between H-score values of total and unphosphorylated β-catenin (r_s = 0.634, p < 0.001), which confirms the presence of an active form of β-catenin in tumor cells.

3.4. APC Exon 11 Genetic Changes in Glioblastoma

Genetic changes of *APC* exon 11 were analyzed in 27 glioblastoma samples that were available for the analysis, nine (33%) of which were homozygous i.e., uninformative. Taking into account informative (heterozygous) samples, 44.44% (8/18) showed one of the two observed genetic changes. More precisely, LOH was detected in 33% (6/18) and the introduction of the restriction site because of mutation in 11.11% (2/18) cases (Figure 6).

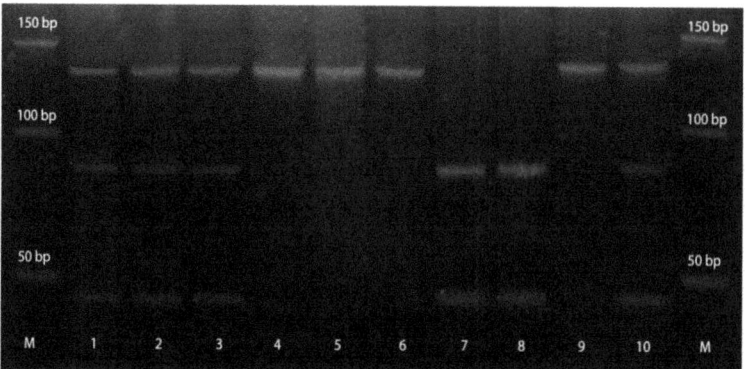

Figure 6. APC exon 11/RsaI/RFLP in glioblastoma samples is demonstrated. Lane M-standard DNA 50 bp ladder (Invitrogen); lanes 1, 2: heterozygous sample (tumor and blood), both alleles, cut and uncut, are visible; lane 3: possible restriction site introduced in tumor sample; lane 4: paired homozygous sample (blood); lanes 5, 6: homozygous sample (tumor and blood), uncut alleles are visible; lanes 7, 8: homozygous sample (tumor and blood), cut alleles are visible; lane 9: LOH, cut allele is missing; lane 10: corresponding informative blood sample, both alleles, cut and uncut, are visible.

Eight glioblastoma samples with genetic change in *APC* exon 11 showed moderate expression of total β-catenin in 62.5% and unphosphorylated β-catenin in 50% of samples. Student t-test revealed a significant difference of total β-catenin expression between groups with and without genetic changes in *APC's* exon 11. Samples with changes had higher H-score values for total β-catenin, compared to the group without changes (t = −2.264, p = 0.038). However, a significant association of unphosphorylated (active) β-catenin H-score values with groups with or without *APC* genetic changes (U = 54.500, p = 0.197) could not be established.

3.5. The Correlations of Molecular Findings and Clinical Parameters

Spearman test revealed a significant positive correlation between *DKK3* methylation status and expression of active pGSK3β-Y216 (r_s = 0.356, p = 0.011), indicating that when the *DKK3* was epigenetically silenced, the expression of the active GSK3β was on the rise. Inactive pGSK3β-S9 protein was significantly positively correlated with the methylation of the GSK3β promoter region (r_s = 0.278, p = 0.050). Additionally, a bivariate correlation between active pGSK3β-Y216 and active (unphosphorylated) β-catenin showed a trend of negative association of the two proteins (r_s = −0.427, p = 0.088). Our analysis also showed that samples with genetic change in *APC* exon 11 were statistically significantly correlated with the increase of total β-catenin expression (r_s = 0.542, p = 0.004). The upregulation of β-catenin expression was noticed in 66% of analyzed samples. Of note is that 55% of the samples with upregulated β-catenin showed methylation in negative regulators of the signaling *DKK1* or *DKK3*.

Finally, no statistical significance was found between molecular findings and clinical parameters ($p > 0.05$), meaning that the analyzed molecular features were independent of the patients' age and sex.

4. Discussion

The Wnt signaling pathway is frequently implicated in the etiology of various cancers and plays important roles in tumor initiation and progression. As recent reports indicate, impairment of negative regulators of Wnt signalization, i.e., DKKs, is often involved in tumor formation and growth [34]. Expression of the *DKK1* and *DKK3* gene is controlled, among other mechanisms, by DNA methylation, a common epigenetic silencing tool, which is increased in many tumors and tumor cell lines. Most research has indicated a DKK1 inhibitory effect in tumors [35–38], but interestingly, some studies showed DKK1's tumor-promoting role [18,39]. Similarly, DKK3 was discovered to be downregulated in various types of malignant tissue [36,40–44], but there are also reports of DKK3 overexpression in hepatocellular and esophageal cancer [45–47].

Our findings on 50 astrocytoma samples revealed promoter methylation of *DKK1* in 38% and *DKK3* in 42.86% of the samples. Methylation of *DKK1* and *DKK3* was relatively constant across different grades (*DKK1*-AII 30%, AIII 45.45%, GBM 37.93%; *DKK3*-AII 44.44%, AIII 36.36%, GBM 44.83%). The remaining portion of astrocytoma samples did not show *DKK1* and *DKK3* promoter methylation; downregulation could be explained by the existence of additional epigenetic regulatory events. In the case of DKK1 and DKK3, these may be post-translational modifications in the histone tails, which are associated with transcriptional repression [35,48]. We also point out other mechanisms here that may contribute to *DKK1* and *DKK3* gene (and consequently DKK1 and DKK3 protein) silencing, such as the mutational burden and various miRNAs, as recently shown in a case of melanoma [49] and colorectal cancer [38,50,51].

A study by Götze et al. [27] suggests that primary and secondary GBMs are characterized by different *DKK1* and *DKK3* gene methylation profiles, helpful to distinguish between glioblastoma subtypes. In their study, promoter methylation of *DKK1* was quite rare in lower-grade astrocytoma but frequent in glioblastoma. Additionally, *DKK1* methylation was more frequently observed in secondary GBM (5/10), whereas none of the primary GBMs showed methylation of the *DKK1* promoter region. These findings suggest that methylation of *DKK1* may be linked to glioma progression and thus might be a potential prognostic marker. Furthermore, this study indicates that methylation of *DKK3* is a rare event in glioma, with no obvious association with the tumor type or grade [27]. Our research showed no significant association between methylation of *DKK1* ($p = 0.767$) or *DKK3* ($p = 0.885$) and the tumor grade or type. However, the frequency of methylation of the two genes was overall substantial, and it was shown that methylation of *DKK1* was higher in pooled grades III and IV (40%) in comparison to AII (30%). No significant association of promoter methylation between *DKK1* and *DKK3* ($p = 0.429$) was found in our study. Mizobuchi et al. [25] showed that DKK3 plays a pivotal role in regulating cell survival in human malignant glioma, promotes apoptosis, and facilitates the degradation of β-catenin. Similarly, there are also reports about a DKK1 pro-apoptotic function in glioma [36].

Apart from epigenetic silencing of negative regulators, aberrant pathway activity may be a result of the mutations in downstream components. Modifications that cause change in GSK3β activity, *CTNNB1* gene mutations targeting sites phosphorylated by GSK3β on β-catenin (S33, S37, and S41), and mutations of proteins that form a destruction complex with GSK3β (for example, APC) may all cause Wnt pathway hyperactivity [9].

The influence of GSK3β on tumor formation and promotion is still controversial. GSK3β can display both pro-oncogenic and tumor-suppressive effects as it has diverse roles in numerous cellular processes that also differ among different cell types [5].

In order to determine the character of the GSK3β role in astrocytoma grades II–IV, we examined the promoter methylation of the *GSK3β* gene and level of expression of active (pY216) and inactive (pS9) form of GSK3β protein. Although the proportion of methylated samples was relatively small in each astrocytoma grade, our results showed that methylation of *GSK3β* decreased with grade. In astrocytoma grade II, 30% of samples had methylated *GSK3β* promoter, followed by 27% of astrocytoma grade III and 10% of glioblastoma. Of note is that the number of unmethylated samples increased with grade, meaning that GSK3β is upregulated in aggressive cases. GBM is primarily diagnosed at older ages, and recent reports suggest that epigenetics, especially DNA methylation, seem to be age-dependent [52].

Immunohistochemical analysis revealed low expression levels of active pGSK3β-Y216 in 4% (2/50), moderate levels in 26% (13/50), and strong levels in 70% (35/50) of samples, which is consistent with the findings on unmethylated promoter. Expression of inactive pGSK3β-S9 was weak in 36% (18/50), moderate in 50% (25/50), and strong in 14% (7/50) of astrocytoma samples in grades II–IV. Wilcoxon test showed significant opposite levels of expression between pGSK3β-S9 and pGSK3β-Y216 protein in astrocytoma cells ($p < 0.001$, $Z = -5.332$), indicating that samples with a higher level of expression of active pGSK3β-Y216 have a lower expression level of inactive pGSK3β-S9 protein. Inactive pGSK3β-S9 protein was significantly positively correlated with methylation of *GSK3β* promoter ($r_s = 0.278$, $p = 0.050$), showing that in methylated cases, phosphorylation events also decrease protein expression. Similarly, Shakoori et al. [53,54] studied the expression of active and inactive forms of GSK3β in colorectal cancer. Although the study included a smaller number of samples, they proved that most patients had elevated expression of pGSK3β-Y216, whereas pGSK3β-S9 was mainly present in non-neoplastic tissues. Contrary to previously mentioned studies, high expression of inactive pGSK3β-S9 is found in skin [55], oral [56], and lung [57] cancers, which suggests tumor-suppressing effects of the enzyme in those malignant tissues.

The pro-oncogenic activity of GSK3β is based on the findings that deregulated GSK3β maintains tumor cell survival, proliferation, and invasion by enhancing machinery for cell motility and migration [58]. Finally, growing evidence marks GSK3β as a potential therapeutic target in cancer [59,60], thus encouraging the development of GSK3β inhibitors for cancer treatment [61]. In glioblastoma multiforme, such inhibitors facilitate apoptosis through inhibition of anti-apoptotic mechanisms in mitochondria and the NFkB pathway that is essential for cell survival [58,62].

Although GSK3β is generally considered a cytosolic protein, it can also be present in the nucleus. Our data showed an elevated level of expression of pGSK3β-Y216 in the cell nuclei of almost every sample of astrocytic brain tumors. It is known that GSK3β nuclear levels increase in response to apoptotic stimuli, and its major role is to affect gene expression by regulating the activity of many transcription factors [63].

The largest number of glioblastomas analyzed for both total and unphosphorylated β-catenin had moderate cytoplasmic expression (56.67% and 60%, respectively); weak expression was noted in 36.66% and 33.33%, respectively; while a strong signal was present in a smaller percentage of samples (6.67% and 6.67% respectively). Overall cytoplasmic accumulation of β-catenin predominated, whereas the expression of total and unphosphorylated β-catenin in the nucleus was observed in only four (13.33%) and five (16.67%) samples, respectively. It seems that strong expression and consequent transfer in the nucleus occurs in a smaller number of glioblastomas. Utsuki et al. [64] and Kahlert et al. [65] also found a small number of samples with nuclear expression, which can be partly explained by the Wnt pathway activity only in a small proportion of glioblastoma cells that have stem cell properties [66]. Another explanation is that the active form of beta-catenin that is transferred to the nucleus lacks specific epitopes and cannot be detected by this antibody. Spearman's correlation showed a statistically significant positive correlation between H-score values of total and unphosphorylated β-catenin ($r_s = 0.634$, $p < 0.001$), thus confirming the presence of an active form of β-catenin in tumor cells. Phosphorylation status and localization of β-catenin are important indicators of the Wnt signaling pathway's activation. Liu et al. [67] studied β-catenin expression in different grades of astrocytoma and noticed significantly higher levels of β-catenin in glioblastoma compared to lower grades and control groups, thus suggesting a role for β-catenin in the progression of malignant gliomas. The study by Sareddy et al. [68] on astrocytoma grade II–IV reports on the positive correlation of β-catenin mRNA and protein levels with the increase of malignancy grades. They also noticed a nuclear and cytoplasmic accumulation of β-catenin in astrocytoma, which is the hallmark of active Wnt/β-catenin signaling. Previous research by our laboratory has shown that tumors of neuroepithelial origin have higher levels of β-catenin expression compared to β-catenin expression levels in healthy brain tissue [69]. Kafka et al. [70] revealed that DVL3, TCF1, and LEF1 expression significantly increased with astrocytoma malignancy grades, suggesting their cooperation with nuclear β-catenin and joint involvement in malignant progression. In the present investigation, the bivariate correlation between unphosphorylated active β-catenin and active pGSK3β-Y216 showed a trend of negative association of the two proteins ($r_s = -0.427$, $p = 0.088$), confirming their mutually dependent relationship. Still, it seems that GSK3β activity toward β-catenin does not depend unambiguously on its phosphorylation status on S9, which appears to be a protective mechanism when GSK3β is aberrantly phosphorylated by some kinases [71,72]. It has been shown that highly active Akt does not fully inhibit GSK3β activity in some cancers and cancer cell lines [53]. However, a more recent study on human colorectal cancer cell lines shows that hyperactive Akt causes GSK3β inhibition and consequential β-catenin accumulation [73]. Recent studies demonstrated that active DKK3 is associated with reduced cytoplasmic and nuclear accumulation of β-catenin in different tumor types [74].

APC is a tumor-suppressor gene and an essential component of the beta-catenin complex that controls cytoplasmic beta-catenin levels. *APC* mutations occur early in gliomagenesis and result in increased beta-catenin levels that lead to the expression of Wnt responsive genes [9]. In our study, genetic change in *APC* exon 11 was present in 44.44% of the informative samples. Our laboratory group previously reported on *APC* exon 11 genetic changes in human brain tumors [75], brain metastases [76], and laryngeal squamous cell carcinoma [77] and found 33.3%, 58.8%, and 41% of samples with LOH or mutation of this gene, respectively. The present investigation also found that samples with changes of the *APC* gene had significantly higher values of total β-catenin H-score, compared to the group without genetic changes ($t = -2.264$, $p = 0.038$). Although the result for unphosphorylated β-catenin was not significant, its elevated expression in glioblastoma indicates the pathway's activity and its association with genetic changes in *APC*. The relatively rare expression of β-catenin in the nucleus may also be explained by work from Morgan et al. [78], where they showed that APC loss alone was insufficient to stimulate nuclear β-catenin translocation, and further dysregulation is required. Another explanation for the rare β-catenin nuclear expression is the finding that most of the C-terminal deletions show the predominant nuclear localization [79], and the antibody that we used in our study was raised against the C-terminal β-catenin epitope.

In conclusion, the results of this study undoubtedly indicate the activation of the Wnt signaling pathway in astrocytoma. Our findings on *DKK1* and *DKK3* demonstrate the importance of methylation in the regulation of Wnt signaling activity but also suggest that additional regulatory mechanisms may be involved. Our findings indicate pro-oncogenic effects of GSK3β on astrocytoma development and progression not necessarily connected to the Wnt destruction complex. It is also evident that large deletions and mutations in the *APC* gene increase the level of β-catenin expression in glioblastomas. This research can provide more data about astrocytoma pathogenesis and help to better understand and improve the management of gliomas.

Supplementary Materials: The following are available online at https://www.mdpi.com/article/10.3390/cancers13112530/s1, Figures S1–S4: M = 50 bp molecular marker; MK-MR = methylated control methylated reaction; MK-UMR = methylated control unmethylated reaction; UMK-MR = unmethylated control methylated reaction; UMK-UMR = unmethylated control unmethylated reaction; S(1–6)-MR = sample (1–6) methylated reaction; S(1–6)-UMR = sample (1–6) unmethylated reaction; NK-MR = negative control methylated reaction; NK-UMR = negative control unmethylated reaction.

Author Contributions: A.K. conceived the idea, designed the study, performed experimental work, contributed to data acquisition and analysis, wrote the manuscript, and revised it for important intellectual content. A.B. contributed to the data interpretation, manuscript editing, and revised the manuscript for important intellectual content. E.B. performed experimental work and participated in data collection, interpretation, and analysis. A.-M.J. performed experimental work and contributed to interpretation of the results. K.P. performed experimental work and participated in tumor sample analysis and results interpretation. P.B. contributed to data acquisition, the interpretation of the results, and manuscript editing. N.N. contributed to data acquisition and participated in tumor sample collection. K.Ž. participated in tumor sample analysis and revised the manuscript for important intellectual content. N.P.-Š. conceived the idea, designed the study, contributed to analysis and interpretation of the results, wrote the manuscript and revised it for important intellectual content, and approved the final version of the manuscript. All authors have read and agreed to the published version of the manuscript.

Funding: This research was funded by the Scientific Centre of Excellence for Basic, Clinical and Translational Neuroscience (project "Experimental and clinical research of hypoxic-ischemic damage in perinatal and adult brain"; GA KK01.1.1.01.0007 funded by the European Union through the European Regional Development Fund).

Institutional Review Board Statement: The study was conducted according to the guidelines of the Declaration of Helsinki and approved by the Ethics Committee of School of Medicine University of Zagreb (Case number: 380-59-10106-17-100/98; Class: 641-01/17-02/01, 23 March 2017), Ethics Committee of University Hospital Center Zagreb (number 02/21/AG, class: 8.1-16/215-2, 02 February 2017), and Ethics Committee of University Hospital Center "Sisters of Charity" (number EP-5429/17-5, 23 March 2017).

Informed Consent Statement: Informed consent was obtained from all subjects involved in the study.

Data Availability Statement: Data supporting reported results are contained within the article. Some of the data presented in this study are available on request from the corresponding author. The data are not publicly available due to privacy issues.

Conflicts of Interest: All authors declare that they have no conflict of interest.

References

1. Perry, A.; Wesseling, P. Histologic Classification of Gliomas. *Handb. Clin. Neurol.* **2016**, *134*, 71–95. [CrossRef] [PubMed]
2. Wesseling, P.; Capper, D. WHO 2016 Classification of Gliomas. *Neuropathol. Appl. Neurobiol.* **2018**, *44*, 139–150. [CrossRef] [PubMed]
3. Louis, D.N.; Perry, A.; Reifenberger, G.; von Deimling, A.; Figarella-Branger, D.; Cavenee, W.K.; Ohgaki, H.; Wiestler, O.D.; Kleihues, P.; Ellison, D.W. The 2016 World Health Organization Classification of Tumors of the Central Nervous System: A Summary. *Acta Neuropathol.* **2016**, *131*, 803–820. [CrossRef]
4. Kristensen, B.W.; Priesterbach-Ackley, L.P.; Petersen, J.K.; Wesseling, P. Molecular Pathology of Tumors of the Central Nervous System. *Ann. Oncol.* **2019**, *30*, 1265–1278. [CrossRef] [PubMed]
5. Glibo, M.; Serman, A.; Karin-Kujundzic, V.; Bekavac Vlatkovic, I.; Miskovic, B.; Vranic, S.; Serman, L. The Role of Glycogen Synthase Kinase 3 (GSK3) in Cancer with Emphasis on Ovarian Cancer Development and Progression: A Comprehensive Review. *Bosn. J. Basic Med. Sci.* **2021**, *21*, 5–18. [CrossRef]
6. Duda, P.; Akula, S.M.; Abrams, S.L.; Steelman, L.S.; Martelli, A.M.; Cocco, L.; Ratti, S.; Candido, S.; Libra, M.; Montalto, G.; et al. Targeting GSK3 and Associated Signaling Pathways Involved in Cancer. *Cells* **2020**, *9*, 1110. [CrossRef]
7. Majewska, E.; Szeliga, M. AKT/GSK3β Signaling in Glioblastoma. *Neurochem. Res.* **2016**, *42*, 918–924. [CrossRef] [PubMed]
8. Domoto, T.; Pyko, I.V.; Furuta, T.; Miyashita, K.; Uehara, M.; Shimasaki, T.; Nakada, M.; Minamoto, T. Glycogen Synthase Kinase-3β is a Pivotal Mediator of Cancer Invasion and Resistance to Therapy. *Cancer Sci.* **2016**, *107*, 1363–1372. [CrossRef] [PubMed]
9. Bugter, J.M.; Fenderico, N.; Maurice, M.M. Mutations and Mechanisms of WNT Pathway Tumour Suppressors in Cancer. *Nat. Rev. Cancer* **2021**, *21*, 5–21. [CrossRef] [PubMed]

10. Zeng, X.; Tamai, K.; Doble, B.; Li, S.; Huang, H.; Habas, R.; Okamura, H.; Woodgett, J.; He, X. A Dual-kinase Mechanism for Wnt Co-receptor Phosphorylation and Activation. *Nature* **2005**, *438*, 873–877. [CrossRef]
11. Baetta, R.; Banfi, C. Dkk (Dickkopf) Proteins. *Arterioscler. Thromb. Vasc. Biol.* **2019**, *39*, 1330–1342. [CrossRef]
12. Zhang, K.; Watanabe, M.; Kashiwakura, Y.; Li, S.A.; Edamura, K.; Huang, P.; Yamaguchi, K.; Nasu, Y.; Kobayashi, Y.; Sakaguchi, M.; et al. Expression Pattern of REIC/Dkk-3 in Various Cell Types and the Implications of the Soluble Form in Prostatic Acinar Development. *Int. J. Oncol.* **2010**, *37*, 1495–1501. [CrossRef] [PubMed]
13. Shi, R.Y.; Yang, X.R.; Shen, Q.J.; Yang, L.X.; Xu, Y.; Qiu, S.J.; Sun, Y.F.; Zhang, X.; Wang, Z.; Zhu, K.; et al. Expression of Dickkopfrelated Protein 1 is Related to Lymphatic Metastasis and Indicates Poor Prognosis in Intrahepatic Cholangiocarcinoma Patients after Surgery. *Cancer* **2013**, *119*, 993–1003. [CrossRef]
14. Begenik, H.; Kemik, A.S.; Emre, H.; Dulger, A.C.; Demirkiran, D.; Ebinc, S.; Kemik, O. The Association between Serum Dickkopf-1 Levels and Esophageal Squamous Cell Carcinoma. *Hum. Exp. Toxicol.* **2014**, *33*, 785–788. [CrossRef] [PubMed]
15. Chen, C.; Zhou, H.; Zhang, X.; Ma, X.; Liu, Z.; Liu, X. Elevated Levels of Dickkopf-1 are Associated with beta-catenin AccumuLation and Poor prognosis in Patients with Chondrosarcoma. *PLoS ONE* **2014**, *9*, e105414. [CrossRef]
16. Rachner, T.D.; Thiele, S.; Göbel, A.; Browne, A.; Fuessel, S.; Erdmann, K.; Wirth, M.P.; Fröhner, M.; Todenhöfer, T.; Muders, M.H.; et al. High Serum Levels of Dickkopf-1 are Associated with a Poor Prognosis in Prostate Cancer Patients. *BMC Cancer* **2014**, *14*, 649. [CrossRef]
17. Shi, Y.; Gong, H.L.; Zhou, L.; Tian, J.; Wang, Y. Dickkopf-1 is a Novel Prognostic Biomarker for Laryngeal Squamous Cell Carcinoma. *Acta Otolaryngol.* **2014**, *134*, 753–759. [CrossRef]
18. Han, S.X.; Zhou, X.; Sui, X.; He, C.C.; Cai, M.J.; Ma, J.L.; Zhang, Y.Y.; Zhou, C.Y.; Ma, C.X.; Varela-Ramirez, A.; et al. Serum Dickkopf-1 is a Novel Serological Biomarker for the Diagnosis and Prognosis of Pancreatic Cancer. *Oncotarget* **2015**, *6*, 19907–19917. [CrossRef]
19. Sun, D.K.; Wang, L.; Wang, J.M.; Zhang, P. Serum Dickkopf-1 Levels as a Clinical and Prognostic Factor in Patients with Bladder Cncer. *Genet. Mol. Res.* **2015**, *14*, 18181–18187. [CrossRef]
20. Shi, X.D.; Yu, X.H.; Wu, W.R.; Xu, X.L.; Wang, J.Y.; Xu, L.B.; Zhang, R.; Liu, C. Dickkopf-1 Expression is Associated with Tumorigenicity and Lymphatic Metastasis in Human Hilar Cholangiocarcinoma. *Oncotarget* **2016**, *7*, 70378–70387. [CrossRef]
21. Watany, M.; Badawi, R.; Elkhalawany, W.; Abd-Elsalam, S. Study of Dickkopf-1 (DKK-1) Gene Expression in Hepatocellular Carcinoma Patients. *J. Clin. Diagn. Res.* **2017**, *11*, Oc32–Oc34. [CrossRef] [PubMed]
22. Jiang, T.; Wang, S.; Huang, L.; Zhang, S. Clinical Significance of Serum DKK-1 in Patients with Gynecological Cancer. *Int. J. Gynecol. Cancer* **2009**, *19*, 1177–1181. [CrossRef]
23. Liu, Z.; Sun, B.; Qi, L.; Li, Y.; Zhao, X.; Zhang, D.; Zhang, Y. Dickkopf-1 Expression is Down-regulated during the Colorectal Adenomacarcinoma Sequence and Correlates with Reduced Microvessel Density and VEGF Expression. *Histopathology* **2015**, *67*, 158–166. [CrossRef]
24. Zhao, Y.P.; Wang, W.; Wang, X.H.; Xu, Y.; Wang, Y.; Dong, Z.F.; Zhang, J.J. Downregulation of Serum DKK-1 Predicts Poor Prognosis in Patients with Papillary Thyroid Cancer. *Genet. Mol. Res.* **2015**, *14*, 18886–18894. [CrossRef]
25. Mizobuchi, Y.; Matsuzaki, K.; Kuwayama, K.; Kitazato, K.; Mure, H.; Kageji, T.; Nagahiro, S. REIC/Dkk-3 Induces Cell Death in Human Malignant Glioma. *Neuro Oncol.* **2008**, *10*, 244–253. [CrossRef]
26. Zhou, Y.; Li, W.; Xu, Q.; Huang, Y. Elevated Expression of Dickkopf-1 Increases the Sensitivity of Human Glioma Cell Line SHG44 to BCNU. *J. Exp. Clin. Cancer Res.* **2010**, *29*, 131. [CrossRef]
27. Götze, S.; Wolter, M.; Reifenberger, G.; Müller, O.; Sievers, S. Frequent Promoter Hypermethylation of Wnt Pathway Inhibitor Genes in Malignant Astrocytic Gliomas. *Cancer Genet.* **2010**, *126*, 2584–2593. [CrossRef]
28. Oka, T.; Kurozumi, K.; Shimazu, Y.; Ichikawa, T.; Ishida, J.; Otani, Y.; Shimizu, T.; Tomita, Y.; Sakaguchi, M.; Watanabe, M.; et al. A Super Gene Expression System Enhances the Anti-glioma Effects of Adenovirus-mediated REIC/Dkk-3 Gene Therapy. *Sci. Rep.* **2016**, *6*, 33319. [CrossRef] [PubMed]
29. Green, M.R.; Sambrook, J. *Molecular Cloning—A Laboratory Manual*, 4th ed.; Cold Spring Harbor Laboratory Press: New York, NY, USA, 2012.
30. Miller, S.A.; Dykes, D.D.; Polesky, H.F. A Simple Salting out Procedure for Extracting DNA from Human Nucleated Cells. *Nucleic Acids Res.* **1988**, *16*, 883–893. [CrossRef]
31. Maehata, T.; Taniguchi, H.; Yamamoto, H.; Nosho, K.; Adachi, Y.; Miyamoto, N.; Miyamoto, C.; Akutsu, N.; Yamaoka, S.; Itoh, F. Transcriptional Silencing of Dickkopf Gene Family by CpG Island Hypermethylation in Human Gastrointestinal Cancer. *World J. Gastroenterol.* **2008**, *14*, 2702–2714. [CrossRef]
32. Zhang, M.; Huang, M.; Cao, B.; Sheng, X.; Li, P. Methylation of the DKK3 Promoter is Associated with Poor Prognosis in Patients with Cervical Adenocarcinoma. *Int. J. Clin. Exp. Pathol.* **2018**, *11*, 788–794. [PubMed]
33. Naghibalhossaini, F.; Zamani, M.; Mokarram, P.; Khalili, I.; Rasti, M.; Mostafavi-pour, Z. Epigenetic and Genetic Analysis of WNT Signaling Pathway in Sporadic Colorectal Cancer Patients from Iran. *Mol. Biol. Rep.* **2012**, *39*, 6171–6178. [CrossRef] [PubMed]
34. Katoh, M.; Katoh, M. Molecular Genetics and Targeted Therapy of WNT-related Human Diseases (Review). *Int. J. Mol. Med.* **2017**, *40*, 587–606. [CrossRef] [PubMed]
35. Aguilera, O.; Fraga, M.F.; Ballestar, E.; Paz, M.F.; Herranz, M.; Espada, J.; García, J.M.; Muñoz, A.; Esteller, M.; González-Sancho, J.M. Epigenetic Inactivation of the Wnt Antagonist DICKKOPF-1 (DKK-1) Gene in Human Colorectal Cancer. *Oncogene* **2006**, *25*, 4116–4121. [CrossRef] [PubMed]

36. Guo, C.C.; Zhang, X.L.; Yang, B.; Geng, J.; Peng, B.; Zheng, J.H. Decreased Expression of dkk1 and dkk3 in Human Clear Cell Renal Cell Carcinoma. *Mol. Med. Rep.* **2014**, *9*, 2367–2373. [CrossRef] [PubMed]
37. Galamb, O.; Kalmar, A.; Peterfia, B.; Csabai, I.; Bodor, A.; Ribli, D.; Krenács, T.; Patai, Á.V.; Wichmann, B.; Barták, B.K.; et al. Aberrant DNA Methylation of WNT Pathway Genes in the Development and Progression of CIMP-negative Colorectal Cancer. *Epigenetics* **2016**, *11*, 588–602. [CrossRef]
38. Wang, W.; He, Y.; Rui, J.; Xu, M.Q. miR-410 Acts as an Oncogene in Colorectal Cancer Cells by Targeting Dickkopf-related Protein 1 via the Wnt/β-catenin Signaling Pathway. *Oncol. Lett.* **2019**, *17*, 807–814. [CrossRef] [PubMed]
39. Shen, Q.; Fan, J.; Yang, X.R.; Tan, Y.; Zhao, W.; Xu, Y.; Wang, N.; Niu, Y.; Wu, Z.; Zhou, J.; et al. Serum DKK1 as a Protein Biomarker for the Diagnosis of Hepatocellular Carcinoma: A Large-scale, Multicentre Study. *Lancet Oncol.* **2012**, *13*, 817–826. [CrossRef]
40. Urakami, S.; Shiina, H.; Enokida, H.; Kawakami, T.; Kawamoto, K.; Hirata, H.; Tanaka, Y.; Kikuno, N.; Nakagawa, M.; Igawa, M. Combination Analysis of Hypermethylated Wnt-antagonist Family Genes as a Novel Epigenetic Biomarker Panel for Bladder Cancer Detection. *Clin. Cancer Res.* **2006**, *12*, 2109–2116. [CrossRef]
41. Yue, W.; Sun, Q.; Dacic, S.; Landreneau, R.J.; Siegfried, J.M.; Yu, J.; Zhang, L. Downregulation of dkk3 Activates Beta-catenin/tcf-4 Signaling in Lung Cancer. *Carcinogenesis* **2008**, *29*, 84–92. [CrossRef]
42. You, A.; Fokas, E.; Wang, L.F.; He, H.; Kleb, B.; Niederacher, D.; Engenhart-Cabillic, R.; An, H.X. Expression of the Wnt Antagonist dkk3 is Frequently Suppressed in Sporadic Epithelial Ovarian Cancer. *J. Cancer Res. Clin. Oncol.* **2011**, *137*, 621–627. [CrossRef]
43. Park, J.M.; Kim, M.K.; Chi, K.C.; Kim, J.H.; Lee, S.H.; Lee, E.J. Aberrant Loss of dickkopf-3 in Gastric Cancer: Can it Predict Lymph Node Metastasis Preoperatively? *World J. Surg.* **2015**, *39*, 1018–1025. [CrossRef]
44. Lorsy, E.; Topuz, A.S.; Geisler, C.; Stahl, S.; Garczyk, S.; von Stillfried, S.; Hoss, M.; Gluz, O.; Hartmann, A.; Knüchel, R. Loss of dickkopf 3 Promotes the Tumorigenesis of Basal Breast Cancer. *PLoS ONE* **2016**, *11*, e0160077. [CrossRef]
45. Pei, Y.; Kano, J.; Iijima, T.; Morishita, Y.; Inadome, Y.; Noguchi, M. Overexpression of Dickkopf 3 in Hepatoblastomas and Hepatocellular Carcinomas. *Virchows Arch.* **2009**, *454*, 639–646. [CrossRef]
46. Fujii, M.; Katase, N.; Lefeuvre, M.; Gunduz, M.; Buery, R.R.; Tamamura, R.; Tsujigiwa, H.; Nagatsuka, H. Dickkopf (dkk)-3 and β-catenin Expressions Increased in the Transition from Normal Oral Mucosal to Oral Squamous Cell Carcinoma. *J. Mol. Histol.* **2011**, *42*, 499–504. [CrossRef]
47. Wang, Z.; Lin, L.; Thomas, D.G.; Nadal, E.; Chang, A.C.; Beer, D.G.; Lin, J. The Role of Dickkopf-3 Overexpression in Esophageal Adenocarcinoma. *J. Thorac. Cardiovasc. Surg.* **2015**, *150*, 377–385. [CrossRef] [PubMed]
48. Valdora, F.; Banelli, B.; Stigliani, S.; Pfister, S.M.; Moretti, S.; Kool, M.; Remke, M.; Bai, A.H.C.; Brigati, C.; Hielscher, T.; et al. Epigenetic Silencing of DKK3 in Medulloblastoma. *Int. J. Mol. Sci.* **2013**, *14*, 7492–7505. [CrossRef] [PubMed]
49. Huo, J.; Zhang, Y.; Li, R.; Wang, Y.; Wu, J.; Zhang, D. Upregulated MicroRNA-25 Mediates the Migration of Melanoma Cells by Targeting DKK3 through the WNT/β-Catenin Pathway. *Int. J. Mol. Sci.* **2016**, *17*, 1124. [CrossRef] [PubMed]
50. Rui, Y.; Hu, M.; Wang, P.; Zhang, C.; Xu, H.; Li, Y.; Zhang, Y.; Gu, J.; Wang, Q. LncRNA HOTTIP Mediated DKK1 Downregulation Confers Metastasis and Invasion in Colorectal Cancer Cells. *Histol. Histopathol.* **2019**, *34*, 619–630. [CrossRef] [PubMed]
51. Guo, J.; Yang, Z.; Zhou, H.; Yue, J.; Mu, T.; Zhang, Q.; Bi, X. Upregulation of DKK3 by miR-483-3p Plays an Important Role in the Chemoprevention of Colorectal Cancer Mediated by Black Raspberry Anthocyanins. *Mol. Carcinog.* **2020**, *59*, 168–178. [CrossRef] [PubMed]
52. Unnikrishnan, A.; Freeman, W.M.; Jackson, J.; Wren, J.D.; Porter, H.; Richardson, A. The Role of DNA Methylation in Epigenetics of Aging. *Pharmacol. Ther.* **2019**, *195*, 172–185. [CrossRef] [PubMed]
53. Shakoori, A.; Ougolkov, A.; Yu, Z.W.; Zhang, B.; Modarressi, M.H.; Billadeau, D.D.; Mai, M.; Takahashi, Y.; Minalmoto, T. Deregulated GSK3beta Activity in Colorectal Cancer: Its Association with Tumor Cell Survival and Proliferation. *Biochem. Biophys. Res. Commun.* **2005**, *334*, 1365–1373. [CrossRef]
54. Shakoori, A.; Mai, W.; Miyashita, K.; Yasumoto, K.; Takahashi, Y.; Ooi, A. Inhibition of GSK-3 Beta Activity Attenuates Proliferation of Human Colon Cancer Cells in Rodents. *Cancer Sci.* **2007**, *98*, 1388–1393. [CrossRef] [PubMed]
55. Ma, C.; Wang, J.; Gao, Y.; Gao, T.W.; Chen, G.; Bower, K.A.; Odetallah, M.; Ding, M.; Ke, Z.; Luo, J. The Role of Glycogen Synthase Kinase 3beta in the Transformation of Epidermal Cells. *Cancer Res.* **2007**, *67*, 7756–7764. [CrossRef] [PubMed]
56. Mishra, R.; Nagini, S.; Rana, A. Expression and Inactivation of Glycogen Synthase Kinase 3 Alpha/Beta and their Association with the Expression of Cyclin D1 and p53 in Oral Squamous Cell Carcinoma Progression. *Mol. Cancer* **2015**, *14*, 20. [CrossRef] [PubMed]
57. Zheng, H.; Saito, H.; Masuda, S.; Yang, X.; Takano, Y. Phosphorylated GSK3beta-ser9 and EGFR are Good Prognostic Factors for Lung Carcinomas. *Anticancer Res.* **2007**, *27*, 3561–3569. [PubMed]
58. Acikgoz, E.; Güler, G.; Camlar, M.; Oktem, G.; Aktug, H. Glycogen Synthase Kinase-3 Inhibition in Glioblastoma Multiforme Cells Induces Apoptosis, Cell Cycle Arrest and Changing Biomolecular Structure. *Spectrochim. Acta Part A Mol. Biomol. Spectrosc.* **2019**, *209*, 150–164. [CrossRef]
59. McCubrey, J.A.; Steelman, L.S.; Bertrand, F.E.; Davis, N.M.; Sokolosky, M.; Abrams, S.L.; Montalto, G.; D'Assoro, A.B.; Libra, M.; Nicoletti, F.; et al. GSK-3 as Potential Target for Therapeutic Intervention in Cancer. *Oncotarget* **2014**, *5*, 2881–2911. [CrossRef] [PubMed]
60. Walz, A.; Ugolkov, A.; Chandra, S.; Kozikowski, A.; Carneiro, B.A.; O'Halloran, T.V.; Giles, F.J.; Billadeau, D.D.; Mazar, A.P. Molecular Pathways: Revisiting Glycogen Synthase Kinase-3β as a Target for the Treatment of Cancer. *Clin. Cancer Res.* **2017**, *23*, 1891–1897. [CrossRef]

61. Sahin, I.; Eturi, A.; De Souza, A.; Pamarthy, S.; Tavora, F.; Giles, F.J.; Carneiro, B.A. Glycogen Synthase Kinase-3β Inhibitors as Novel Cancer Treatments and Modulators of Antitumor Immune Responses. *Cancer Biol. Ther.* **2019**, *20*, 1047–1056. [CrossRef]
62. Kotliarova, S.; Pastorino, S.; Kovell, L.C.; Kotliarov, Y.; Song, H.; Zhang, W.; Bailey, R.; Maric, D.; Zenklusen, J.C.; Lee, J.; et al. Glycogen Synthase Kinase-3 Inhibition Induces Glioma Cell Death through c-MYC, Nuclear Factor-kappaB, and Glucose Regulation. *Cancer Res.* **2008**, *68*, 6643–6651. [CrossRef] [PubMed]
63. Beurel, E.; Grieco, S.F.; Jope, R.S. Glycogen Synthase Kinase-3 (GSK3): Regulation, Actions, and Diseases. *Pharmacol. Ther.* **2015**, *148*, 114–131. [CrossRef]
64. Utsuki, S.; Sato, Y.; Oka, H.; Tsuchiya, B.; Suzuki, S.; Fujii, K. Relationship between the Expression of E-, N-cadherins and Beta-catenin and Tumor Grade in Astrocytomas. *J. Neurooncol.* **2002**, *57*, 187–192. [CrossRef]
65. Kahlert, U.D.; Suwala, A.K.; Koch, K.; Natsumeda, M.; Orr, B.A.; Hayashi, M.; Maciaczyk, J.; Eberhart, C.G. Pharmacologic Wnt Inhibition Reduces Proliferation, Survival, and Clonogenicity of Glioblastoma Cells. *J. Neuropathol. Exp. Neurol.* **2015**, *74*, 889–900. [CrossRef]
66. Tompa, M.; Kalovits, F.; Nagy, A.; Kalman, B. Contribution of the Wnt Pathway to Defining Biology of Glioblastoma. *Neuromolecular Med.* **2018**, *20*, 437–451. [CrossRef] [PubMed]
67. Liu, X.; Wang, L.; Zhao, S.; Ji, X.; Luo, Y.; Ling, F. β-Catenin Overexpression in Malignant Glioma and Its Role in Proliferation and Apoptosis in Glioblastoma Cells. *Med. Oncol.* **2011**, *28*, 608–614. [CrossRef] [PubMed]
68. Sareddy, G.R.; Panigrahi, M.; Challa, S.; Mahadevan, A.; Babu, P.P. Activation of Wnt/β-catenin/Tcf Signaling Pathway in Human Astrocytomas. *Neurochem. Int.* **2009**, *55*, 307–317. [CrossRef]
69. Nikuševa-Martić, T.; Pećina-Šlaus, N.; Kušec, V.; Kokotović, T.; Mušinović, H.; Tomas, D.; Zeljko, M. Changes of AXIN-1 and Beta-catenin in Neuroepithelial Brain Tumors. *Pathol. Oncol. Res.* **2010**, *16*, 75–79. [CrossRef] [PubMed]
70. Kafka, A.; Bačić, M.; Tomas, D.; Žarković, K.; Bukovac, A.; Njirić, N.; Mrak, G.; Krsnik, Ž.; Pećina-Šlaus, N. Different Behaviour of DVL1, DVL2, DVL3 in Astrocytoma Malignancy Grades and their Association to TCF1 and LEF1 Upregulation. *J. Cell. Mol. Med.* **2019**, *23*, 641–655. [CrossRef]
71. Woodgett, J.R. Judging a Protein by more than Its Name: GSK-3. *Sci. STKE* **2001**, *2001*, re12. [CrossRef]
72. Ng, S.S.; Mahmoudi, T.; Danenberg, E.; Bejaoui, I.; de Lau, W.; Korswagen, H.C.; Schutte, M.; Clevers, H. Phosphatidylinositol 3-kinase Signaling does not Activate the Wnt Cascade. *J. Biol. Chem.* **2009**, *284*, 35308–35313. [CrossRef]
73. Yun, S.H.; Park, J.I. PGC-1α Regulates Cell Proliferation and Invasion via AKT/GSK-3β/β-catenin Pathway in Human Colorectal Cancer SW620 and SW480 Cells. *Anticancer Res.* **2020**, *40*, 653–664. [CrossRef] [PubMed]
74. Veeck, J.; Dahl, E. Targeting the Wnt Pathway in Cancer: The Emerging Role of Dickkopf-3. *Biochim. Biophys. Acta* **2012**, *1825*, 18–28. [CrossRef] [PubMed]
75. Nikuševa-Martić, T.; Beroš, V.; Pećina-Šlaus, N.; Pećina, H.I.; Bulić-Jakuš, F. Genetic Changes of CDH1, APC, and CTNNB1 Found in Human Brain Tumors. *Pathol. Res. Pract.* **2007**, *203*, 779–787. [CrossRef] [PubMed]
76. Pećina-Šlaus, N.; Martić, T.N.; Zeljko, M.; Bulat, S. Brain Metastases Exhibit Gross Deletions of the APC Gene. *Brain Tumor Pathol.* **2011**, *28*, 223–228. [CrossRef]
77. Pećina-Šlaus, N.; Kljaić, M.; Nikuševa-Martić, T. Loss of Heterozygosity of APC and CDH1 Genes in Laryngeal Squamous Cell Carcinoma. *Pathol. Res. Pract.* **2005**, *201*, 557–563. [CrossRef] [PubMed]
78. Morgan, R.G.; Ridsdale, J.; Tonks, A.; Darley, R.L. Factors Affecting the Nuclear Localization of β-Catenin in Normal and Malignant Tissue. *J. Cell. Biochem.* **2014**, *115*, 1351–1361. [CrossRef]
79. Dar, M.S.; Singh, P.; Singh, G.; Jamwal, G.; Hussain, S.S.; Rana, A.; Akhter, Y.; Mong, S.P.; Dar, M.J. Terminal Regions of β-catenin are Critical for Regulating Its Adhesion and Transcription Functions. *Biochim. Biophys. Acta* **2016**, *1863*, 2345–2357. [CrossRef]

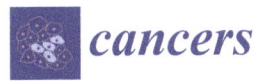

Article

Small Molecule Inhibitors of Microenvironmental Wnt/β-Catenin Signaling Enhance the Chemosensitivity of Acute Myeloid Leukemia

Paul Takam Kamga [1,2,†], Giada Dal Collo [1,3,†], Adriana Cassaro [4,5,†], Riccardo Bazzoni [1], Pietro Delfino [6], Annalisa Adamo [1], Alice Bonato [1], Carmine Carbone [7], Ilaria Tanasi [1], Massimiliano Bonifacio [1] and Mauro Krampera [1,*]

1. Section of Hematology, Stem Cell Research Laboratory, Department of Medicine, University of Verona, 37134 Verona, Italy; Paul.Takam-Kamga@ac-versailles.fr (P.T.K.); g.dalcollo@erasmusmc.nl (G.D.C.); riccardo.bazzoni@univr.it (R.B.); annalisa.adamo@univr.it (A.A.); alice.bonato@icgeb.org (A.B.); ilaria.tanasi@univr.it (I.T.); massimiliano.bonifacio@univr.it (M.B.)
2. EA4340-BCOH, Biomarker in Cancerology and Onco-Haematology, Université de Versailles-Saint-Quentin-En-Yvelines, Université Paris Saclay, 92100 Boulogne-Billancourt, France
3. Department of Immunology, Erasmus University Medical Center, Doctor Molenwaterplein 40, 3015 GD Rotterdam, The Netherlands
4. Department of Oncology, Hematology Unit, Niguarda Hospital, 20162 Milan, Italy; adriana.cassaro@ospedaleniguarda.it
5. Department of Health Sciences, University of Milan, 20146 Milan, Italy
6. Department of Diagnostics and Public Health, University and Hospital Trust of Verona, 37134 Verona, Italy; pietro.delfino@univr.it
7. Fondazione Policlinico Universitario Gemelli, IRCCS, 00168 Roma, Italy; carmine.carbone@univr.it
* Correspondence: mauro.krampera@univr.it; Tel.: +45-045-812-4420; Fax: +45-045-802-7488
† These authors contribute equally to this study.

Received: 5 September 2020; Accepted: 17 September 2020; Published: 21 September 2020

Simple Summary: Considering the pivotal role of Wnt/β-catenin signaling in AML development and persistence, the current study addresses in AML, the prognostic value of Wnt/β-catenin signaling molecules and the anti-leukemic value of Wnt/β-catenin inhibition. In silico analysis of RNAseq data from AML patients and flow cytometric analysis of primary AML samples revealed that higher levels of Wnt/β-catenin pathway is a poor prognostic marker. Next, we found that pharmacological interference, through small molecule inhibitors of Wnt and/or GSK-3 signaling reduces AML cell survival by sensitizing the leukemia cells to chemotherapeutic agents both in vitro and in vivo. Overall, our findings suggested that Wnt-inhibitory therapy could overcome the prognostic significance of patient risk stratification, standing as a therapeutic response for all subgroups of AML.

Abstract: Wnt/β-catenin signaling has been reported in Acute Myeloid leukemia, but little is known about its significance as a prognostic biomarker and drug target. In this study, we first evaluated the correlation between expression levels of Wnt molecules and clinical outcome. Then, we studied—in vitro and in vivo—the anti-leukemic value of combinatorial treatment between Wnt inhibitors and classic anti-leukemia drugs. Higher levels of β-catenin, Ser675-phospho-β-catenin and GSK-3α (total and Ser 9) were found in AML cells from intermediate or poor risk patients; nevertheless, patients presenting high activity of Wnt/β-catenin displayed shorter progression-free survival (PFS) according to univariate analysis. In vitro, many pharmacological inhibitors of Wnt signalling, i.e., LRP6 (Niclosamide), GSK-3 (LiCl, AR-A014418), and TCF/LEF (PNU-74654) but not Porcupine (IWP-2), significantly reduced proliferation and improved the drug sensitivity of AML cells cultured alone or in the presence of bone marrow stromal cells. In vivo, PNU-74654, Niclosamide and LiCl administration significantly reduced the bone marrow leukemic burden acting synergistically with Ara-C, thus improving mouse survival. Overall, our study demonstrates the antileukemic role of Wnt/β-catenin inhibition that may represent a potential new therapeutics strategy in AML.

Keywords: microenvironment; Wnt; AML; drug target

1. Introduction

Acute myeloid leukemia (AML) is the most common acute leukemia in adults; relapse after chemotherapy still represents a critical problem in most patients, with only a 35–40% five-year overall survival rate for non-promyelocytic AML [1,2]. Nevertheless, accurate biomarkers for early diagnosis and response prediction to chemotherapy or allogeneic transplantation are still lacking [3]. The persistence of residual leukemia cells during chemo- or immunotherapy is favored by different components of the bone marrow stromal niche through a redundant panel of molecular pathways, such as Wnt, Notch and Hedgehog, supporting cell survival, proliferation and chemoresistance [4–6]. However, the role of these pathways in the interaction between AML cells and bone marrow microenvironment is not entirely clear yet [7,8].

Wnt/β-catenin signaling is a developmental pathway mostly involved in tissue patterning during embryonic development, through its ability to modulate proliferation, differentiation and motility of embryonic and adult stem cells [9]. The pathway is activated when secreted Wnt proteins (Wnt-1, Wnt-3a, Wnt-3b etc.) bind to the extracellular domain of the frizzled family of receptors and lipoprotein receptor-related protein (LRP) co-receptors. This binding stabilizes β-catenin by disrupting the β-catenin destruction complex consisting in GSK-3 and other proteins. The inactivation of the β-catenin destruction complex promotes the nuclear accumulation of β-catenin, which in turn triggers the expression of several target genes [10]. Deregulation of the pathway can occur in cancer, either as result of gene mutations in components of Wnt/β-catenin pathway or because of the crosstalk between tumor-associated stroma and cancer cell bulk. This deregulation can induce a persistent accumulation of β-catenin in the nucleus, thus favoring cancer growth and dissemination, maintenance of cancer stem cells, and drug resistance [11,12]. Considering the pivotal role of Wnt/β-catenin signaling in several cancers, small molecules inhibitors have been developed as potent anticancer agents, including inhibitors of Frizzled, Porcupine, GSK-3 and disruptors of the β-catenin/TCF/LEF complexes [13].

In AML, a number of studies support the contribution of the canonical Wnt signaling in the maintenance of leukemia stem cells (LSCs) [14]. Indeed, many molecular events contribute to the aberrant expression of the Wnt pathway in AML cells, such as FLT3 signaling, hypermethylation of the secreted frizzled-related proteins, high levels of Frizzled receptors and Wnt ligands [15]. Moreover, preclinical studies have demonstrated that activating the mutation of β-catenin in stromal cells is sufficient to induce AML-like disease in mice [16]. Overall, the canonical Wnt signaling appears relevant for leukemogenesis in AML and therefore drug targetable.

In this work, we demonstrate that pharmacological interference, through small molecules inhibitors of Wnt and/or GSK-3 signaling reduces AML cell survival by sensitizing the leukemia cells to chemotherapeutic agents both in vitro and in vivo. Consequently, combination treatments with small molecules inhibitors of Wnt/GSK3 axis and chemotherapy may represent a novel therapeutic strategy for a better chance of AML cell eradication.

2. Materials and Methods

2.1. Chemicals and Antibodies

The antibodies used for blast cell identification by Flow Cytometry (FACSCanto II, Becton Dickinson, Rutherford, NJ, USA) were: anti-CD45-VioBlue, anti-CD45-APC-Vio770, anti-CD34-PerCP and anti-CD117-APC all from Miltenyi Biotech (Bergsch gradbach, Germany). For Western blot analysis, anti-β-catenin, anti- Ser675-phospho-β-catenin, anti-Ser33/37/Thr41-phospho-β-catenin, anti-non-phopho-β-catenin, anti-GSK-3β, anti-Ser9-phospho-GSK-3β, anti-GSK-3α, anti-Ser21-phospho-GSK-3α anti-Histone H3 antibodies and Alexa 488-conjugated secondary antibodies were from Cell Signaling

(Danvers, MA, USA); anti-GAPDH, and HRP-conjugated secondary antibodies against mouse or rabbit were from Sigma-Aldrich (Darmstadt, Germany). Wnt modulators used for proliferation and vitality assays, i.e., Wnt-3a, PNU-74654, Niclosamide, IWP-2, Lithium Chloride (LiCl), and AR-A014418, were all purchased from Sigma-Aldrich. For the analysis of cell death, Propidium iodide (PI) and FITC-conjugated Annexin V were from Miltenyi Biotechnology. CellTiter 96® AQ$_{ueous}$ One Solution Cell Proliferation Assay (MTS, Eden Prairie, MN, USA) was from Promega (Promega, Milano, Italy). Cytarabine (Ara-C) and Idarubicin (Ida) were provided by the Pharmacy Unit of the University Hospital of Verona.

2.2. Patients, Samples and Cell Lines

All cell samples were collected from AML patients and healthy donors after written informed consent, as approved by the Ethics Committee of Azienda Ospedaliera Universitaria Integrata Verona (N. Prog. 1828, 12 May 2010—'Institution of cell and tissue collection for biomedical research in Onco-Hematology'). In detail, AML blast cells were obtained from bone marrow or peripheral blood samples of patients with AML at diagnosis (>80% of leukemia cells). Samples with less than 80% of blast cells were enriched with CD34$^+$ using MACS CD34 Microbead Kit (MiltenyiBiotec). AML patients characteristics have been described elsewhere [17] and summarized in Table S1. Human bone marrow mesenchymal stromal cells were obtained from bone marrow aspirates of healthy donors (hBM-MSCs, n = 12) and AML patients (hBM-MSCs*, n = 18) after informed consent as previously described [17,18]. Human cell lines HL-60 (acute promyelocytic leukemia cell line), THP1 (acute monocytic leukemia cell line), U937(myeloid histiocytic sarcoma cell line), were grown in complete RPMI-1640 medium (RPMI supplemented with 10% FBS, 1% L-Glutamine solution 200 mM and 1% Penicillin/Streptomycin). HEK-293 (human embryonic kidney cell line) and hBM-MSCs were maintained in complete DMEM. Cell lines were purchased from the American Type Culture Collection. Flow cytometry of membrane marker and cell morphology through Giemsa staining were used to check stability and identity of cell lines as previously described [19]. Cell lines were routinely tested to be Mycoplasma-free.

2.3. Western Blotting

Immunoblotting were performed as previously described [19]. Briefly, Cells were lysed with the RIPA lysis buffer (25 nM Tris pH 7.6, 150 mM NaCl, 1% NP40, 1% Na-deoxycholate, 0.1% SDS). Then, samples were subjected to SDS-PAGE (sodium dodecyl sulfate polyacrylamide gel electrophoresis) followed by protein transfer onto nitrocellulose membrane (GE Healthcare, Chicago, IL, USA), that were subsequently probed with antibodies specific to target proteins.

2.4. Cell Proliferation and Apoptosis and Viability Assays

The IC50 for each drug were obtained by analyzing treated cells with the colorimetric One Solution Cell Proliferation Assay (MTS), as previously described [19,20]. Cell proliferation, cell death and apoptosis were assessed through flow cytometric analysis of AML cells stained with CFSE (carboxyfluorescein succinimidyl ester, proliferation) TOPRO-3 (cell death) and FITC-Annexin V/Propidium Iodide (PI) (apoptosis) as previously described [17–19].

2.5. Xenograft Mouse Model

Animal care was performed in accordance with institution guidelines as approved by the Italian ministry of health. Mice were purchased from Taconic (Germantown, NY, USA). Animal experiments were carried in pathogen-free conditions at the animal facility of the Interdepartmental Centre of Experimental Research Service of the University of Verona. Parameters used for sample size are power of 80%, a signal/noise ratio of 2 and a significance level of 5% ($p \leq 0.05$) using a one-sample t-test power calculation. With a commitment to providing refinement, reduction and replacement (3Rs), application of factorial design to reduce the minimum group size was applied to obtain a minimum group size of 5–8 mice. Xenograft mouse model were generated in NOD/Shi-scid/IL-2Rγnull (NOG, Minnetonka, MN, USA) mice as previously described [17]. Briefly, U937 AML cell line (1×10^6) were injected into the tail vein of totally irradiated (1.2 Gy, ^{137}Cesium source), 8–12-week-old male mice. At day 9 post-injection, mice (randomly allocated) received for 5 days intraperitoneal daily injection of Ara-C (25 mg/Kg) or its vehicle (dimethyl sulfoxide, DMSO). In case of combined treatment, Ara-C or DMSO were associated with each Wnt/GSK-3 inhibitor for the first two days, followed by three days of Ara-C or DMSO. Mice were sacrificed after 2 weeks following the cell line injection, and bone marrow leukemic burden was evaluated as percentage of human hCD45+ cells. No blinding was done. Wnt inhibitors used for mouse experiments were PNU-74654 (0.5 mg/kg), Niclosamide (10 mg/Kg) and LiCl (25 mg/Kg).

2.6. Cell Culture and Co-Culture

To study the capability of hBM-MSCs to support AML cell survival, AML cells were cultured in suspension or on a confluent monolayer of hBM-MSCs with complete RPMI 1640 in 96-well plates: 10^5 AML blast cells or 2×10^4 cells from AML cell lines were cultured in 100 µL of complete RPMI for 48 h. Wnt modulators, Ara-C and Idarubicin were added in co-culture. Co-cultured AML cells were collected and stained with anti-CD45 antibodies conjugated to APC or PerCP and analyzed for proliferation (CFSE dilution) and cell death (TOPRO-3, Annexin V/PI).

2.7. Flow Cytometry Analysis of Wnt Molecules

AML cell lines or AML blast cells identified as CD45+, CD34+, CD38- cells by flow cytometry, were fixed and permeabilized for 30 min at 4 °C. Permeabilized cells were probed with primary antibodies or their specific isotype for 1 h. Subsequently cells were washed and labelled for 30 min with Alexa 488-conjugated secondary antibodies. Protein expression was then analyzed through flow cytometry and expressed as relative median of fluorescence intensity (rMFI), defined as the ratio of the specific antibody fluorescence over the specific isotype fluorescence.

2.8. Gene Reporter

To monitor Wnt/β-catenin transcriptional activity, we transfected THP1 with reporter plasmids encoding for an inducible TCF responsive GFP reporter (Qiagen, Hilden, Germany) as previously described [8] GFP signal was observed through Axiovert Z1 (Zeiss, Sheung Kehen, Germany) and quantitatively measured by flow cytometry. The Wnt pathway activity was determined by normalizing the activity of TCF-GFP to that of CMV-GFP plasmid.

2.9. RNA-seq Analysis

RNA-seq data from 173 AML patients were obtained as part of The Cancer Genome Atlas project (TCGA). Gene expression data in Z-score format were downloaded from the cbioportal R package cgdsr for the TCGA-LAML. Normalized data were used for Z-score calculation. For each mRNA, a sample showing a Z-score higher or lower than the average Z-score for the whole population was considered as expressing highly or lowly, respectively, the corresponding gene, $Z > +/- 1.96; p < 0.05$. This strategy was applied for the gene of the WNT signaling pathways (APC, AXIN1, CTNNB1, FZD4, GSK3A, GSK3B, LRP5, TCF4, WNT3A, WNT5A, WNT5B, WNT10A, WNT10B).

2.10. Statistical Analysis

Statistical analysis was performed using GraphPad Prism software (La Jolla, CA, USA). Mann–Whitney and Kruskal–Wallis were used to compare two groups or more than two groups, respectively. All tests were one-sided. Pearson Chi-square analysis was used to test association among variables. Survival curves were calculated by the Kaplan–Meier Method.

3. Results

3.1. Wnt/GSK-3 Axis Is Functional in AML Cell Lines

We first evaluated in three AML cell lines, HL-60, THP1 and U937, the basal expression and activation of the Wnt molecules, including total β-catenin, pan-phosphorylated β-catenin(Ser33–37/Thr41), Ser675-phospho-β-catenin, active non-phospho-β-catenin, GSK-3β (total and Ser9) and GSK-3α (total and Ser9). These proteins were expressed in all the three cell lines (Table 1). Western immunoblot of nuclear fraction confirmed the activation of the Wnt/β-catenin pathway, since β-catenin was found in the nuclear fraction of lysate for each cell line (Figure S1A). Next, we used a pharmacological approach to confirm the activation of the pathway in AML cell lines by adding Wnt inhibitors (PNU-74654, IWP-2 and Niclosamide) or GSK-3 inhibitors (LICL, AR-A014418) in the culture medium. Cells were treated with increasing concentrations of each inhibitor, then cell viability was assessed through MTS. The samples treated with all the GSK-3 and Wnt inhibitors, except IWP-2, displayed reduction in cell viability in a dose-dependent manner (Figure S1B). As MTS assay cannot discriminate cell death or cell proliferation, cell lines were treated with a single concentration (close to the IC50) of each drug, and then cell death and proliferation were analyzed using TOPRO-3 and CFSE staining. Except Niclosamide, which induced a strong effect, the other Wnt inhibitors PNU-74654 and IWP-2 slightly reduced cell viability, while inducing a significant reduction in cell proliferation (Figure 1A,B). GSK-3 inhibitors, including LiCl and AR-A014418, induced a significant reduction in both cell viability and proliferation (Figure 1A,B) in all the tested cell lines. THP1 cell line, expressing higher levels of Wnt proteins compared to the two other cell lines (Table 1 and Figure S1A,B), was mostly sensitive to Wnt inhibitors (Figure 1A). The use of Wnt ligands, such as Wnt-3a and Wnt-5a, did not modify either cell proliferation or cell survival (Figure S1C).

Table 1. Flow cytometric analysis of Wnt/β-catenin and GSK-3 molecules in AML cell lines. HL-60, THP1 and U937 were probed with specific primary antibodies and labelled with Alexa 488-conjugated secondary antibodies. Data are expressed as relative median of fluorescence intensity and reported as mean ± SEM of 6 independent experiments.

Relative Expression of Wnt Molecules in AML Cell Lines	HL-60	THP1	U937
	Relative median of fluorescence intensity (rMFI) ± SEM		
Total β-catenin	2.466 ± 0.238	6.765 ± 1.508	2.781 ± 0.288
Non-phospho-β-catenin	1.676 ± 0.058	2.360 ± 0.209	1.442 ± 0.0677
Ser675-phospho-β-catenin	3.471 ± 0.202	7.847 ± 1.443	3.398 ± 0.566
Ser33/37/Thr41-phospho-β-catenin	2.135 ± 0.119	3.013 ± 0.395	2.232 ± 0.21
GSK-3α	2.275 ± 0.161	2.654 ± 0.298	2.194 ± 0.18
pGSK-3α (Ser21)	9.355 ± 1.641	1.640 ± 2.678	7.901 ± 1.643
GSK-3β	2.217 ± 0.139	2.456 ± 0.293	1.713 ± 0.064
GSK-3β (Ser 9)	4.600 ± 0.416	9.401 ± 3.046	3.935 ± 0.643

3.2. Wnt Molecules Are Enriched in Patient Samples

To determine whether the Wnt/β-catenin pathway was represented in patient samples, we first used in silico analysis of RNA-seq data from more than 170 AML patients that were part of The Cancer Genome Atlas (TCGA) project on AML [21]. We observed that several genes of the Wnt/GSK-3/β-catenin axis were enriched in AML samples, including *AXIN*, *APC*, *CTNNB1* (BETA-CATENIN), *GSK-3A* and *GSK-3B* (Figure 2). We then used flow cytometric analysis to determine the Wnt expression pattern in a cohort of 60 AML patients admitted to our institution. Consistently with in silico analysis, we observed in primary AML samples, a robust expression of β-catenin (total and phosphorylated forms), GSK-3β (total and Ser9) and GSK-3α (total and Ser21) (Figure 3A). However, the expression levels of each protein were not homogeneous amongst samples. To investigate whether this heterogeneous expression of Wnt molecules could have prognostic significance, the samples were classified according to the expression degree (high versus low) as compared to the mean values of expression for all samples.

Then, we used a Kaplan–Meier analysis to determine patient survival in the two groups, censoring data after 36 months. For all the proteins considered, no significant differences were observed neither in overall survival (OS), nor in progression free survival (PFS). By contrast, when we considered the activation of β-catenin pathway as the ratio between the non-active form (Ser33/37/Thr41 β-catenin) and the total β-catenin, patients with low activation status (high ratio) displayed a better PFS compared to patients presenting high activation status of the pathway (low ratio) (Figure 3B). Pearson analysis showed a positive association between leucocyte count (WBC) and expression levels of pan-phospho-β-catenin (Ser33–37/Thr41), Ser 675-phospho-β-catenin, non-phospho-β-catenin and GSK-3β (Table 2A). A positive association was also found between hemoglobin (Hb) level and active β-catenin (non-phosphorylated), phospho-GSK-3β (Ser 9), pan-phospho-β-catenin and Ser 675-phospho-β-catenin) (Table 2B). The European Leukemia Network (ELN) recommendations for diagnosis and management of AML in adults has proposed the stratification of AML patients according to genetic and molecular characteristics, dividing patients into three risk categories that are relevant for clinical outcomes, i.e., good/favorable, intermediate, poor/adverse [22]. Accordingly, thanks to the cytogenetics and mutational pattern of each patient, we classified patients in these three risk groups, observing that β-catenin, Ser675-phospho-β-catenin and GSK-3α (total and Ser21) were preferentially expressed in adverse and intermediate risk groups (Figure 4). All these observations suggested that Wnt or GSK signaling could be associated with AML chemosensitivity.

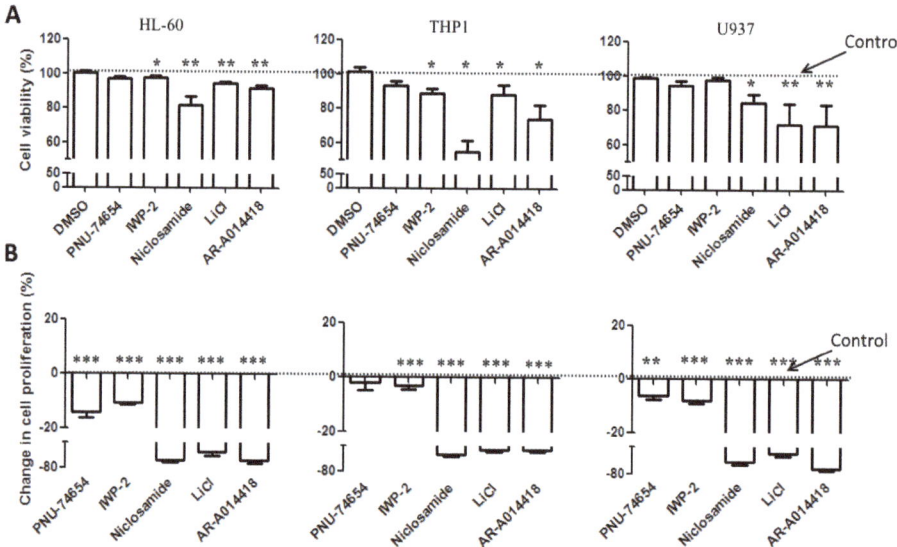

Figure 1. Cell viability and proliferation of AML cell lines cultured in the presence of Wnt and GSK-3 inhibitors. AML cells lines were stained with CFSE and cultured in the presence of either Wnt modulators, including PNU-74654 (15 µM), IWP-2 (15 µM) Niclosamide (1 µM), or GSK-3 inhibitors, including LiCl (10 mM), AR-A014418 (15 µM). After 4 days, cells were stained with TOPRO-3 to exclude dead cells. (**A**) Viable cells (TOPRO-3 negative cells) and CFSE-stained cells were quantified by FACS analysis. (**B**) Relative cell proliferation was expressed as the percentage of CFSE median fluorescence of treated cells compared to the cells treated with DMSO. Data are reported as mean ± SEM of 5 independent experiments. A Mann–Whitney test was used to analyze the differences between means. * $p < 0.05$, ** $p < 0.01$, *** $p < 0.001$. Dot line: control.

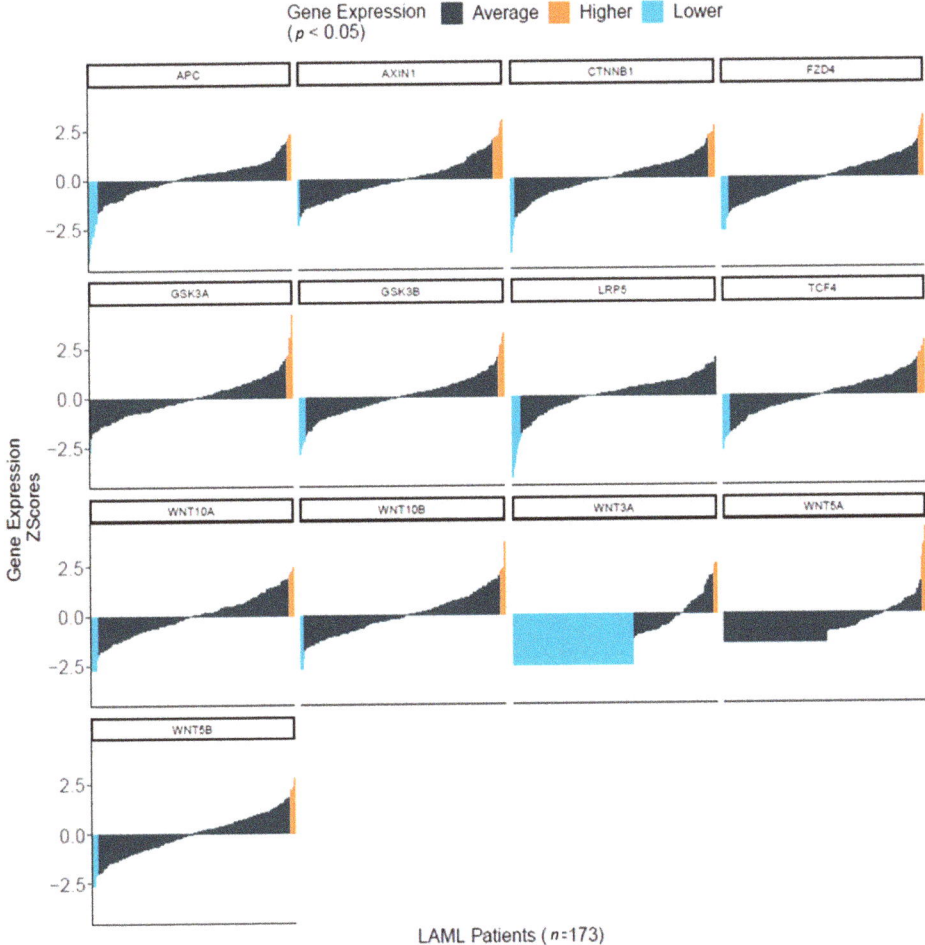

Figure 2. Enrichment of Wnt signaling component in primary AML samples. Wnt signaling expression data from 173 de novo AML samples obtained from The Cancer Genome Atlas RNA-Seq database for AML, Gene expression data in Z-score format were downloaded from the cbioportal R package cgdsr for the TCGA-LAML. Normalized data were used for Z-score calculation. For each mRNA, a sample showing a Z-score higher or lower than the average Z-score for the whole population was considered as having higher or lower expression respectively for the corresponding gene, Z +/− 1.96 ($p < 0.05$).

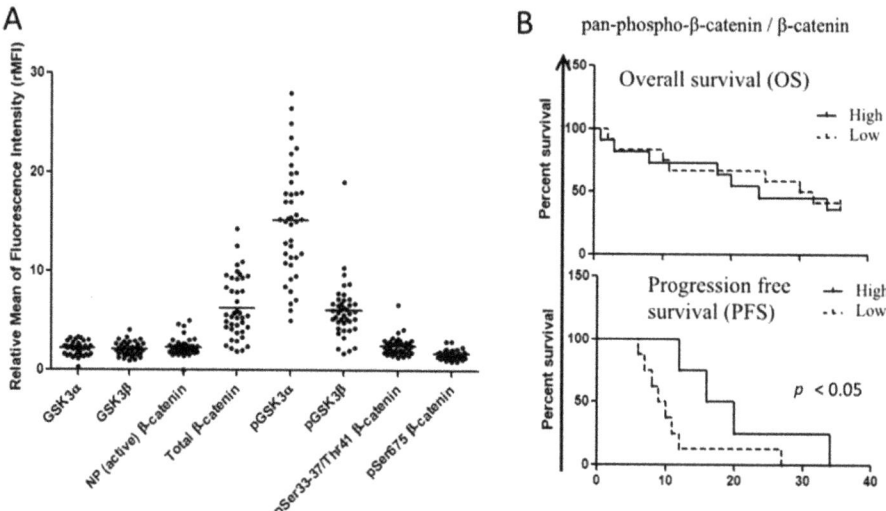

Figure 3. Expression of Wnt signaling in primary AML samples. (**A**) Flow cytometric analysis of Wnt components in AML primary samples ($n = 60$), probed with specific primary antibody and labeled with FITC-conjugated secondary antibodies. Data were expressed as relative median of fluorescence intensity. (**B**) The ratio between inactive Ser33–37/Thr41-phospho-β-catenin and total β-catenin was evaluated for each sample and classified as high ratio or low ratio when they were above and below the mean ratio value for all samples, respectively. Gehan–Breslow–Wilcoxon analysis was used to establish the difference in overall survival and progression-free survival among the groups.

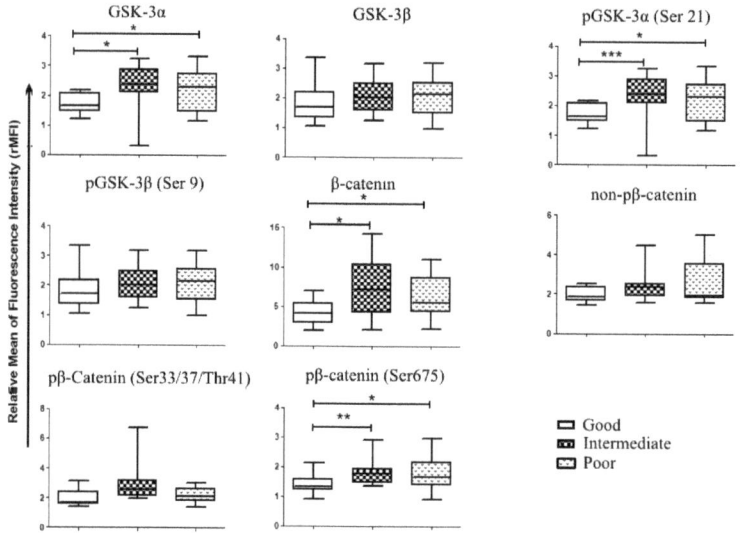

Figure 4. Wnt and GSK-3 expression in primary AML samples according to patient stratification. Patient samples analyzed for Wnt expression, were stratified according to their mutational status and their cytogenetics into 3 risks group as proposed by the European Leukemic Network (ELN)s; favorable risk or good ($n = 11$), intermediate ($n = 12$) and poor ($n = 13$). Mann–Whitney test was used to analyze differences between the two groups * $p < 0.05$, ** $p < 0.01$, *** $p < 0.001$.

Table 2. Correlation between hemogram and Wnt signaling expression in AML blast cells. Spearman analysis was used to assess the correlation between Wnt protein levels in blast cells and parameters of the hemogram, including (**A**) white blood cells (WBC); (**B**) Hemoglobin (Hb), and (**C**) platelets (PLTS). Statistical significance when $p \leq 0.05$.

				(A) White Blood Cells (WBC)				
WBC	GSK3α	GSK3β	Non-Phospho-β-catenin	Total β-Catenin	Phospho-GSK-3α (Ser 21)	Phospho-GSK3β (Ser 9)	Ser33/37/Thr41-Phospho-β-Catenin	Ser675-Phospho-β-Catenin
r	0.1117	0.3236	0.3205	0.2317	0.1109	0.2414	0.4311	0.4106
p value	0.2583	0.0271	0.0284	0.0870	0.2597	0.0780	0.0043	0.0064
				(B) Hemoglobin (Hb)				
Hb	GSK3α	GSK3β	Non-Phospho-β-Catenin	Total β-Catenin	Phospho-GSK-3α (Ser 21)	Phospho-GSK3β (Ser 9)	Ser33/37/Thr41-Phospho-β-Catenin	Ser675-Phospho-β-Catenin
r	−0.02664	−0.02471	0.09962	0.002832	0.1640	0.2041	0.1749	0.2092
p value	0.4387	0.4431	0.2816	0.4935	0.1696	0.1162	0.1538	0.1104
				(C) Platelets (PLTS)				
PLTS	GSK3α	GSK3β	Non-Phospho-β-Catenin	Total β-Catenin	Phospho-GSK-3α (Ser 21)	Phospho-GSK3β (Ser 9)	Ser33/37/Thr41-Phospho-β-Catenin	Ser675-Phospho-β-Catenin
r	0.2725	0.2478	0.4430	0.1463	0.2366	0.3473	0.3730	0.4452
p value	0.0539	0.0726	0.0034	0.1972	0.0824	0.0190	0.0125	0.0033

3.3. hBM-MSCs Express Wnt Molecules but are Insensitive to Pathway Inhibitors

Considering the importance of bone marrow microenvironment in AML onset and recurrence, ex-vivo co-culture of leukemic cells on bone marrow stromal monolayer represents a good tool for evaluating drug sensitivity [23,24]. Bone marrow stromal cells from healthy donors and patients were analyzed for expression of components of Wnt/GSK-3/β-catenin axis. Western blot analysis highlighted that all healthy donors hBM-MSCs (n = 12) and AML-hBM-MSCs (hBM-MSCs*, n = 18) samples expressed Wnt components, suggesting a possible paracrine signal between hBM-MSCs and leukemic cells. The presence of active forms of β-catenin, including non-phospho-β-catenin and Ser675-phospho-β-catenin [25], revealed a constitutive activation of the Wnt/β-catenin pathway in these cells (Figure 5A). To assess whether hBM-MSC and AML cell co-culture induces the activation of Wnt/β-catenin in AML cells, we used THP1 cells expressing the TCF/LEF-GFP reporter gene. Transfected cells seeded on hBM-MSCs displayed enhanced GFP signal (Figure 5B) and the increase in TCF/LEF activity was similar to that observed when cells were challenged with Wnt-3a (Figure 5B). As the inhibition of the pathways could theoretically interfere with some hBM-MSC functions, we assessed hBM-MSC viability through MTS assay with increasing concentrations of Wnt/GSK-3 inhibitors. hBM-MSCs and hBM-MSCs* viability was not altered by Wnt/GSK-3 inhibitors unless at very high concentrations (Figure 5C). We also analyzed immunomodulatory properties and adipogenic or osteogenic differentiation of hBM-MSCs treated with Wnt or GSK-3 inhibitors for 48 h; hBM-MSCs retained the same capability both to suppress stimulated PBMC proliferation (Figure S2A) and to undergo differentiation into osteocyte and adipocytes (Figure S2B).

3.4. Wnt Modulators Enhance Chemosensitivity of AML Cells

We assessed whether Wnt inhibitors could increase AML cell sensitivity to drugs normally used for AML therapy, such as Idarubicin or Ara-C. AML cells were cultured alone or in the presence of hBM-MSCs for 48 h, with or without Wnt modulators and chemotherapeutic agents. Cells were harvested, stained with annexin and analyzed for apoptosis. Idarubicin (0.5 μM) or Ara-C (10 μM) significantly induced the apoptosis of both AML cell lines and AML primary cells, while co-culture with hBM-MSCs led to a significant rescue effect (Figure 6A and Figure S4). The addition of PNU-74654 (15 μM), Niclosamide (1.5 μM), LiCL (15 mM) or AR-A014418 (15 μM) significantly lowered the anti-apoptotic effect on AML cells mediated by bone marrow stromal cells, regardless their origin (hBM-MSCs or hBM-MSCs*) and the ELN risk classification of the AML patients.

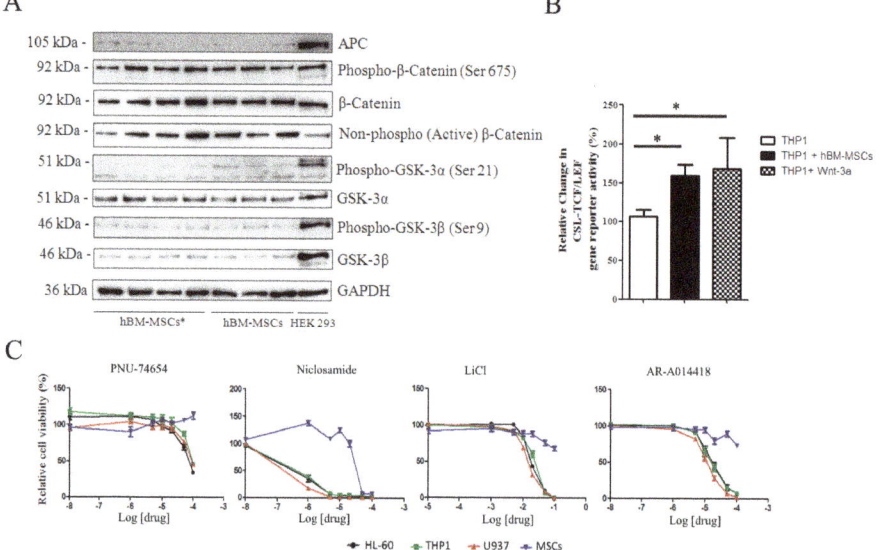

Figure 5. Expression of Wnt and GSK-3 molecules in hBM-MSCs. (**A**) Representative Western blot analysis (Figure S3) of Wnt components in AML-hBM-MSC (hBM-MSCs *) and hBM-MSCs from normal donors. Images are representative of 12 hBM-MSC and 18 hBM-MSC * samples. (**B**) Wnt activity according to GFP signal in THP1 cells expressing the gene reporter CSL-TCF/LEF-GFP. Transfected cells were cultured either alone or in presence of hBM-MSCs or in medium supplemented with Wnt-3a (25 ng/mL). (**C**) hBM-MSC viability in growth medium supplemented with increasing concentrations of Wnt and GSK-3 inhibitors. Data are representative of at least 4 independent experiments. * $p < 0.05$.

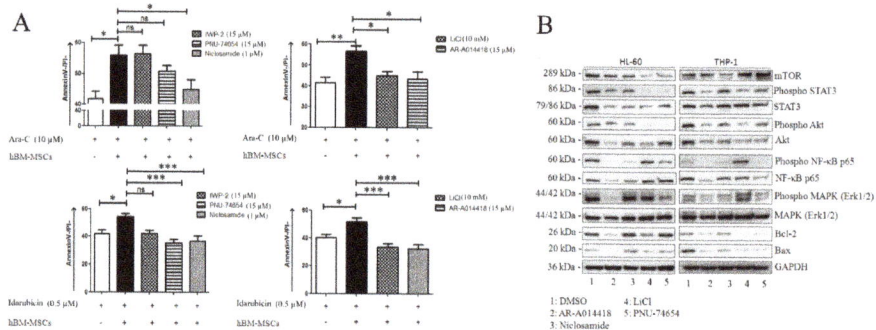

Figure 6. Wnt modulators improve chemosensitivity of AML blasts. (**A**) Primary AML blasts were treated with Ara-C or Idarubicin in presence or absence of hBM-MSCs and Wnt or GSK-3 inhibitors. After 48 h of incubation, cells were collected and stained with AnnexinV/PI to evaluate cell apoptosis. Data are expressed as mean ± SEM of at least 3 independent experiments performed in triplicate: * $p < 0.05$, ** $p < 0.01$, *** $p < 0.001$, ns (not significant). (**B**) Representative Western blot analysis (Figure S5) of HL-60 and THP1 cell lines treated for 48 h with Wnt or GSK-3 inhibitors, including PNU 74,654 (15 µM), IWP-2 (15 µM), Niclosamide (1 µM), LiCl (15 mM) and AR-A014418 (15 µM). Images are representative of at least 3 experiments.

To investigate which microenvironmental prosurvival protein network was affected by Wnt pharmacological inhibition, we first analyzed how the Wnt-GSK axis was modulated in AML cell lines treated with above mentioned inhibitors, observing that the pattern of modulation was cell line-dependent, probably reflecting differential modulation of the pathway according to molecular features of the AML cell/samples (Figure S6). Briefly, Niclosamide and PNU-74654 reduced the levels of Ser675-phospho-β-catenin in the HL-60 cell line, whereas Niclosamide induced reduced levels of both total β-catenin and the pan-phospho-β-catenin in the THP1 cell line. Of note, as previously described, the PNU-74654 treatment induced increased levels of total β-catenin [26]. This effect could be related to the accumulation of the protein in the cytoplasm, because the inhibition of the Tcf/β-catenin complex, PNU-74654, decreased nuclear β-catenin accumulation (Figure S6A) [26]. In contrast, both Wnt and GSK-3 inhibitors were associated with reduced phosphorylation of GSK-3β at Ser 9 (Figure S6B). Then, we analyzed the expression and activation of Bcl-2, mT/Akt and MAP kinase family proteins in THP1 and HL-60 cell lines treated with above mentioned inhibitors. A persistent modulation of Bax, STAT-3, Akt, NF-κB, and ErK 1/2 was clearly evident (Figure 6B).

To assess whether he anticancer effect of Wnt and GSK-3 inhibitors could be operational in vivo, we generated a xenograft model of AML by injecting the U937 cell line in the tail vein of NOG mice, as previously described [17]. Two weeks later, the mice were treated with either Ara-C alone or Ara-C in combination with each inhibitor (except AR-A014418 for its known toxicity). Treatment of engrafted mouse with Ara-C significantly reduced the leukemic burden in mouse bone marrow (Figure 7A), but this effect was stronger when Ara-C was associated with either PNU-74654, Niclosamide, or LiCl. Accordingly, the mean of mouse survival was significantly improved when Ara-C was associated with each inhibitor, i.e., PNU-74654 (33 days), Niclosamide (29 days) and LiCl (33 days), as compared to mice treated with Ara-C alone (mean survival = 26 days) (Figure 7B).

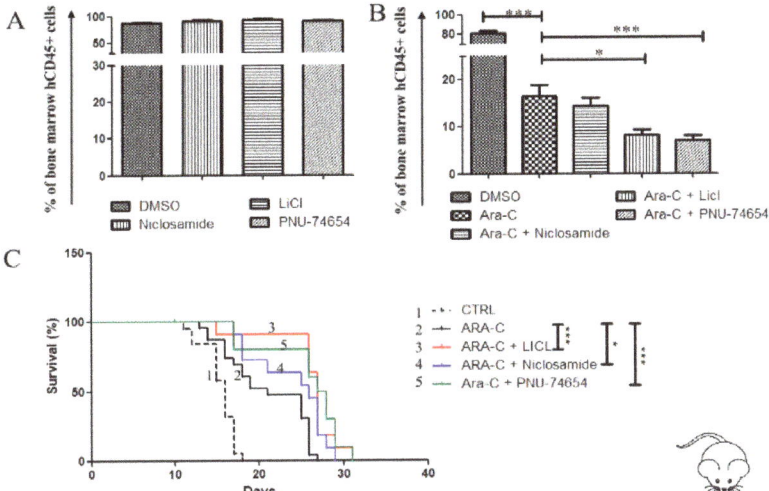

Figure 7. Wnt inhibition reduces bone marrow leukemic burden and prolongs survival of the cell line-based AML xenograftmouse model. (**A**,**B**) Flow cytometry analysis of human CD45+ in bone marrow samples obtained from mice transplanted with AML cell line U937. Starting from day 9 post-engraftment, mice were treated for 2 days with one of the following schedules: DMSO, Ara-C alone (25 mg/Kg), Wnt inhibitor alone, or Wnt inhibitor + Ara-C. Then Ara-C were administered for further 3 days in the groups receiving Ara-C (alone or in combination), while the other groups received DMSO. The following concentrations were used for each inhibitor: PNU-74654 0.5 mg/kg, Niclosamide 10 mg/kg, LiCl 25 mg/kg. The assay was performed with at least 5 mice in each group. Data are reported as mean ± SEM of values obtained from at least 5 mice. (**C**) Survival of mice transplanted with U937, differences in survival curves were analyzed with the Log-rank (Mantel–Cox) Test, * $p < 0.05$, *** $p < 0.001$.

4. Discussion

Targeted treatments using small molecule inhibitors are extensively studied as promising strategies to eradicate drug resistance in cancer and in AML [27]. In this study, we demonstrated—in vitro, ex vivo and in vivo in a murine model—that the use of pharmacological inhibitors of Wnt/β-catenin enhances the effectiveness of chemotherapeutic agents in eradicating AML cells.

The rationale for using pharmacological inhibitors of Wnt signaling as anti-leukemic agents is the evidence of aberrant activation of Wnt pathway in AML samples [28,29]. Through flow cytometric analysis, we confirmed that β-catenin was present in AML primary cell samples in a variable phosphorylated status, including the Ser675-phospho-β-catenin and the (Ser33/37/Thr41)-phospho-β-catenin. Considering the heterogeneity of each AML sample, we did not use Western blot of nuclear fraction as a method to analyze Wnt activation in samples. We took the (Ser33/37/Thr41)-phospo-β-catenin/total β-catenin ratio as a surrogate for assessing Wnt/β-catenin activation, demonstrating that the pathway is constitutively active in a large portion of patients. Besides the robust expression of β-catenin, we also observed a robust expression of different forms of GSK-3 proteins in AML samples. Within the Wnt/β-catenin cascade, GSK-3 is considered as a negative regulator of the pathway [30,31]. Its inhibition is often used as an indirect strategy to stabilize cellular β-catenin [32,33]. Nevertheless, we report here that the use of GSK-3 inhibitors reduced cell viability, similarly to Wnt inhibition. There are at least two pools of GSK-3, one associated with Axin and involved in β-catenin phosphorylation, the other not associated with Axin. Interestingly, Wnt signaling can modulate both β-catenin-associated GSK-3 and β-catenin-independent GSK-3 [30,34]. Evidence from the literature also shows that GSK-3 is not only involved in the Wnt signaling, but also crosstalk with multiple others survival pathways, such as Notch, Hegehog and Akt-related cascades [27,32,34–38]. As the role of GSK-3 cannot be only related to Wnt/β-catenin signaling, we cannot exclude the involvement of a GSK-3-independent Wnt signaling in AML pathogenesis [27,32,34–38]. Interestingly, a previous work has demonstrated that GSK-3 inhibition can improve 1,25-dihydroxyvitamin D3-mediated differentiation of AML cells, suggesting that a combinatorial treatment including GSK-3 inhibitors and anti-leukemic drugs is a promising and safety strategy in AML [39].

Wnt/β-catenin signaling is a multiple step cascade. The importance of each step for cancer development is disease- and cell context-dependent [40,41]. The inhibitors used in this study were chosen for their ability to interfere with specific steps of the pathway, i.e., ligand and receptors (IWP-2 and Niclosamide), GSK-3 (LiCl, AR-A014418), or nuclear transactivation or TCF/LEF complex (PNU-74654 and PKF118-310). While all GSK-3 inhibitors and TCF/LEF inhibitors showed the same activity for each member of Wnt family, IWP-2 failed to reproduce the capability of Niclosamide of reducing AML cell viability and sensitizing them to drugs. This discrepancy can be explained by the mechanisms triggered by each of the inhibitors; in fact, IWP-2 interferes with biogenesis of Wnt ligand, by targeting porcupine, while Niclosamide interferes directly with the co-receptor LRP-6 [13,42].

Our data show that small molecule inhibitors of Wnt or GSK-3 substantially enhance the antitumor effect of Ara-c and Idarubicin in vitro and reduce AML cell survival advantage, thus lowering the leukemic burden in the bone marrow of AML mouse models. The mechanisms involved in Ara-C or Idarubicin-induced cell death include the modulation of many pathways, such as mTor/Akt, Erk, NF-KB, stat3, Bax/Bak etc [17,18,43–45]. Through Western blot analysis, we clearly showed that these proteins were down-regulated in AML cell lines treated with Wnt or GSK-3 inhibitors. These observations are in favor of a synergistic activity between our inhibitors and the chemotherapeutic agents used in this study. We cannot exclude the interaction with other specific mechanisms of drug resistance, but Wnt/β-catenin signaling seems to play a pivotal role in this phenomenon.

The main molecular events related to Wnt pathway activation in AML are both chromosomal translocations and/or mutations of *FLT3* [15]. Enhanced FLT3 signaling is similarly associated to poor prognosis in AML [22]. However, aberrant Wnt signaling was also observed in patients with normal karyotype, i.e., patients classified as an intermediate-risk group according to WHO and ELN classifications [15,46]. We observed a significant expression of total β-catenin, Ser675-phospo-β-catenin, and GSK-3α (total and Ser 21) molecules in intermediate- and adverse-risk patients compared to favorable-risk groups. In addition, we found a significant association between Wnt/β-catenin activation and PFS, suggesting that Wnt/β-catenin signaling could be related to the persistence of residual leukemic cells along the treatment course. Residual resistant cells are mainly found in the bone marrow, as the result of a close interaction between bone marrow microenvironment and AML blast cells and leukemia stem cells. This phenomenon is associated with drug resistance and relapse [47–49]. Several literature data permit to elaborate a model of AML development, according to which Wnt/β-catenin is both involved in the crosstalk between stromal cells and AML cells, and in autocrine signaling amongst AML cells [46,50]. Our co-culture data support this hypothesis, demonstrating through gene reporter assays the presence of enhanced activity of Wnt/β-catenin in AML cells cultured on stromal cell monolayers. In the model of AML leukemogenesis induced by activating mutation in β-catenin, the stromal cell contribution is at least equal to the role played by hematopoietic cells [16]. Thus, Wnt inhibition may sensitize AML cells to therapy by both targeting directly resistant cells and interfering with the stromal cell support towards leukemic cells that is necessary for the persistence and selection of resistant clones [48]. Therefore, Wnt-inhibitory therapy could overcome the prognostic significance of patient risk stratification, standing as a therapeutic response for all subgroups of AML.

5. Conclusions

Overall, our study demonstrates that because of their capabilities to interfere with AML cell growth and chemoresistance, small molecule inhibitors of Wnt and GSK-3 signaling may represent potential candidates for drug development in AML.

Supplementary Materials: The following are available online at http://www.mdpi.com/2072-6694/12/9/2696/s1, Figure S1: Wnt expression and activity in AML cell lines, Figure S2: Differentiation and immunomodulatory capabilities of hBM-MSCs in presence of Wnt and GSK-3 inhibitors, Figure S3: Original Western blot figures (Figure 5), Figure S4: Contribution of Wnt modulators to AML cell lines chemosensitivity, Figure S5: Original Western blot figures (Figure 6), Figure S6: Representative Western blot analysis of HL-60 and THP1 cell lines treated for 48hours with Wnt or GSK-3 inhibitors, Table S1: List of patients and their characteristics.

Author Contributions: Conception and design: P.T.K., A.C., G.D.C. and M.K.; In vitro, in vivo studies, patient's samples management and data acquisition: P.T.K., G.D.C., A.C., R.B., A.A., A.B., C.C., I.T., M.B. and M.K.; Analysis and interpretation of data (e.g., statistical analysis, biostatistics, computational analysis): P.T.K., G.D.C., A.C., P.D. and M.K.; Writing and review of the manuscript: P.T.K., G.D.C., A.C., R.B. and M.K.; Study supervision: P.T.K. and M.K.; Grant and Funding: M.B. and M.K. All authors have read and agreed to the published version of the manuscript.

Funding: This work was supported by: (i) Progetti di Rilevante Interesse Nazionale (PRIN) Italia, Bando 2017; (ii) Fondazione CARIVERONA Italia, Bando 2012.

Acknowledgments: The study was conducted in the Interdepartmental Laboratory of Medical Research (LURM) at the University of Verona, Verona, Italy.

Conflicts of Interest: The material presented in this study is an original research, has not been previously published and has not been submitted for publication elsewhere while under consideration. The authors declare no conflict of interest.

References

1. Kumar, C.C. Genetic abnormalities and challenges in the treatment of acute myeloid leukemia. *Genes Cancer* **2011**, *2*, 95–107. [CrossRef] [PubMed]
2. Döhner, H.; Weisdorf, D.J.; Bloomfield, C.D. Acute Myeloid Leukemia. *N. Engl. J. Med.* **2015**, *373*, 1136–1152. [CrossRef] [PubMed]
3. Marcucci, G.; Mrózek, K.; Bloomfield, C.D. Molecular heterogeneity and prognostic biomarkers in adults with acute myeloid leukemia and normal cytogenetics. *Curr. Opin. Hematol.* **2005**, *12*, 68. [CrossRef] [PubMed]
4. Kamdje, A.H.N.; Bassi, G.; Pacelli, L.; Malpeli, G.; Amati, E.; Nichele, I.; Pizzolo, G.; Krampera, M. Role of stromal cell-mediated Notch signaling in CLL resistance to chemotherapy. *Blood Cancer J.* **2012**, *2*, e73. [CrossRef]

5. Takebe, N.; Miele, L.; Harris, P.J.; Jeong, W.; Bando, H.; Kahn, M.; Yang, S.X.; Ivy, S.P. Targeting Notch, Hedgehog, and Wnt pathways in cancer stem cells: Clinical update. *Nat. Rev. Clin. Oncol.* **2015**, *12*, 445–464. [CrossRef]
6. Zhao, C.; Blum, J.; Chen, A.; Kwon, H.Y.; Jung, S.H.; Cook, J.M.; Lagoo, A.; Reya, T. Loss of beta-catenin impairs the renewal of normal and CML stem cells in vivo. *Cancer Cell* **2007**, *12*, 528–541. [CrossRef]
7. Mikesch, J.-H.; Steffen, B.; Berdel, W.E.; Serve, H.; Müller-Tidow, C. The emerging role of Wnt signaling in the pathogenesis of acute myeloid leukemia. *Leukemia* **2007**, *21*, 1638–1647. [CrossRef]
8. Lee, M.W.; Ryu, S.; Kim, D.S.; Lee, J.W.; Sung, K.W.; Koo, H.H.; Yoo, K.H. Mesenchymal stem cells in suppression or progression of hematologic malignancy: Current status and challenges. *Leukemia* **2019**, *33*, 597–611. [CrossRef]
9. Steinhart, Z.; Angers, S. Wnt signaling in development and tissue homeostasis. *Development* **2018**, *145*, dev146589. [CrossRef]
10. MacDonald, B.T.; Tamai, K.; He, X. Wnt/beta-catenin signaling: Components, mechanisms, and diseases. *Dev. Cell* **2009**, *17*, 9–26. [CrossRef]
11. Scholer-Dahirel, A.; Schlabach, M.R.; Loo, A.; Bagdasarian, L.; Meyer, R.; Guo, R.; Woolfenden, S.; Yu, K.K.; Markovits, J.; Killary, K.; et al. Maintenance of adenomatous polyposis coli (APC)-mutant colorectal cancer is dependent on Wnt/β-catenin signaling. *Proc. Natl. Acad. Sci. USA* **2011**, *108*, 17135–17140. [CrossRef] [PubMed]
12. Macheda, M.L.; Stacker, S.A. Importance of Wnt signaling in the tumor stroma microenvironment. *Curr. Cancer Drug Targets* **2008**, *8*, 454–465. [CrossRef] [PubMed]
13. Krishnamurthy, N.; Kurzrock, R. Targeting the Wnt/beta-catenin pathway in cancer: Update on effectors and inhibitors. *Cancer Treat. Rev.* **2018**, *62*, 50–60. [CrossRef] [PubMed]
14. Wang, Y.; Krivtsov, A.V.; Sinha, A.U.; North, T.E.; Goessling, W.; Feng, Z.; Zon, L.I.; Armstrong, S.A. The Wnt/beta-catenin pathway is required for the development of leukemia stem cells in AML. *Science* **2010**, *327*, 1650–1653. [CrossRef]
15. Gruszka, A.M.; Valli, D.; Alcalay, M. Wnt Signalling in Acute Myeloid Leukaemia. *Cells* **2019**, *8*, 1403. [CrossRef]
16. Kode, A.; Manavalan, J.S.; Mosialou, I.; Bhagat, G.; Rathinam, C.V.; Luo, N.; Khiabanian, H.; Lee, A.; Vundavalli, M.; Friedman, R.; et al. Leukemogenesis Induced by an Activating β-catenin mutation in Osteoblasts. *Nature* **2014**, *506*, 240–244. [CrossRef]
17. Takam Kamga, P.; Collo, G.D.; Resci, F.; Bazzoni, R.; Mercuri, A.; Quaglia, F.M.; Tanasi, I.; Delfino, P.; Visco, C.; Bonifacio, M.; et al. Notch Signaling Molecules as Prognostic Biomarkers for Acute Myeloid Leukemia. *Cancers* **2019**, *11*, 1958. [CrossRef]
18. Takam Kamga, P.; Bassi, G.; Cassaro, A.; Midolo, M.; Di Trapani, M.; Gatti, A.; Carusone, R.; Resci, F.; Perbellini, O.; Gottardi, M.; et al. Notch signalling drives bone marrow stromal cell-mediated chemoresistance in acute myeloid leukemia. *Oncotarget* **2016**, *7*, 21713–21727. [CrossRef]
19. Kamga, P.T.; Dal Collo, G.; Bassi, G.; Midolo, M.; Delledonne, M.; Chilosi, M.; Bonifacio, M.; Krampera, M. Characterization of a new B-ALL cell line with constitutional defect of the Notch signaling pathway. *Oncotarget* **2018**, *9*, 18341–18350. [CrossRef]
20. Takam Kamga, P.; Dal Collo, G.; Midolo, M.; Adamo, A.; Delfino, P.; Mercuri, A.; Cesaro, S.; Mimiola, E.; Bonifacio, M.; Andreini, A.; et al. Inhibition of Notch Signaling Enhances Chemosensitivity in B-cell Precursor Acute Lymphoblastic Leukemia. *Cancer Res.* **2019**, *79*, 639–649. [CrossRef]
21. Grieselhuber, N.R.; Klco, J.M.; Verdoni, A.M.; Lamprecht, T.; Sarkaria, S.M.; Wartman, L.D.; Ley, T.J. Notch Signaling in Acute Promyelocytic Leukemia. *Leukemia* **2013**, *27*, 1548–1557. [CrossRef] [PubMed]
22. Estey, E.H. Acute myeloid leukemia: 2019 update on risk-stratification and management. *Am. J. Hematol.* **2018**, *93*, 1267–1291. [CrossRef] [PubMed]
23. Ding, W.; Nowakowski, G.S.; Knox, T.R.; Boysen, J.C.; Maas, M.L.; Schwager, S.M.; Wu, W.; Wellik, L.E.; Dietz, A.B.; Ghosh, A.K.; et al. Bi-directional activation between mesenchymal stem cells and CLL B-cells: Implication for CLL disease progression. *Br. J. Haematol.* **2009**, *147*, 471–483. [CrossRef] [PubMed]
24. Jin, L.; Tabe, Y.; Lu, H.; Borthakur, G.; Miida, T.; Kantarjian, H.; Andreeff, M.; Konopleva, M. Mechanisms of apoptosis induction by simultaneous inhibition of PI3K and FLT3-ITD in AML cells in the hypoxic bone marrow microenvironment. *Cancer Lett.* **2013**, *329*, 45–58. [CrossRef] [PubMed]

25. Spirli, C.; Locatelli, L.; Morell, C.M.; Fiorotto, R.; Morton, S.D.; Cadamuro, M.; Fabris, L.; Strazzabosco, M. PKA dependent p-Ser-675β-catenin, a novel signaling defect in a mouse model of Congenital Hepatic Fibrosis. *Hepatol. Baltim. Md.* **2013**, *58*, 1713–1723. [CrossRef] [PubMed]
26. Leal, L.F.; Bueno, A.C.; Gomes, D.C.; Abduch, R.; de Castro, M.; Antonini, S.R. Inhibition of the Tcf/beta-catenin complex increases apoptosis and impairs adrenocortical tumor cell proliferation and adrenal steroidogenesis. *Oncotarget* **2015**, *6*, 43016–43032. [CrossRef]
27. Ougolkov, A.V.; Fernandez-Zapico, M.E.; Savoy, D.N.; Urrutia, R.A.; Billadeau, D.D. Glycogen synthase kinase-3beta participates in nuclear factor kappaB-mediated gene transcription and cell survival in pancreatic cancer cells. *Cancer Res.* **2005**, *65*, 2076–2081. [CrossRef]
28. Staal, F.J.T.; Famili, F.; Garcia Perez, L.; Pike-Overzet, K. Aberrant Wnt Signaling in Leukemia. *Cancers* **2016**, *8*, 78. [CrossRef]
29. Tickenbrock, L.; Hehn, S.; Sargin, B.; Choudhary, C.; Bäumer, N.; Buerger, H.; Schulte, B.; Müller, O.; Berdel, W.E.; Müller-Tidow, C.; et al. Activation of Wnt signalling in acute myeloid leukemia by induction of Frizzled-4. *Int. J. Oncol.* **2008**, *33*, 1215–1221. [CrossRef]
30. Wu, D.; Pan, W. GSK3: A multifaceted kinase in Wnt signaling. *Trends Biochem. Sci.* **2010**, *35*, 161–168. [CrossRef]
31. Metcalfe, C.; Bienz, M. Inhibition of GSK3 by Wnt signalling–two contrasting models. *J. Cell Sci.* **2011**, *124*, 3537–3544. [CrossRef] [PubMed]
32. Chen, R.-H.; Ding, W.V.; McCormick, F. Wnt Signaling to β-Catenin Involves Two Interactive Components glycogen synthase kinase-3β inhibition and activation of protein kinase C. *J. Biol. Chem.* **2000**, *275*, 17894–17899. [CrossRef] [PubMed]
33. Xia, M.; Zhao, X.; Huang, Q.; Sun, H.; Sun, C.; Yuan, J.; He, C.; Sun, Y.; Huang, X.; Kong, W.; et al. Activation of Wnt/β-catenin signaling by lithium chloride attenuates d-galactose-induced neurodegeneration in the auditory cortex of a rat model of aging. *FEBS Open Bio* **2017**, *7*, 759–776. [CrossRef] [PubMed]
34. Ding, V.W.; Chen, R.H.; McCormick, F. Differential regulation of glycogen synthase kinase 3beta by insulin and Wnt signaling. *J. Biol. Chem.* **2000**, *275*, 32475–32481. [CrossRef] [PubMed]
35. McCubrey, J.A.; Steelman, L.S.; Bertrand, F.E.; Davis, N.M.; Sokolosky, M.; Abrams, S.L.; Montalto, G.; D'Assoro, A.B.; Libra, M.; Nicoletti, F.; et al. GSK-3 as potential target for therapeutic intervention in cancer. *Oncotarget* **2014**, *5*, 2881–2911. [CrossRef] [PubMed]
36. Zhou, W.; Wang, L.; Gou, S.-M.; Wang, T.-L.; Zhang, M.; Liu, T.; Wang, C.-Y. ShRNA silencing glycogen synthase kinase-3 beta inhibits tumor growth and angiogenesis in pancreatic cancer. *Cancer Lett.* **2012**, *316*, 178–186. [CrossRef]
37. Dong, J.; Peng, J.; Zhang, H.; Mondesire, W.H.; Jian, W.; Mills, G.B.; Hung, M.-C.; Meric-Bernstam, F. Role of glycogen synthase kinase 3beta in rapamycin-mediated cell cycle regulation and chemosensitivity. *Cancer Res.* **2005**, *65*, 1961–1972. [CrossRef]
38. Dal Col, J.; Dolcetti, R. GSK-3beta inhibition: At the crossroad between Akt and mTOR constitutive activation to enhance cyclin D1 protein stability in mantle cell lymphoma. *Cell Cycle Georget. Tex* **2008**, *7*, 2813–2816. [CrossRef]
39. Gupta, K.; Stefan, T.; Ignatz-Hoover, J.; Moreton, S.; Parizher, G.; Saunthararajah, Y.; Wald, D.N. GSK-3 Inhibition Sensitizes Acute Myeloid Leukemia Cells to 1,25D-Mediated Differentiation. *Cancer Res.* **2016**, *76*, 2743–2753. [CrossRef]
40. Zhan, T.; Rindtorff, N.; Boutros, M. Wnt signaling in cancer. *Oncogene* **2017**, *36*, 1461–1473. [CrossRef]
41. Carbone, C.; Piro, G.; Gaianigo, N.; Ligorio, F.; Santoro, R.; Merz, V.; Simionato, F.; Zecchetto, C.; Falco, G.; Conti, G.; et al. Adipocytes sustain pancreatic cancer progression through a non-canonical WNT paracrine network inducing ROR2 nuclear shuttling. *Int. J. Obes.* **2018**, *42*, 334–343. [CrossRef]
42. Lu, W.; Lin, C.; Roberts, M.J.; Waud, W.R.; Piazza, G.A.; Li, Y. Niclosamide suppresses cancer cell growth by inducing Wnt co-receptor LRP6 degradation and inhibiting the Wnt/β-catenin pathway. *PLoS ONE* **2011**, *6*, e29290. [CrossRef] [PubMed]
43. Morgan, M.A.; Onono, F.O.; Spielmann, H.P.; Subramanian, T.; Scherr, M.; Venturini, L.; Dallmann, I.; Ganser, A.; Reuter, C.W.M. Modulation of anthracycline-induced cytotoxicity by targeting the prenylated proteome in myeloid leukemia cells. *J. Mol. Med. Berl. Ger.* **2012**, *90*, 149–161. [CrossRef]

44. Nishioka, C.; Ikezoe, T.; Yang, J.; Yokoyama, A. Inhibition of MEK signaling enhances the ability of cytarabine to induce growth arrest and apoptosis of acute myelogenous leukemia cells. *Apoptosis Int. J. Program. Cell Death* **2009**, *14*, 1108–1120. [CrossRef] [PubMed]
45. Ristic, B.; Bosnjak, M.; Arsikin, K.; Mircic, A.; Suzin-Zivkovic, V.; Bogdanovic, A.; Perovic, V.; Martinovic, T.; Kravic-Stevovic, T.; Bumbasirevic, V.; et al. Idarubicin induces mTOR-dependent cytotoxic autophagy in leukemic cells. *Exp. Cell Res.* **2014**, *326*, 90–102. [CrossRef] [PubMed]
46. Lazzaroni, F.; Giacco, L.D.; Biasci, D.; Turrini, M.; Prosperi, L.; Brusamolino, R.; Cairoli, R.; Beghini, A. Intronless WNT10B-short variant underlies new recurrent allele-specific rearrangement in acute myeloid leukaemia. *Sci. Rep.* **2016**, *6*, 1–14. [CrossRef]
47. Parmar, A.; Marz, S.; Rushton, S.; Holzwarth, C.; Lind, K.; Kayser, S.; Döhner, K.; Peschel, C.; Oostendorp, R.A.J.; Götze, K.S. Stromal niche cells protect early leukemic FLT3-ITD+ progenitor cells against first-generation FLT3 tyrosine kinase inhibitors. *Cancer Res.* **2011**, *71*, 4696–4706. [CrossRef]
48. Behrmann, L.; Wellbrock, J.; Fiedler, W. Acute Myeloid Leukemia and the Bone Marrow Niche—Take a Closer Look. *Front. Oncol.* **2018**, *8*, 444. [CrossRef]
49. Tabe, Y.; Konopleva, M. Role of Microenvironment in Resistance to Therapy in AML. *Curr. Hematol. Malig. Rep.* **2015**, *10*, 96–103. [CrossRef]
50. Toni, F.D.; Racaud-Sultan, C.; Chicanne, G.; Mas, V.M.-D.; Cariven, C.; Mesange, F.; Salles, J.-P.; Demur, C.; Allouche, M.; Payrastre, B.; et al. A crosstalk between the Wnt and the adhesion-dependent signaling pathways governs the chemosensitivity of acute myeloid leukemia. *Oncogene* **2006**, *25*, 3113–3122. [CrossRef]

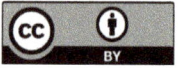
© 2020 by the authors. Licensee MDPI, Basel, Switzerland. This article is an open access article distributed under the terms and conditions of the Creative Commons Attribution (CC BY) license (http://creativecommons.org/licenses/by/4.0/).

MDPI
St. Alban-Anlage 66
4052 Basel
Switzerland
Tel. +41 61 683 77 34
Fax +41 61 302 89 18
www.mdpi.com

Cancers Editorial Office
E-mail: cancers@mdpi.com
www.mdpi.com/journal/cancers